# KEY TO THE MAP

| Chapter | Group |
|---------|-------|
| 3 | African American |
| 4 | Amish |
| 5 | Appalachian |
| 6 | Arab |
| 7 | Chinese |
| 8 | Cuban |
| 9 | Egyptian |
| 10 | Filipino |
| 11 | French Canadian |
| 12 | Greek |
| 13 | Iranian |
| 14 | Irish |
| 15 | Jewish |
| 16 | Mexican |
| 17 | Navajo |
| 18 | Vietnamese |

| Disk | Group |
|------|-------|
| D 1 | Baltic |
| D 2 | Brazilian |
| D 3 | German |
| D 4 | Haitian |
| D 5 | Hindu |
| D 6 | Italian |
| D 7 | Japanese |
| D 8 | Korean |
| D 9 | Polish |
| D 10 | Puerto Rican |
| D 11 | Turks |

# UWEC – IRR Textbook

Date     Student Name(please print)     Semester

_____

_____

_____

_____

_____

_____

_____

_____

# TRANSCULTURAL HEALTH CARE
## A Culturally Competent Approach

**Larry D. Purnell, RN, PhD**
Associate Professor
College of Health and Nursing Sciences
University of Delaware
Newark, Delaware

**Betty J. Paulanka, RN, EdD**
Professor and Dean
College of Health and Nursing Sciences
University of Delaware
Newark, Delaware

F. A. DAVIS COMPANY · Philadelphia

F. A. Davis Company
1915 Arch Street
Philadelphia, PA 19103

Printed in the United States of America

Last digit indicates print number: 10 9 8 7 6

*Nursing Editor:* Alan Sorkowitz
*Production Editor:* Devorah W. Zuckerman
*Cover Designer:* Louis J. Forgione

As new scientific information becomes available through basic and clinical research,
recommended treatments and drug therapies undergo changes. The authors and publisher have done everything possible to make this book accurate, up to date, and in
accord with accepted standards at the time of publication. The authors, editors, and
publisher are not responsible for errors or omissions or for consequences from application of the book, and make no warranty, expressed or implied, in regard to the
contents of the book. Any practice described in this book should be applied by the
reader in accordance with professional standards of care used in regard to the unique
circumstances that may apply in each situation. The reader is advised always to
check product information (package inserts) for changes and new information regarding dose and contraindications before administering any drug. Caution is especially urged when using new or infrequently ordered drugs.

**Library of Congress Cataloging-in-Publication Data**

Transcultural health care : a culturally competent approach / [edited
by] Larry D. Purnell, Betty J. Paulanka.
     p.   cm.
   Includes bibliographical references and index.
   ISBN 0–8036–0208–1 (paper : alk. paper)
   1. Transcultural medical care—United States.   2. Transcultural
medical care—Canada.   3. Minorities—Medical care—United States.
4. Minorities—Medical care—Canada.   I. Purnell, Larry D.
II. Paulanka, Betty J.
   [DNLM: 1. Delivery of Health Care—North America.   2. Ethnic
Groups—North America.   3. Cross-Cultural Comparison.   W 84 DA2 T7
1998]
RA418.5.T73T73   1998
362.1'089—dc21
DNLM/DLC
for Library of Congress                                           97-5282
                                                                      CIP

# Preface

The idea for this textbook, *Transcultural Health Care: A Culturally Competent Approach,* evolved in response to the trend toward a global society, with increasing diversity among health-care clients, students, and staff. Students and providers in all health disciplines need to expand their worldview and explore cultural diversity from a global perspective. Health-care providers, and ultimately their clients, benefit from knowledge of cultural concepts and ethnicity. Individual caregivers must integrate an understanding of their own culture with the institutional culture in which they work in order to gain some perspective on how this interaction affects staff and health-care delivery to clients, families, and the community. As people begin to accumulate knowledge about specific ethnic and cultural groups, they are challenged to look at both the differences and similarities that exist across cultures. By demonstrating an active interest in learning cultural concepts, people increase their respect and sensitivity for diversity, minimize their potential for violating cultural norms, and improve health-care and working relationships among individuals from similar and dissimilar cultures. This book is designed to:

- Introduce a new and evolving conceptual model for learning about culture

- Provide a macroapproach and microapproach to the study of culture

- Describe characteristics of selected ethnocultural groups

Within North America, there are more than 500 American Indian tribes; numerous Asian, Pacific Islander, and Indochinese groups; dozens of Hispanic groups; diverse African-American groups; and numerous northern, central, southern, eastern, and western European groups as well as many others. Space and cost concerns imposed limits on the number of groups selected for inclusion in this textbook and on the accompanying electronic disk. Specific criteria were used for identifying the 16 groups represented in the book and the 11 included in electronic format. Groups included in the book fulfill any of these five criteria:

- The group has a large population in North America, such as Mexican, Irish, and African-Americans.

- The group is relatively new in its migration status, such as Vietnamese, Cubans, and Arabs.

- The group is widely dispersed throughout North America, such as Iranians and Appalachians.

- The group has little written about it in the health-care literature, such as Egyptians and Koreans.

- The group holds minority status, such as the Navajo, a large American Indian group.

Educators who adopt the book for course instruction receive free of charge the 11 chapters that are on disk. These electronic chapters can be used to explore health-care issues relating to cultures not included in the book without leaving the classroom or going to the library. The electronic chapters may be printed out and photocopied (for instructional purposes only) for each student in the class or downloaded in a computer learning lab for students to access. Additionally, students can use the disk on their personal computers; faculty members can create a listserve of students and use the chapters for discussion or course credit. Students can be provided with hard copies of specific chapters to give class presentations or enhance class discussions, or for writing required papers or fulfilling extra credit options. Clinical instructors can have fingertip access to these chapters, using their portable computers to assist in making culturally competent clinical decisions. Because it is impossible to cover all cultures in a small, readily available textbook, this option is both economical and efficient for teaching students on clinical units that provide care to clients from a wide variety of cultures. Those who purchase the book for personal use can obtain the additional chapters in electronic format for a nominal charge by calling the publisher, F. A. Davis, at 1-800-323-3555.

Most chapter authors come from the culture about which they write, others have been selected on the basis of their extensive research on a particular cultural group, and some meet both of these criteria; thus, they write from empirical evidence, ethnographic research, and personal experience. Some of the chapter authors have significant publications to their names, whereas, for others, this is the first publication. A special thanks is extended to all of the authors and to the numerous content reviewers who are from a specific ethnic background or teach cultural content in a college or university setting.

We have strived to portray each culture without stereotyping. The book is now yours. We hope you enjoy it and are as excited about it as we are.

*Larry D. Purnell*
*Betty J. Paulanka*

# About the Contributors

## Chapter 1: Transcultural Diversity and Health Care

## Chapter 2: Purnell's Model for Cultural Competence

**Larry D. Purnell, RN, PhD,** is Associate Professor, College of Health and Nursing Sciences, University of Delaware, in Newark, Delaware. He heads the Masters in Nursing Administration program and teaches courses in transcultural health care. Originally from Appalachia, Dr. Purnell has worked with Mexicans and Mexican-Americans in Chicago, Delaware, and Maryland. Dr. Purnell's transcultural health-care experience spans the globe, including Africa, Australia, the Caribbean, China, Hong Kong, Great Britain, Mexico, Spain, and South America.

**Betty J. Paulanka, RN, EdD,** is Professor and Dean, College of Health and Nursing Sciences, University of Delaware, in Newark, Delaware. She has fostered the development of international nursing courses in both the undergraduate and graduate health programs.

## Chapter 3: African-Americans

**Josepha Campinha-Bacote, RN, PhD, CS, CTN,** is President, Transcultural C.A.R.E. Associates, Transcultural Consultant, Cincinnati, Ohio. Dr. Campinha-Bacote has conducted research on the African-American culture for over 10 years. She has been funded for several research projects, such as "Voodoo Illness in the Southern Africa-American Population," "Misdiagnosis among African-American Psychiatric Patients," and "The Use of Humor and Music Therapy with Dually Diagnosed African-American Clients."

## Chapter 4: The Amish

**Anna Frances (Fran) Z. Wenger, RN, PhD, FAAN,** is Associate Professor and Director, Transcultural and International Nursing Center of the Nell Hodgson Woodruff School of Nursing, Emory University, in Atlanta, Georgia. Dr. Wenger grew up in Pennsylvania and worked in Indiana near two of the three largest Amish settlements in the United States. As a nurse educator, her work in teaching and administration has been complemented by research focused on cultural aspects of health-care promotion. Her doctoral dissertation and many subsequent publications draw upon her participant observation of the Amish in Indiana.

**Marion R. Wenger, PhD,** is a language and culture specialist, Stone Mountain, Georgia. Dr. Wenger has taught college German and linguistics in Indiana and Ohio, near two of the three largest Amish settlements. His doctoral dissertation was based on descriptive research into the German dialect stock, which provides the basis for the first language of most Amish. His views on Amish communication are drawn from personal observation and language teaching among the Amish.

## Chapter 5: Appalachians

**Larry D. Purnell, RN, PhD,** is Associate Professor, College of Health and Nursing Sciences, University of Delaware, Newark, Delaware, where he teaches nursing administration and culture in the undergraduate and graduate programs. Dr. Purnell spent his formative years in Northern Appalachia, where he lived with several families from differing socioeconomic backgrounds. He later returned to Appalachia, where he held positions in nursing service administration and nursing education.

**Mona Counts, RN, PhD, RNC, FNAP,** traces her ancestry to several generations of Appalachians. She has been at the University of West Virginia since 1981, and is currently Professor, School of Nursing, and Chair, Department of Health Promotion/ Risk Reduction, School of Nursing.

## Chapter 6: Arab-Americans

**Patricia AbuGharbieh, RN, MSN,** lived in Amman, Jordan, from 1987 to 1990.She taught nursing in the undergraduate and graduate nursing programs at the University of Jordan in Amman. Currently, she is project coordinator for "Connections," a community-based program for African-Americans with diabetes mellitus, in Erie, Pennsylvania.

## Baltic-Americans *(chapter on disk)*

**Rauda Gelazis, RN, PhD, CS, CTN,** is Associate Professor, Ursuline College, Pepper Pike, Ohio. Dr. Gelazis is a Lithuanian-American who has done research on Lithuanian-Americans and completed her doctoral dissertation on humor, care, and well-being in Lithuanian-Americans. She has taught transcultural nursing and psychiatric mental health nursing for several years. She is an active member of the Lithuanian and Baltic communities in Cleveland, Ohio.

## Brazilian-Americans *(chapter on disk)*

**Marga Simon Coler, RN, EdD, ARNP, CTS, FAAN,** is Professor, Psychiatric and International/Transcultural Nursing, University of Connecticut–School of Nursing. Dr. Coler has collaborated with Brazilian nurses in education and research since the mid 1970s, starting with Project Hope at the Federal University of the State of Pernaumbuco. She subsequently returned to Brazil as a Fulbright Fellow and Visiting Professor at the Federal University of Paraiba and has reviewed funding from PAHQ, CNPQ, National Science Council of Brazil, and Partners of the Americas. With Brazilian colleagues, she has coauthored a reference manual on nursing diagnosis in Portuguese and has published internationally in professional journals in English and Portuguese.

## Chapter 7: Chinese-Americans

**Linda K. Matocha, RN, PhD,** was formerly Associate Professor, College of Health and Nursing Sciences, University of Delaware, where she taught undergraduate and graduate students. Her teaching areas included research methods and family, transcultural, maternal-child, and neonatal ICU nursing. She is currently Visiting Professor,

Beijing Medical University, People's Republic of China, and a consultant in curriculum development for the World Health Organization in China.

## Chapter 8: Cuban-Americans

**Divina Grossman, RN, PhD, ARNP, CS,** is Associate Professor and Chairperson, Adult/Gerontological and Psychiatric Nursing, Florida International University–School of Nursing, and Adjunct Nurse Researcher at the Department of Veterans Affairs Medical Center in Miami, Florida. An immigrant from the Philippines, Dr. Grossman has lived in Miami since 1979. She has been the Chairperson of the Florida Nurses Association (FNA) Task Force on Cultural Diversity since 1993 and was the recipient of the FNA's Mary Cash Award for outstanding contributions to the advancement of cultural diversity in nursing.

## Chapter 9: Egyptian-Americans

**Afaf I. Meleis, RN, PhD, DrPs (hon), FAAN,** is Professor, School of Nursing, Department of Mental Health, Community, and Administrative Nursing at the University of California–San Francisco. Born in Egypt, she came to the United States in the early 1960s to complete graduate education. Dr. Meleis has been professionally involved with health care for Middle Eastern communities in San Francisco and Los Angeles for 30 years.

**Mahmoud Meleis, PhD, PE,** is a nuclear engineer. Born in Egypt, he came to the United States in the early 1960s to complete graduate education. Dr. Meleis was Vice President for the Egyptian Cultural Club of the San Francisco Bay Area for 2 years and has been very involved in the Egyptian-American community in Los Angeles and San Francisco.

## Chapter 10: Filipino-Americans

**Beatriz F. Miranda, RN, MS, FAAN,** is a Gerontological Clinical Nurse Specialist in the Department of Veterans Affairs Medical Center, Lyons, New Jersey. The immediate past president of the Philippine Nurses Association, Ms. Miranda migrated to the United States when the first wave of nurses and physicians were recruited in the 1960s. She participated in the 1994 Health Study of Filipino-Americans in New Jersey funded by a grant from the New Jersey Department of Health, Office of Minority Health.

**Magelende (Melen) R. McBride, RN, PhD,** is Assistant Director and Ethnogeriatric Rehabilitation Clinical Specialist, Stanford Geriatric Education Center–Division of Family and Community Medicine, School of Medicine, Stanford University, where she does curriculum development and coordinates postgraduate geriatric training programs for health professionals. She has extensive experience in the acute and chronic care of middle-aged and older adults, with special emphasis on ethnogeriatrics, rehabilitation, and health promotion. Her research activities focus on multisensory impairment, health promotion, and disease prevention issues of Filipino elders in the United States. She is a member of the Ad Hoc Advisory Committee on Minority Populations for the National Heart, Lung and Blood Institute.

**Zen Spangler, RN, PhD,** is the Director of Nursing Research and Education at the Robert Packer Hospital in Sayre, Pennsylvania. She has conducted several transcultural nursing studies involving Filipino-Americans and was the co-principal investigator of a study of the health status of Filipino-Americans in New Jersey.

## Chapter 11: French Canadians

**Ginette Coutu-Wakulczyk, RN, PhD,** is Assistant Professor, School of Nursing, Faculty of Health Sciences, University of Ottawa, Ontario, Canada. French Canadian, born of parents with a genealogy dating to the early settlers from France, she was raised and educated in the French language from elementary school to the end of her graduate studies. Her cross-cultural experiences include overseas practice in Nigeria.

**Ann C. Beckingham, RN, PhD,** is Professor, School of Nursing, Faculty Health Sciences and Vice-Chair, Continuing Education, McMaster University, Hamilton, Ontario, Canada. With over 20 years' experience in international health, she has been active with the World Health Organization in the Eastern Mediterranean, Southeast Asian, African, and European regions. In addition to her work with gerontology and community nursing, she has published widely and presented numerous papers, seminars, and workshops on cultural diversity.

**Denise Moreau, RN, MSc, PhD (candidate),** is a Lecturer at the School of Nursing, Faculty of Health Sciences, University of Ottawa, Ontario, Canada. A community nurse clinical specialist, she teaches maternity and child-care nursing.

## German-Americans *(chapter on disk)*

**Jessica A. Steckler, RN, EdD (candidate), RNC,** is Associate Director, Lake Area Health Education Center, Veterans Affairs Medical Center, Erie, Pennsylvania. Born and raised in York County, Pennsylvania, Mrs. Steckler, a fifth-generation German-American, grew up in a family that valued its German heritage and preserved its traditions. She has taught various levels of nursing and professional continuing education classes in the predominantly German communities of York and Erie, Pennsylvania.

## Chapter 12: Greek-Americans

**Toni Tripp-Reimer, RN, PhD, FAAN,** is Professor and Director of the Office for Nursing Research Development and Utilization at the University of Iowa, College of Nursing. She is also Director (Principal Investigator) of the National Institutes of Health Funded Gerontological Nursing Interventions Research Center, the Institutional NRSA Training Program in Gerontological Nursing Research, and the Iowa–Veterans Affairs Nursing Research Consortium. She is also editor of the Springer Series, *Advances in Gerontological Nursing.*

**Bernard Sorofman, PhD,** is Associate Professor in the Division of Clinical and Administrative Pharmacy at the University of Iowa College of Pharmacy in Iowa City. Dr. Sorofman is a member of the executive committees of the Iowa Center on Aging and the Center for International, Rural, and Environmental Health as well as a former Fellow of the Kellogg Pharmaceutical Clinical Scientist Program.

## Haitian-Americans *(chapter on disk)*

**Jessie M. Colin, RN, PhD (candidate),** is Assistant Professor of Nursing at Barry University in Miami Shores, Florida. She is a doctoral candidate at Adelphi University,

Garden City, New York, studying the experience of being a Haitian adolescent living in another culture. She is Haitian-American and migrated to the United States as an adolescent. She is cofounder of the Haitian Health Foundation of South Florida, a member of the Haitian-American Nurses Association of Florida, and Chair of the American Nurses Association Commission on Economic and Professional Security.

**Ghislaine Paperwalla, RN, BSN,** is a Research Nurse in Immunology at the Veterans Administration Medical Center in Miami, Florida. Born in Haiti, she immigrated to the United States in 1960. She received her nursing education at Laval University in Canada and at Florida International University. She is president of the Haitian-American Nurses Association of Florida and Vice President of the Haitian Health Foundation of South Florida.

## Hindu-Americans *(chapter on disk)*

**Jayalakshmi Jambunathan, RN, PhD, RNC,** is Associate Professor, College of Nursing, University of Wisconsin in Oshkosh. Born in India, she has resided in the United States for the last 25 years. Frequent visits to her homeland keep her current on Indian health care and health-care practices. Her area of cultural interest is the sociocultural factors affecting depression in Asian women.

## Chapter 13: Iranians

**Juliene G. Lipson, RN, PhD, FAAN,** Professor, University of California–San Francisco, is a nurse-anthropologist and co-director of the Mid-East S.I.H.A. (Study of Health and Adjustment) Project, a health resource center for Middle-Eastern immigrants and those who care for them. She has done research on the health and adjustment of Iranian and Arab immigrants and Afghan refugees since 1982.

**Homeyra Hafizi, RN, MS,** an Iranian immigrant, is Director of Medical/Surgical and Behavioral Health Services, Wuesthoff Memorial Hospital, Rockledge, Florida. She has experience working with culturally diverse clients in San Francisco and at the Mid-East S.I.H.A. Project as language and cultural interpreter for Middle-Eastern immigrants. She has a degree in cross-cultural nursing from the University of California–San Francisco.

## Chapter 14: Irish-Americans

**Sarah A. Wilson, RN, PhD,** is a first-generation Irish-American and is Assistant Professor, Marquette University, College of Nursing in Milwaukee, Wisconsin. A nurse-anthropologist, she teaches community health nursing, culture, and health. Her professional interests are in cultural influences on health, caregivers, hospices, and death and dying.

## Italian-Americans *(chapter on disk)*

**Sandra M. Hillman, RN, PhD,** is Assistant Professor of Nursing Administration at the Medical College of Georgia in Augusta, Georgia. She has been a college teacher for 20 years and is president of her own consulting business, Hillman International Consulting. A third-generation Italian, Dr. Hillman has experienced the Italian culture first-hand in community and home health care.

## Japanese-Americans *(chapter on disk)*

**Nancy C. Sharts-Hopko, RN, PhD, FAAN,** is Professor, College of Nursing, Villanova University, Villanova, Pennsylvania. Dr. Sharts-Hopko served as an Overseas Associate, Presbyterian Church (U.S.A.) in Tokyo, Japan, for over two years, from 1984 to 1986. In that capacity, she worked at St. Lukes College of Nursing, Tokyo, provided counseling to women in the international community, and conducted research on the childbearing experiences of American women in Japan. Dr. Sharts-Hopko continues to serve on the American Council for St. Lukes, Tokyo, a national committee associated with the Episcopal Church.

## Chapter 15: Jewish-Americans

**Janice Selekman, RN, DNSc,** is Professor and Chair, College of Health and Nursing Sciences, University of Delaware, Newark, Delaware. A second-generation Jew of Ashkenazi descent, Ms. Selekman is a member of the Jewish Nurses Council of Hadassah and is on the Board of Directors of the Hillel–Student Center at the University of Delaware.

## Korean-Americans *(chapter on disk)*

**Lauren Regan Sabet, RN, MSN,** spent her undergraduate years at Boston College, where she began her work in International Affairs. Following her acute-care nursing career at the University of California–San Francisco Medical Center, she received her Master of Nursing degree from the University of California–San Francisco. Her education focused on international/cross-cultural nursing, with an advanced degree in community nursing. She is presently working as Human Capital Consultant with Options and Choices, Inc., a health and productivity management consulting company.

## Chapter 16: Mexican-Americans

**Larry D. Purnell, RN, PhD,** is Associate Professor, College of Health and Nursing Sciences, University of Delaware, Newark, Delaware, where he teaches nursing administration and culture in the undergraduate and graduate programs. He has formal and informal experience working with Hispanics in both structured and unstructured settings. He has traveled in Spain, Mexico, Panama, and Puerto Rico and has published two textbooks in Spanish for medical professionals.

## Chapter 17: Navajo Indians

**Olivia Still, RN, MSN,** is a native of the Cherokee Indian tribe and has lived on both Navajo and Zuni Indian reservations. She currently works on the Indian reservation in Tuba City, New Mexico.

**David Hodgins, RN,** has worked with Navajo and Hopi Indians for 6 years at Keana Canyon Hospital and in Tuba City, New Mexico. Half Navajo, he was raised as a Native American on the Hopi Reservation.

## Polish-Americans *(chapter on disk)*

**Martha A. From, EdD, RNC,** is Assistant Professor, Community Health Nursing, Widener University School of Nursing in Chester, Pennsylvania. Dr. From is a first-generation Polish-American who grew up in a Polish Catholic farming community; she maintains her ethnic heritage by practicing Polish rituals and customs. Dr. From has spent time with relatives in Poland and is part of the Kosciuszko Foundation/ UNICEF summer program, teaching English to high school students in Poland.

## Puerto Ricans *(chapter on disk)*

**Teresa C. Juarbe, RN, PhD,** is a consultant in issues related to promotion of health among Latina women in the United States. She is a first-generation Puerto Rican, living in San Jose, California, who immigrated to the United States in 1983.

The author gratefully acknowledges the support and assistance of Mrs. Elizabeth Rolón, San Jose, California. Her Puerto Rican cultural knowledge and experiences were an inspiration for this chapter.

## Turkish-Americans *(chapter on disk)*

**Cara B. Towle, RN, MSN, MA,** is Coordinator of International Clinical Programs—University of California–San Francisco Medical Center. She holds a master's degree in community health nursing administration, with an emphasis on international and cross-cultural nursing. Prior to entering the field of nursing, she earned a master's degree in international/intercultural administration and worked for several years as a foreign student advisor. Ms. Towle has lived in Turkey and is actively involved in the Turkish-American community in California.

**Timur Arslanoglu, BSME, CVT, MSBA (candidate),** has worked as a business consultant for the medical community in the United States and in Turkey. He has served as president of the Turkish-American Association of Northern California. Currently, he is collaborating on a cardiovascular research project in Turkey for the Gladstone Institute at the University of California–San Francisco.

## Chapter 18: Vietnamese-Americans

**Thu T. Nowak, RN,** a native of Viet Nam, came to America in 1970 and pursued her education in nursing at George Mason University. Her career in hospital, community health, and home care has emphasized the application of transcultural health-care principles to minority and refugee populations. Ronald M. Nowak, PhD, assisted in the preparation of the manuscript for this chapter.

# Consultants

**Mohammed S. Alkhalil, DNS**
Jordan University of Science/
　Technology
Irbid, Jordan

**Lynn Assimacopoulos, RN, BSN**
Sioux Falls, South Dakota

**Cynthia Baker, PhD, MN,
　MPhil(Anthropology)**
Associate Professor
University of New Brunswick
Faculty of Nursing
Moncton, New Brunswick, Canada

**Deanna Balantac, RN, MS**
Professor
Division of Nursing
California State University–
　Sacramento
Sacramento, California

**Joanna Basuray, RN, PhD**
Assistant Professor
Department of Nursing
Towson State University
Towson, Maryland

**Patricia Gauntlett Beare, RN, PhD**
Professor
Louisiana State University Medical
　Center
School of Nursing
New Orleans, Louisiana

**Dr. Valerie A. Browne-Krimsley, RN**
Assistant Professor, Coordinator
Department of Nursing
University of Central Florida
Cocoa, Florida

**Kathryn R. Carnaghan-Sherrard, RN,
　BN, MSc(A)**
Faculty Lecturer
McGill University
School of Nursing
Montreal, Quebec, Canada

**Rosie K. Chang, RN, PhD**
Associate Professor (retired)
University of Hawaii
Honolulu, Hawaii

**Rosalind Y. C. Chia, RN, MA**
Head Nurse
Queens Hospital Center
Jamaica, New York

**Elizabeth C. Choi, RN, PhD**
Associate Professor
George Mason University
College of Nursing and Health
　Sciences
Fairfax, Virginia

**Noel J. Chrisman, PhD, MPH**
Professor
University of Washington
School of Nursing
Seattle, Washington

**Monique Cormier-Daigle, BScN, MN**
Director of Education and Research:
　Nursing Sciences
Corporation Hôpitalière Beausejour
Moncton, New Brunswick, Canada

**Rosario T. DeGracia, RN, MSN, C**
Associate Professor
Seattle University
School of Nursing
Seattle, Washington

**Lydia DeSantis, RN, PhD, FAAN**
Professor
University of Miami
Coral Gables, Florida

**Marilyn (Marty) K. Douglas, RN,
　DNSc, CCRN**
Nurse Research and Clinical Nurse
　Specialist, MICU/CCU
Veterans Affairs Medical Center
Palo Alto, California
Assistant Clinical Professor
School of Nursing
University of California, San Francisco
San Francisco, California

# Contents

# Contents for the Computer Disk

**Baltic-Americans: Estonians, Latvians, and Lithuanians**
*Rauda Gelazis*

**Brazilian-Americans**
*Marga Simon Coler*

**German-Americans**
*Jessica A. Steckler*

**Haitian-Americans**
*Jessie M. Colin and Ghislaine Paperwalla*

**Hindu-Americans**
*Jayalakshmi Jambunathan*

**Italian-Americans**
*Sandra M. Hillman*

**Japanese-Americans**
*Nancy C. Sharts-Hopko*

**Korean-Americans**
*Lauren Regan Sabet*

**Polish-Americans**
*Martha A. From*

**Puerto Ricans**
*Teresa C. Juarbe*

**Turkish-Americans**
*Cara B. Towle and Timur Arslanoglu*

# Introduction

Exposure to global diversity and multicultural populations has far-reaching implications for health-care practitioners, delivery of health-care services, and health-care organizations. Many different immigration patterns in the United States have led to a unique multicultural society, reflected locally, regionally, and nationally. Economic, technological, and social changes have prompted a need for modifications in health-care practices to address these changes. Educational and service organizations need to prepare students and staff to provide culturally sensitive, culturally congruent, and culturally competent care to individuals, families, and communities. Health care must reflect a unique understanding of the values of diverse populations and individual acculturation patterns.

As societies become increasingly borderless (real or imagined), consumers of multicultural health information include clients and their families, students, and staff. Organizations are being forced to recognize and pay greater attention to issues related to racial differences, ethnicity, and diversity, when providing care in a multicultural society. Administrators and professionals must meet the needs of their ethnic, racial, and culturally diverse clients and staff.

Culturally specific health information benefits health-care providers by enabling them to offer culturally congruent health interventions, health promotion and disease prevention activities, and teaching strategies. Although physicians, nurses, social workers, nutritionists, technicians, therapists, home health aides, and other health-care providers need similar culturally specific information, the manner in which the information is used differs according to the caregiver's profession, individual experiences, and specific circumstances.

Culture has a powerful influence on one's interpretation of and responses to health care. Clients and staff have the right to be understood, respected, and treated as individuals despite their differences. In addition, they have a right to expect employers and health-care providers to realize that they are different and that their perspectives on and interpretations of health are legitimate. Respect for such differences is demonstrated by incorporating traditional cultural practices for staying healthy into professional prescriptions and interventions. If clients and staff are forced to relinquish their personal ideologies and cultural beliefs, resentment, anger, and noncompliance may result. In some instances, if non-Western medicines and complementary therapies such as traditional Chinese and ayurvedic medicine, acupressure, acumassage, acupuncture, reflexology, rolfing, moxibustion, cupping, and herbal therapies are not incorporated into health-care regimens, prescribed interventions may be ignored. In some cultures, lay and traditional healers are preferred over professional caregivers.

Health-care providers who have specific cultural knowledge can maximize therapeutic interventions by becoming coparticipants or client advocates in diverse health-care settings. The challenge for the health-care provider is to understand the client's perspective. This approach requires that the health-care provider develop an open style of communication, be receptive to learning from multicultural clients, and demonstrate a tolerance for ambiguities inherent in cultural norms, which evolve and are thus continually changing. Whereas many cultural characteristics are readily apparent, others are less obvious and need conscious exploration.

Valuing diversity in health care enhances the delivery and effectiveness of care, both physically and symbolically. Health-care providers need to address their personal views of traditional values, including biases and prejudices about other cultures and ethnic groups. Teaching diversity increases students' sophistication and understanding of the world in which they live. Educators can improve instruction related to diversity by first determining students' knowledge and perceptions of specific ethnic groups. Correcting prior misconceptions is essential so that they do not interfere with learning. Allowing students to see the world differently helps them to develop more creative solutions to simple as well as complex problems. Multicultural education is an important aspect of personal and professional development.

Leadership is a key factor in promoting effective multicultural relationships. Leaders influence policy and practice, creating an organizational culture and setting the tone for cultural competence and sensitivity. Leaders must be role models of holistic health care through their interactions with consumers. Administrative and managerial staff often undergo cultural training and should be viewed as an educational resource for staff.

Cultural diversity permeated North American society before Christopher Columbus' crew came ashore in 1492 and has increased since that time. In 1784, Benjamin Franklin related concerns regarding differences in the values inherent in cultural behaviors. His account of a short dialogue (Kronenberger, 1970) that took place over 200 years ago is an excellent example of individuals from two distinct cultural groups who failed to understand the other's attitudes, beliefs, values, and lifestyle.

> At the treaty of Lancaster, in Pennsylvania, anno 1744, between the Government of Virginia and the Six Nations, the commissioners from Virginia acquainted the Indians by a speech, that there was at Williamsburg a college with a fund for educating youth, and that if the chiefs of the Six Nations would send down half a dozen of their sons to that college, the government would take care that they be well provided for, and instructed in all the learning of the white people.
>
> The Indians' Spokesman replied: . . . We are convinced . . . that you mean to do us good by your proposal and we thank you heartily. But you, who are wise, must know that different nations have different conceptions of things; and you will not therefore take it amiss, if our ideals of this kind of education happen not to be the same as yours. We have some experience of it; several of our young people were formerly brought up at the colleges of northern provinces; they came back to us; they were bad runners, ignorant of every means of living in the woods, unable to bear either cold or hunger, knew neither how to build a cabin, take a deer, nor kill an enemy, spoke our language imperfectly, were therefore neither fit for hunters, warriors, nor counsellors; they were totally good for nothing.
>
> We are however not the less obligated by your kind offer, though we decline accepting it; and, to show our grateful sense of it, if the gentlemen of Virginia will send us a dozen of their sons, we will take care of their education, instruct them in all we know, and make men of them.[1]

Similar experiences have occurred over millennia. Perhaps one of the most important concepts in this eloquent dialogue is that the two differing cultural groups took the time to communicate their individual belief systems. Without this willingness to communicate and understand one another's culture, mutually satisfying relationships are hindered. Lack of communication can threaten the quality of health care provided in a multicultural setting.

When studying culture and ethnicity, one should not overanalyze behaviors and situations that could lead to reductionist language. The complexities of culture strongly influence perceptions. Ultimately, experience working with diverse staff and clients may be the best educational environment for learning about culture.

This textbook presents a framework for collecting health data about individuals or groups from diverse cultural backgrounds in a nonjudgmental way; this assists health-care providers in delivering competently conscious, congruent, and relevant care in diverse settings.

The book is divided into 18 chapters. Chapter 1 provides an overview of culture and ethnicity and defines terms commonly used in the study of culture. Chapter 2

---

1. Kronenberger, L. (1970). *The cutting edge* (pp. 5–6). Garden City, NY: Doubleday & Co.

introduces and explains Purnell's Model for Cultural Competence. Chapters 3 through 18 describe the health-care needs and practices of specific ethnic and cultural groups. The chapters are organized alphabetically by ethnic group, and the format follows Purnell's Model. A list of key words or phrases specific to each culture is offered at the beginning of each chapter. Pictures or graphics representative of the culture, a cultural case study, and a reference list are included.

The book concludes with a glossary incorporating key terms appearing in the chapters and on the accompanying electronic disk. A subject index to this text is provided for easy reference.

# Transcultural Diversity and Health Care

*Larry D. Purnell and Betty J. Paulanka*

---

• Key terms to become familiar with in this chapter are:

| | |
|---|---|
| Acculturate | Ethnocultural |
| Assimilate | Generalization |
| Attitude | Ideology |
| Belief | Refugee |
| Culture | Sojourner |
| Cultural competence | Stereotyping |
| Cultural diversity | Subculture |
| Ethnic | Worldview |
| Ethnocentrism | Values |

## DIVERSITY IN NORTH AMERICA

The world's population reached 5.6 billion persons in 1994 and is expected to approach 7.9 billion by 2020, an increase of 2.3 billion. Ninety percent of this increase will be in developing countries, with 1 billion occurring in Asia alone. A significant number of immigrants to the United States and Canada comes from one of the world's 20 most populous countries. These include Mexico, the Philippines, Vietnam, China, India, Iran, Germany, Turkey, and Egypt. Over 19 million people, or 1 in every 13 residents in the United States, are foreign-born (*Information please: Almanac,* 1995).

California has the most striking mix in population demographics, with 39 percent of the national Asian population, 34 percent of the Hispanic population, and 12 percent of the Native-American population. The rest of the country is expected to mirror this trend, but at a slower pace (Norbeck, 1995). By the year 2000, one-third of all U.S. citizens will be members of minority groups (Department of Veterans Affairs, 1995). By the year 2050, the nation's Asian population is expected to increase from 3 to 11 percent, the black population from 12 to 16 percent, and the Hispanic population from 9 to 21 percent (Norbeck, 1995). Other ethnic groups such as Arabs, Germans, Brazilians, Greeks, Egyptians, and Turks are also increasing.

Long-standing homogeneous areas in the United States, such as Montgomery

County, Maryland, are changing dramatically. Between 1990 and 1994, 9 out of 10 new residents in Montgomery County were members of minority groups (*Washington Post,* 1995). Similar trends are occurring in Canada (*Statistics Canada: Ethnic origins,* 1993). Thus, North America is increasingly becoming a mosaic of many cultures, reflecting a mixture of ideologies, beliefs, and health-care practices.

Original Native-Americans, immigrants, and their descendants have transformed the United States into the world's most powerful nation. The earliest immigrants to North America were primarily from northern European countries, France, and Spain. However, as society has become more diverse, awareness of cultural and ethnic differences between clients and health-care providers has needed to increase. Thus, it is more important than ever for health-care providers to learn about cultural variations in health-care practices.

## CULTURAL CONCEPTS AND TERMS DEFINED

Anthropologists and sociologists have proposed many definitions of culture. For the purposes of this book, **culture** is defined as:

> the totality of socially transmitted behavioral patterns, arts, beliefs, values, customs, lifeways, and all other products of human work and thought characteristics of a population of people that guide their worldview and decision making.

These patterns may be explicit or implicit, are primarily learned and transmitted within the family, are shared by the majority of the members of the culture, and are emergent phenomena that change in response to global phenomena. Culture is largely unconscious and has powerful influences on health and illness.

When individuals of dissimilar cultural orientations meet in a work or therapeutic environment, the likelihood for developing a mutually satisfying relationship is improved if both parties in the relationship attempt to learn about each other's culture. Increasing one's consciousness of **cultural diversity** improves the possibilities for health-care practitioners to provide culturally competent care. **Cultural competence,** as used in this book, means:

1. Developing an awareness of one's own existence, sensations, thoughts, and environment without letting it have an undue influence on those from other backgrounds.

2. Demonstrating knowledge and understanding of the client's culture.

3. Accepting and respecting cultural differences.

4. Adapting care to be congruent with the client's culture. Cultural competence is a conscious process and not necessarily linear.

One progresses from unconscious incompetence (not being aware that one is lacking knowledge about another culture) to conscious incompetence (being aware that one is lacking knowledge about another culture); then to conscious competence (learning about the client's culture, verifying generalizations about the client's culture, and providing culturally specific interventions); and finally to unconscious competence (automatically providing culturally congruent care to clients of a diverse culture). Unconscious competence is difficult to accomplish. Most health-care providers can expect to reach only the conscious competence stage of cultural development. To be even minimally effective, culturally competent care must have the assurance of continuation after the original impetus is withdrawn; it must be integrated into and valued by the culture that is to benefit from the interventions.

Developing mutually satisfying relationships with diverse cultural groups involves good interpersonal skills and the application of knowledge and techniques learned from the physical, biologic, and social sciences as well as the humanities. An understanding of one's own culture and personal values and the ability to detach oneself from "excess baggage" associated with personal views are essential to cultural competence. Even then, traces of ethnocentrism may unconsciously pervade one's attitudes and behavior. **Ethnocentrism,** the universal tendency of human beings to think that their ways of thinking, acting, and believing are the only right, proper, and natural ways, can be a major barrier to providing culturally conscious care. Ethnocentrism perpetuates an attitude that beliefs that differ greatly from one's own are strange, bizarre, or unenlightened, and therefore wrong. **Values** are principles and standards that have meaning and worth to an individual, family, group, or community. The extent to which one's cultural values are internalized influences the tendency toward ethnocentrism. The more one's values are internalized, the more difficult it is to avoid the tendency toward ethnocentrism.

## Attitude, Belief, and Ideology

Within the definition of culture are the terms attitude, belief, and ideology. **Attitude** is a state of mind or feeling with regard to some matter of a culture. A **belief** is something that is accepted as true, especially as a tenet or a body of tenets accepted by people in an ethnocultural group. Attitudes and beliefs do not have to be proven; they are unconsciously accepted as truths. **Ideology** consists of the thoughts and beliefs that reflect the social needs and aspirations of an individual or ethnocultural group.

## Worldview, Subcultures, and Ethnicity

**Worldview** is the way individuals or groups of people look at the universe to form values about their lives and the world around them. Worldview includes cosmology, relationships with nature, moral and ethical reasoning, social relationships, magicoreligious beliefs, and aesthetics.

Any **generalization** made about the behaviors of any individual or large group of people is almost certain to be an oversimplification. When a generalization relates less to the actual observed behavior than to the motives thought to underlie the behavior (that is, the *why* of the behavior), it is likely to be oversimplified. Thus, generalizations can lead to **stereotyping,** an oversimplified conception, opinion, or belief about some aspect of an individual or group of people.

Within all cultures are subcultures and ethnic groups that may not hold all the values of their dominant culture. **Subcultures, ethnic** groups, or **ethnocultural** populations are groups of people who have experiences different from those of the dominant culture by virtue of status, ethnic background, residence, religion, education, or other factors that functionally unify the group and act collectively on each member with a conscious awareness of these differences. Subcultures differ from the dominant ethnic group and share beliefs according to the primary and secondary characteristics of diversity.

Primary and secondary characteristics of diversity affect how people view their culture. Primary characteristics include nationality, race, color, gender, age, and religious affiliation. Secondary characteristics include socioeconomic status, length of time away from the country of origin, education, occupation, military status, urban versus rural residence, marital status, parental status, physical characteristics, sexual orientation, and women's issues. In addition, the reason for immigration influences a person's worldview. For example, people who immigrate generally **acculturate** more willingly, that is, modify their own culture as a result of contact with another culture, and **assimilate,** that is, gradually adopt and incorporate the characteristics of the prevailing culture, than people who immigrate unwillingly or as sojourners. **Sojourners,** who immigrate with the intention of remaining in their new homeland only a short time, or **refugees,** who think they may return to their home country, may not have the need to acculturate or assimilate. Undocumented individuals (illegal aliens) may have a worldview different from those who have arrived legally on a work visa or as "legal immigrants."

## TRANSCULTURAL HEALTH CARE

The debate regarding the precise definition of the terms *transcultural, crosscultural,* and *intercultural* continues. Many authors and texts define the terms differently. This book uses the terms interchangeably to mean "crossing," "spanning," or "interacting" with a culture other than one's own. When people interact with persons from a culture different from their own, they are engaged in *cultural diversity.* Awareness of the differences and similarities among ethnocultural groups results in a broadened multicultural worldview.

## DIVERSITY FOR THE HEALTH PROFESSIONS

People may wear the same brand and style of clothes, drive the same make of automobile, and watch the same television shows but still be worlds apart in cultural and ethnic backgrounds that define their basic heritage and values. The more dissimilar in appearances individuals are, the easier it becomes for others to realize they may have differing beliefs, attitudes, and ideologies. Unfortunately, this observation does not necessarily enhance better acceptance of individual differences. Increased similarity in the appearance of culturally diverse individuals challenges others to be more consciously aware of differences underlying ethnocultural diversity.

The mass media, professional organizations, the workplace, and educational institutions from elementary schools to colleges and universities have addressed the need for individuals to become knowledgeable about and sensitive to cultural diversity. Health-care personnel provide care to people of diverse cultures in numerous settings. Long-term-care facilities, acute care facilities, clinics, the community, and the client's home are common examples of settings in which health-care providers encounter culturally diverse clients and staff. Although physicians, nurses, nutritionists, therapists, technicians, morticians, home health aides, and other caregivers need similar culturally specific information, the manner in which the information is used may differ significantly based on the discipline, individual experiences, and specific circumstances of the client. Each discipline has its own unique knowledge to support its ways of knowing, techniques, roles, norms, values, ideologies, attitudes, and beliefs, which interlock to make a reinforced and supportive system within its defined practice. Thus, an understanding of ethnocultural diversity is essential for all health-care providers.

Before the 1960s, many health-care facilities and places of business openly discriminated against people of color and selected ethnic backgrounds. Organizational practices of discrimination often segregated these ethnic groups into separate settings or locations. After the civil rights movement of the 1960s, a surge of individual and political support developed for treating all people equally regardless of their color, race, ethnicity, culture, religion, gender, and more recently sexual orientation and disability. Today, each subgroup has the right to be respected for its unique individuality.

Perhaps no other professional group in society has recognized the impact of cultural diversity on its work as much as the health profession. Nursing has always stressed the importance of providing *culturally conscious* care that respects individual differences and incorporates unique values and lifestyles into the delivery of health care. Health-care professionals, their teachers, and their students have supported the concept of holistic care and recognized the necessity of understanding the client's background to provide comprehensive care that respects personal values and individuality.

In 1983, the National League for Nursing (NLN) developed criteria to guide nursing programs in providing curricula that respect cultural, racial, and ethnic diversity. In June 1993, the NLN adopted *Resolution No. 2: Equity in nursing for members of racial and ethnic minorities.* This resolution addresses the need for an agenda that promotes racial and ethnic sensitivity and equity throughout the community and among educational programs accredited by the NLN (*Resolution No. 2,* 1993).

## RESOURCES FOR CULTURAL DIVERSITY

In 1899, the International Council of Nurses was started and now publishes the *International Journal of Nursing Studies* and the *International Nursing Review* (International Council of Nurses, 1991). The Council on Nursing and Anthropology was initiated in 1969 to include cultural content in nursing curricula, help improve care for underserved and ethnic populations, and encourage relevant research. In 1974, the Transcultural Nursing Society was founded by Madeline Leininger, a nurse anthropologist, to promote interest in transcultural nursing and to prepare nurses to optimize their competence in transcultural nursing care (Transcultural Nursing Society, 1993). The society publishes the *Journal of Transcultural Nursing,* which started in 1989. Other journals that address cultural and ethnic diversity issues include the *Western Journal of Medicine: Cross Cultural Issues,* the *Journal of Cultural Diversity,* and the *Journal of Multicultural Nursing.* The Consortium for International Nursing Education, founded in 1993, publishes the newsletter *Broadened Horizons.* The American Academy of Nursing, several state Organizations of Nurse Executives, and the American Association of Colleges of Nursing have position statements regarding diversity issues in a multicultural society and the health-care arena.

In addition to cultural societies and journals, several resource centers and publishers have literature focusing on cultural diversity. The REACH (Respecting Ethnic and Cultural Heritage) Center in Seattle, Washington, has a series of publications and resources for promoting and understanding diversity among elementary school and high school students. Sage Publications in Thousand Oaks, California, and Intercultural Press in Yarmouth, Maine, have books, videos, and other resources for learning about different cultures.

Articles on transcultural research are becoming a common feature in many health-related journals. Health-care professionals engage in basic research for practical applications and in applied research for investigation of cultural issues surrounding the delivery of health care.

Research is needed to examine individual behavioral responses to a multitude of health-care problems experienced during normal health processes, such as pregnancy, birth, death, and human growth and development. Research is also needed to identify new information on the biologic, physical, physiological, spiritual, sociological, and psychological differences within, between, and among cultural groups and subgroups. This information can be used to support the development of specific interventions designed to address unique cultural differences.

Even though much research has been completed on cultural diversity issues, a significant time gap often exists between the identification of findings and the dissemination of information and testing of new hypotheses. The limited dissemination of research findings inhibits widespread acceptance of new interventions for enhancing acceptance of culturally diverse health-care practices. Computer information technology and online networks help to narrow this gap and enhance the dissemination of research findings in a timely manner.

# THEORIES AND CONCEPTUAL MODELS FOR CULTURAL DIVERSITY

In the 1960s, nurses and other health-care theorists began to develop theoretical and conceptual frameworks for assessing, planning, and implementing culturally competent interventions. Since that time, a few culturally based theoretical and conceptual frameworks have been developed for use by health professionals. Each theoretical and conceptual framework has its own advantages. While these frameworks provide excellent experiences for class participation, discussions, mind expansion, and abstract critical thinking, many are difficult for health-care professionals to operationalize and incorporate into their daily practice. Because of the complexities of some of these theories, the average person requires 8 to 10 hours of instruction to understand them.

Some of the more popular transcultural theoretical and conceptual frameworks are Leininger's Sunrise Model, which is designed for nursing (Leininger, 1988), and Murdock's Outline of Cultural Material, which is designed for community assessment (Murdock, 1971). Tripp-Reimer, Brink, and Saunders' (1984) model is more specific to nursing; Giger and Davidhizar's (1991) model is used across subspecialties in nursing; Fong's (1985) model uses the CONFHER (Communication style, Orientation, Nutrition, Family relationships, Health beliefs, Education, and Religion) model, which lists seven areas for assessing a client's background; and Campinha-Bacote's (1991) model, which can be used across disciplines, includes cultural knowledge, awareness, skill, desire, and encounters. Other cultural models are geared toward intercultural adjustment and learning, understanding and coping with cross-cultural stress, the role of culture assimilator training, and a developmental model of intercultural sensitivity (Paige, 1986).

This book uses Purnell's Model for Cultural Competence, which includes an easy-to-use and easy-to-understand organizing framework for practicing health-care providers in all professions. The organizing framework can be used regardless of one's ethnic or cultural background and understanding of conceptual models. This model and its organizing framework are described in Chapter 2.

## *References*

Campinha-Bacote, J. (1991). *The process of cultural competence: A culturally competent model of care* (2nd ed.). Wyoming, OH: Transcultural C.A.R.E. Associates.

*Diversity in the workplace* (1995). Washington, DC: Department of Veterans' Affairs.

Fong, C. M. (1985). Ethnicity and nursing practice. *Topics in Clinical Nursing, 7*(3), 1–10.

Giger, J. and Davidhizar, R. (1991). *Transcultural nursing.* St. Louis: C. V. Mosby.

*Information please: almanac* (48th ed.) (1995). New York: Houghton Mifflin.

International Council of Nurses (1991). *Nursing voice worldwide.* Geneva, Switzerland: Author.

Leininger, M. M. (1988). Leininger's theory of nursing: Culture care diversity and universality. *Nursing Science Quarterly, 1*(4), 152–160.

Murdock, G. (1971). *Outline of cultural materials* (4th ed.). New Haven: Human Relations Area Files.

National League for Nursing (1983). *Criteria for the evaluation of baccalaureate and higher degree programs in nursing.* New York: Author. NLN Publication No. 15-125-1A.

National League for Nursing (June 1993). *Resolution No. 2: Equity in nursing for members of racial and ethnic minorities.* New York: Author.

Norbeck, J. (1995). Who is our consumer? Shaping nursing programs to meet emerging needs. *Journal of Professional Nursing, 11*(6), 325–331.

Paige, M. R. (1986). *Cross-cultural orientation: New conceptualizations and applications.* Lanham, MD: University Press of America.

*Statistics Canada: Ethnic origins* (1993). Ottowa, Canada: Minister of Industry, Science, and Technology.

Transcultural Nursing Society, Madonna University College of Nursing and Health. (1993). *The Transcultural Nursing Society Newsletter.* Livonia, MI: Author.

Tripp-Reimer, T., Brink, P., & Saunders, J. (1984). Cultural assessment: Content and process. *Nursing Outlook, 32*(2), 32.

*U.S. Immigration population at postwar high* (August 8, 1995). Washington Post, A1, A8.

# Purnell's Model for Cultural Competence

*Larry D. Purnell* and *Betty J. Paulanka*

---

• Key terms to become familiar with in this chapter are:

| | |
|---|---|
| Community | Health |
| Family | Person |
| Global society | |

Western academic and health-care organizations stress structure, systematization, and formalization when studying complex phenomena such as culture and ethnicity. Given the complexity of individuals, Purnell's evolving Model for Cultural Competence provides a comprehensive, systematic, and concise framework for learning culture. The empirical framework of the model can assist health-care providers, managers, and administrators in all health disciplines to provide holistic, culturally competent therapeutic interventions, health promotion, health maintenance, disease prevention, and health teaching across educational and practice settings.

The purposes of this model are to:

1. Provide a framework for all health-care providers to learn inherent concepts and characteristics of culture

2. Define circumstances that affect one's cultural worldview in the context of historical perspectives

3. Provide a model that links the most central relationships of culture

4. Interrelate characteristics of culture to promote congruence and facilitate the delivery of consciously competent care

5. Provide a framework that reflects human characteristics such as motivation, intentionality, and meaning

6. Provide a structure for analyzing cultural data

7. View the individual, family, or group within a unique ethnocultural environment

## OVERVIEW OF THE MODEL

The model (Fig. 2–1) is a circle, with an outlying rim representing global society, a second rim representing community, a third rim representing family, and an inner rim representing the person. The interior of the circle is divided into 12 pie-shaped wedges depicting cultural domains and their concepts. The dark center of the circle represents unknown phenomena. Along the bottom of the model is an erose line representing the nonlinear concept of cultural consciousness.

## Macroaspects of the Model

The macroaspects of this interactional model include the metaparadigm concepts of a global society, community, family, person, and conscious competence. Fields of inquiry incorporated in the model include biology, anthropology, sociology, economics, geography, history, ecology, physiology, psychology, political science, pharma-

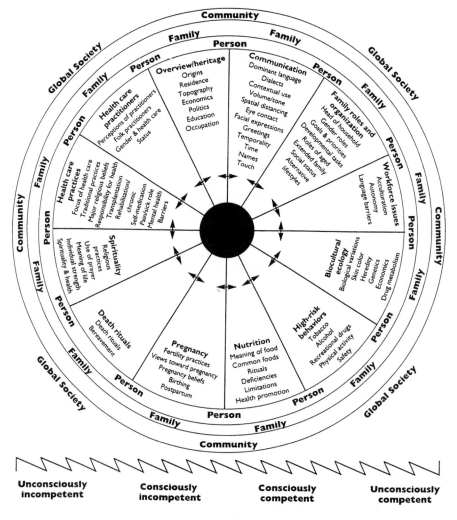

**Figure 2–1.** Purnell's Model for Cultural Competence. (See text for explanation.)

cology, and nutrition as well as theories from communication, family development, and social support. The model can be used in clinical practice, education, research, and the administration and management of health-care service.

Phenomena related to a **global society** include world communication and politics; conflicts and warfare; natural disasters and famines; international exchanges in business, commerce, and information technology; advances in the health sciences; space exploration; and the increased ability for people to travel around the world and to interact with diverse societies. Global events that are widely disseminated by television, radio, satellite transmission, newsprint, and information technology affect all societies, either directly or indirectly. Such events create chaos and consciously and unconsciously force people to alter their lifeways and worldviews.

In its broadest definition, **community** is a group of people having a common interest or identity and living in a specified locality. Community includes the physical, social, and symbolic characteristics that cause people to connect. Bodies of water, mountains, rural versus urban living, and even railroad tracks help people to define their physical concept of community. Economics, religion, politics, age, generation, and marital status delineate the social concepts of community. Sharing a specific language or dialect, lifestyle, history, dress, art, or musical interest are symbolic characteristics of community. People actively and passively interact with the community, necessitating adaptation and assimilation for equilibrium and homeostasis in their worldview. Individuals may willingly change their physical, social, and symbolic community when it no longer meets their needs.

**Family** is two or more people who are emotionally involved with each other. They may, but not necessarily do, live in close proximity to each other. Family may include physically and emotionally close and distant consanguineous relatives and physically and emotionally close and distant non-blood-related significant others. Family structure and roles change according to age, generation, marital status, relocation or immigration, and socioeconomic status, necessitating each person to rethink individual beliefs and lifeways.

**Person** is a biopsychosociocultural human being who is constantly adapting. Human beings adapt biologically and physiologically with the aging process; psychologically in the context of social relationships, stress, and relaxation; socially as they interact with the changing community; and ethnoculturally within the broader global society.

The concept of health, which permeates all metaparadigm concepts of culture, is defined globally, nationally, regionally, locally, and individually. Thus, people can speak about their personal health status or the health status of the nation or community. Health can also be subjective or objective in nature. **Health**, as used in this book, is a state of wellness as defined by people within their ethnocultural group and generally includes physical, mental, and spiritual states because group members interact with the family, community, and global society.

## Microaspects of the Model

On a microlevel, the model has an organizing framework consisting of 12 domains and their concepts, which are common to all cultures. These 12 domains are interconnected with each other and have implications for health. The utility of this organizing framework comes from its concise structure, which can be used in any setting, applied to a broad range of empirical experiences, and can foster inductive and deductive reasoning in the assessment of cultural domains. Once cultural data are analyzed, the practitioner can fully adopt, modify, or reject health-care treatment regimens according to their respect for the client's needs and, ultimately, whether they improve the quality of the client's health-care experiences and personal existence.

## THE TWELVE DOMAINS OF CULTURE

The 12 domains essential for assessing the ethnocultural attributes of an individual, family, or group are as follows:

1. Overview, inhabited localities, and topography

2. Communication

3. Family roles and organization

4. Workforce issues

5. Biocultural ecology

6. High-risk health behaviors

7. Nutrition

8. Pregnancy and childbearing practices

9. Death rituals

10. Spirituality

11. Health-care practices

12. Health-care practitioners

## Overview, Inhabited Localities, and Topography

The domain overview, inhabited localities, and topography includes concepts related to country of origin, current residence, the effects of the topography of country of origin and current residence on health, economics, politics, reasons for migration, educational status, and occupations. These concepts are interrelated. For example, economic and political conditions may affect one's reason for migration, and educational attainment is usually interrelated with employment choices. Sociopolitical and socioeconomic conditions influence individual behavioral responses to health and illness.

Becoming knowledgeable about a different culture includes becoming familiar with the heritage of its people and their part of the world. Salient historical events, such as discrimination in the country of origin, affect culture and influence value systems, beliefs, and explanatory frameworks used in everyday life. Given the primary and secondary characteristics of diversity (see Chapter 1), generalizations and stereotypes may not be part of a specific individual's beliefs or value system.

### *Heritage and Residence*

A common practice for many immigrants is to relocate to an area that has an established population with similar ideologies that can provide initial support, serve as cultural brokers, and orient them to their new culture and health-care system. For example, many Vietnamese immigrants have settled in Arlington, Virginia, Irish in Boston, Germans in Pennsylvania, Mexicans in Texas and California, Jews and Italians in New York, Chinese in California, Polish in Illinois, and Cubans in Florida. Thus, these cities have Chinatowns, Polonias, Jewish settlements, Little Italies, and other ethnic enclaves. When immigrants settle and work exclusively in predominantly ethnic communities, primary social support is enhanced, but acculturation and assimilation into the wider society may be hindered. In contrast, the earlier immigrant Vietnamese refugee population had no group to offer initial support, yet many had an unplanned precipitous departure, with dangerous escapes from their homeland by land and sea, (Hinton et al., 1993; Muecke, 1983), making their adjustment in their new homeland particularly difficult.

An awareness of the geographic residence of an ethnocultural group increases opportunities for collaborating with health-care providers in these communities. Collaboration is essential for health promotion, health maintenance, disease prevention, treatment, and health teaching.

Table 2–1 lists the approximate population and predominant residence in the United States and Canada of the cultural and ethnic groups presented in this book. Conflicting demographic and population statistics for each of these groups may exist depending on the reference and methods used for collecting data.

### Reasons for Migration and Associated Economic Factors

The social, economic, religious, and political forces of the country of origin play an important role in the development of the ideologies and the worldview of individuals, families, and groups and are often a major motivating force for emigration. For example, political oppression (Jews), religious persecution (Germans), famines (the Irish), environmental disasters (earthquakes in Peru), economics (lack of job opportunities in Brazil), and personal ideologies (Cubans) are reasons that some individuals and groups choose to relocate. Most people immigrate to this country in the hopes of a better life; however, this ideology is personally defined by the individual or group. Understanding the reason for a person's immigration, whether voluntary, sojourner, refugee, or undocumented status, provides clues to the person's acculturation patterns.

Most newer immigrants within the last few decades have had existing ethnic enclaves in the United States to assist them with acculturation. However, those groups who do not have established enclaves, such as Iranians and Vietnamese, may need extra help in adjusting to their new homeland's language, access to health-care services, living accommodations, and employment opportunities. People who move across cultures voluntarily are likely to experience less difficulty with acculturation than people who are forced to emigrate to a new culture (Berry, 1990). Some individuals immigrate with the intention of remaining in this country only a short time, making money and returning home, whereas others immigrate with the intention of relocating permanently. Therefore, it is imperative for the health-care provider to assess the reasons behind the individual's migration to understand the implications for culturally competent care.

### Educational Status and Occupations

The value placed on formal education differs among cultural and ethnic groups and is often related to their socioeconomic status in their homeland, their reasons for emigrating, or their ability to emigrate. For example, Iranian-Americans and Egyptian-Americans place a high value on education, and those who earn an advanced degree are placed in high esteem. Others, such as some newer Mexican-Americans, do not stress formal education because it was not needed for employment in their homeland. Consequently, they may become engulfed in poverty, which further limits their potential for formal educational opportunities and planning for the future.

Primary learning styles also vary among individuals from different cultures. For example, Arab education emphasizes theory, but little attention is given to practical application. As a result, Arab students are more proficient at tests requiring rote learning than at those requiring conceptualization and analysis. Being familiar with the individual's personal educational values and learning modes allows for health-care providers, educators, and employers to adjust teaching strategies for clients,

Table 2–1 • **U.S. and Canadian Populations and Predominant U.S. Residence of Ethnic/Cultural Groups Covered**

| Ethnic/Cultural Group | Population of Country of Origin | Population in the United States | Predominant Residence in the United States | Population in Canada |
|---|---|---|---|---|
| African-Americans | Multiple countries | 27,100,000 | 54% in South Louisiana, Georgia, Virginia, Mississippi, Indiana, Illinois, Michigan, Tennessee, New York, New Jersey, and Washington, D.C. | 224,620 |
| Amish | Unknown | 130,000 | Pennsylvania, Indiana, and Ohio | Not listed as such |
| Appalachian | England, Scotland, Wales, and Germany | 23,000,000 | Georgia, Alabama, Mississippi, Virginia, West Virginia, North Carolina, South Carolina, Kentucky, Tennessee, Ohio, Maryland, New York, and Pennsylvania | Not listed as such |
| Arab | Multiple Mediterranean countries | 3,000,000 | New York, Washington, D.C., Massachusetts, New Jersey, Pennsylvania, Michigan, Ohio, Texas, Illinois, and California | 144,050 |
| Baltic | Estonia 1,500,000<br>Latvia 2,800,000<br>Lithuania 3,500,000 | 26,762<br>75,745<br>811,865 | New York, Washington, Illinois, Oregon, Massachusetts, Pennsylvania, Ohio | 39,610 |
| Brazilian | 155,000,000 | 3,000,000 | Massachusetts, New York, New Jersey, Florida, California, and Michigan | 2,525 |
| Chinese | 1,300,000,000 | 1,505,000 | New York, California | 586,645 |
| Cuban | 11,100,000 | 860,000 | New York, Florida | 660 |
| Egyptian | 58,900,000 | 1,000,000 | New York, California, Washington, D.C., and Illinois | 18,950 |

**Table 2–1 • U.S. and Canadian Populations and Predominant U.S. Residence of Ethnic/Cultural Groups Covered** (*Continued*)

| Ethnic/Cultural Group | Population of Country of Origin | Population in the United States | Predominant Residence in the United States | Population in Canada |
|---|---|---|---|---|
| Filipino | 68,700,000 | 1,450,000 | California, Hawaii, Alaska, New York, New Jersey, Illinois, and Texas | 157,250 |
| French Canadian | 6,146,000 | 2,167,000 | Northeastern United States | 6,146,000 |
| German | 81,200,000 | 58,000,000 | Pennsylvania, Indiana, New York, Maryland, Virginia, Midwest, Texas, and Ohio | 911,560 |
| Greek | 10,400,000 | 1,400,000 | Utah, Colorado, Nevada, New Hampshire, Connecticut, Massachusetts, Illinois, Michigan, Ohio, Wisconsin, New York, and Pennsylvania | 151,150 |
| Hatian | 7,000 | 365,000 | New York, Illinois, Massachusetts, Florida, California | 22,805 |
| Hindu | 911,600,000 | 786,000 | California, New York, and the Midwest | 324,840 |
| Iranian | 61,200,000 | 1,000,000 | Half in California; the rest are scattered | 38,915 |
| Irish | 3,600,000 | 38,700,000 | Massachusetts, New York, Pennsylvania, Ohio, Illinois, and Michigan | 725,600 |
| Italian | 57,200,000 | 14,660,000 | New York, New Jersey, Pennsylvania, Virginia, Maryland, and Lower Mississippi Valley | 750,055 |
| Japanese | 121,000,000 | 1,004,645 | California, Hawaii, Oregon, Washington | 48,595 |
| Jewish | 18,153,000 | 5,789,000 | New York, New Jersey, Florida, Massachusetts, and Maryland | 245,840 |

**Table 2-1 • U.S. and Canadian Populations and Predominant U.S. Residence of Ethnic/Cultural Groups Covered** (*Continued*)

| Ethnic/Cultural Group | Population of Country of Origin | Population in the United States | Predominant Residence in the United States | Population in Canada |
|---|---|---|---|---|
| Korean | 67,600,000 | 626,000 | California, New York, and Washington State | 44,095 |
| Mexican | 91,800,000 | 12,000,000 | California, Texas, Illinois, Arizona, Colorado, and Florida | 8,015 |
| Navajo | Native-American | 200,000 | Arizona, Utah, and New Mexico | Not listed as such |
| Polish | 38,600,000 | 9,366,000 | Illinois, Florida, Texas, California, New Jersey, New York, and Ohio | 272,810 |
| Puerto Rican | 3,000,000 | 2,400,000 | New York, Connecticut, Florida, Illinois | Not listed as such |
| Turks | 61,800,000 | 85,000 | New York, California, New Jersey, and Florida | 8,525 |
| Vietnamese | 73,100,000 | 615,000 | California, Texas, Virginia, New York, Pennsylvania | 84,005 |

*Sources:* Data from *Information please: Almanac.* Boston: Houghton Mifflin, 1995. *Statistics Canada: Ethnic origins.* 1993. *U.S. statistical abstracts, 1995;* and *Gale Publishing encyclopedia of multicultural Americans, I,* p. 46 and *II,* pp. 868, 881. Detroit, MI: Gale Publishing.

students, and employees. Educational materials and explanations must be presented at a level consistent with the client's educational capabilities and within their cultural framework and beliefs.

Immigrants bring job skills from their native homelands and traditionally seek employment in the same or similar trades. Sometimes these job skills are inadequate for the available jobs in the new society; thus, immigrants are forced to take low-paying jobs and join the ranks of the working poor and economically disadvantaged. Most immigrants in America include persons employed in a broad variety of occupations and professions; however, experiential and educational limitations and language abilities of more recent immigrants often restrict employment possibilities. More importantly, experiential backgrounds sometimes encourage employment choices that are identified as high risk for chronic diseases, such as exposure to pesticides and chemicals. Others may work in factories that manufacture hepatotoxic chemicals, in industries with pollutants that increase the risk for pulmonary diseases, and in crowded conditions with poor ventilation that increase the risk for tuberculosis or other respiratory diseases. In some immigrant populations, the country of origin has lost many of its professional and well-educated people, who have difficulty finding work comparable to what they did in their homeland (Lipson & Haifizi, 1997), resulting in a "brain drain" for the host country and underemployment in their new environment (Ronaghy, et al., 1975).

Being knowledgeable about an individual's current and previous work background is essential for health screening. For example, newer immigrants who worked in malaria-infested areas (Egypt, Italy, Turkey, and Vietnam) may need health screening for malaria. Those who worked in mining industries in their homeland (Irish and Polish) may need screening for respiratory diseases. Those who lived in overcrowded and unsanitary conditions (Vietnamese refugees, Brazilian and Turkish immigrants) may need to be screened for infectious diseases such as tuberculosis, parasitosis, and respiratory diseases.

Box 2–1 identifies guidelines for assessing the cultural domain overview, inhabited localities, and topography.

## Communication

Perhaps no other domain has the complexities of communication. Communication is interrelated with all other domains and depends on verbal language skills that include the dominant language, dialects, and the contextual use of the language as well as paralanguage variations such as voice volume, tone, intonations, reflections, and willingness to share thoughts and feelings. Other important communication characteristics include nonverbal communications such as eye contact, facial expressions, use of touch, body language, spatial distancing practices, and acceptable greetings; temporality in terms of past, present, or future orientation of worldview; clock versus social time; and the degree of formality in the use of names. Commu-

---

Box 2–1
## Overview, Inhabited Localities, and Topography

**Overview, Inhabited Localities, and Topography**

1. Identify the part of the world from which this cultural or ethnic group originates and describe the climate and topography of the country.

**Heritage and Residence**

2. Identify where this group predominantly resides and include approximate numbers.

**Reasons for Migration and Associated Economic Factors**

3. Identify major factors that motivated this group to emigrate.

4. Explore economic or political factors that have influenced this group's acculturation and professional development in America.

**Educational Status and Occupations**

5. Assess the educational attainment and value placed on education by this ethnic group.

6. Identify occupations that individuals in this group predominantly seek on immigration.

nication styles may vary between insiders (family and close friends) and outsiders (strangers and unknown health-care providers). Hierarchical relationships, gender, and some religious beliefs affect communication.

## Dominant Language and Dialects

The health-care provider must be aware of the dominant language and the difficulties that dialects may cause when communicating in the client's native language. For example, Mexico has as many as 50 different dialects within its borders, China has 55, and the Philippines has 87. Even though the health-care provider might be fluent in the dominant language, other dialects may pose a communication barrier. Dialects that vary widely may pose substantial problems for health-care providers and interpreters in performing health assessments and in obtaining accurate health data, in turn increasing the difficulty of making an accurate diagnosis.

When speaking in a nonnative language, health-care providers must select words that have relatively pure meanings, be certain of the voice intonation, and avoid the use of regional slang and jargon to avoid being misunderstood. Minor variations in pronunciation may change the entire meaning of a word or a phrase and result in inappropriate interventions. For example, in the Spanish language, there are two forms of the verb "to be" (*ser* and *estar*). Using the incorrect form can cause a miscommunication, as evidenced by the following situation. A school nurse, who spoke limited Spanish, telephoned the mother of an 8-year-old boy with diarrhea. The nurse used the phrase *es enfermo* meaning "he is sick" (a permanent condition) instead of *esta enfermo* meaning "he is sick" (a temporary situation). This subtle distinction in language translation increased the mother's concern and anxiety over her child's illness and resulted in her thinking something was seriously wrong with him.

In the Vietnamese language, although vowels may appear to be the same, pronunciation varies radically depending on associated marks indicating tone and accent. These marks give the word a totally different meaning. Given the difficulty of obtaining the precise meaning of words in a language, it is best for the health-care provider to obtain someone who can interpret the meaning and message, not just translate the individual words. Some prudent guidelines for communicating with non-English-speaking clients include:

1. Use interpreters rather than translators. Translators just restate the words from one language to another. An interpreter decodes the words and provides the meaning behind the message.

2. Use dialect-specific interpreters whenever possible.

3. Use interpreters trained in the health-care field.

4. Give the interpreter time alone with the client.

5. Provide time for translation and interpretation.

6. Be aware that interpreters may affect the reporting of symptoms, insert their own ideas, or omit information.

7. Avoid the use of relatives who may distort information or not be objective.

8. Avoid using children as interpreters, especially with sensitive topics.

9. Use same-age and same-gender interpreters whenever possible.

10. Maintain eye contact with both the client and interpreter to elicit feedback and read nonverbal cues.

11. Remember that clients can usually understand more than they can express; thus, they need time to think in their own language. They are alert to the health-care

provider's body language, and they may forget some or all of their English in times of stress.

12. Speak slowly without exaggerated mouthing, allow time for translation, use active rather than passive tense, wait for feedback, and restate the message. Do not rush; do not speak loudly. Use a reference book with common phrases such as *Roget's International Thesaurus* or *Taber's Cyclopedic Medical Dictionary*.

13. Use as many words as possible in the client's language and nonverbal communication when unable to understand the language.

14. If an interpreter is unavailable, the use of a translator may be acceptable. The difficulty with translation is omission of parts of the message, distortion of the message, including transmission of information not given by the speaker, and messages not being fully understood.

15. *Note:* Social class differences between the interpreter and the client may result in the interpreter's not reporting information that he or she perceives as superstitious or unimportant.

Those with limited English ability may have inadequate vocabulary skills to communicate in situations where strong verbal skills are required or where highly abstract levels of verbal skills are required, such as in the psychiatric setting. Additional techniques that might be helpful when communicating with diverse clients include being tactful, using a considerate approach, gaining trust and respect by listening attentively, addressing the client by formal name, and showing genuine warmth and openness to get the client to divulge full information. When giving directions, be explicit. Do not use complex sentences with conjunctions. Give directions in sequential procedural steps (for example, first, second, third).

Before trying to engage in more sensitive areas of the health interview, the healthcare practitioner may need to start with safer topics to establish trust, use an open-ended format rather than yes or no closed-response questions, and elicit opinions and beliefs. An awareness of nonverbal behaviors helps to establish a mutually satisfying relationship.

The context within which a language is spoken is an important aspect of communication. German, English, and French languages are low in context, and most of the message is explicit, requiring many words to express a thought (Kaplan, 1989). Chinese and Native-American languages are highly contextual, with most of the information either in the physical context or internalized, resulting in the use of fewer words with more emphasis on unspoken understandings.

Voice volume and tone are important paralanguage aspects of communication. European-Americans and African-Americans may be perceived as being loud and boisterous because their volume carries to those nearby. European-Americans and African-Americans generally talk loudly in comparison with the Chinese and Hindus. Their loud voice volume may be interpreted by Chinese or Hindus as reflecting anger when, in fact, a loud voice is merely being used to express their thoughts in a dynamic manner. In contrast, westerners witnessing impassioned communication among Arabs may interpret the excited speech pattern and shouting as anger, but emotional communication is part of the Arab culture and is usually unrelated to anger. Thus, health-care providers must be cautious about voice tones when interacting with diverse cultural groups so their intentions are not misunderstood.

## Cultural Communication Patterns

Communication includes the willingness of individuals to share their thoughts and feelings. As a group, European-Americans are more willing to share their thoughts and feelings among family, friends, and strangers on almost any topic; in fact, sharing is encouraged. In some cultural groups, such as the Japanese, individuals are expected to be shy, withdrawn, and diffident—at least in public (Mattson & Lew, 1991)—whereas in others, such as Jewish and Italian, individuals are expected to be more flamboyant and assertive (Alland, 1971). Most Appalachians and Mexican-Americans willingly share their thoughts and feelings among family members and close friends but may not easily share thoughts, feelings, and health information with "outside" health-care providers until after they get to know them (Giger & Davidhizar, 1995). By engaging in small talk and inquiring about family members before addressing the client's health concerns, health-care providers can help establish trust and in turn encourage more open communication and sharing of important health information.

Touch, a method of nonverbal communication, has substantial variations among cultures. Among Egyptian-Americans, touch between opposite sexes is accepted in private and only between husband and wife, parents and children, and adult brothers and sisters; it is less readily accepted from strangers. Mexican-Americans, even though they frequently touch family members and friends, tend to be modest during health-care examinations by the opposite gender (Thayer, 1988). Being aware of individual practices regarding touch is essential for effective health assessments.

Personal space needs to be respected when working with multicultural clients and staff. European-American, Canadian, and British conversants tend to place at least 18 inches of space between themselves and the person to whom they are talking (Watson, 1980). Turks and Arabs require little personal space when talking with each other (Watson, 1980). They are quite comfortable standing closer to each other than European-Americans would; in fact, they interpret physical proximity as a valued sign of emotional closeness. Middle Eastern clients, who stand very close and stare during a conversation, may offend health-care practitioners. These clients may interpret European-American health-care providers as being cold because they stand so far away (Lipson & Meleis, 1985). To the German, who views space as sacred, even the distance between pieces of furniture is not conducive to easy conversation. Doors are used to protect privacy and require a knock and an invitation before entering. In fact, one should not even look into the room because this is perceived as an intrusion of privacy. An understanding of personal space and distancing characteristics can enhance the quality of communication among individuals.

Maintaining direct eye contact without staring is an expectation among European-Americans regardless of class or social standing of the conversants. A person who does not maintain eye contact may be perceived as not listening, not being trustworthy, or not caring. To the contrary, maintaining sustained eye contact in Bolivia is considered rude. Among Mexicans, Cubans, Puerto Ricans, Iranians, Egyptians, Italians, and Greeks, sustained eye contact between a child and an older adult is believed to cause the folklore illness "evil eye" or "bad eye." In Vietnam, a person of lower social class or status should avoid eye contact with superiors or those with a higher educational status (Hoang, Erickson, & Erickson, 1982). Thus, eye contact must be interpreted within its cultural context to optimize relationships and health assessments.

Facial expressions vary among cultures. For example, Jewish, Italian, and Hispanics smile more than other ethnic groups (Eibl-Eibesfelt, 1972), whereas the Cofan Indians of Ecuador rarely smile because showing their teeth may be interpreted as a sign of aggression (personal communication, Purnell, January 1986).

Preferred greetings and acceptable body language also vary among cultural groups. An expected practice for European-American males is to extend their hand when greeting someone for the first time. In Finland, it is considered rude and impolite to converse with hands in the pockets (Lammi, 1989). In the United States, confidence and competence are associated with a relaxed posture; however, in Korea and Japan, confidence and competence are more closely associated with slightly tense postures (Krebs & Kunimoto, 1994).

In Iran, beckoning is done by waving the fingers with the palm down, whereas extending the thumb, like thumbs-up, is considered a vulgar sign. Among the Vietnamese, signaling for someone to come by using an upturned finger is a provocation, usually done to a dog (Nguyen, 1985). Among the Navajo it is considered rude to point; rather the Navajo shift their lips toward the desired direction.

## Temporal Relationships

Temporal relationships, people's worldview in terms of past, present, and future orientation, vary among cultural groups. For example, the German culture is regarded as a past-oriented society. The past is important to Germans; therefore, laying a proper foundation by beginning presentations with historical background information can enhance communication with this group (Friday, 1989). The European-American culture is more future-oriented, and persons are encouraged to sacrifice for today and work to save and invest in the future. Puerto Rican, Mexican-American, Brazilian, French Canadian (Paquet, 1989), and Chinese cultures are more present-oriented (Tripp-Reimer & Lively, 1988), placing great importance on the here and now, not something that may occur in the future or has occurred in the past. Among Brazilians, punctuality, especially in social situations, is not taken seriously. However, for persons in many societies, temporality is balanced among past, present, and future in the sense of respecting the past, valuing and enjoying the present, and saving for the future.

Differences in temporal orientation can cause concern or misunderstanding among health-care providers. For example, in a future-oriented culture, a person is expected to delay purchase of nonessential items to afford prescription medications. However, in less future-oriented cultures, the person buys the nonessential item because it is readily available and defers purchasing the prescription medication. The attitude is why not buy it now when the prescription medication can be purchased *mañana* (tomorrow or later).

Expectations for punctuality can cause conflicts between health-care providers and clients, even if one is cognizant of these differences. Specifically, Americans, British, and Germans are seen as being very punctual with appointments and reporting to work on time (Orque, Block, & Monrroy, 1983). Trains and transportation systems are expected to be on time. If an appointment is made for 9 A.M., the person is there at 8:45. Conversely, Filipinos may be more relaxed regarding punctuality in social situations but adhere more strictly to clock schedules in business situations (Orque, Block, & Monrroy, 1983). When visiting friends or meeting for strictly social engagements, Filipinos may be less structured, but one is expected to appear within a reasonable time frame.

For immigrants from rural settings, time may be even less important. These individuals may not even own a timepiece or be able to tell time. The European-American culture has difficulty with a less punctual time concept, and as a result, health-care practitioners may become concerned when people are late or do not report for appointments. These details must be carefully explained to individuals when such situations occur. Being late for appointments should not be misconstrued as a sign of irresponsibility or not valuing one's health.

## Format for Names

Names are important to individuals, and their format differs among cultures. The American name David Thomas Jones denotes a man whose first name is David, his middle name is Thomas, and his family surname is Jones. Friends would call him by his first name, David, and in the formal setting, he would be called Mr. Jones. Cambodians use the opposite position in sequencing names. For example, the name Pak Pourin denotes a woman whose last name is Pak and whose first name is Pourin.

Friends would address her as Pourin, and in a formal situation, she would be addressed as Mrs. Pak.

Hispanics may have a more complex system for denoting their full name. For example, a married woman may take her husband's surname while maintaining both her parents' last names, resulting in an extended name such as La Señora Roberta Rodriguez de Malena y Perez. In this example, Mrs. Rodriguez has the first name of Roberta, her husband's surname Rodriguez, her mother's maiden name Malena, and her father's surname Perez. Friends would address her as Roberta, whereas in the formal setting she would be called Mrs. Rodriguez. Such extensive naming formats can create a challenge for health-care workers keeping a medical record when they are unaware of differences in ethnic recording of names.

Box 2–2 identifies guidelines for assessing the cultural domain communications.

# Family Roles and Organization

The cultural domain family roles and organization affects all other domains and defines relationships among insiders and outsiders. This domain includes concepts related to the head of the household and gender roles, family goals and priorities, and developmental tasks of children and adolescents, roles of the aged and extended family members, individual and family social status in the community, and acceptance of alternative lifestyles such as single parenting, nontraditional sexual orientations, childless marriages, and divorce. Family structure in the context of the larger society determines acceptable roles, priorities, and the behavioral norms for its members.

## Head of Household and Gender Roles

An awareness of family dominance patterns is important for determining with whom to speak when health-care decisions have to be made. Patriarchal family households include Appalachian (Murdock, 1971), Italian, and Filipino (Manio & Hall, 1987); matriarchal households include African-American (Covell & Turnbull, 1982) and Navajo. Others are more egalitarian (for example, European-American). In the Appalachian culture, the father is responsible for deciding when to seek health care for a family member, but paternal grandmothers may have a significant influence on final decisions (Tripp-Reimer, 1982). Among Mexican-Americans and newer Italian immigrants, the male may still consider it rude if a health-care provider directs questions about a child's illness to the mother instead of him.

In some societies, such as Iranian, very specific roles are outlined for men and women, whereas in others, such as among African-Americans, these roles are less well-defined. Among European-Americans, it is acceptable for women to have a career orientation and for men to assist with child care, household domestic chores, and cooking responsibilities. With many women working outside the home and parents working part-time and nonday work schedules, the high cost of child care has led to men's taking a more active role in child care.

## Prescriptive, Restrictive, and Taboo Behaviors for Children and Adolescents

Every society has prescriptive, restrictive, and taboo practices for children and adolescents. Prescriptive beliefs are those things that the children or teenagers *should do* to have harmony with the family and a good outcome in society. Restrictive practices are those things that children and teenagers *should not* do to have a positive

Box 2–2
# Communications

## Dominant Language and Dialects

1. Identify the dominant language of this group.

2. Identify dialects that may interfere with communication.

3. Explore contextual speech patterns of this group. What is the usual volume and tone of speech?

## Cultural Communication Patterns

4. Explore the willingness of individuals to share thoughts, feelings, and ideas.

5. Explore the practice and meaning of touch in their society: within the family, between friends, with strangers, with members of the same sex, with members of the opposite sex, and with health-care providers.

6. Identify personal spatial and distancing characteristics when communicating on a one-to-one basis. Explore how distancing changes with friends versus strangers.

7. Explore the use of eye contact within this group. Does avoidance of eye contact have special meanings? How does eye contact vary among family, friends, and strangers? Does eye contact change among socioeconomic groups?

8. Explore the meaning of various facial expressions. Do specific facial expressions have special meanings? Do persons tend to smile a lot? How are emotions displayed or not displayed in facial expressions?

9. Are there acceptable ways of standing and greeting outsiders?

## Temporal Relationships

10. Explore temporal relationships in this group. Are individuals primarily past-, present-, or future-oriented? How do individuals see the context of past, present, and future?

11. Identify how differences in the interpretation of social time versus clock time are perceived.

12. Explore how time factors are interpreted by this group. Are individuals expected to be punctual in terms of jobs, appointments, and social engagements?

## Format for Names

13. Explore the format for a person's names.

14. How does one expect to be greeted by strangers and health-care practitioners?

outcome. Taboo practices are those things that, if done, are likely to cause significant concern or negative outcomes for the child, teenager, family, or community at large.

A prescriptive practice among Haitians includes periodic purging with laxatives to clean the blood and to ensure the child's health. Thus, health-care practitioners need to incorporate health teaching that emphasizes the recognition of the signs and symptoms of dehydration and teach interventions for dehydration in each age group (DeSantis, 1988; Thomas & DeSantis, 1995). The Cuban-American ethnocultural health belief that fat children are healthy children encourages early introduction of food supplements, solid food, and prolonged bottle feeding, which in some cases results in infants being so obese that they cannot sit or stand (DeSantis, 1988). Anticipatory guidance from health-care practitioners may be advantageous to help prevent the detrimental effects of obesity in these infants and children.

Adolescents have their own subculture with its own values, beliefs, and practices that may not be in harmony with those of their major ethnic group. It may be especially important for adolescents to be in harmony with peers and conform with the prevalent choice of clothing, hair styles, and adornment. Thus, role conflicts can become a considerable source of family strain as traditional ethnic beliefs are influenced by the perceived American values of individuality, independence, self-assertion, and egalitarian relationships (Nguyen, 1985). Thus, many teens may experience a cultural dilemma with exposure outside the home and family.

Restrictive practices among Iranian teens discourage the expression of anger toward parents or teachers, although anger is expressed toward peers. Silence is preferred toward those in authority because respect for authority figures is stronger than the aggressive impulse. As a result, Iranian adolescents often find themselves caught in a dilemma—pulled between parents' attempts to maintain control and instill ethnocultural knowledge and values, and their own desire to be like American teens (Lipson & Haifizi, 1997).

Many Puerto Rican adolescents are expected to refrain from having sexual discussions because this topic is considered taboo (Cordasco & Bucchione, 1973). As outsiders, health-care practitioners in school health can have a significant role in providing factual information regarding issues related to sexuality. Expressing an openness to discuss these sensitive issues in a group or one-on-one format within their cultural context may assist teens to learn more about sexuality and primary prevention.

Health-care providers can assist adolescents and family members to work through these cultural differences by helping them resolve personal conflicts in ways that convey respect for the family's culture. Discussing personal parenting practices and providing information about disease, illness, and treatment in culturally congruent ways encourages individuals to explore alternative beliefs while continuing to value their own culture.

### Family Goals and Priorities

In most societies, young adulthood is the time when persons work on Erikson's developmental tasks of intimacy versus isolation and generativity versus stagnation. Family goals and priorities center on raising and educating the children. During this stage in the European-American culture, young adults make a personal commitment to a spouse or significant other and seek satisfaction through productivity in career, family, and civic interests (Friedman, 1986).

The cultural significance of children is another important aspect to be considered. The European-American culture places a high value on children, and many laws have been enacted to protect children who are seen as the "future of the society." In most Asian cultures, children are desirable and highly valued as a source of family strength (Manio & Hall, 1987), and family members are expected to care for each other (Chen & Yang, 1986).

The definition of aging varies among cultures and can be defined by age in years, functional abilities, or social mores. In the Korean culture, persons are considered old and expected to retire at the age of 60 regardless of their health status. This amount of time allows them to have completed the 60 cycles of the Chinese lunar calendar. Within Brazilian-American society, the aged live with one of their children, are included in family activities, and usually accompany their children's family on vacation. The European-American culture, which emphasizes youth, beauty, thinness, independence, and productivity, contributes to some societal views of the aged as being less important and tends to minimize the problems of the elderly. A contrasting view among some European-Americans emphasizes the importance of the elderly in society.

Occasionally, lifestyle dictates the fate of the elderly. Because of the rigorous lifestyle of the Cofan Indians in the Amazon Basin of South America, all persons are expected to be contributing members of society. Thus, when an elderly person is no longer able to keep up with the rest of the tribe in terms of travel and basic production, the person may be left behind when the group moves to a new location (personal observation, Purnell, January 1986).

Chinese and Appalachian cultures have great reverence for the wisdom of the elderly, and families eagerly make space for them to live with extended families. Children are expected to care for elders when the elders are unable to care for themselves. A great embarrassment may occur to family members when they cannot take care of their elderly family members. Helping the ethnic family to network and find social support, resources, or acceptable long-term-care facilities within the community is a useful strategy for the health-care provider.

The concept of extended family membership varies among societies. The extended family is extremely important in the Mexican-American culture and health-care decisions may not be made unless the entire family is consulted (Murillo, 1978). The extended family may include biologic relatives and nonbiologic members who may be considered brother, sister, aunt, or uncle. In some Asian cultures, the influence of grandparents in decision making is considered more important than that of the parents (Manio & Hall, 1987). An accepted practice among Brazilian-Americans is for the grandparents to raise the grandchildren so that the parents may pursue work-related goals. The parental role among African-American families is often assumed by grandparents, aunts, and cousins (Boyd-Franklin, 1989), and fellow church members are frequently considered important members of the extended family (Levin & Taylor, 1993). A common practice in such cultures is for several generations of a family to live in the same household. The health-care provider can have a significant impact on the health status of the extended family in acute, long-term, primary, or home health care.

Status in some cultures, such as the Hindu, is connected with a specific and rigid caste system in which people are born into a social class and are unable to move in and out of their caste, regardless of changes in their socioeconomic status. However, in other societies, such as among Koreans, not as much attention is given to one's heritage; educational accomplishments give one status. In European-American society, with hard work, a person can climb the socioeconomic scale and gain respect; however, the person can easily fall from high socioeconomic status just as quickly. By using health teachers of the same socioeconomic status as the client, the health-care provider can capitalize on the client's cultural beliefs regarding status when teaching health promotion and disease prevention.

## Alternative Lifestyles

The traditional American family is nuclear, with a married man and woman living together with one or more unmarried children. However, in some cultures, the traditional family is extended, with parents, unmarried children, married children with their children, and grandparents all sharing the same living space.

The American family is becoming a more varied community. It includes unmarried people, both men and women living alone, single people of the same or different gender living together with or without children, single parents with children, and blended families consisting of two parents who are remarried, with children from their previous marriages and additional children from their current marriage.

The sexual revolution of the 1960s marked the beginning of a sharp increase in divorce rates (passing the one million mark by 1975 and hitting an all-time high of 5.8 per 1000 marriages in 1979). Today, 60 percent of first marriages are likely to end in divorce (*Information please: Almanac,* 1995). In some societies, divorce continues to carry a stigma. High levels of marital instability challenge norms and create new patterns of family life. Rates for unmarried adults living together have increased to 2.9 million households, with 58 percent of them between the ages of 25 and 44 and 28 percent under the age of 25. Nearly one-third of these households have children under the age of 15. Between 1970 and 1991, interracial married couples increased from 310,000 to 994,000 (although *CNN News* on July 25, 1995, reported 2 million). These couples include blacks married to whites (231,000) and the remainder, blacks and whites married to "others." The number of female single parents approaches almost 10 million, an increase of 39 percent over the last decade, and 26 percent of children are born to unmarried mothers (*Information please: Almanac,* 1995).

The newest category of family, domestic partnerships, is sanctioned by over 25 cities or counties in the United States (for example, New York City, San Francisco, Boston, and Minneapolis) and grants some of the rights of traditional married couples to unmarried heterosexual, homosexual, elderly, and disabled couples who share the traditional bond of the family. In Denmark, homosexual marriages are legal, and survivors of same-sex partnerships are granted the right to survivor benefits and the right to inherit their partner's pension but are not granted the right to adopt children. Courts in New York, New Jersey, Vermont, Minnesota, and California allow gay and lesbian couples to adopt children (*Information please: Almanac,* 1995).

Among more rural subcultures, same-sex couples living together may not be as accepted or recognized in the community as they are in larger cities. As gay parents have become more visible, lesbian and gay parenting groups have arisen in many cities across the United States and offer information, support, and guidance resulting in more lesbians' and gay men's considering parenthood through adoption and artificial insemination.

Homosexuality is permitted in some form or another in almost every society. Three generalizations about homosexual behavior include:

1. Social attitudes toward homosexual activity vary widely (Ford & Beach, 1951).

2. Homosexual behavior occurs in societies that deny its presence (Ford & Beach, 1951).

3. More men than women engage in homosexual activity (Brink, 1987; Ford & Beach, 1951).

Homosexual behavior carries a stigma in most societies, with the exception of Oceania (Micronesia, Melanesia, and Polynesia), where male homosexuality is believed to be a necessary step to manhood and is required in puberty transition rituals. However, young Oceanian men are expected to marry women and have children, even though they are permitted to continue having homosexual affairs (Herdt, 1981; Read, 1952). To be gay or lesbian is considered immoral and is not accepted by most elements of the monotheist religions (Orthodox Judaism, Christianity, and Islam). To discover a gay son or lesbian daughter is akin to a catastrophic event for Egyptian-Americans. In Iran and some provinces of China, a lesbian or gay may be killed.

When the health-care provider needs to provide assistance and make a referral for a gay, lesbian, or bisexual, a number of options are available. Some referral agencies are local, whereas others are national with local or regional chapters. Many are ethnically or religiously specific. National resources include the AIDS Action Council; National AIDS Hotline; Gay and Lesbian Medical Association; National AIDS Bereavement Center; National Gay and Lesbian Task Force for students, faculty, and staff in colleges and universities; AIDS National Interfaith Network; National Center for Lesbian Rights; NOW Lesbian Rights; We Are Families; and the National Lesbian and Gay Health Association. Ethnically and religiously specific support groups include Salud and Hola Gay for Hispanics, Asians Together, Dignity USA for gay Catholics, Telos for Baptists, Bet Mishpachah for Jewish gays and lesbians, and Unitarians for Lesbian and Gay Concerns ("Gay resources," *1995*).

Box 2–3 identifies guidelines for assessing the cultural domain family roles and organization.

---

Box 2–3
## Family Roles and Organization

### Head of Household and Gender Roles

1. Identify the perceived head of the household. How does this change during different developmental aspects of life?

2. Describe gender-related roles of men and women in the family system.

### Prescriptive, Restrictive, and Taboo Behaviors

3. Identify prescriptive, restrictive, and taboo behaviors for children.

4. Identify prescriptive, restrictive, and taboo behaviors for adolescents.

### Family Roles and Priorities

5. Describe family goals and priorities emphasized by this culture.

6. Explore developmental tasks in this group.

7. Explore the status and role of the aged in the family.

8. Explore the roles and importance of extended family members.

9. Describe how one gains social status in this cultural system. Is there a caste system?

### Alternative Lifestyles

10. Describe how alternative lifestyles and nontraditional families such as single parents, blended families, communal families, same-sex families, and so forth, are viewed by this society.

## Workforce Issues

A fourth domain of culture is workforce issues. Differences and conflicts that occur among a homogeneous culture in health-care organizations may be intensified in a multicultural workforce. Factors that affect these issues include language barriers, degree of assimilation and acculturation, and issues related to autonomy. Moreover, concepts such as gender roles, cultural communication styles, health-care practices from the country of origin, and selected concepts from all other domains affect workforce issues in a multicultural work environment.

### *Culture in the Workplace*

By the year 2000, 75 percent of people entering the job market will be women and persons of color, and one-third of all U.S. citizens will be members of minority groups (*Diversity in the workplace*, 1995). By the year 2080, minorities will constitute 51.1 percent of the population (Crow, 1993). Native-Americans, blacks, Asian-Americans, and Hispanic-Americans will be the most populous groups (*Information please: Almanac,* 1995). The challenge of managing a multicultural workforce requires employers and employees to understand diversity and view it as an asset to create harmony and productivity in the work environment.

Clinical professionals trained in their home countries now occupy a significant share of technical and laboratory positions in U.S. hospitals. Service workers such as food preparation workers, nurses' aides, orderlies, housekeepers, and janitors represent the most culturally diverse component of the hospital workforce. These unskilled and semiskilled positions are among the most attainable for new immigrants (Motwani, Hodge, & Crampton, 1995). Although information regarding a multicultural workforce in nonacute health-care facilities could not be found, one might expect such a workforce to mirror the labor needs of the acute health-care environment.

Minority groups employed as professionals are underrepresented among all health-care professions (Price & Cordell, 1994). Of registered nurses (RNs) in the United States, 90 percent come from white backgrounds, whereas only 10 percent come from nonwhite racial or ethnic backgrounds. Black RNs make up 4 percent of the population, Asian-Pacific islanders account for 3.4 percent, Hispanics 1.4 percent, and Native-Americans and Alaskan Natives 0.4 percent. RNs of ethnically or racial diverse backgrounds most often practice in the Middle Atlantic, South Atlantic, East South Central, and Pacific states (*Today's registered nurses: Numbers and demographics,* 1994). The California Organization of Nurse Executives' 1991 position paper recommends employing nurses with culturally diverse backgrounds in numbers proportionate to their culturally diverse clients.

Foreign-educated physicians have increased in the United States (Mark & Smith, 1987) and represent almost 20 percent of licensed physicians (Motwani, Hodge, & Crampton, 1995). In 1976, the Health Professions Training Assistance Act placed restrictions on the number of graduates from foreign medical schools allowed to practice in the United States and initiated a certification process to recognize their credentials. This was done at the request of the Graduate Medical Educational National Advisory Committee and the Department of Health and Human Services.

The educational level of health-care professionals in some countries may not be comparable to the educational requirements of health-care professionals in the United States. The vast array of health providers such as radiologic technicians, physical therapists, occupational therapists, social service workers, electrocardiogram technicians, and respiratory therapists in America may not be familiar to all health-care professionals. In Mexico, some Latin American countries, and some developing countries, nursing education is offered primarily at the high-school level. In the Philippines and Australia, a baccalaureate degree in nursing may not be seen as equivalent to the baccalaureate degree awarded in the United States. In Australia, all baccalaureate programs are 3 years in length, and in Great Britain, most nurses are trained at the diploma level with an apprenticeship. Moreover, not all nursing programs include psychiatric, community, or obstetric nursing content in their curricula.

Concerns surface about the amount of additional training needed for some foreign graduates before sitting for the licensing examination when these professionals immigrate to the United States. Often the sponsoring organization pays for the additional education. Some American-educated nurses see this as unfair because they paid for their own education and receive the same salary as foreign-educated nurses.

In previous decades, American health-care facilities relied on the importation of nurses from Puerto Rico, the Philippines, Canada, England, and other foreign countries to supplement their numbers in the American workforce. Some of these nurses assimilate into the workforce more easily than others. For example, some British and Australian nurses have initial difficulty with defensive charting done in the United States because in their socialized health-care system, clients are not likely to bring litigation (Purnell & Galloway, 1995).

Many health-care organizations, such as those in New York City, which employ the majority of their workers from over 200 ethnic groups, are addressing multicultural issues in the workforce. To address conflicts among the multicultural workforce, the New York State Nurses' Association sponsors workshops supported by the American Nurses' Association and New York Council on Human Rights, with varying degrees of success (Ketter, 1995). Other educational and health-care facilities, such as the Veterans Affairs Medical Centers, have initiated cultural sensitivity and cultural diversity workshops to address multicultural workforce issues.

Timeliness and punctuality are two culturally based attitudes that can create serious problems in the multicultural workforce. In some situations, conflicts may arise over the issue of reporting to work on time or on an assigned day. Respect for time and personal responsibility for meeting time demands in other countries is often in direct opposition to the European-American ethic for punctuality.

In regard to learning styles, many Native-Americans have a spiral and circular thought pattern that moves from concept to concept without being linear or sequential; therefore, they have difficulty placing information in a stepwise methodology (Crow, 1993). The Western system places a high value on the ability to categorize information using linear, sequential thought processes. When a person is unaware of the value given to such behaviors, individuals may see each other as disorganized, scattered, and faulty in their cognitive patterns, resulting in increased difficulty in written and verbal communications.

The personality styles of Filipinos may cause them to appear as noncaring, and clients may object to their attitude (Burner, Cunningham, & Hatter, 1990; Martin, Wimberley, & O'Keese, 1994). To overcome these obstacles, one hospital in New Jersey instituted cultural sensitivity workshops to help personnel better understand each other (Martin, et al., 1994). When professionals of differing cultures clash, both sides need to develop an understanding of their diverse perspectives.

Health-care administration and management initiatives to support a diverse work environment include cultural competence and diversity workshops, cultural celebrations, a specific orientation to the United States' changing health-care system, provision of cultural brokers as mentors or preceptors to assist new immigrants in learning about the American workforce, and identification of ways to work more effectively with employees of diverse backgrounds. Orientation classes may need to include the difference in the length of clients' hospital stays in the United States as compared with those in the employee's country of origin; the greater diversity in health professions; the authority of insurance companies; concerns related to malpractice; and different nursing-care delivery modes, such as team nursing, primary nursing, case management, and functional nursing.

### *Issues Related to Autonomy*

Cultural differences related to assertiveness influence how health-care practitioners view each other. Specifically, Asian nurses may not be as assertive with physicians as American nurses, which may cause concerns and problems in the American workforce (Martin, Wimberley, & O'Keese, 1994). The concept of the nurse being dependent on physicians and male administrators is inseparable from the Muslim concept of a woman as subject to the authority of husbands, fathers, and elder brothers (Harner, et al., 1994). Polish nursing is seen as a vocation, and, therefore, Polish nurses may be unprepared for the level of sophistication and autonomy of American nursing. Educational training for nurses in Pakistan is culturally different from training in America. In Pakistan, "nurses are not socially or culturally prepared to assume the role of decisionmaker, risk taker, teacher, or change agent" (Harner, et al., 1994).

Foreign graduates unaccustomed to American levels of autonomy may accept and be more assertive if their duties are placed in the perspective of legal and professional requirements. Organizational orientation programs for foreign graduates may need to focus on legal and ethical requirements of proper documentation as well as specific institutional approaches, an overview of dominant American practices, quality improvement issues, informed consent procedures, and client autonomy.

The Commission on Graduates of Foreign Nursing Schools administers a screening examination for temporary work visas to foreign graduates seeking work. This examination assesses the ability to write and comprehend the English language. It cannot, however, examine the specific nuances of selected language barriers that may cause difficulties in the workplace. The ability to take physicians' prescriptions over the telephone is an area where problems typically develop. The newer immigrant health-care professional may have passed the state's professional licensing examination but still need extra time in translating the message and formulating a reply.

When individuals speak in their native language at work, it may become a source of contention for both clients and medical personnel (Burner, Cunningham, & Hatter, 1990; Martin, Wimberley, & O'Keese, 1994). For example, Filipinos do not want to exclude or offend others, but it is easier to speak in their native language to articulate ideas, feelings, and humor among themselves. The outspoken, fast-moving behaviors of American nurses may be seen as "crass" (Martin, Wimberley, & O'Keese, 1994). Negative interpretations of behaviors can be detrimental to working relationships in the health-care environment. Given a limited aural language ability, some foreign graduates may need to have care instructions written or procedures demonstrated. In addition, health-care employers should provide classes and workshops for all employees who work with multicultural clients and personnel and English as a Second Language classes to improve communication among the multicultural workforce.

Box 2–4 identifies guidelines for assessing the cultural domain workforce issues.

# Biocultural Ecology

The domain biocultural ecology identifies specific physical, biologic, and physiological variations in ethnic and racial origins. These variations include skin color and physical differences in body habitus; genetic, hereditary, endemic, and topographic diseases; psychological makeup of individuals; and the biologic differences that affect the way drugs are metabolized by the body. No attempt is made here to explain or justify any of the numerous and conflicting views on the genetic and environmental reasons for variations. If readers are interested in the controversial anthropological, genetic, and biologic perspectives on such variations, they are referred to Alland (1971), Breslin (1993), and Brown (1984). In this book, observations of physical and genetic variations are identified. These observations may be more accurate

---

Box 2–4
# Workforce Issues

### Culture in the Workplace

1. Identify specific workforce issues affected by immigration, e.g., education.
2. Describe specific multicultural considerations when working with this culturally diverse individual or group in the workforce.
3. Explore factors influencing patterns of acculturation in this cultural group.
4. Explore native health-care practices and their influence in the workforce.

### Issues Related to Autonomy

5. Identify cultural issues related to professional autonomy, superior or subordinate control, religious issues, and gender in the workforce.
6. Identify language barriers with concrete interpretations of the language.

---

with some individuals than with others. Frequently, intraethnic variations are greater than interethnic variations.

## *Skin Color and Other Biologic Variations*

Skin coloration is an important concern for health-care providers. The health-care provider must assess jaundice and blood oxygenation levels differently in dark-skinned people than in light-skinned people. For example, to assess anemia in dark-skinned people, the provider should examine the oral mucosa and capillary refill at the nail bed. Jaundice is more easily determined in Asian persons by assessing the sclera rather than relying on the change in skin color. The health-care provider must establish a baseline skin color (ask a family member or someone known to the individual), use direct sunlight if possible, observe areas with the least amount of pigmentation, palpate for rashes, and compare skin in corresponding areas. For Polish, Irish, and Germans with fair skin, prolonged exposure to the sun places them at an increased risk for skin cancer.

Variations in body habitus occur among ethnic and racially diverse individuals. For example, the long bones of many blacks are significantly longer and narrower than those of whites (Giger & Davidhizar, 1995), and Asians have narrower shoulders and wider hips when compared to blacks. Additional racial variations include flat nose bridges among Koreans and other Asians, which may be overlooked by opticians when fitting and dispensing eyeglasses. Many Vietnamese children are commonly small by American standards, not fitting the published growth curves (Felice, 1986). Mandibular tori occur in about 40 percent of Asians as compared with only seven percent of European-Americans (Overfield, 1977), making the fitting of dentures more difficult. Such biocultural data provide important information for the health-care practitioner when assessing health problems geared to the unique attributes of peoples of diverse cultures. Given diverse gene pools, this type of information is often difficult to obtain.

## Diseases and Health Conditions

Endemic diseases are those diseases that occur continuously in a specific racial or ethnic group. Health-care providers should assess newer immigrants for diseases common in their homelands. For example, immigrant populations from Egypt may display liver impairment, portal hypertension, esophageal varices, and renal impairment due to bilharzia infection (Markell, Vage, & John, 1992) and infectious blindness and scleral infections due to endemic trachoma (Lane, 1987). An awareness of at-risk populations for specific endemic diseases allows the health professional to provide culturally appropriate screening and education for disease prevention and health promotion.

The topography of a given country or region may provide the health-care practitioner with essential clues to symptoms requiring investigation. For instance, as mentioned earlier, people who emigrate from mosquito-infested tropical areas such as those in Brazil, Turkey, and Vietnam may present with chills, fever, lassitude, and splenic enlargement, which are consistent with malaria (Guerrero, Chin, & Collins, 1982). Air pollution, which increases the risk for respiratory diseases, may be a significant risk factor for any group that emigrates from or lives in a large city. Knowledge of specific risk factors related to the topography of the client's country of origin and current residence enhances the diagnostic process and ensures accurate assessments.

Some ethnic groups have an increased genetic susceptibility to specific diseases and conditions. For instance, the predicted incidence of diabetes mellitus varies among specific cultural groups. The incidence of diabetes mellitus among blacks is at least 1.6 times greater than that in European-Americans (Roseman, 1985), Native-Americans are 1.9 to 3 times more likely to have diabetes than the general population (Freeman et al., 1989), and more than 65 percent of Pima Indians over the age of 30 have noninsulin-dependent diabetes (Department of Health, 1995). Limited gene pools among the Amish populations result in a greater proportion of genetic defects such as dwarfism and muscular dystrophy (Thayer, 1993). Cystic fibrosis is the most common fatal hereditary illness among French Canadians (DeBraekeleer, 1991). Sickle cell anemia occurs more commonly among blacks, and Tay-Sachs disease occurs predominantly in French Canadians (DeBraekeleer, 1991) and Jews of eastern European (Ashkenazi) descent. Ethnic-specific genetic counseling, newborn screening, symptom recognition, and treatment protocols enhance health-care delivery for such diverse populations.

## Variations in Drug Metabolism

Information regarding drug metabolism among racial and ethnic groups has important implications for health-care practitioners when prescribing medications. Besides the effects that smoking and nutritional status have on drug metabolism, studies have identified alterations in drug metabolism among diverse racial and ethnic groups. For example, Chinese are more sensitive to the cardiovascular effects of propranolol than their European-American counterparts (Zhou, et al., 1989). Native-American and Eskimo Indians have a 90 percent risk of developing peripheral neuropathy while taking the drug isoniazid, compared with a 40 percent risk in European-Americans, who inactivate the drug more rapidly (Vessel, 1972). Health-care providers need to investigate the literature for ethnic-specific studies regarding variations in drug metabolism, communicate these findings among colleagues, and educate their clients regarding these side effects.

Box 2–5 identifies guidelines for assessing the cultural domain biocultural ecology.

Box 2–5
# Biocultural Ecology

### Skin Color and Biologic Variations

1. Identify the skin color and physical variations for this group.

2. Explore any special problems or concerns the skin color may pose for health-care practitioners.

3. Identify biologic variations in body habitus or structure.

### Diseases and Health Conditions

4. Identify specific risk factors for individuals related to the topography or climate.

5. Identify any hereditary or genetic diseases or conditions that are common with this group.

6. Identify any endemic diseases specific to this cultural or ethnic group.

7. Identify any diseases or health conditions for which this group has increased susceptibility.

### Variations in Drug Metabolism

8. Identify specific variations in drug metabolism, drug interactions, and related side effects.

## High-Risk Behaviors

Although variations in high-risk behaviors are shared among cultures, some groups may not place a high value on certain high-risk health behaviors such as using tobacco, alcohol, and recreational drugs; lack of physical activity; increased calorie consumption; and nonuse of safety measures such as seat belts, helmets, and safe driving practices.

The incidence of cigarette smoking has been declining in the United States over the last 25 years but continues to remain steady among Mexican-American populations, is increasing among Puerto Ricans and Cuban-Americans (Escobedo & Remington, 1989), and remains high among Greeks (Wilson, et al., 1993).

Alcohol consumption crosses almost all cultural and socioeconomic groups. Even in cultures where alcohol consumption is "tabooed, it is not ignored" (Al-lssa & Dennis, 1970, p. 544). When drinking is culturally approved, it is typically done more by men than women and is more often a social rather than a solitary act. The group in which drinking is most frequently practiced is usually composed of same-age and social peers (Al-lssa & Dennis, 1970). Ethnocultural studies of alcohol use provide important data on health-care problems related to alcoholism in specific groups. For example, nonwhite Hispanics, as compared with white Hispanics, consume alcoholic beverages to make themselves more emotionally fluid and socially extroverted (Perez-Stable, Marin, & Marin, 1994). Among French Canadians, alcohol abuse is highest among men in the 20- to 24-year age bracket (Mosian, 1991). When assessing clients' alcohol and recreational drug use, the health-care provider must place these high-risk behaviors within the context of their cultural group.

### Health-care Practices

A lack of health promotion and safety practices may be a major threat to the health of some persons. For example, obesity is greater among Amish women than non-Amish women in Ohio (Fuchs, et al., 1992). Weight gain among the Amish may be related to the importance of food in the culture and the higher rates of pregnancy throughout childbearing years (Wenger, 1996). Health-care providers can assist overweight clients in reducing calorie consumption by identifying healthy choices among culturally preferred foods, altering preparation practices, and reducing portion size.

The ethnocultural practice of self-care using folk and magicoreligious practices before seeking professional care may also have a negative impact on the health status of some persons. Overreliance on these practices may mean that the health condition is in a more advanced stage when a consultation is sought. Such delays make treatment more difficult and prolonged.

The cultural domain of high-risk behaviors is one area where health-care providers can make a significant impact on the client's health status. Risk factors can be controlled through ethnic-specific interventions aimed at health promotion and health-risk prevention through educational programs in schools, business organizations, churches, and recreational and community centers as well as through the use of one-on-one and family counseling techniques. Taking advantage of public communication technology can enhance participation in these programs if they are geared to the unique needs of the individual, family, or community.

Box 2–6 identifies guidelines for assessing the cultural domain high-risk behaviors.

---

Box 2–6
## High-Risk Behaviors

**High-Risk Behaviors**

1. Identify specific high-risk behaviors common among this group.

2. Explore behaviors related to the use of alcohol, tobacco, and recreational drugs and other substances among this group.

**Health-care Practices**

3. Identify the typical health-seeking behaviors of this group.

4. Assess the level of physical activity in their lifestyle.

5. Assess the use of safety measures such as seat belts and helmets.

# Nutrition

The cultural domain nutrition includes more than having adequate food for satisfying hunger. It also includes the meaning of food to the culture; common foods and rituals; nutritional deficiencies and food limitations; and the use of food for health promotion, restoration, and disease prevention.

## *Meaning of Food*

Food and its absence, hunger, have diverse meanings among cultures and individuals. Cultural beliefs, values, and types of foods available influence what people eat, avoid, or alter to make food congruent with cultural lifeways; and food offers cultural security and acceptance (Leininger, 1988). Food is not only necessary as a means of survival and relief from hunger but also plays a significant role in socialization. It has symbolic meaning for peaceful coexistence and is used to promote healing. It denotes caring or lack of caring, closeness, kinship, and solidarity, and it may be used as an expression of love or anger (Leininger, 1988).

## *Common Foods and Food Rituals*

To assist the health-care practitioner in becoming knowledgeable about ethnocultural dietary practices, each of the groups discussed in this book has a section devoted to specific foods, ingredients in selected native food dishes, and preparation practices. Becoming knowledgeable about a client's ethnic food patterns is essential for providing culturally competent dietary counseling. The health-care practitioner may be considered professionally negligent when prescribing an American diet to a Hispanic or an Asian client whose food choices and meal times may be different.

Given the intraethnic variations of diet, it is important for health professionals to inquire about the specific diet of their clients. The Irish diet has the potential for being high in fats and cholesterol, and the Korean, Chinese, and Filipino diets may be high in sodium owing to their practice of preserving food in salt. Culturally congruent dietary counseling, such as changing amounts and preparation practices while including ethnic food choices, can reduce risks for cardiovascular disease and cancer of the nasopharynx, stomach, and esophagus. Whenever possible, determining a client's dietary practices should be accomplished during the intake interview.

Eating and drinking are often ritualistic behaviors in many cultures where offering food, drink, or both is a common practice as soon as one enters a home or participates in a social engagement. Widely known cultural food rituals include British afternoon tea and the American morning coffee break. Rituals related to mealtime may have a significant impact on some Hispanic groups, especially for those with diabetes mellitus. Expecting the client to eat on an American mealtime schedule and selecting American foods from an exchange list may be unrealistic for clients of different cultural backgrounds. Counseling about food-group requirements, intake restrictions, and exercise must respect cultural behaviors and individual lifestyles.

Special occasions and holidays among many cultures are frequently associated with ethnic foods. For example, in the United States, hot dogs are consumed at sports events, turkey is served at Thanksgiving, and a goose is commonly served in rural communities on New Year's Day. Many religious groups are required to fast at specific holiday seasons, such as Ramadan for Muslims and Lent for Catholics. However, health-care providers may need to remind clients that fasting is not required during times of illness or pregnancy.

Some religious and ethnic groups have taboos for certain foods and methods of preparation. For example, when in the home of a kosher Jewish client, the caregiver should not use cooking items, dishes, or silverware without knowing which are used for meats and which are used for dairy. An assessment of food rituals needs to be individually determined so that these rituals can be incorporated into dietary planning to assist clients in developing culturally accepted healthy food choices.

### Dietary Practices for Health Promotion

The nutritional balance of a diet is recognized by most cultures throughout the world. Most cultures have their own distinct theories of nutritional practices for health promotion and disease prevention. Common folklore practices and selected diets are recommended during periods of illness and for prevention of illness or disease. For example, many societies such as Iranian, Mexican, Puerto Rican, Chinese, and Vietnamese subscribe to the "hot and cold" theory of food selection to prevent illness and maintain health. Although each of these ethnic groups has its own specific name for the hot and cold theory of foods, the overall belief is that the body needs a balance of opposing foods.

In the Western health-care system, diets low in sodium and fats are prescribed for the prevention and treatment of heart conditions. Diets high in fat are recognized as increasing risks for the development of cardiovascular disease and some types of cancer. Many societies are becoming more health-conscious about reducing fat in their diets. Some Asian cultures prepare very spicy foods, which increase the incidence of stomach cancer, ulcers, and gastrointestinal bleeding. A thorough history and assessment of dietary practices can be an important diagnostic tool to guide health promotion. Although school lunch programs, Meals on Wheels, and church meal plans are programs through which the health-care provider can encourage and support families in attaining better nutrition, these programs may still not provide good nutrition.

### Nutritional Deficiencies and Food Limitations

Because of limited socioeconomic resources or limited availability of their native foods, immigrants may eat something that was not available in their home country and incur health problems on arrival in a new environment. This is more likely to occur when individuals immigrate to a country where they do not have native foods readily available and do not know which new foods contain the necessary and comparable nutritional ingredients. Consequently, they do not know which foods to select for balancing their diet. Widespread nutritional deficiencies of many types have occurred with recent immigrants from Southeast Asia, in part because of the time spent in refugee camps, but also because of changes in food habits when immigrating to America (Mattson & Lew, 1991). Among Hindu, the consumption of a single grain such as rice may result in a poor intake of lysine and other essential amino acids.

Enzyme deficiencies exist among some ethnic and racial groups. For example, many Vietnamese-Americans have lactose intolerance and are unable to drink milk or eat dairy products to maintain their calcium needs. By consuming soups and stews made with pureed bones and cooked to an edible consistency, this deficiency can be overcome (Burtis, Davis, & Martin, 1988). For persons with glucose-6-phosphate dehydrogenase deficiency, such as Greek-Americans, the consumption of fava beans can induce hemolysis, resulting in an acute anemic crisis (Reipl, et al., 1993). In general, the wide availability of foods in this country reduces the risks of these disorders as long as immigrants have the means to obtain nutritious foods. Recent emphasis on cultural foods has resulted in small businesses selling ethnic foods and spices to the general public. The health-care provider's task is to determine how to assist the client and identify alternative foods to supplement the diet when these stores are not accessible financially or geographically.

Box 2–7 identifies guidelines for assessing the cultural domain nutrition.

Box 2–7
## Nutrition

**Meaning of Food**

1. Explore the meaning of food to this group.

**Common Foods and Food Rituals**

2. Identify foods, preparation practices, and major ingredients commonly used by this group.
3. Identify specific food rituals.

**Dietary Practices for Health Promotion**

4. Identify dietary practices used to promote health or to treat illness in this cultural group.

**Nutritional Deficiencies and Food Limitations**

5. Identify enzyme deficiencies or food intolerances commonly experienced by this group.
6. Identify large-scale or significant nutritional deficiencies experienced by this group.
7. Identify native food limitations in America that may cause special health difficulties.

# Pregnancy and Childbearing Practices

The cultural domain pregnancy and childbearing practices includes culturally sanctioned and unsanctioned fertility practices; views toward pregnancy; and prescriptive, restrictive, and taboo practices related to pregnancy, birthing, and postpartum.

More traditional, folklore, and magicoreligious beliefs surrounding fertility control, pregnancy, childbearing, and postpartum practices exist in this cultural domain than in any other. The reason may be the mystique that surrounds the processes of conception, pregnancy, and birthing. Ideas about conception, pregnancy, and childbearing practices are handed down from generation to generation and are acculturated into the society without validation or being completely understood. For some, the success of modern technology in inducing pregnancy in postmenopausal women and others who desire children through in vitro fertilization and the ability to select a child's gender raises serious ethical questions about parenting.

## Fertility Practices and Views toward Pregnancy

Commonly used methods of fertility control in North America include natural ovulation methods, birth control pills, foams, Norplant, the morning-after pill, intrauterine devices, sterilization, vasectomy, prophylactics, and abortion. Although not all of these methods are acceptable to all people, many women use a combination of fertility control methods. The most extreme examples of fertility control are sterilization and abortion. Sterilization in North America is now strictly voluntary; however, some countries still perform involuntary sterilization to control birth rates and to control conception in retarded or deformed persons. Abortion remains a controversial issue in North America and in other countries. For example, in Chile, women are encouraged to have as many children as possible, and abortion is illegal (Geissler, 1993). However, in China, abortion is commonly used as a means of limiting family size because of "China's one couple, one child law" (Lawson & Lin, 1994).

Although few comprehensive research studies exist regarding the fertility control practices of diverse ethnic, cultural, and racial groups, some are notable. Herold, et al. (1989) studied the use of fertility control methods among Catholic Puerto Rican women and found that the incidence of pregnancy is higher for Catholic Puerto Ricans than for non-Catholic Puerto Ricans. However, contraception use is widespread among the Puerto Rican population regardless of social contexts such as socioeconomic levels, rural versus urban residence, and educational level.

Mosher and Goldscheider (1984) studied 14,000 married women in the United States from Protestant, Catholic, and Jewish backgrounds including white and non-white women. Their data showed a dramatic increase in surgical sterilization (from 9 to 23 percent) between 1955 and 1970, with a sharper increase in the use of sterilization among males. This finding implies a much higher use of sterilization in the United States than is found in other industrialized countries. Sterilization increased threefold during this same time among Catholics and doubled among Protestants and Jews. Jewish couples were also more likely to use contraception than Protestants or Catholics. Male sterilization among black couples in all religious groups is rare. Differences in contraceptive choices by race are larger than those by religion. Furthermore, this same study implies that black couples with no religious affiliation were the group least likely to use contraception.

Fertility practices and sexual activity, both sensitive topics for many women, especially teenagers, is one area in which "outsider" health-care practitioners may be more effective than health-care providers known to the client. Using videos in the native language and videos and pictures of native ethnic people, material written at the individual's level of education, and providing written instructions in both English and the native language are some of the ways health-care providers can promote better understanding of and compliance with practices related to family planning. Health-care providers should avoid family planning discussions on the first encounter; such information may be better received on subsequent visits when some trust has developed (Hoang, Erickson, & Erickson, 1982). Approaching the subject of family planning obliquely may make it possible to discuss these topics more successfully.

Because pregnancy is not considered an illness in many societies, the idea of seeking advice from a health professional during pregnancy may not be a common practice. However, pregnant women commonly seek advice from elders and family members (Mattson & Lew, 1991). Although pregnancy is not typically seen as an illness in the Polish-American culture, a high value is placed on prenatal care.

## *Prescriptive, Restrictive, and Taboo Practices in the Childbearing Family*

Most societies have prescriptive, restrictive, and taboo beliefs for maternal behaviors and the delivery of a healthy baby. Such beliefs affect sexual and lifestyle behaviors during pregnancy, birthing, and the immediate postpartum period. Prescriptive practices are those things that the mother should do to have a good outcome (healthy baby and pregnancy). Restrictive belief practices are those things that the mother should not do to have a positive outcome (healthy baby and delivery). Taboo practices are those things that, if done, are likely to harm the baby or mother.

A prescriptive belief among Polish-Americans is that women are expected to seek preventive care, eat well, and get adequate rest to have a healthy pregnancy and baby. The health-care provider should encourage the use of these practices through culturally congruent dietary counseling. A restrictive belief among the Navajo is that clothes should not be purchased for the infant before birth because preparing for the infant is forbidden by Indian tradition. When an expectant woman does not prepare for the birth of her baby, it does not mean that she does not care about herself or her baby. A taboo belief among some blacks is that a pregnant woman should not reach over her head because the baby may be born with the cord around its neck.

According to Andrade (1980), a restrictive belief among some Latin-American families is that allowing the father to be present in the delivery room and seeing the mother or baby before they have been cleaned can cause harm to the baby or mother. Because the father is absent from the delivery room or does not want to see the mother or baby immediately after birth does not mean that he does not care about them. However, in the European-American culture, in which the father is often encouraged to take prenatal classes with the expectant mother and provide a supportive role in the delivery process, fathers with opposing beliefs may feel guilty if they do not comply.

In the Japanese culture, the postpartum woman is prescribed a prolonged period of recuperation in the hospital, something that may not be feasible in the United States due to the shortened length of confinement in the hospital after delivery (Sharts-Hopko, 1995). A prescriptive postpartum practice among Haitian women includes initial infant feedings of a preparation (lok) that contains a laxative to hasten the expulsion of meconium. Even though the health-care practitioner may not be successful in getting the mother to cease this practice, educational emphasis can be placed on the prevention of dehydration and nutritional requirements for growth and development (DeSantis, 1988; Thomas & Desantis, 1995). Among the Vietnamese, the head is considered sacred, and it is taboo to touch the head of the mother or the infant. Even removal of vernix from the infant's head can cause distress.

The health-care provider must respect cultural beliefs associated with pregnancy and the birthing process when making decisions related to the health care of pregnant women, especially those practices that do not cause harm to the mother or baby. Most cultural practices can be integrated into preventive teaching in a manner that promotes compliance.

Box 2–8 identifies guidelines for assessing the cultural domain pregnancy and childbearing practices.

# Death Rituals

The cultural domain death rituals includes how the individual and the society view death and euthanasia, rituals to prepare for death, and bereavement and burial practices. Death rituals of ethnic and cultural groups are the least likely to change over time and may cause concerns among health-care personnel in regard to client care and multicultural staff. To avoid cultural taboos, health professionals must become knowledgeable about unique practices related to death, dying, and bereavement.

## Death Rituals and Expectations

A ritual among Orthodox Jews is to bury their deceased before sundown the next day and have postdeath rituals that last for several days. Because the Jewish person should be buried whole, an amputated limb may be buried in the future gravesite. The health-care provider should respect this practice by assisting the amputee or closest family member in making arrangements for burial.

Other groups have elaborate ceremonies in commemoration of the dead, such as a *velorio* among Mexican-Americans (Robs, 1981), which may last for days. To some

Box 2–8
# Pregnancy and Childbearing Practices

**Fertility Practices and Views Toward Pregnancy**

1. Explore cultural views and practices related to fertility control.

2. Identify cultural practices and views toward pregnancy.

**Prescriptive, Restrictive, and Taboo Practices in the Childbearing Family**

3. Identify prescriptive, restrictive, and taboo practices related to pregnancy, such as foods, exercise, intercourse, and avoidance of weather-related conditions.

4. Identify prescriptive, restrictive, and taboo practices related to the birthing process, such as reactions during labor, presence of men, position for delivery, preferred types of health practitioners, or place of delivery.

5. Identify prescriptive, restrictive, and taboo practices related to the postpartum period, such as bathing, cord care, exercise, foods, and roles of men.

persons, these rituals look like a celebration. In Greek Orthodox society, there are successive stages of mourning (Eisenbruch, 1984) that include memorial services 40 days after burial and then at three months and six months, with yearly rituals thereafter.

When approaching death, Muslims may wish to face Mecca and recite passages from the *Holy Qur'an;* the health-care provider needs to determine the direction of Mecca and position the bed accordingly. Whether in the hospital, extended-care facility, or at home in the community, the furniture may need to be rearranged to accomplish this important ritual.

## *Responses to Death and Grief*

The expression of grief in response to death varies intraethnically as well as interethnically. In the East Indian Hindu culture, loved ones are expected to suffer the grief of death in silence with little display of emotion (Miller & Supersad, 1991). Bereavement time for Chinese may be a week or longer depending on the relationship of the family member to the deceased and the degree of acculturation. The family of a deceased Chinese-American may need extra leave time to fulfill their cultural obligations. These variations in the grieving process may cause confusion for health-care providers, who may perceive some clients as overreacting and others as not caring. The behaviors associated with the grieving process must be placed in the context of the specific ethnocultural belief system in order to provide culturally competent care. Caregivers should encourage ethnically specific bereavement practices when providing support to family and friends. Bereavement support strategies include being physically present, encouraging a reality orientation, openly acknowledging the family's right to grieve, assisting them to express their feelings, encouraging interpersonal relationships, promoting interest in a new life, and making referrals to other staff and clergy as appropriate (Stuart & Sundeen, 1995).

Box 2–9 identifies guidelines for assessing the cultural domain death rituals.

Box 2–9
## Death Rituals

**Death Rituals and Expectations**

1. Identify culturally specific death rituals and expectations.

2. Explain the purpose of death rituals and mourning practices.

3. What are specific burial practices, such as cremation?

**Responses to Death and Grief**

4. Identify cultural expectations of responses to death and grief.

5. Explore the meaning of death, dying, and the afterlife.

## Spirituality

The domain spirituality involves more than formal religious beliefs related to faith and affiliation and the use of prayer. For some persons, religion has a strong influence over and shapes nutrition practices, health-care practices, and other cultural domains. Spirituality includes all behaviors that give meaning to life and provide strength to the individual.

Spirituality, a component of health related to the essence of life, is a vital human experience that gives life to the physical organism. In contrast to its purely material aspects, spirituality relates more to the soul than to the body (Hill & Smith, 1985) and is characterized by meaning, hope, (Clark, et al., 1991), purpose, love, trust, forgiveness, and creativity (Carson, 1989). Spirituality is patterned unconsciously from a person's worldview: central assumptions, concepts, and premises that are assumed true and have neither been questioned, reasoned, nor necessarily proved, and that permeate every aspect of the person's life (Crow, 1993). Persons who subscribe to a particular religion may deviate somewhat from the majority view or position. Emblen and Halstead (1993) identified five common interventions that the health professional can use to meet the client's spiritual needs: prayer, scripture, presence, listening, and referral.

### Dominant Religion and Use of Prayer

A person's religious beliefs may have a profound effect on health-care practices. Among Hindus, Jews, Catholics, and Islamics, religion may be the primary focus underlying the manner in which certain health services and practices such as seeking or limiting methods of birth control are practiced. Dietary rules in the Jewish faith include specific methods for slaughtering animals and strict proscriptions against mixing meat and milk at the same meal.

The health-care practitioner who is aware of the client's religious practices and spiritual needs is in a better position to promote culturally competent health care. The practitioner must demonstrate an appreciation of and respect for the dignity and spiritual beliefs of clients by avoiding negative comments about religious beliefs and practices. Clients may find considerable comfort in speaking with religious leaders in times of crisis and serious illness.

Prayer takes different forms and has different meanings. Some persons pray on a daily basis and may have altars in the home. Others may consider themselves to be devoutly religious and only say prayers on special occasions or in times of crisis or illness. Among the Amish, faith-related behavior includes corporate worship and prayer and singing, which helps build conformity and maintain harmony within the group (Kraybill, 1989). The health-care provider may need to make special arrangements for persons to say prayers in accord with their belief system.

### Meaning of Life and Individual Sources of Strength

What gives meaning to life varies among and within cultural groups. To some persons, their formal religion may be the most important facet of fulfilling spirituality needs, whereas in others, religion may be replaced as a driving force by other life forces and worldviews. Among Mexican-Americans, family is extremely important in helping to meet the spiritual needs of individuals. For example, the condition *susto,* "lost soul," has symptoms that include loss of appetite, disinterest in surroundings, neglect of normal duties, and disinterest in family members and friends. A specific example is the case of a Guatemalan woman who suffered from *susto* (Rubel, 1978); her soul was returned to her when her husband and other relatives returned from a migrant work camp.

A person's inner strength comes from different sources. Among the Navajo, the inner self is dependent on being in harmony with one's surroundings. For Christians, a belief in God may give personal strength. Prayer is a significant source of individual strength for Moslems who pray five times a day. Knowing these beliefs allows health-care providers to assist individuals and families in their quest for strength and self-fulfillment.

### Spiritual Beliefs and Health-care Practices

Wellness spirituality brings fulfillment from a lifestyle of purposive and pleasurable living that embraces free choices, purpose in life, satisfaction in life, and self-esteem (Pilch, 1988). For example, when Navajo Indians are not in harmony with their surroundings and experience insomnia from anxieties, the Blessingway Ceremony, ritual dancing, and herbal treatments combined with prayers and song are performed for total body healing and the return of spirits to the body (Wilson, et al., 1993). Practices that interfere with a person's spiritual life can hinder physical recovery and promote physical illness.

Health-care providers should inquire if the person wants to see a member of the clergy even if they have not been active in church. Religious emblems should not be removed as they provide solace to the person and removing them may increase or cause anxiety. A thorough assessment of spiritual life is essential for the identification of solutions and resources that can support other treatments.

Box 2–10 identifies guidelines for assessing the cultural domain spirituality.

## Health-care Practices

Health-care practices, another domain of culture, are interconnected with all other domains of culture. The focus of health care, such as acute or preventive, includes traditional, magicoreligious, and biomedical beliefs; individual responsibility for health; self-medicating practices; and views toward mental illness, chronicity, rehabilitation, and organ donation and transplantation. In addition, responses to pain and the sick role are shaped by specific ethnocultural beliefs. Significant barriers to health care may be shared among cultural and ethnic groups.

Box 2–10
## Spirituality

### Religious Practices and Use of Prayer

1. Identify the influence of the dominant religion of this group on health-care practices.

2. Explore the use of prayer, meditation, and other activities or symbols that help individuals reach fulfillment.

### Meaning of Life and Individual Sources of Strength

3. Explore what gives meaning to life for individuals.

4. Identify the individual's sources of strength.

### Spiritual Beliefs and Health-care Practices

5. Explore the relationship between spiritual beliefs and health practices.

## Health-seeking Beliefs and Behaviors

A wide variety of healing and medical practices among and across diverse populations have maintained the health status of people for centuries. For example, Navajo beliefs about health are intimately connected with traditional beliefs and values of having a harmonious relationship with all living things. The Navajo attempt to create harmony between self, society, and the world, believing that illness is "not simply disease but manifests [itself] as a karmic relationship associated with improper thought and behavior affecting self and others, plants, animals, and environment" (Bell, 1994, p. 237). Among Mexican-Americans, good health is a divine province from God, and a person has little control on the overall outcome of being healthy or ill.

American health-care practices are undergoing a change in focus from treatment based on curative and restorative interventions to increased personal responsibility through education aimed at health promotion and disease prevention. Differences among cultures regarding their acceptance of this concept may vary significantly. For example, Guatemala has only acute-care health practices, and the government opposes interventions geared to preventive health-care practices (Heggenhougen, 1984). Countries such as the United States, Canada, Great Britain, and Australia have strong biomedical health-care practices with much emphasis on technology (Leininger, 1990). Arab countries, with their focus on acute-care interventions, favor intrusive treatments, regarding them as more effective. Intramuscular injections are preferred over pills, and intravenous injections are preferred over intramuscular ones (Meleis, 1981).

Most countries engage in immunization practices. Immunization practices for children were developed largely as a result of the influence of the World Health Organization. Specific immunization schedules and the age at which they are prescribed are highly variable among countries and can be obtained from the World Health Organization. Some religious groups, such as Christian Scientists, do not believe in immunizations. Beliefs such as this that restrict optimal health to children have resulted in court battles with varied outcomes.

Some societies do not have the sophisticated technology and resources needed to facilitate health promotion. For example, Pap smears are new in Egypt, and mammograms are not offered, encouraged, or even known in some societies. Thus, the health-care provider's first step may be to assess a person's previous knowledge and experience related to preventive and acute-care practices.

### Responsibility for Health Care

The health-care delivery system of the country of origin may shape the client's and employee's beliefs regarding personal responsibility for health care. For example, Amish want to be actively involved in decisions regarding health-care options and are expected to help themselves before seeking advice from outsiders (Wenger, 1991). Great Britain and Canada have free health care at the point of entry to the health-care system, with reimbursement coming from the government. Persons who did not need health insurance in their native country may not realize the importance of having health insurance in the United States. A large number of the working poor cannot afford to purchase basic economic essentials for the family and thus cannot even consider the purchase of health insurance when the government or the employer does not provide it. Health-care providers should not assume that clients who do not have health insurance or practice health prevention do not care about their health. The health-care provider must assess each client individually and provide culturally congruent education regarding health promotion and disease prevention activities.

A potential high-risk behavior in the self-care context includes self-medicating practices. Self-medicating behavior in itself may not be harmful, but when combined with prescription medications or used to the exclusion of prescription medications, it may be detrimental to the person's health. A common practice with prescription medications is for people to take medicine until the symptom disappears and then discontinue the medicine prematurely. This practice commonly occurs with antihypertensive medications and antibiotics.

Each country has some type of control over the purchase and use of medications. The United States is more restrictive than many countries and provides warning labels and directions for the use of over-the-counter medications. In Turkey, which has the highest consumer over-the-counter purchase of medications, pharmacists may be consulted before physicians for fever-producing and pain-reducing medicines (Aksit, 1993). In Guatemala, a person can purchase antibiotics, intravenous fluids, and a variety of medications over the counter; most stores sell medications, and vendors sell drugs in street corner shops and on public transportation systems (Miralles, 1989). People who are accustomed to purchasing medications over the counter in their native country frequently see no problem in sharing their medications with family and friends. To help prevent contradictory or exacerbated effects of prescription medication and treatment regimens, the health-care provider should ask about the client's self-medicating practices. One cannot ignore the ample supply of over-the-counter medications in American pharmacies or the numerous television advertisements for self-medication.

### Folk Practices

Many societies practice a blend of folklore, traditional, and biomedical health-care practices. Some societies favor traditional, folklore, or magicoreligious health-care practices over biomedical practices. In this country, interest has increased in traditional and complementary health practices. The United States government has an Office of Alternative Medicine at the National Institutes of Health that has awarded millions of dollars in grants to bridge the gap between traditional and nontraditional therapies.

As an adjunct to biomedical treatments, many people use acupressure, acumassage, other traditional treatments, and herbal therapies. Examples of the use of folk medicines include covering a boil with axle grease, wearing copper bracelets for arthritic pain, mixing wild turnip root and honey for sore throats, and drinking herbal teas. Native-American traditions include ceremonial dances and song. The Chinese subscribe to the "Ying and Yang" theory of treating illnesses, and Hispanic populations adhere to the hot and cold theory of foods for treating illnesses and disease. Traditional schools of pharmacy in Brazil grow, sell, and teach courses on folk remedies. Most Americans practice folk medicine in some form, which includes the use of family remedies passed down from previous generations.

An awareness of combined practices when treating or providing health education to individuals and families helps ensure that therapies do not contradict each other, intensify the treatment regimen, or cause an overdose. At other times, they may be harmful, conflict with, or potentiate prescription medications. It is essential to inquire about the full range of therapies being used, such as food items, teas, herbal remedies, nonfood substances, over-the-counter medications, and medications prescribed or loaned by others. Many times these traditional, folklore, and magicoreligious practices are and should be incorporated into the plan of care for the individual client. However, the health-care provider must ask the individual about these practices so that conflicting treatment modalities are not used. If the clients perceive that the health-care provider does not accept their beliefs, they may be less compliant with prescriptive treatment.

## Barriers to Health Care

Access to health care includes more than having health-care resources available and the economic means for obtaining them. Geographic barriers to health care exist in areas such as Appalachia. Transportation services may not be available, or rivers and mountains may make it difficult for people to obtain needed health-care services when no health-care provider is available in their immediate region. Many Appalachians live in isolated areas where numbers of health professionals are inadequate to provide needed services. Kentucky was one of the first states to adopt the practice of nurses delivering primary care in areas that lack physicians. Current trends and legislation supporting health-care reform, and the increased use of advanced practice nurses may help remove some of these barriers.

Additional barriers to health care include subjective beliefs in relation to the cost of health care, lack of insurance, adverse subjective beliefs and attitudes from caregivers, home responsibilities (no child care available), unavailability of clinic hours that coincide with clients' work hours (making it difficult to schedule appointments), fear of work reprisals, caregivers' judgments of noncompliance (deviant behaviors), lack of client motivation, inability to effectively communicate their needs in the English language, fear of being criticized for traditional practices, lack of knowledge and availability of resources, self-medicating practices, and dependency on family and friends. Health-care providers can help reduce some of these barriers by calling an area ethnic agency or church for assistance, establishing an advocacy role, involving professionals and lay people from the same ethnicity as the client, and using cultural brokers.

## Cultural Responses to Health and Illness

Beliefs regarding pain are one of the oldest culturally related research areas in health care. A 1969 study revealed that Irish-Americans are stoic in their responses to pain, and Jewish-Americans and Italian-Americans are more vocal (Zborowski, 1969). The Navajo regard pain and discomfort as a way of life (Bell, 1995), and many Filipinos view pain as part of life and as an opportunity to atone for past transgressions; thus, they may be tolerant and stoic with the pain experience (Mattson & Lew, 1991). Astute observations and careful assessments must be completed to determine the level of pain a person can tolerate. Health-care practitioners must investigate the meaning of pain to each person within a cultural explanatory framework to interpret diverse behavioral responses and provide culturally competent care. The health-care provider may need to offer and encourage pain medication and to explain that it will help the healing progress more rapidly. Combined research needs to be conducted in the area of ethnic pain experiences and management.

The manner in which mental illness is perceived and expressed by a cultural group has a direct effect on how individuals present themselves and consequently on how health-care providers interact with these persons. In some societies, mental illness may be seen by many as not being as important as physical illness. Mental illness is culture-bound; what may be perceived as a mental illness in one society may not be considered a mental illness in another. The landmark study by Jewell (1952) demonstrated how a Navajo Indian was misdiagnosed with schizophrenia when, in actuality, the Navajo was reacting in a manner expected of him in his culture.

Among Asian-Americans such as Japanese, Chinese, Filipino, Asian Indian, and Koreans; Pacific Islanders such as Hawaiians, Samoans, and Guamanians; and Indochinese such as Vietnamese, Cambodians, and Laotians, having a mental illness or an emotional difficulty is considered a disgrace and taboo (Yamamoto et al., 1993). As a result, the family is likely to keep the mentally ill person at home as long as they can (Louie, 1985). This practice may be reinforced by the belief that all persons are expected to contribute to the household for the common good of the family, and when a person is unable to contribute, further disgrace occurs.

Filipinos may not readily accept professional mental health care but are open to support and advice from family and friends. In Korea, mentally disturbed children are stigmatized, and the lack of supportive services may cause families to abandon their loved ones because of the cost of chronic care and their desire and desperate need for support. Such children are kept from the public eye in hope of saving the family from stigmatization. Korean-Americans may hold these same values.

Culturally congruent mental health services for these clients include:

1. Avoid emphasizing the independence of children and adolescents on the first encounter.

2. Explore the cultural normative approach to shame and guilt (Sue & Sue, 1990).

3. Maintain formality and conversational distance (Chung, 1992; Yamamoto, 1986).

4. Do not expect an open public discussion of emotional problems (Sue & Sue, 1990).

5. Expect somatization of emotional problems (Ho, 1992; Hughes, 1993).

6. Consider the first session a crisis because of the delay in seeking treatment (Fujii, Fukushima, & Yamamoto, 1993; Gaw, 1993).

7. Avoid discussion of hospitalization and seek alternative care services if possible (Fujii, Fukushima, & Yamamoto, 1993; Yamamoto, 1986).

8. Provide concrete and tangible advice. The Asian client does not expect psychotherapy on the first session (Sue & Sue, 1990).

9. On the first encounter, avoid sensitive issues such as sexual practices (Gaw, 1993; Kim, 1993).

The physically and mentally handicapped may be treated differently in diverse cultures. In previous decades in America, physically handicapped individuals were seen as being less desirable than those who did not have a handicap. If the handicap was severe, the person was sometimes hidden from the public's view. In 1992, the Americans with Disabilities Act became effective, protecting handicapped individuals from discrimination.

In the United States, rehabilitation and occupational health services focus on returning the individual to a productive lifestyle in society as soon as possible. Among Greek-Americans and Egyptian-Americans, rehabilitation programs that include drastic changes in lifestyles are more appealing when they are convinced that programs are scientifically supported. To establish rapport, health-care practitioners working with clients suffering from chronic disease must avoid assumptions regarding health beliefs and provide rehabilitative health interventions within the scope of cultural customs and beliefs. Failure to respect and accept the clients' values and beliefs can lead to misdiagnosis, lack of cooperation, and alienation of clients from the health-care system.

Germans accept people with disabilities and are receptive to the concept of rehabilitation, which is a strong component of U.S. and German psychiatric facilities (Wuerth, 1993). Rapid return to previous roles is paramount. However, many developing countries do not have provisions for rehabilitative services, are not financially able to provide rehabilitative services, and may not see them as important (Kronfol & Bashshar, 1989).

Sick role behaviors are culturally prescribed and vary among ethnic societies. Unlike the European-American practice of fully disclosing the health condition to the client, the Filipino family prefers to be informed of the bad news, and they in turn slowly break the news to the sick family member. The sick role may not be readily accepted by Italian-Americans and Polish-Americans, resulting in some persons' keeping their illness hidden from their family until it reaches a more advanced stage. Given the ethnocultural acceptance of the sick role, the health-care provider must assess each client and family individually and incorporate culturally congruent therapeutic interventions to return the client to an optimal level of functioning.

## Blood Transfusions and Organ Donation

Some societies do not subscribe to health-care practices that are common in North America. For example, the Jehovah's Witness does not believe in blood transfusions, and Christian Scientists, Orthodox Jews, Greeks, and some Spanish-speaking societies may not participate in organ donation because they believe the body will not be whole on resurrection (Miralles, 1989). The health-care provider may need to assist the client in obtaining a religious leader to support them in making a decision regarding organ donation or transplantation.

Some persons will not sign donor cards because the concept of organ donation and transplantation is not a familiar one in their homeland. Health-care professionals should provide information regarding organ donation on an individual basis, be sensitive to individual and family concerns, explain procedures involved with organ donation and procurement, answer questions factually, and explain involved risks. A key to successful marketing approaches for organ donation is cultural awareness (Randall, 1991).

Box 2–11 identifies guidelines for assessing the cultural domain health-care practices.

Box 2–11

# Health-care Practices

### Health-seeking Beliefs and Behaviors

1. Identify predominant beliefs that influence health-care practices.

2. Describe the influences of health promotion and prevention practices.

### Responsibility for Health Care

3. Describe the focus of acute-care practice (curative or fatalistic).

4. Explore who assumes responsibility for health care in this culture.

5. Describe the role of health insurance in this culture.

6. Explore behaviors associated with the use of over-the-counter medications.

### Folklore Practices

7. Explore combinations of magicoreligious beliefs, folklore, and traditional beliefs that influence health-care behaviors.

### Barriers to Health Care

8. Identify barriers to health care such as language, economics, and geography for this group.

### Cultural Responses to Health and Illness

9. Explore cultural beliefs and responses to pain that influence interventions. Does pain have a special meaning?

10. Describe beliefs and views about mental illness in this culture.

11. Differentiate between the perceptions of mentally and physically handicapped in this culture.

12. Describe cultural beliefs and practices related to chronicity and rehabilitation.

13. Identify cultural perceptions of the sick role in this group.

### Blood Transfusion and Organ Donation

14. Describe the acceptance of blood transfusions, organ donation, and organ transplantation among this group.

# Health-care Practitioners

The domain health-care practitioners includes the status, use, and perceptions of traditional, magicoreligious, and biomedical health-care providers and is interconnected with communications, family roles and organization, and spirituality. In addition, the gender of the health-care provider may be significant for some persons.

## *Traditional Versus Biomedical Care*

Most people combine the use of biomedical health-care practitioners with traditional practices, folk healers, and magicoreligious healers. The health-care system abounds with individual and family folklore practices for curing or treating specific illnesses. An estimated 70 to 90 percent of all care is delivered outside the perimeter of the formal health-care arena (Kleinman, Eisenberg, & Good, 1978). Many times herbalist-prescribed therapies are handed down from family members and may have their roots in religious beliefs. Traditional and folk practices often contain elements of historically rooted beliefs (Bushy, 1992).

The health-care provider should recognize and respect differences in gender relationships when providing culturally competent care. For example, Mexican-Americans are traditionally seen as being modest, even with health-care providers and, as a result, may feel uncomfortable and refuse care provided by someone from the opposite gender. Since any open display of affection is tabooed, Hindu women may be especially modest and generally seek out female health-care providers for gynecologic examinations. Health-care providers need to respect their modesty by providing adequate privacy and assigning a same-gender caregiver whenever possible. In providing care to a Hasidic male client, the care provider should only touch him when providing care. Therapeutic touch is inappropriate with these clients.

## *Status of Health-care Providers*

Health-care practitioners are looked on differently among ethnocultural groups. Individual perceptions of selected practitioners may be closely associated with previous contact and experiences with health-care providers. In many Western societies, health-care providers, especially physicians, are viewed with great respect, although recent studies show that this is declining among some groups.

Within the Iranian culture, the physician may rely more on physiological cues than technology for a diagnosis. When physicians order many tests or ask clients what they think the problem is, the client may view them as incompetent (Lipson & Meleis, 1983). Based on status and power differences, Iranian-immigrant physicians may misunderstand the assertive behaviors of American nurses, and Iranian nurses may be considered not as assertive as they should be in the American culture.

Many Middle Easterners perceive older male physicians as being of higher rank and more trustworthy than younger health professionals (Lipson & Meleis, 1983). Chinese-Americans are taught from very early ages to have respect for elders and to show deference to nurses and physicians, regardless of gender or age (Louie, 1985).

Physicians who practice in remote areas of Appalachia and are from foreign countries may be mistrusted, not for gender or profession, but for hierarchical relationships, communication styles, and because they are considered outsiders. To promote acceptance of the health-care provider and to obtain full cooperation, the health professional needs to ask clients what they consider to be the problem before devising a plan of care.

Evidence suggests that respect for professionals is correlated with their educational level. For example, Project 2000 in Great Britain proposes that requiring baccalaureate nursing programs to move from hospitals to a university setting will raise the status of women in British society and elevate the standards of nursing practice.

Box 2–12
## Health-care Practitioners

### Traditional Versus Biomedical Care

1. Explore the roles of traditional, folklore, and magicoreligious practitioners and their influence on health practitioners.

2. Describe the acceptance of health-care practitioners in providing care to each gender. Does the age of the practitioner make a difference?

### Status of Health-care Providers

3. Explore perceptions of health-care practitioners with this group.

4. Identify the status of health-care providers in this society.

5. Describe how different health-care practitioners view each other.

In Australia, paramedics and policemen are held in higher regard than nurses. In most cultures, the nurse is expected to defer to physicians. In Jordan, the nurse is viewed more as a domestic than as a professional person, and it is only the physician who commands respect (AbuGharbieh, 1993).

Nurses in the United States are held in high regard compared to nurses in some other countries. The higher regard for nurses in the United States may be related to factors such as the completion of high school or an equivalency examination before entering a nursing program, the rigorous licensing examination required before practicing the profession, and the impact of nursing interventions on health-care outcomes. Some countries do not have programs leading to a master's or doctoral degree in nursing.

In some cultures, folklore and magicoreligious health-care providers may be deemed superior to biomedically educated physicians and nurses. It may be that folk, traditional, and magicoreligious health-care providers are well-known to the family and provide more individualized care. In such cultures, practitioners take time to get to know the client as a person and engage in small talk totally unrelated to the health-care problem to accomplish their objectives. Establishing satisfactory interpersonal relationships is essential for improving health care and education in these ethnic groups.

Box 2–12 identifies the guidelines for assessing the cultural domain health-care practitioners.

## References

AbuGharbieh, P. (1993). Culture shock in Jordan. *Nursing Health Care: Nursing Worldwide, 14*(10), 534–540.

Alland, A. (1971). *Human Diversity.* New York: Columbia Press.

Al-lssa, I., & Dennis, W. (1970). *Cross-cultural studies of behavior.* New York: Holt Rinehart & Winston.

Andrade, S. J. (1980). Family planning practices of Mexican Americans. In M. B. Melville (Ed.), *Twice a minority: Mexican American women* (pp. 92–98). St. Louis: Mosby.

Askit, B. (1993). Rural health seeking: Under fives in Siva, Van, and Ankara. In P. Stirling (Ed.), *Culture and economy: Changes in Turkish villages* (pp. 23–34). Cambridge, England: Eothen.

Bell, R. (1994). Prominence of women in Navajo

healing beliefs and values. *Nursing Health Care, 15*(1), 232–242.

Berry, J. W. (1990). Psychology of acculturation: Understanding individuals moving between cultures. In R. Breslin (Ed.), *Applied cross-cultural psychology* . Newberry Park, CA: Sage Publications, 232, 253.

Boyd-Franklin, N. (1989). *Black families therapy: A multisystems approach.* New York: Guilford Press.

Brislin, R. (1993). *Understanding culture's influence on behavior.* New York: Harcourt Brace.

Brink, P. (1987). Cultural aspects of homosexuality. *Holistic Nursing Practice, 1*(4), 12–20.

Brown, S. C. (1984). *Objectivity and cultural divergence.* London: Cambridge University Press.

Burner, O. Y., Cunningham, P., & Hatter, H. S. (1990). Managing a multicultural nursing staff in a multicultural environment. *Journal of Nursing Administration, 20*(6), 30–34.

Burtis, J., Davis, J., & Martin, S. (1988). *Applied nutrition and diet therapy.* Philadelphia: W. B. Saunders.

Bushy, A. (1992). Cultural considerations for primary health care: Where do self-care and folk medicine fit? *Holistic Nursing Practice, 6*(4), 10–18.

California Organization of Nurse Executives. (1991, August). Position Paper. Sacramento, CA: Author.

Carson, V. (1989). *Spiritual dimensions of nursing practice.* Philadelphia: W. B. Saunders.

Chen, C. L., & Yang, D. C. V. (1986). The self image of Chinese-American adolescents: A cross-cultural comparison. *International Journal of Social Psychiatry, 42*(4), 19–26.

Chung, D. (1992). Asian cultural communications: A comparison with mainstream American culture. In D. K. Chung, K. Murase, & F. Ross-Sheriff (Eds.), *Social work practice with Asian Americans* (pp. 27–44). Newbury Park, CA: Sage Publications.

Clark, C., et al. (1991). Spirituality: Integral to quality care. *Holistic Nursing Practice, 5*(3), 67–76.

Cordasco, F., & Bucchione, E. (1973). *Puerto Rican adolescents on the United States mainland.* Totowa, NJ: Powman & Littleford.

Covell, K., & Turnbull, W. (1982). The long term effects of father absence in childhood on male university students' sex role identity and personal adjustment. *Journal of Genetic Psychology, 141*(3), 271–276.

Crow, K. (1993). Multiculturalism and pluralistic thought in nursing education: Native American world view and the nursing academic world view. *Journal of Nursing Education, 32*(5), 198–204.

DeBraekeleer, M. (1991). Deleterious genes. In G. Bouchard & M. DeBraekeleer (Eds.), *History of a genome: Population and genetics in Eastern Quebec.* Quebec: Institut Quebecois de Recherche sur la Culture, 343, 363.

Department of Health and Human Services,

Indian Health Services Clinical Support Center, (1995). *Indian health service: Primary care provider, 20*(8). Phoenix, AZ: Author.

DeSantis, L. (1988). Cultural factors affecting infant and newborn diarrhea. *Journal of Pediatric Nursing, 3*(6), 391–398.

*Diversity in the workplace.* (1995). Washington, DC: Veterans Health Association Management Support Office.

Eibl-Eiberfelt, I. (1972). Similarities and differences in expressive movements. In H. Hinde (Ed.), *Nonverbal communications* (pp. 297–312). Cambridge, England: Cambridge University Press.

Eisenbruch, M. (1984). Cross-cultural aspects of bereavement. II: Ethnic and cultural variations in the development of bereavement practices. *Culture, Medicine, and Psychiatry, 8,* 315–347.

Emblen, J. D., & Halstead, L. (1993). Spiritual needs and interventions: Comparing the views of patients, nurses, and chaplains. *Clinical Nurse Specialist, 7*(4), 175–182.

Escobedo, L. G., & Remington, P. L. (1989). Birth cohort analysis of prevalence of cigarette smoking among Hispanics in the United States. *Journal of American Medical Association, 261*(1), 66–69.

Felice, M. (1986). Reflections on caring for Indochinese children and youths. *Developmental and Behavioral Pediatrics, 7*(2), 124–130.

Ford, C., & Beach, F. (1951). *Patterns of sexual behavior.* New York: Harper.

Freeman, W. L., Hosey, G. M., Diehr, P., & Goohdes, D. (1989). Diabetes in American Indians of Washington, Oregon, and Idaho. *Diabetes Care, 12,* 282–288.

Friday, R. (1989). Contrasts in discussion behaviors of German and American managers. *International Journal of Intercultural Relations, 13*(42), 429–446.

Friedman, M. M. (1986). *Family nursing: Theory and assessment* (2nd ed.). Norwalk, CT: Appleton-Century-Crofts.

Fuchs, J., Levinson, R., Allen, A., et al. (1992). Update on the search for DNA markers linked to manic-depressive illness in the Old Order Amish. *Journal of Psychiatric Research, 26*(4), 305–308.

Fujii, J., Fukushima, S., & Yamamoto, J. (1993). Psychiatric care of Japanese Americans. In A. Gaw (Ed.), *Culture, ethnicity, and mental illness* (pp. 305–345). Washington, DC.: American Psychiatric Press.

Gaw, C. (1993). Psychiatric care of Chinese Americans. In A. Gaw (Ed.): *Culture, ethnicity, and mental illness* (pp. 245–280). Washington, DC: American Psychiatric Press.

"Gay resources" (June 16, 1995). *The Washington Blade: The Gay Weekly of the Nation's Capital,* p 103.

Geissler, E. M. (1993). Pocket guide to cultural assessment. St. Louis: Mosby.

Giger, J. N., & Davidhizar, R. E. (1995). *Transcultural nursing: Assessment and intervention.* St. Louis: Mosby.

Guerrero, I., Chin, W., & Collins, W. (1982). A survey of malaria in Indochinese refugees arriving in the United States, 1980. *American Journal of Tropical Medicine and Hygiene, 31*(5), 897–901.

Harner, R., Burns, J., Marshall, P., & Karmaliani, R. (1994). Community-based nursing education in Pakistan. *Journal of Continuing Education in Nursing, 25*(3), 130–132.

Heggenhougen, H. K. (1984). Will primary health care efforts be allowed to succeed? *Social Science Medicine, 19*(3), 217.

Herdt, G. (1981). *Guardians of the flutes: Idioms of masculinity.* New York: McGraw-Hill.

Herold, J. M., Westhoff, C. F., Warren, C. W., & Seltzer, J. (1989). Catholicism and fertility in Puerto Rico. *American Journal of Public Health, 79*(9), 1258–1262.

Hill, L., & Smith, N. (1985). *Self-care nursing.* Norwalk, CT: Appleton-Century-Crofts.

Hinton, W., Chen, Y., Nang, D., et al. (1993). DSM-III-R disorders in Vietnamese refugees. *Journal of the American Medical Association, 181*(2), 113–122.

Ho, M. (1992). *Minority children and adolescents in therapy.* Newbury Park, CA: Sage Publications.

Hoang, G., Erickson, S., & Erickson, R. (1982). Guidelines for providing medical care for Southeast Asian refugees. *Journal of American Medical Association, 248*(6), 710–714.

Hughes, C. (1993). Culture in clinical psychiatry. In A. Gaw (Ed.), *Culture, ethnicity, and mental illness* (pp. 347–357). Washington, DC: American Psychiatric Press.

*Information please: Almanac 1995.* (1995). Boston: Houghton Mifflin.

Jewell, D. (1952). A case of a "psychotic" Navajo Indian male. *Human Organization, 11,* 32–36.

Kaplan, R. B. (1989). Cultural thought patterns in inter-cultural education. In J. S. Wurzel (Ed.), *Toward multiculturalism: Readings in multicultural education* (pp. 207–221). Yarmouth, ME: Intercultural Press.

Ketter, J. (April, 1995). Workforce conflicts subject of multi-cultural workshops. *The American Nurse.* Washington, DC: The American Nurses Association.

Kim, L. (1993). Psychiatric care of Korean Americans. In A. Gaw (Ed.), *Culture, ethnicity, and mental illness* (pp. 347–357). Washington, DC: American Psychiatric Press.

Kleinman, A., Eisenberg L., & Good B. (1978). Clinical lessons from anthropologic and cross-cultural research. *Annals of Internal Medicine, 88*(2), 251–258.

Kraybill, D. (1989). *The riddle of Amish culture.* Baltimore, MD: Hopkins University Press.

Krebs, G., & Kunimoto, Y. (1994). *Effective communication in multicultural health care settings.* Thousand Oaks, CA: Intercultural Press.

Kronfol, N. M., & Bashshar, R. (1989). Lebanon's health care policy: A case study in the evolution of a health system under stress. *Journal of Public Health Policy, 10*(3), 377.

Lammi, U. K. (1989). Functional capacity and associated factors in elderly Finnish men.

*Scandinavian Journal of Social Medicine, 17*(1), 67.

Lane, S. (1987). *A biocultural study of trachoma in an Egyptian hamlet.* Unpublished doctoral dissertation, University of California, San Francisco.

Lawson, J., & Lin, V. (1994). Health status differentials in the People's Republic of China. *American Journal of Public Health, 84*(5), 737–741.

Leininger, M. E. (1988). Transcultural eating patterns and nutrition: Transcultural nursing and anthropological perspectives. *Holistic Nursing Practice, 3*(1), 16–25.

Leininger, M. E. (1990). The significance of cultural concepts in nursing. *Journal of Transcultural Nursing, 2*(1), 22–26.

Levin, J., & Taylor, R. (1993). Gender and age differences in religiosity among Black Americans. *The Gerontologist, 33,* 16–23.

Lipson, J. G., & Meleis, A. I. (1985). Culturally appropriate care: The case of immigrants. *Topics in Clinical Nursing, 7*(3), 48–56.

Lipson, J., & Haifizi, H. (1997). Iranian Americans. In L. Purnell & B. Paulanka (Eds.), Transcultural health care: A culturally competent approach. Philadelphia: F. A. Davis.

Louie, K. B. (1985). Providing health care to Chinese clients. *Topics in Clinical Nursing, 7*(3), 18–25.

Manio, E. B., & Hall, R. R. (1987). Asian family traditions and their influence in transcultural health care delivery. *Children's Health Care, 15*(3), 172–177.

Mark, B. A., & Smith, H.S. (1987). *Essentials of finance in nursing.* Rockville, MD: Aspen.

Markell, E., Vage, M., & John, D. (1992). *Medical parasitology.* Philadelphia: W. B. Saunders.

Martin, K., Wimberley, D., & O'Keese, K. (1994). Resolving conflict in a multicultural nursing department. *Nursing Management, 25*(1), 49–51.

Mattson, S., & Lew, L. (1991). Culturally sensitive prenatal care for Southeast Asians. *Journal of Obstetric, Gynecological, and Neonatal Nurses, 12*(1), 48–54.

Meleis, A. (1981). The Arab-American in the health care system. *American Journal of Nursing, 81*(12), 1180–1183.

Miller, W. S. & Supersad, J. W. (1991). East Hindu Americans. In J. N. Giger & R. E. Davidhizar (Eds.), *Transcultural nursing: Assessment and intervention* (pp. 437–464). St. Louis: Mosby.

Miralles, M. A. (1989). *A matter of Life and death: Health seeking behaviors of Guatemalan refugees in South Florida.* New York: AMS Press.

Mosher, W. D., & Goldscheider, C. (1984). *Studies in Family Planning, 15*(3), 101–111.

Mosian, C. (1991). Portrait of alcohol and drug consumption in Quebec: Principle data of the national survey on alcohol and other drugs. *Collection: Donnees statistiques et indicateurs.* Quebec: Ministerie de la Sante et des Services Sociaux.

Motwani, J., Hodge, J., & Crampton, S. (1995).

Managing diversity in the health care industry: A conceptual model and an empirical investigation. *Holistic Care Supervisor, 13*(3), 16–23.

Muecke, M. (1983). In search of healers: Southeast Asian refugees in the American health care system. *Western Journal of Medicine, 139*(6), 835–840.

Murdock, G. (1971). *Outline of cultural materials.* New Haven: Human Relations Area Files.

Murillo, N. (1978). The Mexican American family. In R. A. Martinez (Ed.), *Hispanic culture and health care: Fact, fiction, folklore (pp 3–18).* St Louis: C. V. Mosby.

Nguyen, D. (1985). Culture shock: A review of Vietnamese culture and its concept of health and disease. *Western Journal of Medicine, 142*(3), 409–412.

Overfield, T. (1977). Biological variation. *Nursing Clinics of North America, 12*(1), 19–27.

Orque, M., Block, B. & Monrroy, L. (1983). *Ethnic nursing care: A multicultural approach.* St. Louis: Mosby.

Paquet, J. (1989). *Health and social inequality: Cultural gap.* Quebec: Institut Quebecois de Recherche sur la Culture.

Perez-Stable, E. J., Marin, G. & Marin, B. V. (1994). Behavioral risk factors: A comparison of Latinos and Non-Latino Whites in San Francisco. *American Journal of Public health, 84*(6), 971–976.

Pilch, J. (1988). Wellness spirituality. *Health Values, 12*(3), 28–30.

Price, J., & Cordell B. (1994). Cultural diversity and patient teaching. *Journal of Continuing Education in Nursing, 25*(4), 163–166.

Purnell, L., & Galloway, W. (1995). What to do if called upon to testify. *Accident and Emergency Nursing, 17*(4),246–249.

Randall, T. (1991). Key to organ donation may be cultural awareness. *Journal of the American Medical Association, 285*(2), 176–178.

Read, K. (1952). The Nama cult of the central highland. *New Guinea, 23,* 1–25.

Reipl, R., Schreiner, J., Muller, B., Hildemann, S., & Loeschke, K. (1993). Broad beans as a cause of acute hemolytic anemia. *Deutsche Medizinische Wochenschrift, 118,* 932–935.

Robs, H. M. (1981). Cultural view regarding death and dying. *Topics in Clinical Nursing,* 1–16.

Ronaghy, H. (1975). Migration of Iranian nurses to the United States: A study of one school of nursing in Iran. *International Nursing Review, 22,* 87–88.

Roseman, J. M. (1985). Diabetes in Black Americans. *Diabetes in America.* Washington, DC: U.S. Department of Health and Human Services.

Sharts Hopko, N. (1995). Birth in the Japanese context. *Journal of Obstetrical Gynecological, and Neonatal Nursing, 24,* 343–350.

Stuart, G. & Sundeen, S. (1995). *Principles and practices in psychiatric nursing* (6th ed.). St. Louis: Mosby Year Book.

Sue, D. W., & Sue, D. (1990). *Counseling the culturally different: Theory and practice* (2nd ed.). New York: John Wiley.

Thayer, S. (1988, March). Close encounters. *Psychology Today,* pp. 31–36.

Thayer, S. (1993). The epidemiology of Amish communities. In J. Dow, W. Enninger, & J. Raith (Eds.), *Amishland.* Des Moines, IA: Iowa State University.

Thomas, J. & DeSantis, L. (1995). Feeding and weaning practices of Cuban and Haitian immigrant mothers. *Journal of Transcultural Nursing, 6*(2), 34–42.

*Today's registered nurses: Numbers and demographics.* (1994). Washington, DC: American Nurses' Association.

Tripp-Reimer, T. (1982). Barriers to health care: Variations in interpretation of Appalachian client behaviors by Appalachian and non-Appalachian health professionals. *Western Journal of Nursing Research, 4*(2), 179–191.

Tripp-Reimer, T., & Lively, (1988). Cultural considerations in therapy. In C. K. Beck, R. P. Rawlins, & S. Williams (Eds.), *Mental health/psychiatric nursing* (pp. 185–199). St. Louis: C. V. Mosby.

Vessel, E. (1972). Therapy-pharmacogenetics. *New England Journal of Medicine, 287*(18), 904–909.

Watson, O. M. (1980). *Proxemic behavior: A cross cultural study.* The Hague, Netherlands: Mouton.

Wenger, A. F. Z. (1991). The culture care theory and the Old Order Amish. In M. M. Leininger (Ed.), Culture care diversity and universality: A theory of nursing. New York: National League for Nursing.

Wenger, A. F. Z. (1996). Cultural context, health, and health care decision making. *Journal of Transcultural Nursing, 7*(1), 3–14.

Wilson, A., Bekiaris, J., Gleeson, S., Papasavva, C. Wise, M., & Hawe, P. (1993). The good heart, good life survey: Self-reported cardiovascular disease risk factors, health knowledge, and attitudes among Greek-Australians in Sydney. *Australian Journal of Public Health, 17,* 215–221.

Wuerth, U. (1993). An open psychiatric unit in the U. S. and Germany. *Journal of Psychosocial Nursing, 31*(3), 29–33.

Yamamoto, J. (1986). Therapy for Asian Americans and Pacific Islanders. In C. Wilkinson (Ed.), *Ethnic psychiatry* (pp. 89–141). New York: Plenum.

Yamamoto. J., Silva, J. Justice, L., Chang, C., & Leong,. G. (1993). Cross-cultural psychotherapy. In A. Gaw (Ed.), *Culture, ethnicity, and mental illness* (pp. 101–124). Washington, DC: American Psychiatric Press.

Zborowski, M. (1969). *People in pain.* San Francisco: Jossey- Bass.

Zhou, H. H., Koshakji, R. J. P., Silberstein, D. J., Wilkinson, G. R., & Wood, A. J. J. (1989). Racial differences in drug response: Altered sensitivity to and clearance of propranolol in men of Chinese descent as compared with American Whites. *New England Journal of Medicine, 320,* 565–570.

# African-Americans

*Josepha Campinha-Bacote*

---

• Key terms to become familiar with in this chapter are:

| | |
|---|---|
| African-Americans | Laying on of hands |
| Augmented families | Low blood |
| Black English | *Nguzo Sabo* |
| Colored | Pidgin |
| The dozens | Secondary members |
| Falling out | Speaking in tongues |
| Fatback | Soul food |
| Geophagia | Subfamilies |
| Gullah | Witchcraft |
| High blood | |

## OVERVIEW, INHABITED LOCALITIES, AND TOPOGRAPHY

### Overview

African-Americans are one of the largest ethnic groups in the United States. U.S. African-Americans are mainly of African ancestry; however, many have non-African ancestors as well. In fact, African-Americans encompass a gene pool of over 100 racial strains (Goddard, 1990). African-Americans have been identified as "Negro," "colored," "black," and "Black American." Depending on their cohort group, some African-Americans may prefer to identify themselves differently. For example, younger blacks may prefer the term **African-American**, whereas elderly African-Americans use the terms *Negro* and **colored**. In contrast, middle-aged African-Americans refer to themselves as *black*. These different descriptors can cause confusion when attempting to use the politically correct term for this ethnic group. In addition, we still see such organizational titles as the National Black Nurses Association and the National Association for the Advancement of Colored People, which clearly depict the differences in how African-Americans prefer to be identified. Therefore, it is culturally sensitive to ask African-Americans what they prefer to be called.

Much diversity exists among African-Americans, and health-care providers must be aware of intraethnic variation among this ethnic group. Intraethnic variation implies that there is more variation within an ethnic group than across ethnic groups.

Factors such as religious affiliation, educational status, occupation, socioeconomic status, and geographic location are but a few variables that contribute to intraethnic variation within the African-American population. Thus, the health-care provider must assess and plan interventions for African-Americans on an individual basis.

## Heritage and Residence

African-Americans are largely the descendants of African slaves brought into this country between 1619 and 1860 (Branch & Paxton, 1976). The literature is saturated with conflicting reports of the exact number of slaves that arrived in this country. Varying estimates reveal a range from 3.5 to 24 million slaves who landed in America during the entire slave trade era (Curtin, 1969). The largest group of slaves transported to the United States came from the West Coast of Africa.

In 1990, about half of the nation's 29,067,430 African-Americans lived in the South. Based on the 1990 census, African-Americans are concentrated in large cities, with more than one million living in both New York City and Chicago. African-American majorities reside in 11 major cities: Atlanta, Georgia; Washington, D.C.; Baltimore, Maryland; Jackson, Mississippi; Gary, Indiana; Newark, New Jersey; Detroit, Michigan; Memphis, Tennessee; Birmingham, Alabama; Richmond, Virginia; and New Orleans, Louisiana.

## Reasons for Migration and Associated Economic Factors

Involuntary migrants (slaves) were concentrated in the South. After the Civil War, more African-Americans migrated from southern rural areas to northern urban areas. World War II was a major catalyst in fostering this migration to urban and northern areas. Urban and northern areas provided African-Americans with greater economic opportunities, which brought African-Americans and European-Americans into close contact for the first time. Jaynes and Williams (1989) reported that during the 1940s, a net out-migration from the South totalled approximately 1.5 million African-Americans (15 percent of the South's black population).

## Educational Status and Occupations

Before 1954, educational opportunities were compromised for African-Americans. School systems were segregated and blacks were victims of inferior facilities. In 1910, almost one third of all blacks were illiterate (Blum, et al., 1981). However, in 1954, the Supreme Court decision in Brown v. Board of Education of Topeka ruled against the segregation of blacks and whites in the public school systems.

Poverty too has had an impact on African-American communities in ways that often cause a ripple effect in terms of social consequences (Lander & Gourdine, 1992), such as poorly educated individuals and high dropout rates from school. In some urban areas, the dropout rate among African-Americans has been reported as high as 61 percent (Hammack, 1986).

Despite these devastating statistics, most African-American families place a high value on education. Hines and Boyd-Franklin (1982) stated that education is viewed by the African-American family as the process most likely to ensure work security and social mobility. Families often make great sacrifices so at least one child can go to college.

African-Americans are not well-represented in managerial and professional positions; however, they represent a large segment of blue-collar workers employed in service occupations (Minorities and Women in the Health Fields, 1990). One reason for this disproportionate representation in professional and managerial positions is thought to be discrimination in employment and job advancement. In 1961, President Kennedy established the Committee on Equal Employment Opportunity to protect minorities against discrimination in employment. However, most African-Americans still believe that job discrimination is a major variable contributing to problems they encounter in obtaining a better job or successful career mobility.

The majority of African-Americans in the working class do not typically advance to the higher-class levels (Goddard, 1990). Because they are overrepresented in the working class, they experience increased exposure to hazardous occupations, resulting in occupation-related diseases and illness. For example, Michaels (1983) reported that African-American males are at a higher risk for developing cancer, which is related to their high representation in the steel and tire industries. Health-care providers must assess African-American clients for occupation-related diseases such as cancer and stress-related diseases such as hypertension.

# COMMUNICATIONS

## Dominant Language and Dialects

The dominant language spoken among African-Americans is English. However, many people have referred to the informal language of African-Americans as **Black English.** This term is incorrect because Black English is not a language, but rather a dialect in which pronunciation of words may be different. For example, some African-Americans may pronounce *th* as "de." Therefore, *these* may be pronounced as "dese." Health-care professionals must not stereotype African-Americans as speaking only in Black English because most African-Americans are articulate and competent in the formal English language.

**Pidgin** is another form of communication found in the African-American population. Pidgin dates to the slavery era, in which African slaves from different tribes were forced to develop their own form of communication among themselves. *Pidgin* is a form of communication that occurs when two peoples do not have a common language (Bloch, 1983) and are forced to develop a third language (pidgin), which is a combination of their respective languages.

Sometimes a pidgin becomes the first language of a group of speakers; then it is a creole language. **Gullah** is a creole language that is spoken by African-Americans who live on or near the Sea Islands off Georgia and South Carolina. After the Civil War, these sea islands, such as Sapelo Island and Hilton Head Island, were left to the freed slaves, who developed their own culture. Today, their descendants still speak Gullah, a dialect derived from several West African languages. Health-care providers must refrain from assuming the client who uses a dialect is poorly educated or lacks intelligence.

## Cultural Communication Patterns

African-Americans are highly verbal and express their feelings openly to trusted friends or family. What transpires within the family is viewed as private and not appropriate for discussion with strangers (Bourjolly, 1994). A common phrase that reflects this perspective is, "Don't air your dirty laundry." The volume of African-Americans' voices is usually louder than those in other cultures. Health-care providers must not misunderstand this attribute as reflecting anger, when, in fact, they are merely expressing their thoughts in a dynamic manner.

Humor is one form of communication found among African-Americans. Humor serves as a tool for the release of hostile and angry feelings. Robinson (1977) stated that some African-American comedians use wit and humor as a force in easing racial tension. **The dozens,** a social game in which African-Americans use humor, is a joking relationship between two African-Americans in which each in turn is, by custom, permitted to tease or make fun of the other. Often times the joking is loud and can be mistaken as aggressive communication if not understood within the context of the African-American culture.

African-American speech is dynamic and expressive. Body movements are involved when communicating to others. Facial expressions can be very demonstrative in nature. Touch is another form of nonverbal communication seen when African-Americans are interacting with relatives and extended family. African-Americans are reported to be comfortable with a closer personal space than other ethnic groups, (Reynolds, 1992). Maintaining direct eye contact with some African-Americans can be misinterpreted as an aggressive behavior. Health-care providers must consider these nonverbal behaviors when providing care to African-American clients.

## Temporal Relationship

In general, African-Americans are more present- than past- or future-oriented. However, the past and future play a role in specific subgroups of African-Americans. Specifically, the past plays an important role with elderly African-Americans. Storytelling is an example of an oral tradition found among African-Americans, which strongly draws on their rich history and heritage. Other subgroups of African-Americans are more future-oriented. The value that is placed on education is an example of the future orientation.

African-Americans are relaxed about time. It is more important to make an appointment than to be on time for the appointment. What they see as important is the fact that they are there, even though they may arrive one to two hours late. Therefore, flexibility in timing appointments may be necessary for African-Americans, who have a circular sense of time rather than the dominant culture's linear sense of time (Olsen & Frank-Stromborg, 1994).

## Format for Names

African-Americans prefer to be greeted formally as Mr., Mrs., or Miss. They prefer their surname, because the "family name" is highly respected and connotes pride in their family heritage. However, African-Americans do not use such formal names when they interact among themselves. It is not uncommon for an African-American youth to call an unrelated African-American who lives in the community uncle, aunt, or cousin. The health-care provider should greet the African-American client by the last name and appropriate title.

## FAMILY ROLES AND ORGANIZATION

### Head of Household and Gender Roles

Traditionally, the head of the household in the African-American family is the mother. This matriarchal family system is rooted in the era of slavery when many families were separated and the fathers were sold to other plantations. The mother was expected to care for the children.

Today, it is not uncommon to see African-American families reflecting a patriarchal system. However, a high percentage of African-American households are still headed by a female single parent. Ladner and Gourdine (1992) stated that "single parenting and poverty are viewed as the causal factor in dis-stabilizing the African American family" (p. 208).

Because African-American families are pluralistic in nature, gender roles and childrearing practices vary widely depending on ethnicity, socioeconomic class, rural versus urban location, and educational achievement. Because of dual employment of many middle-class African-American families, cooperative teamwork is needed. Many family tasks such as cooking, cleaning, child care, and shopping are shared, requiring flexibility and adaptability of roles. Many middle-class African-American families may be more egalitarian in structure than European-American middle-class families (Willie & Greenbelt, 1978). Because many African-American families, especially those with a single head of household, are matrifocal in nature, the health-care provider must recognize women's importance in decision making and disseminating health information.

## Prescriptive, Restrictive, and Taboo Roles for Children and Adolescents

Given African-Americans' strong work and achievement orientation, they value self-reliance and education for their children. Here a dichotomy might exist. Because many do not expect to get full benefit from their efforts because of discrimination, families tend to be more protective of their children and act as a buffer between their children and the outside world (McAdoo, 1983). Respectfulness, obedience, conformity to rules, and good behavior are stressed for children. In violence-ridden communities, mothers try to keep young children off the streets. As children enter the teenage years, this becomes increasingly futile and a mother may give up, disengage, and let them have their freedom (Friedman, 1986; Rainwater, 1971). Adolescents are assigned household chores as part of their family responsibility and are encouraged to seek employment for pay when old enough, thereby learning survival skills (Willie, 1976).

Although premarital teenage pregnancy is not condoned, it is accepted in the family after the fact. Lower-socioeconomic-class African-American adolescents have sexual experiences and marry at a younger age than African-American adolescents from middle-class families (Rainwater, 1971).

## Family Roles and Priorities

African-American families come out of various backgrounds, share a wide range of characteristics, and are found throughout all socioeconomic levels (Spurlock & Lawrence, 1985). However, one in three African-Americans lives in a household with an income below the poverty level (Jaynes & Williams, 1989), which has a pronounced effect on their goals and priorities. African-Americans are very concerned about the future of their children and express the same wishes for their children as the wider society. Most African-American families want their children to achieve the "American Dream" (Ladner & Gourdine, 1992). However, they view their options for improving their condition as more limited.

African-American values, goals, and priorities are seen from an Afrocentric framework. An Afrocentric worldview incorporates *Nguzo Sabo* as the guidelines for living. *Nguzo Sabo* encompasses the seven principles of *Umojo* (unity), *Kujichagula* (self-determination), *Ujima* (collective work and responsibility), *Nia* (purpose), *Imani* (faith), *Ujamaa* (cooperative economics), and *Kuumba* (creativity) (Phillips, 1988).

The elders in an African-American community are valued and treated with respect. The role of the grandmother is one of the most central roles in the African-American family (Boyd-Franklin, 1989). Grandmothers are frequently the economic support of African-American families, and they often play a critical role in child care. It is not uncommon to see African-American children raised by grandparents.

Boyd-Franklin (1989) stated that the extended family is essential in understanding the lives of African-American families. There are several African-American extended-family models. Billingsley (1968) divided African-American extended families into four major types: (1) subfamilies, (2) families with secondary members, (3) augmented families, and (4) nonblood relatives. **Subfamilies'** members are considered to be relatives such as nieces, nephews, cousins, aunts, and uncles. **Secondary members** consist of peers of the primary parents, older relatives of the primary parents, and parents of the primary parents. In an **augmented family,** the head of household is raising children who are not his or her own relatives. *Nonblood relatives* are individuals who are unrelated by blood ties but who are part of the family in terms of involvement and function.

Social status is important within the African-American community. Certain occupations receive higher esteem than others. For example, African-American physicians and dentists tend to have a privileged position (Boyd-Franklin, 1989). Ministers and clergy also receive respect within the African-American community.

African-Americans who move up the socioeconomic ladder often find themselves caught between two worlds. They have their roots in the African-American community, but at times they find themselves interacting more within the European-American community. Other African-Americans negatively refer to these individuals as "oreos." Oreo is a derogatory term that means "black on the outside, but white on the inside."

Sports and entertainment figures such as Michael Jordan, Mohammed Ali, Michael Jackson, Magic Johnson, and Whitney Houston are given special social status within the African-American community. These sports and entertainment figures serve as role models, particularly for socioeconomically deprived African-American children.

## Alternative Lifestyles

A single head of household is accepted without associated stigma in African-American families. When women are unable to provide emotional and physical support, maternal grandmothers and aunts readily provide assistance and frequently raise the children as their own (Boyd-Franklin, 1989). In addition, extended and augmented families may take responsibility for children.

Lesbian and gay relationships undoubtedly occur as frequently among African-Americans as in other ethnic groups. Acceptance of same-sex relationships varies between and among families. Personal disclosure to friends and family may jeopardize relationships, thereby forcing some to remain closeted. The high incidence of acquired immunodeficiency syndrome (AIDS) is associated with high-risk sexual activity and intravenous drug use common to all ethnic populations in America.

## WORKFORCE ISSUES

### Culture in the Workplace

African-American men are more at risk for developing hypertension and stress-related diseases because they are more likely to be employed in low-paying, insecure, dead-end jobs that create stress (Waitzman & Smith, 1994). In fact, Waitzman and Smith's study of 1982 working-age men over a 7- to 13-year period found a pattern of downward job mobility for African-American men.

African-Americans adhere strongly to the work ethic. However, a study conducted by Stevens, Hall, and Meleis (1992) of ethnically diverse female clerical workers reveals that African-American women experience racial tension within the work role. *Ethnic or racial tension* is defined as "negative workplace atmosphere motivated by prejudicial attitudes about cultural background and/or skin color" (Stevens, Hall, & Meleis, 1992, pp. 759–760).

Although an African-American axiology reflects a strong emphasis on spirituality, there is an economics-driven emphasis on materialism. African-Americans feel a need to acculturate into mainstream society to survive in the workforce. Bell and Evans (1981) identify four different interacting styles within the African-American culture. The *acculturated interpersonal* style occurs when African-American people make a conscious or subconscious decision to reject the values, beliefs, practices, and general behaviors associated with their own ethnic group. Acculturated African-Americans become sensitive to punctuality, timeliness, and adoption of other values of European-Americans. In contrast, the *culturally immersed* African-American rejects all values and behaviors except those held by his or her own culture. This person is often labeled "militant" or "difficult to work with." In the *traditional interacting* style, African-Americans neither reject nor accept their ethnic identity. They do not disclose and are referred to as the "easy-to-get-along-with" African-American. Their motto is "Don't rock the boat." The *bicultural interacting* style demonstrates the pride that African-Americans have for their identity, history, and cultural traditions, while still feeling comfortable in the mainstream. The bicultural African-American's values integrate living and ethnic diversity.

## Issues Related to Autonomy

Some African-American men may experience a difficult time in taking direction from a European-American supervisor or boss. This difficulty stems from the era of slavery when African-Americans were considered the property of their master. Many African-Americans continue to be frustrated at their lower-level positions and the absence of African-American leadership in many workplaces.

Because the dominant language of African-Americans is English, they usually have no difficulty communicating verbally with others in the workforce. However, some persons may view African-Americans who speak Black English, Gullah, or other African dialects exclusively as poorly educated or unintelligent. This misinterpretation may affect employment and job promotion where verbal skills are more valued. In addition, nonverbal communications of African-Americans are sometimes misunderstood and are often labeled as being more aggressive than assertive because of intonation and body movements.

## BIOCULTURAL ECOLOGY

### Skin Color and Other Biologic Variations

Goddard (1990) stated that African-Americans encompass a gene pool of over 100 racial strains. Therefore, skin color among African-Americans can vary from a light-colored to a very dark-colored skin tone. Assessing the skin of most African-American clients requires different clinical skills. For example, pallor in dark-skinned African-Americans can be observed by the absence of the underlying red tones that give the brown and black skin its "glow" or "living color" (Roach, 1981). Brown-skinned African-Americans appear more yellowish brown, whereas darker-skinned African-Americans appear as an ashen-gray color.

To assess such conditions as inflammation, cyanosis, jaundice, and petechiae may require natural light and the use of different assessment skills. Health-care professionals cannot rely solely on their usual observation skills. African-Americans exhibiting inflammation must be assessed by palpation of their skin for warmth, edema, tightness, or induration. To assess for petechiae in dark-skinned blacks, the health-care professional needs to observe the oral mucosa or conjunctiva. Jaundice is assessed more accurately in dark-skinned persons by observing the sclera of the eyes and the palms of hands and feet, which may have a yellow discoloration.

African-Americans have a tendency toward the overgrowth of connective tissue components connected with the protection against infection and repair after injury (Henderson & Primeaux, 1981). Keloid formation is one example of this tendency toward overgrowth of connective tissue. Polednak (1974) noted that diseases such as lymphoma and systemic lupus erythematosus occur in African-Americans secondary to this overgrowth of connective tissue.

Bone density is a biologic variation noted among African-Americans. African-Americans have a higher bone density than that of European-Americans, Asians, and Hispanics. In addition, their long bones are longer. African-Americans also experience a lower incidence of osteoporosis.

Certain skin conditions are gender-specific among some African-Americans. Pseudofolliculitis ("razor bumps") is more common among African-American males, whereas melasma ("mask of pregnancy") is more common among darker-skinned African-American females during pregnancy.

Birthmarks are more prevalent in African-Americans. Birthmarks occur in 20 percent of the African-American population as compared to the one to three percent in other ethnic groups (Giger & Davidhizar, 1995). One example is mongolian spots, which disappear over time and are found more commonly in African-American newborns. In addition, African-American newborns of all socioeconomic levels have a lower birthweight than European-American newborns but are more neurologically advanced (Pratt, Jones, & Seigal, 1977).

## Diseases and Health Conditions

Because African-Americans are concentrated in large inner cities, they are at risk for being victims of violence. In fact, the leading cause of death among young African-American males is homicide. This violence has been referred to as "black-on-black" violence. Gangs are also more prevalent in larger cities, which only increases the likelihood of the occurrence of violence in African-American communities. Living in urban industrial areas exposes African-Americans to pollution, which puts them at an increased risk for developing respiratory diseases. Thus, essential preventive services should include health promotion activities and screening for respiratory diseases related to pollution.

In the United States, African-Americans lead the nation in poverty rates (Crew, 1994), and hypertension continues to be their most serious health problem (Smith, 1992). Approximately 5 million of the 20 million African-Americans residing in the United States are hypertensive (Mallorey, 1988). They also suffer higher mortality and morbidity related to hypertension and at an earlier age (Gregory & Clark, 1992). For example, African-Americans are 3.2 times more likely to develop kidney failure related to hypertension than European-Americans (Funkhouser & Moser, 1990).

African-Americans' average life span is 6.5 years shorter than that of European-Americans (*Health status*, 1990). Cancer, cardiovascular diseases, cirrhosis, diabetes, accidents, homicide, and infant mortality have been identified as the largest contributing factors to the high death rates among African-Americans.

Sickle cell disease is the most common genetic disorder among the African-American population. However, sickle cell disease is also found in persons from geographic areas where malaria is endemic, such as the Caribbean, the Middle East, the Mediterranean region, and Asia (Hauser, et al., 1992). Sickle cell disease represents several hemoglobinopathies that include sickle cell anemia, sickle cell hemoglobin C disease, and sickle cell $\beta$-thalassemia. In addition to sickle cell disease, glucose-6-phosphate dehydrogenase deficiency, which interferes with glucose metabolism, is another genetic disease found in African-Americans.

African-Americans represent 13 percent of the U.S. population; however, they represent 30 percent of the reported cases of AIDS (DiClemente, 1992). In addition, African-Americans experience high cancer rates and lower survival rates for selected primary cancer sites. Specifically, mortality rates for European-Americans with colorectal cancer declined 12.3 percent from 1973 to 1989; however, it increased 7 percent for African-Americans. In addition, African-Americans experienced poorer 5-year survival rates than other groups (Elixhauser & Ball, 1994). Elixhauser and Ball cited the following two reasons for this lower survival rate:

1. African-Americans report later for treatment.

2. Tumors are deeper within the colon of African-Americans, making them more difficult to detect during digital examination.

In summary, health conditions for most African-Americans are below average. In the United States, African-Americans lead the nation in poverty rates (Crew, 1994). The influence of this high poverty rate greatly affects their overall health status. Health-care providers must provide culturally congruent health education, institute prevention practices, and screen African-American populations for hypertension and signs and symptoms of cancer.

## Variations in Drug Metabolism

Most clinical drug trials are conducted on European-American men. More recently, clinical trials have included European-American women. However, specific ethnic groups, regardless of gender, continue to be an underrepresented group in research studies regarding clinical drug trials. African-Americans are among the underrepresented groups.

Although African-Americans are less responsive to beta-blockers, especially propranolol, they respond better to monotherapy in the treatment of hypertension (Levy, 1993). The pathophysiology of hypertension in African-Americans is related to volume expansion, decreased renin, and increased intracellular concentration of sodium and calcium.

Eye color is another genetic variation related to difference in response to a specific drug. Kalow (1984) reported that light eyes dilate wider in response to mydriatic drugs than do dark eyes. This difference in response to a mydriatic drug must be taken into consideration in treating African-Americans.

Cultural factors, such as a health-care professional's personal beliefs about a specific ethnic group, may also account for how a drug is used (Levy, 1993). For example, African-Americans are at a higher risk of misdiagnosis for psychiatric disorders and therefore are given inappropriate drugs. According to Adebimpe (1981), diagnostic statistics reveal high frequencies for the diagnosis of psychosis and low frequencies for the diagnosis of depression in African-American clients. African-Americans also receive higher doses of neuroleptics more frequently and are given high-potency depot neuroleptics more often than European-Americans.

Side effects of psychotropic and antidepressant drugs vary among ethnic groups. Campinha-Bacote (1991) reported that African-American psychiatric clients experience a higher incidence of extrapyramidal effects with haloperidol decanoate than European-Americans. African-Americans are also more susceptible to tricyclic antidepressant (TCA) delirium than European-Americans. Strickland, et al. (1991) reported that for a given dose of a TCA, African-Americans show higher blood levels and a faster therapeutic response. As a result, African-Americans experience more toxic side effects from a TCA than do European-Americans. Health-care providers must make extended efforts to observe African-American clients for extrapyramidal side effects related to tricyclics and other psychotropic medications.

## HIGH-RISK BEHAVIORS

Early unprotected intercourse among African-American teens places them at risk for becoming pregnant and contracting sexually transmitted diseases (Jaynes & Williams, 1989). Ladner and Gourdine (1992) noted that African-American teenagers also represent a group at risk for developing AIDS, addiction to crack, or both. In addition, homicide is a major cause of death and disability among African-American adolescents. Jaynes and Williams (1989) reported that 8000 African-Americans are victims of homicide each year.

African-American have a higher rate of smoking when compared with European-Americans. Although African-Americans experience a higher prevalence of smoking, they do not smoke as heavily as European-Americans (Michaels, 1993). Gregory and Clark (1992) concurred that African-Americans smoke fewer cigarettes but added that they suffer from more smoke-related illnesses, such as lung cancer. The mortality rate per 100,000 people for lung cancer is 95 for African-American males and 70 for European-American males (Jaynes & Williams, 1989). It has been projected "that beyond 1995, African-American females will have the highest prevalence of tobacco smoking" (Shervington, 1994, p. 337).

Goddard (1990) stated that "alcohol use and abuse is so common in the African-American community that it appears to have become acceptable behavior with little or no stigma attached to it" (p. 205). One reason for this "acceptable behavior" is the number of liquor stores, which reflect the most common form of small business in the African-American community (Goddard, 1990). In addition, there are more advertisements for alcohol and tobacco targeted to the African-American community.

The mortality rate from cirrhosis of the liver, which is closely related to alcohol consumption, is nearly twice the rate for African-Americans than for European-Americans (Jaynes & Williams, 1989). Harper and Dawkins (1977) reported that African-Americans who consume alcohol tend to be group drinkers and drink more frequently and heavily during weekends. Community health workers can have a significant impact on these detrimental practices by providing health education at community affairs located in African-American communities.

## Health-care Practices

Because a significant proportion of blacks are poor and may live in inner cities, they tend to concentrate on day-to-day survival. Health care often takes second place to basic needs of the family, such as food and shelter. In addition, the role of the family has an impact on the health-seeking behaviors of blacks. African-Americans have strong family ties and when an individual becomes ill, that individual is taught to seek health care from the family before seeking care from health-care professionals (Plawecki & Plawecki, 1990). This cultural practice may contribute to the failure of blacks to seek treatment at an early stage. Screening programs may best be initiated in community and church activities where the entire family is present.

## NUTRITION

### Meaning of Food

Food is used as a way to celebrate special events, holidays, and birthdays. Food is a symbol of both health and wealth and is usually offered to persons when they enter or leave an African-American household. One is expected to accept the "gift" of food. Health-care providers must be sensitive to the meaning attached to food, because if persons reject the food, they are also perceived as rejecting the giver of the food. Food may have a negative meaning attached to it when referred to in conjunction with perceived **witchcraft** (Snow, 1993). It is thought that witchcraft promotes intentional poisoning through food. Thus, many African-Americans find it important to watch carefully what they eat and who gives them food.

It is common for African-Americans to view individuals who are at an ideal body weight as "not having enough meat on their bones." African-Americans believe that it is important to have meat on your bones to be able to afford to lose weight during times of sickness. Therefore, obesity is seen as positive in this ethnic group.

Food is considered to be important for building blood, for influencing the blood count, or for bringing **high blood** down (Roberson, 1983). Most African-Americans relate high blood and **low blood** to the amount or volume of blood. Therefore, a person with low blood may benefit from eating meats, especially rare meats, which are thought to build blood (Roberson, 1983). In addition, a diet of liver, greens, eggs, fruits, and vegetables are also considered to be a remedy for low blood. However, a person with high blood should avoid or reduce salt intake, pork, red meats, and fried foods. Eating foods such as vinegar, lemon, and garlic are recommended to help "bring blood down."

## Common Foods and Food Rituals

African-American diets are frequently high in fat and fried foods. Blacks eat more animal fat, less fiber, and fewer fruits and vegetables. Their diet is referred to as **soul food,** which is high in sodium and fat. The term soul food comes from the need for African-Americans to "express the group feeling of soul" (Bloch, 1983, p. 95). Salt pork (**fatback** or "fat meat") is a key ingredient of their diet. Salt pork is inexpensive and therefore more frequently purchased.

A significant variation seen in eating patterns among African-American infants is the age at which they are introduced to solid food. African-American parents are encouraged by their elders to begin feeding solid foods at an early age (usually before two months). Formula is mixed in a thick solution with cereal and is given to the infant in a bottle (Snow, 1993). African-American believe giving only formula is starving the baby and that the infant needs "real food" to sleep through the night. Health-care providers working with family planning and child-care clinics can provide factual knowledge regarding the deleterious effects of giving infants solid foods at an early age.

## Dietary Practices for Health Promotion

Some African-Americans believe that too much red meat causes high blood (Andrews & Boyle, 1995), which is thought to cause strokes. Some foods such as milk, vegetables, and meats are referred to as "strength foods." Religious affiliations bring about different dietary habits. Black Muslims have diets similar to Kosher diets (no pork or pork products). Muslims also refuse pork-based insulin. They consider these products to be filthy. There is also a belief that "you are what you eat" (Spector, 1991, p. 194).

## Nutritional Deficiencies and Food Limitations

Lactose intolerance occurs in 75 percent of the African-American population. Low levels of thiamine, riboflavin, vitamins A and C, and iron seen among African-Americans are mostly associated with a poor diet secondary to a low socioeconomic status.

African-Americans' major food preferences are generally available in the United States. "Southern food" is a common preference among European-American subcultures as well as African-Americans.

# PREGNANCY AND CHILDBEARING PRACTICES

## Fertility Practices and Views Toward Pregnancy

Oral contraceptives are the most popular choice of birth control among the African-American inner-city population (Snow, 1993). However, some African-Americans feel that methods of fertility control recommended by physicians can have a dangerous effect on the body. Therefore, it is common for African-American women to use such traditional methods as water and vinegar douches or to have intercourse only during the middle of the month when it is "safe" (Snow, 1993).

There are many views within African-American communities regarding the issue of pregnancy versus abortion. Some African-Americans are directly opposed to abortion because of religious, moral, cultural, or Afrocentric beliefs (Boyd-Franklin, 1989). However, the high rate of teen pregnancy among African-Americans has contributed to this view not being universally embraced.

## Prescriptive, Restrictive, and Taboo Practices in the Childbearing Family

The family support network, especially the grandmother and maternal relatives, is the primary advisor for the pregnant woman (Bryant, 1982). This family network guides many of the practices and beliefs of the pregnant woman, including the common practice of **geophagia.** One theory of geophagy, the eating of earth or clay among some pregnant African-American women, is that this natural craving alleviates several mineral deficiencies. However, geophagy can lead to a potassium deficiency, constipation, and anemia. It is believed that the unborn "needs" this supplement. Although geophagy is a common practice among many African-Americans, some are unaware that the practice exists. Other food cravings are also common. It is believed that if the pregnant mother does not consume her specific craving, it "marks the baby" (Snow, 1993). Some African-Americans claim that the baby signals the mother what it wants via a food craving, and if the mother does not consume the specific food, the child is marked (birthmarked) with that particular food. Roberson (1983) cited the consumption of other nonfood substances, such as cornstarch, baking soda, baking powder, plaster, ashes, and ice. Health-care providers need to provide factual information regarding the consequences of eating nonfood substances that may be harmful to the mother or fetus.

Certain practices are taboo during pregnancy. Some believe that pregnant women should not take pictures because it may cause a stillbirth, nor have their picture taken because it captures their soul. Some also believe that it is not wise to reach over their heads if they are pregnant because the umbilical cord will wrap around the baby's neck. Another taboo concerns the purchase of clothing for the infant. It is thought to be bad luck to purchase clothes for the unborn baby.

Snow (1993) reported several home practices related to initiating labor in pregnant African-American women. Taking a ride over a bumpy road, ingesting castor oil, eating a heavy meal, or sniffing pepper are all thought to induce labor. If a baby is born with the amniotic sac over its head or face, it is thought to have special powers (Hand, 1980; Snow, 1974). The amniotic sac is referred to as a "veil." In addition, a child who is born after a set of twins, born with a physical condition, or is the seventh-born son is also thought to have received special powers from God.

The postpartum period for the African-American woman is greatly extended. It is believed that during the postpartum period the mother is at greater risk than the baby. She is cautioned to avoid cold air and encouraged to get adequate rest to restore the body to normal. Postpartum practices for child care can involve the use of a belly band or a coin. These objects, when placed on top of the infant's umbilical area, are believed to prevent the umbilical area from protruding outward.

# DEATH RITUALS

## Death Rituals and Expectations

A strong tie exists between the world of the living and the world of the dead in the African-American community (Jules-Rosette, 1980). For a majority of African-Americans, death does not end the connection between people, especially family. Relatives who communicate with the deceased's spirit is one example of this endless connection.

Snow (1993) studied African-American families in the southern states and noted interesting rituals regarding spirits of the deceased. If one passes an infant over the casket of the deceased who has died a sudden or violent death, this protects the infant from the deceased victim's "haunting spirits."

Some African-Americans believe in "voodoo death," which is a belief that illness or death may come to an individual via a supernatural force (Campinha-Bacote, 1992). Voodoo is more commonly known as "root work," "hex," "fix," "conjuring," "tricking," "mojo," "witchcraft," "spell," "black magic," or "hoodoo" (Campinha-Bacote, 1986). However, Western medicine has a different explanation of voodoo death. Lex (1974) gave a comprehensive explanation of voodoo death in her three phases of "tuning." She noted that in the third stage, both the parasympathetic and sympathetic nervous systems are stimulated. This view is in contrast to Cannon's (1957) and Richter's (1957) explanations of "magical death." Cannon explained magical death in terms of the response of the autonomic nervous system to extreme emotion. Richter believed that this is due to an excessive response in the parasympathetic nervous system related to feelings of helplessness.

## Responses to Death and Grief

African-Americans believe that the body must be kept intact after death (Callender, et al., 1982). It is not uncommon to hear an African-American say, "I came into this world with all my body parts, and I'll leave this world with all my body parts!"

One response to hearing about a death of a family member or close member in the African-American culture is **falling out,** which is manifested by sudden collapse and paralysis and the inability to see or speak (Westermeyer, 1985). However, the individual's hearing and understanding is still intact. Health-care providers must be knowledgeable about the African-American culture to recognize this condition as a cultural response to the death of a family member and not a medical condition requiring emergency intervention.

Some African-Americans are less likely to express grief openly and publicly (Jacobs, 1990). However, they do express their feelings openly during the funeral. Funeral services encourage emotional expression and catharsis by incorporating religious songs into the ceremony as well as by providing visual confrontation of the body (Markides & Mindel, 1987). Eulogies are extremely important at funerals.

# SPIRITUALITY

## Religious Practices and Use of Prayer

Religion and religious behavior is an integral part of the African-American community (Fig. 3–1). African-American churches have played a major role in the devel-

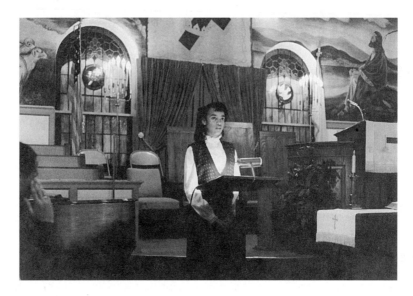

**Figure 3–1.** Spirituality is a significant force for promoting well-being among many African-Americans.

opment and survival of African-Americans (Brown & Gary, 1994). As clearly stated by Lincoln (1974):

> To understand the power of the Black Church, it must first be understood that there is no disjunction between the Black Church and the Black community . . . whether one is a church member or not is beside the point in any assessment of the importance and meaning of the Black Church (pp. 115–116).

African-Americans take their religion seriously, and they expect to receive a message in preaching that helps them in their daily lives (Roberson, 1983). Brown and Gary (1994) found that religious involvement is associated with positive mental health.

Most African-Americans expect to take an active part in religious activities. Participation may involve group singing, creating original words to songs, spontaneous testimony of a personal spiritual view, or expression of deep emotion (Roberson, 1985). Roberson further stated that singers may be encouraged with cries of "sing it, sister" or "that's all right" (p. 89).

The majority of African-American Christians are affiliated with the Baptist and Methodist denominations (Locke, 1992). However, many other denominations and distinct religious groups are represented in African-American communities within the United States. These include African Methodist Episcopal, Jehovah's Witnesses, Church of God in Christ, Seventh Day Adventists, Pentecostal, Apostolic, Presbyterian, Lutheran, Roman Catholic, Nation of Islam, and several other Islamic sects (Boyd-Franklin, 1989).

African-Americans strongly believe in the use of prayer for all situations they may encounter. They also use prayer for the sake of others who are experiencing problems. "Prayers reflect the trust and faith one has in God" (Roberson, 1985, p. 106). The Bible is used as a source of prayers for healing.

African-Americans also believe in the **laying on of hands** while praying. It is believed that certain individuals have the power to heal the sick and ill by placing hands on the sick. African-Americans may pray in a language that is not understood by anyone but the person reciting the prayer. This expression of praying is referred to as **speaking in tongues.**

## Meaning of Life and Individual Sources of Strength

A majority of African-Americans' inner strength comes from trusting in God. Some African-Americans believe that whatever happens is "God's will." Because of this belief, African-Americans may be perceived to have a fatalistic view of life. Snow (1993) reported that African-Americans trust in "Doctor Jesus." They believe that sickness and pain are a form of weakness that comes directly from Satan. Therefore, having faith in God is a major source of inner strength.

## Spiritual Beliefs and Health-care Practices

Roberson (1985) stated that spiritual beliefs form a foundation for the health belief system in African-Americans. African-Americans consider themselves as spiritual beings, and sickness is viewed as a separation between God and man. God is thought to be the Supreme Healer. Health-care practices center on religious and spiritual activities such as going to church, praying daily, and speaking in tongues.

# HEALTH-CARE PRACTICES

## Health-seeking Beliefs and Behaviors

According to Snow (1974), many African-Americans may be pessimistic about human relationships and believe that it is more natural to do evil than to do good (Snow, 1974). Snow concluded that some African-Americans' belief system emphasizes three major themes:

1. The world is a very hostile and dangerous place to live.

2. The individual is open to attack from external forces.

3. The individual is considered to be a helpless person who has no internal resources to combat such an attack and therefore needs outside assistance.

Because most African-Americans tend to be suspicious of health-care professionals, they may see a physician or nurse only when absolutely necessary.

## Responsibility for Health Care

The African-American population believes in natural and unnatural illnesses. Natural illness occurs in response to normal forces from which persons have not protected themselves. Unnatural illness is the belief that harm or sickness can come to you via a person or spirit. In treating an unnatural illness, African-Americans seek clergy, a folk healer, or pray directly to God. In general, health is viewed as harmony with nature, whereas illness is seen as a disruption in this harmonic state due to demons, "bad spirits," or both.

Individuals commonly use home remedies, consult a folk healer (root doctor), and still receive treatment from a Western health-care professional. Powers (1982) found that clients experiencing voodoo illness sought care from local root doctors as well as from physicians. Powers concluded that if nursing staff are unaware that the individual is receiving care from both folk and orthodox health-care systems, the care they render may be ineffective. To render services that are culturally acceptable to African-Americans, health-care providers must become partners with the African-

American community. Strategies such as focus groups can provide health-care professionals with insight into health-care practices acceptable to African-Americans.

African-Americans may use several home remedies in maintaining their health and treating specific health conditions. When taking prescribed medication, it is common for African-Americans to take the medication differently from the way it is prescribed. For example, in treating hypertension, African-Americans may take their antihypertensive medication on an "as-needed" basis. This self-medicating practice may contribute to the high mortality and morbidity among African-Americans from hypertension.

## Folk Practices

African-Americans, like most ethnic groups, engage in folk medicine. The history of African-American folk medicine has its origin in slavery. Slaves had a limited range of choices in obtaining health care. Although they were expected to inform their masters immediately when they were ill, slaves were reluctant to submit themselves to the harsh prescriptions and treatments of 18th and 19th century European-American physicians (Savitt, 1978). They preferred self-treatment or treatment by friends, older relatives, or "folk doctors." This led to a dual system—"white medicine" and "black medicine" (Savitt, 1978). Williams (1975) and Snow (1993) studied hundreds of folk practices used by African-Americans. For example, many believe alcoholism can be cured by drinking a glass half-filled with an alcoholic beverage and half-filled with fish blood. This is believed to give an undesirable taste and cause nausea and vomiting when subsequent alcoholic drinks are taken (Williams, 1975).

## Barriers to Health Care

African-Americans are less likely to have access to and to use health-care services, including preventive care (Bourjolly, 1994). They experience barriers related to health-care services due to economic factors. Needed health-care services may not be affordable for those in lower socioeconomic groups. Although some services may be accessible and available for African-Americans, they may not be culturally relevant. For example, a health-care professional may prescribe a strict American Diabetic Association diet to a newly diagnosed African-Americans client without taking into consideration the dietary habits of this ethnic group. Therefore, therapeutic interventions developed by health-care professionals may be underutilized.

Underwood (1994) identified several barriers to health care that African-Americans and other ethnically diverse populations perceive. One major barrier is that the history of discrimination and abuse against African-Americans causes some to believe that their lives are not valued by most health-care professionals, who may provide differential care according to race. Another barrier is that some African-Americans fear that some providers take risks with their lives when rendering care. Finally, there is a general distrust of health-care professionals, practitioners, and the health-care system.

## Cultural Responses to Health and Illness

Pain is often perceived by African-Americans as a sign of illness or disease. Many times they may not take regularly prescribed medication unless they experience pain. One example is in the treatment of hypertension. African-Americans may take their antihypertensive drug or diuretic only when they experience head or neck pain. This cultural practice interferes with successful and effective treatment of hypertension.

Some African-Americans believe that suffering and pain is inevitable and must be endured. Their spiritual and religious foundations contribute to their high tolerance level for pain. Prayers and the laying on of hands are thought to free the person from all suffering and pain. Persons who still experience pain are considered to have little faith.

Low educational levels among African-Americans may prohibit their exposure to information about the etiology and treatment of mental illness. Some African-Americans hold a stigma against mental illness. The high frequency of misdiagnosis among African-Americans contributes to their reluctance to trust mental health professionals. Adebimpe (1981) reported that over the years, a major diagnostic issue has been the high frequency of the diagnosis of schizophrenia among African-American clients. Mukhejee, et al. (1983) stated that African-Americans are more likely to report hallucinations when suffering from an affective disorder, which may lead to the misdiagnosis of schizophrenia.

Close family and spiritual ties within the African-American family allow one to enter the sick role with ease. Extended and nuclear family members willingly care for sick persons and assume their role responsibilities without hesitation. Sickness and tragedy bring African-American families together, even in the presence of family conflict.

## Blood Transfusion and Organ Donation

Blood transfusions are acceptable unless the African-American client belongs to a religious group, such as Jehovah's Witnesses, where this practice is not permitted. A lower level of organ donation among African-Americans is related to social practices, religious beliefs, and cultural expectations. Plawecki and Plawecki (1992) reported five reasons for the low level of organ donation among African-Americans: (1) lack of information about kidney transplantation, (2) religious fears and superstitions, (3) distrust of health-care providers, (4) fear that donors would be declared dead prematurely, and (5) racism (African-Americans prefer to give their organs to other African-Americans).

## HEALTH-CARE PRACTITIONERS

### Traditional Versus Biomedical Care

Physicians are recognized as heads of the health-care team, with nurses taking lesser importance. However, as nurses are becoming more educated, they are being held in higher regard. Most health professionals have a healthly respect for each group's discipline and consult them in their specialty areas.

Among the African-American community, folk practitioners can be spiritual leaders, grandparents, elders of the community, or voodoo doctors or priests. Voodoo doctors are consulted for specific illnesses. Another reason for consulting voodoo doctors is to remove a hex. An individual may place a hex on a person because of resentment of achievement, sexual jealousy, love, or envy (Ness & Wintrob, 1981). Hexed persons usually are victimized by someone they know personally. A hex can be placed on the victim by using a piece of the individual's hair, fingernails, blood, or some other personal belonging of the victim. The victim usually seeks help from a voodoo or conjure doctor to have the hex removed with magicoreligious powers.

While some individuals may prefer a health provider of the same gender for urologic and gynecologic conditions, generally gender is not a major concern in selection of a health-care provider. Men and women can provide personal care to the opposite sex. On occasion, young men prefer that personal care be given by another man or older women. The health-care provider should respect these wishes when possible.

## Status of Health-care Providers

Folk practitioners are generally not regarded with high esteem by Western professionals. However, as homeopathic and alternative medicine increases in importance in preventive health, these practitioners are likely to gain more respect. Folk practitioners are respected in the African-American community and frequently used by African-Americans of all socioeconomic levels. Many African-Americans perceive health-care professionals as outsiders, whom they resent for telling them what their problems are or telling them how to solve them (Underwood, 1994). Generally, most African-Americans are suspicious and cautious of health-care practitioners they have not heard of or do not know. Because interpersonal relationships are highly valued in this group, it is important to initially focus on developing a sound trusting relationship.

### CASE STUDY

Robert Collins is a 49-year-old African-American man. He resides in the inner city of Detroit, Michigan, with his extended family. He has five children aged 26, 18, 16, 14, and 10. His elderly mother, three of his children (aged 16, 14 and 10), two grandchildren, and his sick sister-in-law compose the household membership.

Mr. Collins completed the 11th grade and maintains employment in a steel factory. Although he works more than 40 hours a week, his income places him at the poverty level. He can not afford to purchase health insurance.

Mr. Collins' 18-year-old daughter, Chole, is pregnant for the third time and is a single parent. Mr. Collins is caring for her other two children. Chole is going to night school to complete her high school education.

The Collins family goes to church every Sunday and is actively involved in the church. Mrs. Collins was diagnosed with cancer, and she is receiving spiritual healing from her pastor and church for this illness. Mr. Collins is extremely concerned about his wife's health and has increased his tobacco use.

### STUDY QUESTIONS

1. Name one occupation-related disease for which Mr. Collins is at risk.

2. Identify one family member who is likely to be caring for the younger children in the family.

3. Describe three beliefs that Chole may have about her pregnancy.

4. Discuss the role that spirituality plays in this family.

5. Identify two religious or spiritual practices that Mrs. Collins may be engaging in.

6. Because Mrs. Collins has cancer, discuss possible thoughts she may have regarding death and dying.

7. Identify two diseases common among African-Americans males.

8. Identify the dropout rate among black teens in the inner city.

9. Name one tobacco-related disease found in the African-American population.

10. Name two dietary health risks for African-Americans.

11. Define the seven principles of *Nguzo Sabo*.

12. Identify five characteristics to consider when assessing the skin of African-American persons.

13. Name two skin conditions common among African-Americans.

## References

Adebimpe, V. (1981). Overview: White norms in psychiatric diagnosis of Black American patients. *American Journal of Psychiatry, 138*(3), 279–285.

Andrews, M., & Boyle, J. (1995). *Transcultural concepts in nursing care.* Glenview, IL: Scott, Foresman & Co.

Bell, P., & Evans, J. (1981). *Counseling the black client.* MN: Hazelden Education Materials.

Billingsley, A. (1968). *Black families in white america.* NJ: Prentice-Hall.

Bloch, B. (1983). Nursing care of black patients. In M. Orque, D. Bloch, & L. Monrroy (Eds). *Ethnic nursing care.* (pp. 82–108). St. Louis: C. V. Mosby.

Blum, J., Morgan, E., Rose, W., Schlesinger, A., Stampp, K., & Woodward, C. (1981). *The national experience.* New York: Harcourt Brace Jovanovich.

Bolton, L. (1993). President's message. *NBNA News, 17*(2), 1–27.

Bourjolly, J. (1994). Cancer support groups for African Americans. *Innovations in Oncology Nursing, 10*(4), 103–104.

Boyd-Franklin, N. (1989). *Black families in therapy.* New York: Guilford Press.

Branch, M. & Paxton, P. (1976). *Providing safe nursing care for ethnic people of color.* NY: Appleton-Century-Crofts.

Bryant, C. (1982). The impact of kin, friends, and neighbors networks on infant feeding practices. *Social Science Medicine, 16,* 1759–1765.

Brown, D. & Gary, L. (1994). Religious involvement and health status among African American males. *Journal of the National Medical Association, 86*(11), 825–831.

Callender, C., Bayton, J., Yeager, C., & Clark, J. (1982). Attitudes among blacks toward donating kidneys for transplantations: A pilot project. *Journal of the National Medical Association, 74,* 807–809.

Campinha, J. (1986). *Consideration of the cultural belief systems of individuals experiencing conjure illness by public health nurses and emergency room nurses: An exploratory study.* Unpublished doctoral dissertation, University of Virginia, Charlottesville, VA.

Campinha-Bacote, J. (1991). Community mental health services for the underserved: A culturally specific model. *Archives of Psychiatric Nursing, 5*(4), 29–35.

Campinha-Bacote, J. (1992). Voodoo illness. *Perspectives in Psychiatric Nursing, 28*(1), 11–19.

Cannon, W. (1957). Voodoo death. *Psychosomatic Medicine, 19*(3), 183–190.

Crew, K. (1994). Blacks as high-risk smokers. *Health Values, 18*(1), 4143.

Curtin, P. (1969). *The Atlantic slave trade.* Milwaukee: University of Wisconsin Press.

DiClemente, R. (1992). Confronting the challenge of AIDS in the African-American community. *Ethnicity and Disease, 2*(4), 358–360.

Elixhauser, A. & Ball, J. (1994). Black/White differences in colorectal tumor location in a national sample of hospitals. *Journal of the National Medical Association, 86*(6), 449–458.

Friedman, M. (1986). *Family nursing: Theory and assessment.* East Norwalk, CT: Prentice-Hall.

Funkhouser, S. & Moser, D. (1990). Is healthcare racist? *Advances in Nursing Science, 12*(2), 47–55.

Giger, J. & Davidhizar, R. (1995). *Transcultural nursing: Assessment and intervention* (2nd ed.). St. Louis: C. V. Mosby.

Goddard, L. (1990). *An Afrocentric model of prevention for African-American high risk youth.* CA: Institute for the Advanced Study of Black Family Life and Culture.

Gregory, S. & Clark, P. (1992). The "big three" cardiovascular risk factors among Americans, Blacks and Hispanics. *Journal of Holistic Nursing, 8*(1), 76–88.

Hammack, F. (1986). Large school systems dropout reports: An analysis of definition, procedures, and findings. *Teachers College Record, 87*(3), 324–341.

Hand, D. (1980). *Magical medicine: The folklorist and ritual of the people of Europe and America.* Berkeley, CA: University of California Press.

Harper, F. D. & Dawkins, M. P. (1977). Alcohol abuse in the Black community. *Black Scholar, 8*(6), 23–31.

Hauser, B., Plawecki, H., Carr, J., Smith, M., Plawecki, J.(1992). A holistic approach to vaso-occlusive pain crisis in children with sickle cell disease. *Journal of Holistic Nursing, 10*(1), 62–75.

*Health status of the disadvantaged* (1990). (DHHS Publication No. HRSA-HRS-P-DV-90-1). Washington, DC: U.S. Department of Health and Human Services, Public Health Service, Health Resources and Services Administration, Bureau of Health Professions, Division of Disadvantaged Assistance.

Henderson, G. & Primeaux, M. (1981). *Transcultural health care.* Menlo Park, CA: Addison-Wesley.

Hines, P. & Boyd-Franklin, N. (1982). Black families. In M. McGoldrick, J. Pearce, & J. Giordano (Eds.), *Ethnicity and family therapy.* (pp. 84–105). New York: Guilford Press.

Jacobs, C. (1990). Healing and prophecy in the Black spiritual churches: A need for reexamination. *Medical Anthropology, 12*(4), 349–370.

Jaynes, D. & Williams, R. (1989). *A common destiny: Blacks and American society.* Washington, DC: National Academy Press.

Jules-Rosette, B. (1980). Creative spirituality from Africa to America: Cross-cultural influences in contemporary religious forms. *Western Journal of Black Studies, 4,* 273–285.

Kalow, W. (1984). Pharmaco-anthropology outline: Problems and nature of case history. *Federation Proceedings, 43*(8), 2314–2318.

Ladner, J. & Gourdine, R. (1992). Adolescent pregnancy in the African American community. In R. Braithwaite & S. Taylor (Eds.) *Health issues in the black community.* (pp. 206–221). San Francisco: Jossey-Bass.

Levy, R. (1993). Ethnic and racial differences in response to medicines: Preserving individualized therapy in managed pharmaceutical programs. *Pharmaceutical Medicine, 7,* 139–165.

Lex, B. (1974). Voodoo death: New thoughts on an old explanation. *American Anthropologist, 76,* 818–823.

Lincoln, C. (1974). *The Black church since Frazier.* New York: Schocken Books.

Locke, D. (1992). *Increasing multicultural understanding.* Newbury Park, CA: Sage Publications.

Mallorey, D. (1988). Compliance and health beliefs in the African American female hypertensive client. *Journal of the National Black Nurses Association, 2*(1), 38–45.

Markides, K. & Mindel, C. (1987). *Aging and ethnicity.* Beverly Hills: Sage Publications.

McAdoo, H. (1983). The black family. In H. I. McCubbin & C. R. Figlel (Eds.), *Stress and the family: Coping with normative transition I* (pp. 178–187). New York: Brunswick.

Michaels, D. (1993). Occupational cancer in the black population: The health effects of job discrimination. *Journal of the National Black Medical Association, 75,* 1014–1018.

*Minorities and women in the health fields.* (1990). (DHHS Publication No. HRSA-P-DV-90-3). U.S. Department of Health and Human Services, Bureau of Health Professions, Division of Health Professions Analysis.

Mukherjee, S., Shukla, S., Woodle, J., Rosen, A., & Olarte, S. (1983). Misdiagnosis of schizophrenia in bipolar patients: A multiethnic comparison. *American Journal of Psychiatry, 140,* 1571–1574.

Ness, R. & Wintrob, R. (1981). Folk healing: A description of synthesis. *American Journal of Psychiatry, 138*(11), 1477–1481.

Olsen, S. & Frank-Stromborg, M. (1994). Cancer prevention and screening activities reported by African-American nurses. *Oncology Forum, 21*(3), 487–494.

Phillips, F. (1988). *NTU psychotherapy: An Afrocentric* approach. Unpublished manuscript, Progressive Life Center, Washinton, DC.

Plawecki, H. & Plawecki, J. (1990). Cultural aspects of caring for Mexican-American clients. *Journal of Holistic Nursing, 8*(1), 37–45.

Plawecki, H. & Plawecki, J. (1992). Improving organ donation rates in the black community. *Journal of Holistic Nursing, 10*(1), 34–46.

Polednak, A. (1974). Connective tissue responses in negroes in relation to disease. *American Journal of Physical Anthropology, 41,* 49–51.

Powers, B. (1982). The orthodox and black American folk medicine. *Advances in Nursing Science, 4*(3), 35–47.

Pratt, M., Jones, Z., & Seigal, N. (1977). National variances in prematurity (1973–1974). In D. M. Reed & F. J. Stanley (Eds.), *The epidemiology of prematurity* (pp. 53–74). Baltimore: Urban & Schwarzenberg.

Rainwater, L. (1971). Crucible of identity: The negro lower-class family. In J. Bracey, A. Meier, & A. Rudwick (Eds.), *Black matriarchy: Reality or myth?* (pp. 76–109). Belmont, CA: Wadsworth.

Reynolds, C. (1992). An administrative program to facilitate culturally appropriate care for the elderly. *Holistic Nursing Practice, 6*(3), 34–42.

Richter, C. (1957). On the phenomenon of sudden death in animals and man. *Psychosomatic Medicine, 23*(3), 191–198.

Roach, L. (1981). Color changes in dark skin. In G. Henderson & M. Primeaux (Eds). *Transcultural health care.* Menlo Park, CA: Addison-Wesley.

Roberson, M. (1983). *Folk health beliefs and practices of rural black Virginians.* Unpublished doctoral dissertation, University of Utah. Salt Lake City, Utah.

Roberson, M. (1985). The influence of religious beliefs on health choices of Afro-Americans. *Topics in Clinical Nursing, 7*(3), 57–63.

Robinson, V. (1977). *Humor and the health professions.* Thorofare, NJ: Charles B. Slack.

Savitt, T. (1978). *Medicine and slavery*. Chicago: University of Illinois Press.

Shervington, D. (1994). Attitudes and practices of African-American women regarding cigarette smoking: Implications and interventions. *Journal of the National Medical Association, 86*(5), 337–342.

Smith, E. (1992). Hypertension management with church-based education: A pilot study. *Journal of National Black Nurses Association, 6*(1), 19–28.

Snow, L. (1974). Folk medical beliefs and their implications for care of patients. *Annals of Internal Medicine, 81,* 82–96.

Snow, L. (1993). *Walkin' over medicine.* Boulder, CO: Westview Press.

Spector, R. (1996). *Cultural diversity in health and illness.* Norwalk, CT: Appleton & Lange.

Spurlock, J. & Lawrence, L. (1985). The black child. In J. Flaskerud (Ed.), *Community Mental Health Nursing.* (pp. 248–256). Norwalk, CT: Appleton-Century-Crofts.

Stevens, P., Hall, J., & Meleis, A. (1992). Examining vulnerability of women clerical workers from five ethnic/racial groups. *Western Journal of Nursing Research, 14*(6), 754–774.

Strickland, T. L., Ranganath, V., Lin, K-M, Poland, R.E., Mendoza, R., & Smith, M.W. (1991). Psychopharmacologic considerations in the treatment of black American populations. *Psychopharmacology Bulletin, 27*(4), 441–448.

Underwood, S. (1994) Increasing the participation of minorities and other at-risk groups in clinical trials. *Innovations in Oncology Nursing, 10*(4), 106.

Waitzman, N. & Smith, K. (1994). The effects of occupational class transitions on hypertension: Racial disparities among working-age men. *American Journal of Public Health, 84*(6), 945–950.

Westermeyer, J. (1985). Psychiatric diagnosis across cultural boundaries. *American Journal of Psychiatry, 142*(7), 798–805.

Williams, R. (1975). *The textbook of black-related disease.* New York: McGraw-Hill.

Willie, C. (1976). *A new look at black families.* Bayside, NY: General Hall.

Willie, C. & Greenblatt, S. (1978). Four classic studies of power relationships in black families: A review and look to the future. *Journal of Marriage and Family, 40,* 691–689.

# The Amish

*Anna Frances Z. Wenger and Marion R. Wenger*

• Key terms to become familiar with in this chapter are:

| | |
|---|---|
| *Aagwachse* | *Demut* |
| *Abnemme* | *Freindschaft* |
| *Abwaarde* | *Gelassenheit* |
| *Achtgewwe* | Old Order Amish |
| Anabaptist | *Ordnung* |
| *Brauche* | Settlement |
| *Braucher* | Visiting |
| *Daadihaus* | Warm hands |
| *Deitsch* | |

## OVERVIEW, INHABITED LOCALITIES, AND TOPOGRAPHY

### Overview

As dusk gathers on the hospital parking lot, a man first ties his horse to the hitching rack and then helps a matronly figure wrapped in a shawl as dark as his own greatcoat down from the carriage. On their mother's heels, a flurry of children dressed like undersized replicas of their parents turn their wide eyes toward the fluorescent-lit glass facade of the reception area, a glimmering beacon from the world of high-technology health care. Their excitement is muted by their father's soft-spoken rebuke in a language more akin to German than English, and in a hush, the Amish family crosses a cultural threshold—into the workaday world of health-care professionals.

This Amish family appears to come from another time and place. Those familiar with the health-care needs of the Amish know the profound cultural distance they have bridged in seeking professional help (Huntington, 1993; Wenger & Wenger, 1988). Others only marginally acquainted with Amish ways may ask why this group dresses, acts, and talks like visitors to the North American cultural scene of the 1990s. Amish are "different" by intention and by conviction. That is to say, for most of the ways in which they depart from the norm for contemporary American culture, they cite a reason related to their understanding of the biblical mandate to live a life separated from a world they see as unregenerate or sinful (Hostetler, 1993; Kraybill, 1993).

As noted in the general introduction to cultural diversity in Chapter 1, dissimilar appearance, behavior, or both may signal deeper underlying differences, but noting them does not of necessity lead to better acceptance or deeper understanding of attitudes and behaviors. Appearances can be misleading. For example, the Amish family's arrival at the hospital by horse and carriage might suggest a general taboo on modern technological conveniences. In fact, most Amish homes are not furnished with electric and electronic labor-saving devices and appliances. But that does not preclude their openness to using state-of-the-art medical technology if it were perceived as necessary to promoting their health (Huntington, 1993).

This minority group's exotic features of dress and language may disguise true motivations regarding health-seeking behaviors, which they share in common with the larger, or majority, culture. To enable such clients to attain their own standard of health and well-being, health-care professionals need to look beyond the superficial appearance and to listen more carefully to the cues they provide (Wenger, 1991b).

## Heritage and Residence

It is as important to locate the Amish topographically according to cultural and religious coordinates as by the geographical areas they inhabit. The hospital visit scenario just portrayed could have taken place in any one of a number of towns across the American Midwest and the Eastern Seaboard, but the basic circumstances surrounding the interaction with professional caregivers and the cultural assumptions underlying it are the same. For the Amish, seeking help from health-care professionals requires them to go outside their own people and, in so doing, to cross over a significant "permeable boundary," which delimits their community in cultural-geographic terms (Huntington, 1987; Wenger, 1988; Wenger, 1994).

Today's Amish live in rural areas in a band of over 20 states stretching westward from Pennsylvania, Ohio, and Indiana as far as Montana, with some scattered *settlements* as far south as Florida and as far north as the province of Ontario, Canada. About 75 percent of their estimated total population of over 130,000 is concentrated in Pennsylvania, Ohio, and Indiana (Kraybill, 1993). The *Old Order Amish*, so-called for their strict observance of traditional ways that distinguishes them from other, more progressive "plain folk," are the largest and most notable group among the Amish. As such, they constitute an ethnoreligious cultural group in modern America with roots in the Europe of the Reformation era.

## Reasons for Migration and Associated Economic Factors

The Amish emerged after 1693 as a variant of one stream of the *Anabaptist* movement that originated in Switzerland in 1525 and spread to neighboring German-speaking lands. The Amish embraced, among other essential Anabaptist tenets of faith, the baptism of adult believers as an outward sign of membership in a voluntary community with an inner commitment to live peaceably with all. The Amish parted ways with the larger Anabaptist group, now known as Mennonites, over the Amish propensity to strict avoidance of those community members whom they excluded from fellowship in their church (Bender & Smith, 1956; Nolt, 1992; Hostetler, 1993).

Anabaptists were disenfranchised and deported and their goods expropriated for their refusal to bear arms as a civic service and to accept the authority of the state church in matters of faith and practice. Their attempts at radical discipleship in a "free church," following the guidelines of the early church as set forth in the New Testament, resulted in conflict with Catholic and Protestant leaders. After experiencing severe persecution and martyrdom in Europe, the Amish and related groups immigrated to America in the 17th and 18th centuries. There are no Amish living in Europe today, the last survivors having been assimilated into other religious groups (Hostetler, 1993). As a result, the Amish, unlike many other ethnic groups in America, have no larger reference group in their former homeland to whom their customs, language, and lifeways can be compared.

Denied the right to hold property in their homelands, the Amish sought not only religious freedom but also the opportunity to buy farmland where they could live out their beliefs in peace. In their communities, the Amish have transplanted and preserved a way of life that bears the outward dress of preindustrial European peasantry. In modern industrial America, they have persisted in social isolation based on religious principles, a paradoxically separated life of Christian altruism. Living for others entails a caring concern for members of their ingroup, a community of mutuality, but also calls them to reach out to others in need outside their immediate Amish household of faith (Hostetler, 1993).

Although the Amish value inner harmony, mutual caring, and a peaceable life in the country, it would be a mistake to see Amish society as an idyllic, pastoral folk culture, frozen in time and serenely detached from the dynamic developments all around them. Since the mid-19th century, Amish communities have experienced inner conflicts and dissension as well as outside pressures to conform and modernize (Hostetler, 1993). Over time, the Amish have continued to adapt and change, but at their own pace, accepting innovations selectively (Olshan, 1991; Kraybill & Olshan, 1994).

One cost of controlled, deliberate change has been the loss of some members through factional divisions over "progressive" motivations, both religious and material. The influence of revivalism led to religious reform variants, which introduced Sunday schools, missions, and worship in meetinghouses instead of homes. Others who were impatient to use modern technology such as gasoline-powered farm machinery, telephones, electricity, and automobiles also split off the main body of the most conservative traditionalists, now called the Old Order Amish. Some variant groups were named after their factional leaders (for example, Egli and Beachy Amish), some were called Conservative Amish Mennonites, and others the New Order Amish. Today, these progressives stand somewhere between the parent body, the Mennonites, and the Old Order (technically Old Order Amish Mennonites), hereafter simply referred to as the Amish (Hostetler, 1993). This latter group, which has been widely researched and reported on, provides the observational basis for this present culture study.

## Educational Status and Occupations

The controversy over schooling of Amish children is a good example of a policy issue that attracts public attention. Amish parents assume primary responsibility for childrearing, with the constant support of the extended family and the church community to reinforce their teaching. On the family farm, parents and older siblings model work roles for younger siblings. Corporate worship and community religious practices nurture and shape their faith. Learning how to live and to prepare for death is more important in the Amish tradition than acquiring special skills or knowledge through formal education or training (Hostetler & Huntington, 1992).

The mixed-grade, one-room schoolhouses (Fig. 4–1) typical of pre-1945 rural America were acceptable to the Amish because the schools were more amenable to local control. With the introduction of consolidated high schools, however, the Amish resisted secondary education, particularly compulsory schooling mandated by state and federal agencies, and raised objections both on principle and on scale. To illustrate the latter, the amount of time required by secondary education and the

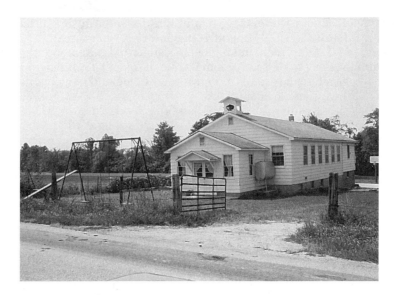

**Figure 4–1.** A one-room Amish schoolhouse in Indiana. (Photograph by Joel Wenger.)

distances required to bus students out of their home communities were cited as problems. But probably more crucial was the understanding that the high school promised to socialize and instruct the young in a value system that was antithetical to the Amish way of life. For example, in the high school, individual achievement and competition were promoted, rather than mutuality and caring for others in a communal spirit. On pragmatic grounds, Amish parents objected to "unnecessary" courses in science, advanced math, and computer technology, which seemed to have no place and little relevance in their tradition (Meyers, 1993).

The Amish response to this perceived threat to their culture was to build and operate their own private elementary schools. Their right to do so was litigated but finally upheld in the U.S. Supreme Court in 1972 with the *Wisconsin* v. *Yoder* ruling. Today, school-aged children are encouraged to attend only eight grades, but Amish parents actively support local private and public schools. Because English serves a useful function as the contact language with the outside world, Amish schools all use English as the language of instruction, with the strong support of parents, as elementary schooling offers the best opportunity for Amish children to master the language. But within Amish homes and communities, use of English is discouraged in favor of the vernacular **Deitsch,** or Pennsylvania German. Because all Amish except preschool children are literate in their second language, American English, language usage helps to define their cultural space (Hostetler, 1993).

The Amish rejection of higher learning for their children means that only the rare individual may pursue professional training and still remain Amish. Health-care professionals, by definition, are seen as outsiders who mediate information on health promotion, make diagnoses, and propose therapies across cultural boundaries. To the extent that they do so with sensitivity and respect for Amish cultural ways, they are respected in turn and valued as an important resource by the Amish.

Throughout the three centuries of Amish history in America, their principal and preferred occupations have been agricultural work and farm-related enterprises (Fig. 4–2). So naturally they settled on good farm land in their earliest immigration to America over 250 years ago. Those who work away from the home farm (for example, young women who have learned quantity cookery at the many church and family

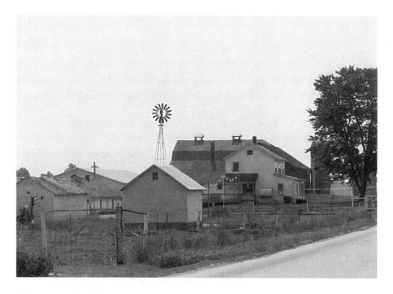

**Figure 4–2.** An Amish farm. The windmill in the background is usually used to pump water. (Photograph by Joel Wenger.)

get-togethers) may find jobs in a restaurant or use skills learned in household chores to work for wages in child care or housecleaning. Young men who bring craft skills from the farm may practice carpentry or cabinetmaking in the construction industry. Jobs away from home increase contacts with non-Amish and test the strength of the many sociocultural bonds that tie the young person to the Amish culture. Given the enticements of the majority culture to change, perhaps it is remarkable that so many Amish find their way back to full membership in the culture that nurtured them (Hostetler & Huntington, 1993; Meyers, 1994a; Meyers, 1994b).

## COMMUNICATIONS

### Dominant Languages and Dialects

Like most people, Amish vary in their language usage depending on the situation and persons addressed. American English is only one of three language varieties in their repertoire. For the Amish, English is the language of school, of written and print communications, and above all, the language used in contacts with most non-Amish outsiders, especially business contacts.

The first language of the majority of Amish is *Deitsch,* an amalgamation of several upland German dialects that emerged from the interaction of immigrants from the Palatinate and Upper Rhine areas of modern France, Germany, and Switzerland. Their regional linguistic differences were resolved in an immigrant language better known in English as "Pennsylvania German." Amish immigrants who later moved more directly from the Swiss Jura and environs to Midwestern states (with minimal mixing in transit with *Deitsch*-speakers) call their home language *Düütsch,* a related variety with marked Upper Alemannic features. Today, *Deitsch* and *Düütsch* both show a strong admixture of vocabulary borrowed from English, while the basic structure remains clearly German. Both have practically the same functional distribution (Wenger, 1970).

*Deitsch* is spoken in the home and in conversation with fellow Amish and relatives, especially during **visiting,** a popular social activity by which news is disseminated orally. It is important to note that *Deitsch* is primarily a spoken language. Some written material has been printed in Pennsylvania German, but Amish seldom encounter it in this form (Haag, 1982). Even Amish publications urging the use of *Deitsch* in the family circle are printed in English, by default the print replacement for the vernacular, the spoken language ("What Is in a Language?" 1986).

Health-care providers can expect all their Amish clients of school age and older to be fluently bilingual. They can readily understand spoken and written directions and answer questions presented in English, although their own terms for some symptoms and illnesses may not have exact equivalents in *Deitsch* and English. Amish clients may be more comfortable consulting among themselves in *Deitsch,* but generally they intend no disrespect for those who do not understand their mother tongue.

Although of limited immediate relevance for health-care considerations, the third language used by the Amish deserves mention in this cultural profile to complete the scope of their linguistic repertoire. Amish proficiency in English varies according to the type and frequency of contact with non-Amish, but it is on the increase. The use of Pennsylvania German is in decline outside the Old Order Amish community. Its retention by Amish, despite the inroads of English, has been related to their religious communities' persistent recourse to *Hochdeitsch,* or Amish High German, their so-called third language, as a sacred language (Huffines, 1994).

Amish do not use Standard Modern High German, but an approximation, which gives access to texts printed in an archaic German with some regional variations. Rote memorization and performance for certain ceremonial and devotional functions, and for selected texts from the Luther Bible, the Ausbund hymnal, and devotional literature are a part of public and private prayer and worship among the Amish. Such restricted nonproductive use of a third language hardly justifies the term "trilingual," because it does not comprise a fully developed range of discourse. However, Amish High German provides a situational-functional complement to their other two languages (Enninger & Wandt, 1982). Its retention is one more symbol of a consciously separated way of life that reaches back to its European heritage.

Within a highly contextual subculture like the Amish, the base of shared information and experience is proportionately larger. As a result, less overt verbal communication is required than in the relatively low-contextual American culture, and more reliance is placed on implicit, often unspoken understandings (Hall, 1976). Amish children and youth may learn adult roles in their society more through modeling, for example, than through explicit teaching. The many and diverse kinds of multigenerational social activities on the family farm provide the optimal framework for this kind of enculturation. Although this may facilitate the transmission of traditional, or accepted, knowledge and values within a high-context culture, this same information network may also impede new information imparted from the outside, which entails some behavior changes. Wenger (1988, 1991) suggested that nurses and other health-care providers should consider role modeling as a teaching strategy when working with Amish clients. Later on, a brief example of the promotion of inoculation is presented to illustrate how public health workers can use culture-appropriate information systems to achieve fuller cooperation among the Amish.

In a final note on language and the flow of verbal information, health-care providers should be aware that much of what passes for "general knowledge" in our information-rich popular culture is screened, or filtered out of, Amish awareness (Hostetler, 1993). The Amish have severely restricted their own access to print media, permitting only a few newspapers and periodicals. They have also rejected the electronic media, beginning with radio and television, but also including entertainment and information applications of film and computers. On the other hand, the Amish are openly curious about the world beyond their own cultural horizons, particularly regarding various literature that deals with health and quality-of-life issues. They especially value the oral and written personal testimonial as a mark of the efficacy of a particular treatment or health-enhancing product or process. Wenger (1988, 1994) identified testimonials from Amish friends and relatives as a key source of information in making choices about health-care providers and products.

## Cultural Communication Patterns

Fondness and love for family members is held deeply but privately. Some nurses have observed the cool, almost aloof behavior of Amish husbands who accompany their wives to a maternity center, but it would be premature to assume that it reflects a lack of concern. The expression of joy and suffering is not entirely subdued by dour or stoic silence, but Amish are clearly not outwardly demonstrative or exuberant. Amish children, who can be as delightfully animated as any other children at play, are taught to remain quiet throughout a worship service lasting more than 2 hours. They grow up in an atmosphere of restraint and respect for adults and elders. But privately, Amish are not so sober as to lack a sense of humor and appreciation of wit.

Beyond language, much of the nonverbal behavior of Amish is also symbolic. Many of the details of Amish garb and customs were once general characteristics without any particular religious significance in Europe, but in the American setting, they are closely regulated and serve to distinguish the Amish from the dominant culture as a self-consciously separate ethnoreligious group (Kraybill, 1989).

It is precisely in the domain of ideas held to be normative for the religious aspects of Amish life that they find their English vocabulary lacking. The key source texts in *Hochdeitsch* and the oral interpretation of them in *Deitsch* are crucial to an understanding of two German values, which have an important impact on Amish nonverbal behavior. **Demut,** German for humility, is a priority value, the effects of which may be seen in details such as the height of the crown of an Amish man's hat, as well as in very general features such as the modest and unassuming bearing and demeanor usually shown by Amish in public. This behavior is reinforced by frequent verbal warnings against its opposite, *Hochmut,* pride or arrogance, which is to be avoided (Hostetler, 1993).

The second term, ***Gelassenheit,*** is embodied in behavior more than it is verbalized. *Gelassenheit* is treasured not so much for its contemporary German connotations of passiveness, even of resignation, as for its earlier religious meanings, denoting quiet acceptance and reassurance, encapsulated in the biblical formula "godliness with contentment" (1 Tim. 6:5). The following Amish paradigm for the good life flows from the calm assurance found through inner yielding and forgoing one's ego for the good of others:

1. One's life rests secure in the hands of a higher power.

2. A life so divinely ordained is therefore a good gift.

3. A godly life of obedience and submission will be rewarded in the life hereafter (Bender & Smith, 1956; Kraybill, 1989).

A combination of these inner qualities, an unpretentious, quiet manner, and modest outward dress in plain colors lacking any ornament, jewelry, or cosmetics, presents a striking contrast to contemporary fashions, both in clothing styles and in personal self-actualization. Amish public behavior is consequently seen as deliberate, rather than rash, deferring to others instead of being assertive or aggressive, avoiding confrontational speech styles, and public displays of emotion in general.

Health-care workers should greet Amish clients with a handshake and a smile. The same greeting is used by Amish both among themselves and with outsiders, but little touching follows the handshake. Younger children are touched and held with affection, but older adults seldom touch socially in public. Therapeutic touch, on the other hand, appeals to many Amish and is practiced informally by some individuals who find communal affirmation for their gift of *warm hands.* This concept is discussed further in the section on health-care practices.

In public, the avoidance of eye contact with non-Amish may be seen as an extension on smaller scale of the general reserve and measured larger body movements related to a modest and humble being. But in one-on-one clinical contacts, Amish clients can be expected to express openness and candor with unhesitating eye contact. Although they, as a people, have a reputation for honesty and forthrightness, they may withhold important medical information from medical professionals by neglecting to mention folk and alternative care being pursued at the same time. When questioned, some Amish admit to being less than candid about using multiple therapies, including herbal and chiropractic remedies, because they believe that "the doctor wouldn't be interested in them." Making choices among folk, alternative, and professional health-care options does not necessarily indicate a lack of confidence or respect for the latter, but rather reflects the belief that one must be actively involved in seeking the best health care available (Wenger, 1994).

Personal distancing in normal interaction is one aspect of the moderate, restrained public behavior described earlier. Among their own, Amish personal space may be collapsed on occasions of crowding together for group meetings or travel. In fact, Amish are seldom found alone, and a solitary Amish person or family is the exception rather than the rule. But Amish are also pragmatic, and in larger families, physical intimacy cannot be avoided in the home where childbearing and care of the ill and dying are accepted as normal parts of life. Once health-care professionals recognize that Amish prefer to have such caregiving within the home and family circle, professionals will want to protect modest Amish clients who feel exposed in the clinical setting.

## Temporal Relationships

So much of current Amish life and practice has a traditional dimension reminiscent of a rural American past that it is tempting to view the Amish culture as "backward-looking." In actuality, Amish self-perception is very much grounded in the present, and historical antecedents or reasons for current consensus have often been lost to common memory. On the other hand, as will be seen in the discussion of spirituality, the Amish existential expression of Christianity focused on today is clearly seen as a preparation for the afterlife. So one may say that Amish are also future-oriented, at least in a metaphysical sense, although not as relates to modern progressive or futuristic thought.

After generations of rural life guided by the natural rhythms of daylight and seasons, the Amish can manage the demands of clock time in the dominant culture. They are generally punctual and conscientious about keeping appointments, although they may be somewhat inconvenienced by not owning a telephone or car.

Because the predominant mode of transportation for the Amish is horse and carriage, travel to the doctor's office, a clinic, or a hospital requires the same adjustment as any other travel outside their rural community to shop, trade, or attend a wedding or funeral. The latter three reasons for travel are important means of reinforcing relationship ties, and on such occasions Amish may use hired or public transportation. Taking time out of normal routines for extended trips related to medical treatments is not uncommon, such as a visit to radioactive mines in the Rocky Mountains or a laetrile clinic in Mexico to cope with cancer (Wenger, 1988).

## Format for Names

Using first names with Amish people is appropriate, particularly because generations of intermarriage have resulted in a large number of Amish who share only a limited number of surnames. So it is preferable to use John or Mary during personal contacts rather than Mr. or Mrs. Miller, for example. In fact, within Amish communities with so many Millers, Lapps, Yoders, and Zooks, given names like Mary and John are overused to the extent that individuals have to be identified further by nicknames, residence, a spouse's given name, or a patronymic, which may reflect three or more generations of patrilineal descent. For example, a particular John Miller may be known as "Red John," or "Gap John," or "Annie's John," or "Sam's Eli's Roman's John," (Hostetler, 1993). The patronymics also illustrate the cultural value placed on intergenerational relationships and help to create a sense of belonging that embraces several generations. Thus, one can see that medical record-keeping can be a challenge where an extensive Amish clientele is served.

## FAMILY ROLES AND ORGANIZATION

### Head of Household and Gender Roles

From the time of marriage, the young Amish man's role as husband is defined by the religious community to which he belongs. Titular patriarchy is derived from the Bible: man is the head of the woman as Christ is the head of the church (I Cor. 3). This patriarchal role in Amish society is balanced or tempered by realities within the family, where the wife and mother is accorded high status and respect for her vital contributions to the success of the family. Practically speaking, husband and wife may share equally in decisions regarding the family farming business. In public, the wife may assume a retiring role, deferring to her husband, but in private they are typically partners (Huntington, 1988).

Traditionally, the highest priority for the parents is childrearing, a charge laid on them by the church. With a completed family of seven children, the Amish mother must contribute physically and emotionally to the burgeoning growth in Amish population. She also has an important role in providing for family food and clothing needs, as well as a major share in child nurturing. Amish society expects the husband and father to contribute guidance, provide role modeling, and discipline the children. This shared task of parenting takes precedence over other needs, including economic or financial success in the family business. On the family farm, all must help out as needed, but in general, field and barn work and animal husbandry are primarily the work of men and boys, whereas food production and preservation, clothing production and care, and management of the household are mainly the province of women (Huntington, 1988).

## Prescriptive, Restrictive, and Taboo Behaviors for Children and Adolescents

Children and youth represent a key to the vitality of the Amish culture. Babies are welcomed as a gift from God, and the high birth rate is one factor in their growth in population. Another is the surprisingly high retention of youth, an estimated 75 percent or more, who choose as adults to remain in the Amish way. Before and during elementary school years, parents are more directive as they guide and train their children to assume responsible, productive roles in Amish society.

Young people over age 16 years may be encouraged to work away from home to gain experience, but their wages are still sent home to the parental household. Some experimentation with non-Amish dress and behavior among Amish teenagers is tolerated during this period of relative leniency, but the expectation is that an adult decision to be baptized before marriage will call young people back to the discipline of the church, as they take on fully adult roles. Additional behavioral expectations of children and adolescents are covered elsewhere in this chapter.

## Family Roles and Priorities

The Amish family pattern is referred to as the *freindschaft,* the dialectical term used for the three-generational family structure. This kinship network includes consanguine relatives consisting of the parental unit and the households of married children and their offspring. All members of the family personally know their grandparents, aunts, uncles, and cousins, with many Amish knowing their second and third cousins as well.

Individuals are identified by their family affiliation (Huntington, 1989). Children and young adults may introduce themselves by giving their father's first name or both parent's names so they can be placed geographically. Families are the units that make up church districts, and the size of church districts are measured by the number of families, rather than by the number of church members.

This extended family pattern has many functions. Families visit together frequently, thus learning to anticipate caring needs and preferences. Health-care information often circulates through the family network, even though families may be geographically dispersed. Wenger (1988) found that informants referred to *freindschaft* when discussing the factors influencing the selection of health-care options. "The functions of family care include maintaining *freindschaft* ties, bonding family members together intergenerationally, and living according to God's will by fulfilling the parental mandate to prepare the family for eternal life" (Wenger, 1988, p. 134). For detailed descriptions of the Amish family, see Hostetler (1993) and Huntington (1988).

As grandparents turn over the primary responsibility for the family farm to their children, they continue to enjoy respected status as elders, providing valuable advice and sometimes material support and services to the younger generation. Many nuclear families live on a farm with an adjacent grandparents' cottage, which promotes frequent interactions across generations. Grandparents provide child care and help in rearing grandchildren and, in return, enjoy the respect generally paid by the next generations. This emotional and physical proximity to older adults also facilitates eldercare within the family setting. In an ethnonursing study on care in an Amish community, Wenger (1998) reported that an informant discussed the reciprocal benefits of having her grandparents living in the attached **daadihaus** and her own parents living in a house across the road. Her three-year-old daughter could go across the hall to spend time with her great-grandfather, which the mother reported was good for him in that he was needed, while the small child benefited from learning to know her great-grandfather, and the young mother gained some time to do chores. There is no set retirement age among the Amish, and grandmothers also continue in an active role as advisors and assistants to younger mothers (Tripp-Reimer, et al., 1988).

Assuming full adult membership and responsibility means the willingness to put group harmony ahead of personal desire. In financial terms, it also means an obligation to help others in need in the brotherhood. This mutual aid commitment also provides a safety net, which allows Amish to rely on others for help in emergencies. Consequently, Amish do not need federal pension or retirement support; they have their own informal "social security" plan. Amish of varying degrees of affluence enjoy approximately the same social status, and extremes of poverty and wealth are uncommon. Property damage or loss and unusual health-care expenses are also covered to a large extent by an informal brotherhood alternative to commercial insurance coverage. The costs of high-technology medical care present a new and severe test of the principle of mutual aid, which grows out of "helping out," almost synonymous with the Amish way of life (Hostetler, 1993).

## Alternative Lifestyles

There is little variation from the culturally sanctioned expectations for parents and their unmarried children to live together in the same household while maintaining frequent contact with the extended family. Unmarried children live in the parents' home until marriage, which usual takes place between the ages of 20 years and 30 years. Some young adults may move to a different community to work and would then live as a boarder with another Amish family.

Singleness is not stigmatized, although almost all Amish do marry. Single adults are included in the social fabric of the community with the expectation that they will want to be involved in family-oriented social events. Persons of the same gender do not live together except in situations where their work may make it more convenient. For example, two female schoolteachers may live together in an apartment or in a home close to the Amish school where they teach.

There are no available statistics on the incidence of homosexuality in Amish culture. Isolated incidents of homosexual practice may come to the attention of health professionals, but homosexual lifestyles do not fit with the deeply held values of Amish family life and procreation.

Pregnancy before marriage does not usually occur, and it is viewed as a situation to be avoided. When it does occur, in most Amish families, the couple would be encouraged to consider marriage. If they are not yet members of the church, they need to be baptized and to join the church before marriage can occur. While not condoning pregnancy before marriage, the families and the Amish community support the young pregnant couple. If the couple chooses not to marry, the young girl is encouraged to keep the baby and her family helps raise the child. Abortion is an unacceptable option. Adoption by an Amish family is an acceptable alternative.

## WORKFORCE ISSUES

### Culture in the Workplace

In every generation except the present one, Amish have worked almost exclusively in agriculture and farm-related tasks. Their large families were ideally suited to labor-intensive work on the family farm. As the number of family farms has been drastically curtailed because of competition from agribusinesses that use mechanized and electronically controlled production methods, few options are available for Amish youth (Hostetler, 1993).

Traditionally, the Amish have placed a high value on hard work, with little time off for leisure or recreation. Productive employment for all is the ideal, and the intergenerational family provides work roles appropriate to the age and abilities of each person. But prospects began to narrow with the increased concentration of family farms in densely settled Amish communities as their population increased.

In addition, several cultural factors combine to limit the horizon of opportunity for young Amish to adapt to new work patterns. Amish children, who are encouraged to attend school only through eight grades, lack a basis for vocational training in work areas other than agriculture. Amish avoidance of compromising associations with "worldly" organizations such as labor unions restricts them to nonunion work, which often pays lower hourly rates. Work off the family farm, at one time a good option for unmarried youth, has become an economic necessity for some parents, although it is considered less acceptable for social reasons. Fathers who "work away," sometimes called "lunchpail daddies," have less contact with children during the workday, which in turn has an impact on the traditional father's modeling role and places more of the responsibility for childrearing on stay-at-home mothers. This shift in traditional parental roles is the source of some concern, although the effects are not yet clear (Meyers, 1983).

## Issues Related to Autonomy

As described previously, external and internal factors have converged in the late 20th century to cause doubt about the continued viability of compact Amish farming communities. Exorbitant land prices triggered group outmigrations and resettlement in states to the West. The declining availability of affordable prime arable land in and around the centers of highest Amish population density is due in part to their non-Amish neighbors' land-use practices, especially in areas of suburban sprawl. A powerful internal force is at work as well in the population growth rate among the Amish, now well above the national average. So, contrary to popular notions that such a "backward" subculture is bound to die out, the Amish today are thriving. Population growth continues even without a steady influx of new immigrants from the European homeland or significant numbers of new converts to their religion or way of life (Kraybill, 1993).

The resulting pressures to control the changes in their way of life while maintaining its religious basis, particularly the high value placed on in-group harmony, have challenged the Amish to develop adaptive strategies. One outcome is an increasingly diversified employment base, with a trend toward cottage industries and related retail sales, as well as toward wage labor to generate cash needed for higher taxes and increasing medical costs. Another recent development includes a shift from traditional multigenerational farmsteads, as some retirees and crafts workers employed off the farm have begun to relocate on the edge of country towns. In summary, pressures to secure a livelihood within the Amish tradition have heightened awareness of the tension field within which the Amish coexist with the surrounding majority American culture (Hostetler, 1993).

Because English is the language of instruction in schools and is used with business contacts in the outside world, there is generally no language barrier for the Amish in the workplace. English vocabulary that is lacking in their normative ideas for religious aspects of Amish life is rarely a concern in the workplace.

## BIOCULTURAL ECOLOGY

### Skin Color and Other Biologic Variations

Most Amish are descendants of 18th-century South German and Swiss immigrants; therefore, their physical characteristics vary as do those of most Europeans, with skin variations ranging from light to olive tones. Hair and eye colors vary accordingly. No specific health-care precautions are relevant to this group.

### Diseases and Health Conditions

Since 1962, several hereditary diseases have been identified among the Amish. The major findings of the genetic studies have been published by Dr. Victor McKusick of the Johns Hopkins University (McKusick, 1978). Because Amish tend to live in settlements with relatively little domiciliary mobility, and because they keep extensive genealogical and family records, genetic studies are more easily done than with more mobile cultural groups. Many years of collaboration between the Amish and a few geneticists from the Johns Hopkins Hospital have resulted in mutually beneficial projects (Hostetler, 1993). The Amish received printed community directories, and geneticists compiled computerized genealogies for the study of genetic diseases that continue to benefit society in general.

The Amish are essentially a closed population with exogamy occurring very rarely. However, they are not a singular genetically closed population. The larger and older communities are consanguineous, meaning that within the community the people are related through bloodlines by common ancestors. Several consanguine groups have been identified where relatively little intermarriage occurs between the groups. "The separateness of these groups is supported by the history of the immigration into each area, by the uniqueness of the family names in each community, by the distribution of blood groups, and by the different hereditary diseases that occur in each of these groups" (Hostetler, 1993, p. 328). These diseases are one of the indicators of distinctiveness among the groups.

Hostetler (1993) cautions that although inbreeding is more prevalent in Amish communities than in the general population, inbreeding does not inevitably result in hereditary defects. Through the centuries in some societies, marriages among first and second cousins were relatively common without major adverse effects. However, in the Amish gene pool there are several recessive tendencies that in some cases are limited to specific Amish communities where the consanguinity coefficient (degree of relatedness) is high for the specific genes. Four of at least 12 recessive diseases should be noted (Hostetler, 1993; McKusick, 1978; Troyer, 1994).

Dwarfism has long been recognized as obvious in several Amish communities. Ellis-van Creveld syndrome, known in Europe and named for a Scottish and a Dutch physician, is especially prevalent among the Lancaster County, Pennsylvania, Amish (McKusick, et al., 1964). This syndrome is characterized by short stature and an extra digit on each hand, with some persons having a congenital heart defect and nervous system involvement resulting in a degree of mental deficiency. The Lancaster County Amish community, the second largest Amish settlement in the United States, is the only one where Ellis-van Creveld Syndrome is found. The lineage of all affected persons has been traced to a single ancestor, Samuel King, who immigrated in 1744 (Troyer, 1994).

Cartilage hair hypoplasia, also a dwarfism syndrome, has been found in nearly all Amish communities in the United States and Canada and is not unique to the Amish (McKusick, et al., 1965). This syndrome is characterized by short stature and fine, silky hair. There is no central nervous system involvement and therefore no mental deficiency. However, most affected persons have deficient cell-mediated immunity, thus increasing their susceptibility to viral infections (Troyer, 1994).

Pyruvate kinase anemia, a rare blood cell disease, was described by Bowman and Procopio in 1963. The lineage of all affected persons can be traced to Jacob Yoder (known as "Strong Jacob"), who immigrated to Mifflin County, Pennsylvania, in 1792 (Hostetler, 1993; Troyer, 1994). This same genetic disorder was found later in the Geauga County, Ohio, Amish community. Notably, the families of all affected persons had migrated from Mifflin County, Pennsylvania, and were from the "Strong Jacob" lineage. Symptoms usually appear soon after birth, with the presence of jaundice and anemia. Transfusions during the first few years of life and eventual removal of the spleen can be considered cures.

Hemophilia B, another blood disorder, is disproportionately high among the Amish, especially in Ohio. Ratnoff (1958) reported on an Amish man who was treated for a ruptured spleen. It was discovered that he had grandparents and 10 cousins who were bleeders; five of the cousins had died from bleeding. Research studies on causative mutations indicated a strong probability that a specific mutation may account for much of the mild hemophilia B in the Amish population (Ketterling, et al., 1991).

Through the vigilant and astute observations of some public health nurses known to this author, a major health-care problem was noted in a northern Indiana Amish community. A high prevalence of phenylketonuria (PKU) in the Elkhart/Lagrange Amish settlement was found (Martin, Davis, & Askew, 1965). Affected persons are unable to metabolize the amino acid phenylalanine, resulting in high blood levels that cause severe brain damage if untreated. Through epidemiologic studies, the Health Department found 1:62 Amish to be affected, whereas the ratio in the general population was 1:25,000 at that time. Through the leadership of these nurses, the county and the state improved case funding for PKU and health-care services for affected families throughout Indiana.

In recent years, a biochemical disorder called glutaric aciduria has been studied. Dr. Holmes Morton, a Harvard-educated physician who has chosen to live and work among the Amish in Lancaster County, Pennsylvania, made house calls, conducted research at his own expense because funding was not forthcoming, and established a clinic in the Amish community to screen, diagnose, and educate people to care for persons afflicted with the disease (Allen, 1989). By observing the natural history of glutaric aciduria type I, the researchers postulated that the onset or progression of neurological disease in Amish clients can be prevented by screening individuals at risk; restricting dietary protein; and thus limiting protein catabolism, dehydration, and acidosis during illness episodes (Morton, et el., 1991).

Dr. Morton was well received in the Amish community, with many persons referring friends and relatives to him. When he noted the rapid onset of the symptoms and the high incidence among the Amish, he did not wait for them to come to his office. He went to their homes and spent evenings and weekends driving from farm to farm, talking with families, running tests, and compiling genealogical information (Wolkomir & Wolkomir, 1991). In 1991, he built a clinic with the help of donations, in part the result of an article in the *Wall Street Journal* about the need for this nonprofit clinic. Hewlett-Packard donated the needed spectrometer costing $80,000, local companies provided building materials, and an Amish couple donated the building site. Although volunteers helped to build the clinic, a local hospital provided temporary clinic space lease-free because the community recognized the very important contribution Morton was making, not only to the Amish and the advancement of medical science but also to the public health of the community.

A county-wide screening program is now in place. Health-care professionals are alert to the recognition of the onset of symptoms. Research continues on this metabolic disorder and its relationship to cerebral palsy in the Amish population and the biochemical causes and methods of prevention of spastic paralysis in the general population. However, education remains a highly significant feature of any community health program. Nurses and physicians need to plan for family and community education about genetic counseling, screening of newborns, recognition of symptoms during aciduric crises in affected children, and treatment protocols.

Extensive studies of manic-depressive illnesses have been conducted in the Amish population, the first reported by Egeland and Hostetler in 1983. At first, there seemed to be evidence of a link between the Harvey-*ras*-1 oncogene and the insulin locus on chromosome 11. Studies on non-Amish families (Detera-Wadleigh, et al., 1987; Hodgkinson, et al., 1987) and more extensive studies on Amish families have revealed new information on the genome, although the locus for the bipolar disorder has not yet been found (Ginns, et al., 1992, Kelso, et al., 1989; Kelso, et al. 1993; Law, et al., 1992; Pauls, et al., 1992).

The incidence of alcohol and drug abuse, which can complicate psychiatric diagnoses, is much lower among the Amish than in the general North American population, thus contributing to the importance of the Amish sample. Although the incidence of bipolar affective disorder is not found to be higher in the Amish, some large families with several affected members continue to contribute to medical science by being subjects in the genetic studies. Because the Old Order Amish descend from 30 pioneer couples whose descendants have remained genetically isolated in North America, have relatively large sibships with multiple living generations, and generally live in close geographic approximation, they are an ideal population for genetic studies (Kelsoe, et al., 1989).

## Variations in Drug Metabolism

No drug studies specifically related to the Amish were found in the literature. However, given the genetic disorders common among selected populations of Amish, this is one area where more research needs to be conducted.

## HIGH-RISK BEHAVIORS

Amish are traditionally agrarian and prefer a lifestyle that provides intergenerational and community support systems to promote health and mitigate against the prevalence of high-risk behaviors. As mentioned in the previous section, genetic studies using Amish populations are seldom confounded by use of alcohol and other substances. However, health professionals should be alert to potential alcohol and recreational drug use in some Amish communities, especially among young unmarried men. There tends to be tolerance for young adult men to stray from the Amish lifeways and "sow their wild oats" before becoming baptized church members and before marriage. Although this may be considered a high-risk behavior, it is not prevalent in all communities, nor is it promoted in any. Parents confide in each other and sometimes in trusted outsiders that this errant behavior causes many heartaches, although at the same time they try to be patient and keep contact with the youth so they may choose to espouse Amish lifeways.

Another lifestyle pattern that poses potential health risks is nutrition. Amish tend to eat high-carbohydrate and high-fat foods with a relatively high intake of refined sugar. Wenger (1994) reported that in an ethnonursing study on health and health-care perceptions, informants talked about their diet being too high in "sweets and starches" and knowing they should eat more vegetables. The prevalence of obesity was found to be greater among Amish women than for women in general in the State of Ohio (Fuchs, et al., 1990). In this major health-risk survey of 400 Amish adults and 773 non-Amish adults in Ohio, it was found that the pattern of obesity in Amish women begins in the 25-year-old and older cohort, with the concentration occurring between the ages of 45 and 64. Explanations for the propensity for weight gain among the Amish may be related to the central place [that] is assigned to the consumption of food in their culture and the higher rates of pregnancy throughout their childbearing years (Wenger, 1994, p.105). Typical nutritional patterns for this ethnoreligious culture is discussed further in a later section of this chapter.

## Health-care Practices

Most Amish are physically active, largely owing to their chosen agrarian lifestyle and farming as a preferred occupation. Physical labor is valued, and men as well as women and children help with farm work. Household chores and gardening, generally considered to be women's work, require physical exertion, particularly because Amish do not choose to use electrically operated appliances in the home and machinery such as riding lawn mowers that conserve human energy. Nevertheless, many women do contend with a tendency to be overweight. In recent years, it is not

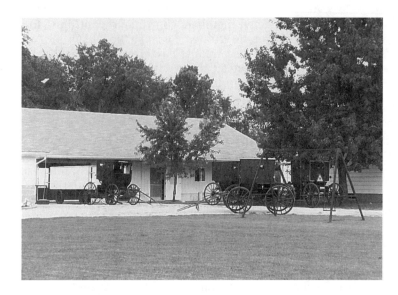

**Figure 4–3.** Amish buggies parked outside a home. Note the reflective safety triangle attached to the back of the rightmost buggy in the picture. These are usually required by law in areas that have large Amish populations. (Photograph by Joel Wenger.)

uncommon to find Amish women seeking help for weight control from Weight Watchers and other similar weight-control support groups.

Farm and traffic accidents are an increasing health concern in communities with a dense Amish population. In states such as Indiana with relatively high concentrations of Amish who drive horse-drawn vehicles (Fig. 4–3), blinking red lights and large red triangles are required by law to be attached to their vehicles. Jones (1990) reported on a study of trauma by examining hospital records of Amish clients admitted to one hospital in mideastern Ohio. Transportation-related injuries were the largest group, with many of those involving farm animals. Falls from ladders and down hay holes resulted in orthopedic injuries but no deaths. Amish families need to be encouraged to monitor their children who operate farm equipment and transportation vehicles and to teach them about safety factors. Concern about accidents is evident in Amish newsletters, many of which have a regular column reporting accidents and asking for prayers or expressing gratitude that the injuries were not more severe, that God had spared the person, or that the community had responded in caring ways (Wenger, 1988).

## NUTRITION

### Meaning of food

The Amish include the serving of food in most social situations. Food is recognized for its nutritional value. Most Amish prefer to grow their own produce for economic reasons and because for generations they have been aware of their connections with the earth. They believe that God expects people to be the caretakers of the earth and to make it flourish.

Food also has a significant social meaning. Because visiting has a highly valued cultural function, many occasions occur during most weeks for Amish to visit family, neighbors, and friends, especially those within their church district. Some of these visits are planned when snacks or meals are shared, sometimes with the guests helping to provide the food. Even if guests come unexpectedly, it is customary in most Amish communities for snacks and drinks to be offered.

## Common Foods and Food Rituals

Typical Amish meals include meat; potatoes, noodles, or both; a cooked vegetable; bread; something pickled (for example, pickles, red beets); cake or pudding; and coffee. Beef is usually butchered by the family and then kept in the local commercially owned freezer for which they pay a rental storage fee. Some families also preserve beef by canning, and most families have chickens and other fowl, such as ducks or geese, which they raise for eggs and for meat. Amish families still value growing their own foods and usually have large gardens. A generation ago, this was an unquestioned way of life, but an increasing number of families living in small towns and working in factories and construction own insufficient land to plant enough food for the family's consumption.

Snacks and meals in general tend to be high in fat and carbohydrates. A common snack is large, home-baked cookies about 3 inches in diameter. Commercial non-Amish companies have recognized large soft cookies as a marketable commodity and have advertised their commercially made products as "Amish" cookies, even though no Amish are involved in the production. Other common snacks are ice cream (store-bought or home-made), pretzels, and popcorn.

When Amish gather for celebrations such as weddings, birthdays, work bees, or quiltings, the tables are usually laden with large varieties of foods. The selection, usually provided by many people, includes several casseroles, noodle dishes, white and sweet potatoes, some cooked vegetables, few salads, pickled dishes, pies, cakes, puddings, and cookies. Hostetler (1993) provides a detailed ethnographic description of the meaning and practices surrounding an Amish wedding including the food preparation, the wedding dinner and supper, and the roles and functions of various key persons in this most important rite of passage that includes serving food.

In communities where tourists flock to learn about the Amish, many entrepreneurs have used the Amish love of wholesome simple foods to market their version of Amish cookbooks, food products, and restaurants that more aptly reflect the Pennsylvania German or Dutch influence of communities such as Lancaster County, Pennsylvania. Many of these bear little resemblance to authentic Amish foods, and some even venture to sell "Amish highballs" or "Amish sodas" (Hostetler, 1993). Some Amish families help to satisfy the public interest in their way of life by serving meals in their homes for tourists and local non-Amish. But most Amish view their foods and food preparation as commonplace and functional, not something to be displayed in magazines and newspapers. Because many Amish are wary of outsiders' undue interest, health professionals need to discuss nutrition and food as a part of their lifeways to promote healthy nutritional lifestyles.

In Amish homes, a "place at the table" is symbolic of belonging (Hostetler, 1993). Seating is traditionally arranged with the father at the head and boys seated youngest to oldest to his right. The mother sits to her husband's left with the girls also seated youngest to oldest or placed so that an older child can help a younger one. The table is the place where work, behavior, school, and other family concerns are discussed. During the busy harvesting season, preference is given to the men and boys who eat and return to the fields or barn. At mealtimes, all members of the household are expected to be present unless they are working away from home or are visiting at a distance, making it difficult to return home.

Sunday church services, which for the Old Order Amish are held in their homes or barns, are followed by a simple meal for all who attended church (Fig. 4–4). The church benches, which are transported from home to home wherever the church service is to be held, are set up with long tables for serving the food. In many communities, some of the benches are built so they can quickly be converted into tables.

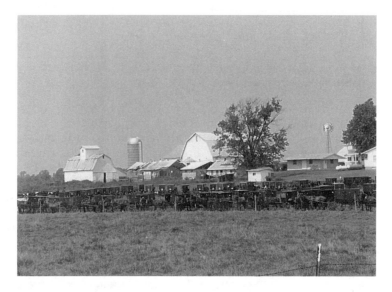

**Figure 4–4.** Buggies parked in a field on an Amish farm where people have gathered for a Sunday church service and noon meal. (Photograph by Joel Wenger.)

Meals become ritualized so the focus is not on what is being served but rather on the opportunity to visit together over a simple meal. In one community, an Amish informant who had not attended services because of a complicated pregnancy told the researcher that she missed the meal, which in that community consisted of bread, butter, peanut butter, apple butter, pickles, pickled red beets, soft sugar cookies, and coffee (Wenger, 1988).

## PREGNANCY AND CHILDBEARING PRACTICES

### Fertility Practices and Views toward Pregnancy

Children are viewed as a gift from God and are welcomed into Amish families. Estimates place the average number of live births per family at seven (Hostetler & Huntington, 1992). The Amish fertility pattern has remained constant throughout this century, while many others have declined. Household size varies from those families having no children to marriage pairs with 15 or more children (Huntington, 1988). Even in large families, the birth of another child brings joy because of the core belief that children are "a heritage from the Lord," and another member of the family and community means another person to help with the chores (Hostetler, 1993).

Ericksen and Klein (1981) suggested that the production of children has a different meaning in Old Order Amish culture than in the dominant American culture. In a study on women's roles and family production, the authors suggested that women in Amish culture enjoy high status despite the apparent patriarchal ideology because of their role as producers of children and producers of food. Large numbers of children benefit small labor-intensive farms and, with large families, comes an apparent need for large quantities of food. Interpretation of this pragmatic view of fertility should always be moderated with recognition of the moral and ethical core cultural belief that children are a gift from God, given to a family and community to nurture in preparation for eternal life.

Scholars and researchers of long-term acquaintance with Old Order Amish agree that the pervasive Amish perception of birth control is that it interferes with God's will and thus should be avoided (Hostetler, 1993; Hostetler & Huntington, 1992; Kraybill, 1989). Nevertheless, fertility control does exist, although the patterns are not well known and very few studies have been reported (Ericksen, et al., 1979). Evidence that "marital fertility declines faster among Amish women who marry early compared with those who marry late indicates that among married women some fertility control occurs" (p. 275). The authors suggested that these results may also indicate the use of sterilization and abstinence. Wenger (1980) discussed childbearing with two Amish couples in a group interview, and they conceded that some couples do use the rhythm method. In referring to birth control, one Amish father stated, "It is not discussed here, really. I think Amish just know they shouldn't use the pill" (Wenger, 1980, p. 5). Three physicians and three nurses were interviewed, and they reported that some Amish do ask about birth control methods, especially those with a history of difficult perinatal histories and those with large families. Some Amish women do use intrauterine devices, but this practice is uncommon. Most Amish women are reluctant to ask physicians and nurses and, therefore, should be counseled with utmost care and respect because this is a topic that generally is not discussed, even among themselves. Approaching the subject obliquely may make it possible for the Amish woman or man to sense the health professional's respect for Amish values and thus encourage discussion. "When you want to learn more about birth control, I would be glad to talk to you" is a suggested approach.

## Prescriptive, Restrictive, and Taboo Practices in the Childbearing Family

Amish tend to have their first child later than do non-Amish. In a retrospective chart review examining pregnancy outcomes of 39 Amish and 145 non-Amish at a rural hospital in southern New York State, it was found that Amish had their first child an average of one year later than non-Amish (Lucas, et al., 1991). The Amish had a narrower range of maternal ages and had proportionately fewer teenage pregnancies. All subjects received prenatal care, with the Amish receiving prenatal care from Amish lay-midwives during the first trimester.

In some communities, Amish have been reputed to be reluctant to seek prenatal health care. Those professionals who gain the trust of the Amish learn that Amish want the best perinatal care, which fits with their view of children being a blessing. However, they may choose to use Amish and non-Amish lay-midwives who promote childbearing as a natural part of the life cycle. Although many may express privately their preference for perinatal care that promotes the use of nurse-midwifery and lay-midwifery services, home deliveries, and limited use of high technology, they tend to use the perinatal services available in their community. In ethnographic interviews with informants, Wenger (1988) found that grandmothers and older women tended to report more preference for hospital deliveries than did younger women who have been influenced by the increasing general interest in childbirth as a natural part of the life cycle and de-emphasis on the medicalization of childbirth. Some Amish communities, especially those in Ohio and Pennsylvania, have a long-standing tradition of using both lay-midwifery and professional obstetric services, often simultaneously (Armstrong & Feldman, 1986; Heikes, 1985; Hostetler, 1993; Kaiser, 1986).

In Ohio, the Mt. Eaton Care Center developed as a community effort in response to retirement of an Amish lay-midwife known as Bill Barb (identified by her spouse's name as discussed in the Communications section). She provided perinatal services, including labor and birth, with the collaborative services of a local Mennonite physician who believed in providing culturally congruent and safe health-care services for this Amish population. At one point in Bill Barb Hochstetler's 30-year practice, the physician moved a trailer with a telephone onto Hochstetler's farm so that he could be called in case of an emergency (Huntington, 1993). Other sympathetic physicians also delivered babies at Bill Barb's home. After state investigation, which coincided with her intended retirement, Hochstetler's practice was recognized to be in a legal grey area. The Mt. Eaton Care Center became a reality in 1985 after careful negotiation with the Amish community, Wayne County Board of Health, Ohio Department of Health, and local physicians and nurses. Physicians and professional nurses and nurse-midwives, who are interested in Amish cultural values and health-care preferences, provide low-cost, safe, low-technology perinatal care in a homelike atmosphere.

Because Amish want family involvement in perinatal care, outsiders may infer that they are open in their discussion of pregnancy and childbirth. In actuality, most Amish women do not discuss their pregnancies openly and make an effort to keep others from knowing about them until physical changes are obvious. Mothers do not inform their other children of the impending birth of a sibling, preferring for the children to learn of it as "the time comes naturally" (Wenger, 1988). This fits with the Amish cultural pattern of learning through observation that assumes intergenerational involvement in life's major events. Armstrong and Feldman (1986) and Kaiser (1986) relate anecdotal accounts of children being in the house, though not physically present, during birth. Fathers are expected to be present and involved, although some may opt to do farm chores that cannot be delayed, such as milking cows.

Amish women do participate in prenatal classes, often with their husbands. The women are interested in learning about all aspects of perinatal care but may choose not to participate in sessions when videos are used. Prenatal class instructors would do well to inform them ahead of time when videos or films will be used, so they can decide whether to attend. For some Amish where the **Ordnung** (the set of unwritten rules prescribed for the church district) is more prescriptive and strict, the persons may be concerned about being disobedient to the will of the community. Even though the information on the videos may be acceptable, the type of media is considered unacceptable.

Amish have no major taboos or requirements for birthing. Men may be present, and most husbands choose to be involved. However, they are likely not to be demonstrative in showing affection verbally nor physically. This does not mean they do not care; culturally it is inappropriate to show affection openly in public. The laboring woman cooperates quietly, seldom audibly expressing discomfort.

Given the Amish acceptance of a wide spectrum of health-care modalities, the nurse or physician should be aware that the woman in labor may be using herbal remedies to promote labor. Knowledge about and a respect for Amish health-care practices alerts the physician or nurse to a discussion about simultaneous treatments that may be harmful or helpful. It is always better if these discussions can take place in a low-stress setting before labor and birth.

As in other hospitalizations, the family may want to spend the least allowable time in the hospital. This is generally related to the belief that birth is not a medical condition and because most Amish do not carry health insurance. In their three-generational family and as a result of their cultural expectations for caring to take place in the community, many persons are willing and able to assist the new mother during the postpartum period. Visiting families with new babies is expected and generally welcomed. Older siblings are expected to help care for the younger children and to learn how to care for the newborn. The postpartum mother resumes her family role managing, if not doing, all the housework, cooking, and child care within a few days after childbirth. For a primiparous mother, her mother often comes to stay with the new family for several days to help with care of the infant and give support to the new mother.

The day the new baby is first taken to church services is considered special. People who did not visit the home want to see the new member of the community. The baby is often passed among the women to hold as they become acquainted and admire the newcomer.

# DEATH RITUALS

## Death Rituals and Expectations

As was noted previously with other health-care practices, Amish customs related to death and dying have dual dimensions. On the one hand, they may be seen as hold-overs from an earlier time when, for most Americans, major life events such as birth and death occurred in the home. On the other hand, Amish retention of such largely outdated patterns is due to distinctively Amish understandings of the individual within and as an integral part of the family and community.

Today, when 70 percent of elderly Americans die in hospitals and nursing homes, some still reflect nostalgically on death as it should be, as in fact it used to be, in the circle of family and friends, a farewell with familiarity and dignity (Boehm, 1995). In Amish society today, this is still a reality in most cases. As physical strength declines, the expectation is that the aging and ill will be cared for by family in the home. Hostetler's brief observation that Amish prefer to die at home (1993) is borne out by research findings. Tripp-Reimer and Schrock (1982) reported from their comparative study of the ethnic aged that 75 percent of the Amish surveyed expressed a preference for living with family, 25 percent preferred living at home with assistance, and none would choose to live in a care facility, even if bedfast.

Clearly, these preferences are motivated by more than a wish to dwell in the past or an unwillingness to change with the times. The obligation to help others, in illness as in health, provides the social network that undergirds Amish practices in the passage from life to death. In effect, it is a natural extension of caregiving embraced as a social duty with religious motivation. The Amish accept literally the biblical admonition to "bear . . . one another's burdens," and this finds expression in communal support for the individual, whether suffering, dying, or bereaved. In Hostetler's description (1993), life's most intensely personal and private act becomes transformed into a community event.

Visiting in others' homes is for Amish a normal and frequent reinforcement of the bonds that tie individuals to extended family and community. As a natural extension of this social interaction, visiting the ill takes on an added poignancy, especially during an illness believed to be terminal. Members of the immediate family are offered not only verbal condolences, but many supportive acts of kindness as well. Others close to them prepare their food and take over other routine household chores to allow them to focus their attention and energy on the comfort of the ailing family member (Hostetler, 1993; Kraybill, 1989).

## Responses to Death and Grief

Ties across generations, as well as across kinship and geographic lines, are reinforced around death as children witness the passing of a loved one in the intimacy of the home. Death brings many more visitors into the home of the bereaved, and the church community takes care of accommodations for visitors from a distance as well as funeral arrangements. The immediate family is thus relieved of responsibility for decision making, which otherwise may add distraction to grief. In some Amish settlements, a wakelike "sitting up" through the night provides an exception to normal visiting patterns. The verbal communication with the bereaved may be sparse, but the constant presence of supportive others is tangible proof of the Amish commitment to community. The return to normal life is eased through these visits by the resumption of conversations (Hostetler, 1993).

Apart from the usual number of visitors who come to pay their respect to the deceased and survivors, the funeral ceremony is as simple and unadorned as the rest of Amish life. A plain wooden coffin is frequently built by a local Amish cabinet-maker. In the past, interment was in private plots on Amish farms, contrasting with the general pattern of burial in a cemetery in the churchyard of a rural church. Because Amish worship in their homes and have no church buildings, they also have no adjoining churchyards. An emerging pattern is to bury in a community cemetery, sometimes together with other Mennonites.

Grief and loss are keenly felt, although verbal expression may seem muted as if to indicate stoic acceptance of suffering. In fact, the meaning of death as a normal transition is embedded in the meaning of life from the Amish perspective. Parents are exhorted to nurture their children's faith because life in this world is seen as a preparation for eternal life (Hostetler, 1993). In the following section, some aspects of Amish spirituality and expression of faith are explored.

## SPIRITUALITY

### Religious Practices and Use of Prayer

Amish settlements are subdivided into church districts similar to rural parishes with 30 to 50 families in each district. Local leaders are chosen from their own religious community and are generally untrained and unpaid. Authority patterns are congregationalist, with local consensus directed by local leadership, designated as bishops, preachers, and deacons, all of which are male. No regional or national church hierarchy exists to govern internal church affairs, although a national committee may be convened to address external institutions of government regarding issues affecting the broader Amish population (Hostetler, 1993; Olshan, 1993).

In addition to Sunday services, silent prayer is always observed at the beginning of a meal, and in many families, a prayer also ends the meal. Children are taught to memorize prayers from a German prayer book for beginning and ending meals and for silent prayer. The father may say an audible amen or merely lift his bowed head to signal the time to begin eating.

### Meaning of Life and Individual Sources of Strength

Outsiders, who are aware of the Amish detachment from the trappings of our modern materialistic culture, may be disappointed to discover in their "otherworldliness" something less than a lofty spirituality. Amish share the earthy vitality of many rural peasant cultures and a pragmatism born of immediate life experiences, not distilled from intellectual pursuits such as philosophy or theology. Amish simplicity is intentional, but even in austerity, there is a relish of life's simpler joys rather than a grim asceticism.

If death is a part of life and a portal to a better life, then individuals are well advised to consider how their lives prepare them for life after death. Amish share the general Christian view that salvation is ultimately individual, preconditioned on one's confession of faith, repentance, and baptism. These public acts are undertaken in the Amish context as part of preparing to assume fully one's adult role in a community of faith. In contrast with the ideals of American individualism, however, the Amish surrender much of their individuality as the price of full acceptance as members of that community. In practical, everyday terms, the religiously defined community is inextricably intertwined with a social reality, which gives it its distinctive shape (Hostetler, 1993).

The importance of conformity for Amish to the will of the group can hardly be exaggerated. To maintain harmony within the group, individuals often forgo their own wishes. In terms of faith-related behavior, this "going along with" the local congregational group is sometimes criticized by outsiders as an expression of religiosity, rather than spirituality. The frequent practice of corporate worship, including prayer and singing, helps to build this conformity. It is regularly tested in "counsel" sessions in the congregational assembly where each individual's commitment to the corporate religious contract is reviewed before taking communion (Kraybill, 1989).

## Spiritual Beliefs and Health-care Practices

As seen in earlier sections on communication among Amish and their socioreligious provenance, many symbols of Amish faith point to the separated life, which they live in accordance with God's will. Over time, they have chosen to embody their faith rather than verbalize it. As a result, they seldom proselytize among non-Amish and nurture among themselves a noncreedal, often primitive form of Christianity that emphasizes "right living." Their untrained religious leaders offer unsophisticated views of what that entails based on their interpretation of the Bible. Most members are content to submit to the congregational consensus on what right living means, with the assumption that it is based on submission to the will of a loving, benevolent God, an aspect of their spirituality that is seldom articulated (Kraybill, 1989).

Although the directives of religious leaders are normative for many types of decisions, this appears not to be the case for health-care choices (Wenger, 1991b). When choosing among health-care options, families usually seek counsel from religious leaders, friends, and extended family, but the final decision resides with the immediate family. Health-care providers need to be aware of the Amish cultural context and may need to adjust the normal routines of diagnosis and therapy to fit Amish clients' socioreligious context.

## HEALTH-CARE PRACTICES

### Health-seeking Beliefs and Behaviors

Amish believe that the body is the temple of God and that human beings are the stewards of their bodies. This fundamental belief is based on the Genesis account of creation (Hostetler, 1993). Medicine and health care should always be used with the understanding that it is God who heals. Nothing in the Amish understanding of the Bible forbids them from using preventive or curative medical services. A prevalent myth among health-care professionals in Amish communities is that Amish are not interested in preventive services. Although it is true that many times the Amish do not use mainstream health services at the onset of recognized symptoms, they are highly involved in the practices of health promotion and illness prevention.

### Responsibility for Health Care

Amish believe that it is their responsibility to be personally involved in promoting health. As in most cultures, health-care knowledge is passed from one generation to the next through women. In the Amish culture, men are involved in major health-care decisions and often accompany the family to the chiropractor, physician, or hospital. Grandparents are frequently consulted about treatment options. In one situation, a scheduled consultation for a four-year-old was postponed until the maternal grandmother was well enough after a cholecystectomy to make the 3-hour automobile trip to the medical center.

A usual concern regarding responsibility for health care is payment for services. Many Amish do not carry any insurance, including health insurance. However, in most communities, there is some form of agreement for sharing losses caused by natural disasters as well as catastrophic illnesses. Some have formalized mutual aid, such as the Amish Aid Society. Wenger (1988) found that her informants were opposed to such formalized agreements and wanted to do all they could to live healthy and safe lives, which they believed would benefit their community in keeping with their Christian calling. Many hospitals have been astounded by the Amish practice of paying their bills despite financial hardship. Because of this generally positive community reputation, hospitals have been willing to set up payment plans for the larger bills. For a brief though comprehensive discussion on compulsory welfare and Amish beliefs and practices involving government programs such as social security, see Hostetler (1993), pages 270 to 273.

Active participation was found to be a major theme in Wenger's (1991b, 1994, 1995) study on cultural context, health, and care. The Amish want to be actively involved in health-care decision making, which is a part of daily living. "To do all one can to help oneself" involves seeking advice from family and friends, using herbs and other home remedies, and then choosing from a broad array of folk, alternative, and professional health-care services. One informant, who visited an Amish healer while considering her physician's recommendation that she have a computed axial tomography (CAT) scan to provide more data on her continuing vertigo, told the researcher, "I will probably have the CAT-scan, but I am not done helping myself and this [meaning the healer's treatment] may help and it won't hurt." In this study, health-care decision making was found to be influenced by three factors: (1) type of health problem, (2) accessibility of health-care services, and (3) perceived cost of the service. For a full description of these and other related factors, see Wenger (1994, 1995). When the Amish use professional health-care services, they want to be partners in their health care and want to retain their right to choose from all culturally sanctioned health-care options.

Caring within the Amish culture is synonymous with being Amish (Wenger, 1991b, 1991c). "It's the Amish way" translates into the expectation that members of the culture be aware of the needs of others and thus fulfill the biblical injunction to bear one another's burdens. Caring is a core value related to health and well-being. Care is expressed in culturally encoded expectations that they can best describe in their dialect as **abwaarde**, meaning "to minister to someone by being present and serving when someone is sick in bed." A more frequently used term for helping is **achtgewwe,** which means "to serve by becoming aware of someone's needs and then to act by doing things to help." Helping others is expressed in gender-related and age-related roles, *freindschaft* (the three-generational family), church district, community (including non-Amish), Amish settlements, and worldwide (Wenger & Wenger, 1988). No outsiders or health-care providers can be expected to understand fully this complex caring network, but health-care providers can learn about it in the local setting by establishing trust in relationships with their Amish clients.

When catastrophic illness occurs, the Amish community responds by being present, helping with chores, and relieving family members to be with the afflicted person in the acute-care hospital. Some do opt to accept medical advice regarding the need for high-technology treatment, such as transplants, or for other high-cost interventions. The client's family seeks prayers and advice from the bishop and deacons of their church and their family and friends, but the decision is generally a personal or family one.

Amish engage in self-medication. Although most Amish regularly visit physicians and use prescription drugs, they also use herbs and other nonprescription remedies, often simultaneously. When discussing the meaning of health and illness, Wenger (1988, 1994) found that her Amish informants considered it their responsibility to investigate their treatment options and to stay personally involved in the treatment process rather than to relegate their care to the judgment of the professional physician or nurse. Consequently, they seek testimonials from other family members and friends about what treatments work best. They may also seek care from Amish healers and other alternative-care practitioners who may suggest nutritional supplements. One informant told how she would take "blue cohosh" pills with her to the hospital when she was in labor because she believed that they would speed up the labor.

Because of the Amish practice of self-medication, it is essential that health-care providers inquire about the full range of remedies that are being used. For the Amish client to be candid, the provider must develop a context of mutual trust and respect. Within this context, the Amish client can feel assured that the professional wants to consider and negotiate the most advantageous yet culturally congruent care for them.

## Folk Practices

The Amish, like many other cultures, have an elaborate health-care belief system that includes traditional remedies passed from one generation to the next. They also use alternative health care that is shared by other Americans, though often not sanctioned by medical and other health-care professionals. Although the prevalence of specific health-care beliefs and practices, such as use of chiropractic, Western medical and health-care science, reflexology, iridology, osteopathy, homeopathy, and folklore, is influenced mainly by *freindschaft* (Egeland, 1967; Wenger, 1991b), variations depend on geographic region and the conservatism of the Amish community.

Herbal remedies include those handed down by successive generations of mothers and daughters. One elderly grandmother showed the researcher the cupboard where she kept some cloths soaked in a herbal remedy and shared the recipe for it (Wenger, 1988). She stated that the cupboard was where she remembers her grandmother keeping those same remedies when her grandmother lived in the *daadihaus,* the grandparent's cottage attached to the family farmhouse where her daughter and son-in-law live. She also confided that, although she prepared the herb-soaked cloths for her daughters when they married, she thinks they opt for more modern treatments, such as herb pills and prescription drugs. This is a poignant example of the effect of modern health care on a highly contextual culture.

"Of all Amish folk health care, **brauche** has claimed the most interest of outsiders, who are often puzzled by its historical origins and contemporary application" (Wenger, 1991a, p. 87). *Brauche* is a folk-healing art that was practiced in Europe around the time of the Amish immigration to America. It was not unique to the Amish but was a common healing art used among Pennsylvania Germans (Yoder, 1972). As with some other European practices, the Amish have retained *brauche* in some communities. In other communities, the practice is considered suspect, and it has been the focus of some church divisions.

*Brauche* is sometimes referred to as sympathy curing or powwowing. It is unrelated to American Indian powwowing, and the use of this English term to refer to the German term *brauche* is unclear. In most literary descriptions of sympathy curing, it refers to the use of words, charms, and physical manipulations for treating some human and animal maladies. In some communities, the Amish refer to brauche as "warm hands," the ability to feel when a person has a headache or a baby has colic. Informants describe situations where some persons can "take" the stomach ache from the baby into their own bodies in what is described by researchers as transference. Wenger (1991b, 1994) stated that all informant families volunteered information about *brauche,* using that term or "warm hands" to describe folk healing. One informant asked the author if she could "feel" it, too.

A few folk illnesses have no Western scientific equivalents. The first is **ab-nemme,** which refers to a condition where the child fails to thrive and appears puny. Specific treatments given to the child may include incantations. Some of the older people remember these treatments, and some informants remember having been taken to a healer for the ailment. The second is **aagwachse** or livergrown, meaning "hide-bound" or "grown together," that was once a common ailment among Pennsylvania Germans (Hostetler, 1993). Symptoms include crying and abdominal discomfort that is believed to be caused by jostling in rough buggy rides. Wenger (1988) reported accompanying an informant with her newborn baby to an Amish healer, and the woman carried the baby on a pillow because she believed the baby to be suffering from *aagwachse.* As stated previously, Amish clients are more likely to discuss folk beliefs and practices with professionals if the nurse or physician gives cues that it is acceptable to do so.

## Barriers to Health Care

Most barriers to health care have been covered elsewhere in this chapter. They include delay in seeking professional health care at the onset of symptoms, occasional overuse of home remedies, and a prevailing preception that health-care professionals are not interested in or may disapprove of the use of home remedies and other alternative treatment modalities. Additionally, some families may live at a great distance from professional health-care services, making travel by horse and buggy difficult or inadvisable. Because in some Amish communities such as the Old Order Amish telephones are not permitted in the home, there may be delays in communication with Amish clients. Finally, the cost of health care without health insurance can deter early access to professional care, which could result in more complex treatment regimens.

## Cultural Responses to Health and Illness

The Amish are unlikely to display pain and physical discomfort. The health-care provider may need to remind the Amish client that medication is available for pain relief if they choose to accept it.

Community for the Amish means inclusion of persons who are chronically ill or "physically or mentally different." Amish culture approaches these differences as a community responsibility. Children with mental or physical differences are sometimes referred to as "hard learners," who are expected to go to school and be incorporated into the classes with assistance from other student "scholars" and parents. A culturally congruent approach is for the family and others to help engage those with differences in work activities, rather than to leave them sitting around and getting more anxious or depressed.

Hostetler (1993) stated "that Amish themselves have developed little explicit therapeutic knowledge to deal with cases of extreme anxiety" (p. 332). They do seek help from trusted physicians, and some are admitted to mental health centers or clinics. However, the mentally ill are generally cared for at home whenever possible. Studies of clinical depression and manic-depressive illness were discussed in the section on biologic ecology.

As previously mentioned, when persons are sick, other family members take on additional responsibilities. Little ceremony is associated with being sick, and persons know that to be healthy means to assume one's role within the family and community. Caring for the sick is highly valued, but at the same time, receiving help is accompanied by feelings of humility. Amish newsletters abound with notices of thanks from persons who were ill. A common expression is, "I am not worthy of it all." A care set identified in one research study is that giving care is a privilege and an obligation and that receiving care involves both expectation and humility (Wenger, 1991b). The sick role is mediated by very strong values related to giving and receiving care.

The Amish culture also sanctions time out for illness when sick persons are relieved of their responsibilities by others who minister to their needs. A good analogy to the communal care of the ill is found in the support offered by family and church at the time of bereavement, as noted in the section on dying. The informal social support network is an important factor in the individual's sense of well-being. An underlying expectation, however, is that healthy persons will want to resume active work and social roles as soon as their recovery permits. With reasonable adjustments for age and physical ability, it is understood that a healthy person is actively engaged in work, worship, and social life of the family and community (Wenger, 1994). Work and rest are kept in balance, but for the Amish, the accumulation of days or weeks of free time or time off for vacation outside the framework of normal routines and social interactions is a foreign idea.

## Blood Transfusion and Organ Donation

There are no cultural or religious rules or taboos that prohibit Amish from accepting blood transfusions or organ transplantation and donation. In fact, with the genetic presence of hemophilia, blood transfusion has been a necessity for some families. Anecdotal evidence is available regarding persons who have received heart and kidney transplants, although no research reports or other written accounts were found. Thus, some Amish may opt for organ transplantation after the family seeks advice from church officials, extended family, and friends, but the final decision is generally made by the patient or immediate family.

## HEALTH-CARE PRACTITIONERS

### Traditional Versus Biomedical Care

Amish usually refer to their own healers by name rather than by title, although some say *brauch-doktor* or **braucher.** In some communities, both men and women provide these services. They may even specialize, with some being especially good with bedwetting, nervousness, women's problems, or livergrown. Some set up treatment rooms and people come early in the morning and wait long hours to be seen. They do not charge fees but do accept donations. A few also treat non-Amish clients. In some communities, Amish folk healers use a combination of treatment modalities, including physical manipulation, massage, *brauche,* herbs and teas, and reflexology. A few have taken short courses in reflexology or therapeutic massage.

In a few cases, their practice has been reported to the legal authorities by persons in the medical profession or others who were concerned about the potential for illegal practice of medicine. Huntington (1993) chronicled several cases, including those of Solomon Wickey and Joseph Helmuth, both in Indiana. Both men continue to practice with some carefully designed restrictions.

### Status of Health Care Providers

For the Old Order Amish, health-care practitioners are always outsiders because thus far this sect has been unwilling to allow their members to attend medical, nursing, or other health-related professional schools or to seek higher education in general. Therefore, the Older Order Amish must learn to trust persons outside their culture for health care and medically related scientific knowledge. Hostetler (1993) contends that the Amish live in a state of liminality when securing health-care services. They rely on their own tradition to diagnose and sometimes treat illnesses, while simultaneously seeking technical and scientific services from health-care professionals.

Most Amish consult within their community to learn about physicians, dentists, and nurses with whom they can develop trusting relationships. For more information on this practice, see the Amish informants' perceptions of caring physicians and nurses in Wenger's chapter and article on health and health-care decision making

(1994, 1995). Amish prefer professionals who discuss their health-care options, giving consideration to cost, need for transportation, family influences, and scientific information. They also like to discuss the efficacy of alternative methods of treatment, including folk care. When asked, many Amish, like other persons from diverse cultures, claim that professionals do not want to hear about nontraditional health-care modalities that do not reflect dominant American health-care values.

Amish hold all health-care providers in high regard. Health is integral to their religious beliefs, and care is central to their worldview. They tend to place trust in people of authority when they fit their values and beliefs. Because Amish are not sophisticated in their knowledge of physiology and scientific health care, the health-care professional who gains their trust should bear in mind that because the Amish respect authority, they may unquestioningly follow orders. Therefore, health-care providers should make sure that their clients understand instructions. Role modeling and other concrete teaching strategies are recommended to enhance understanding.

## CASE STUDY

Elmer and Mary Miller, both 35 years old, live with their five children in the main house on the family farmstead in one of the largest Amish settlements in Indiana. Aaron and Annie Schlabach, aged 68 and 70, live in the attached grandparents' cottage. Mary is the youngest of their eight children, and when she married, she and Elmer moved into the grandparents' cottage with the intention that Elmer would take over the farm when Aaron wanted to retire.

Eight years ago they traded living space, and now Elmer continues to help with the farm work, despite increasing pain in his hip, which the doctor advises should be replaced. Most of Mary and Elmer's siblings live in the area, though not in the same church district or settlement. Two of Elmer's brothers and their families recently moved to Tennessee, where farms are less expensive and where they are helping to start a new church district.

Mary and Elmer's fifth child, Melvin, was born 6 weeks prematurely and is 1 month old. Sarah, aged 13; Martin, aged 12; and Wayne, aged 8, attend the Amish elementary school located 1 mile from their home. Lucille, aged 4, is staying with Mary's sister and her family for a week because baby Melvin was having respiratory problems, and their physician told the family he will need to be hospitalized if he does not get better within 2 days.

At the doctor's office, Mary suggested to one nurse, who often talks with Mary about "Amish ways," that Menno Martin, an Amish man who "gives treatments," may be able to help. He uses "warm hands" to treat people and is especially good with babies because he can feel what is wrong. The nurse noticed that Mary carefully placed the baby on a pillow as she prepared to leave.

Elmer and Mary do not carry any health insurance and are concerned about paying the doctor and hospital associated with this complicated pregnancy. In addition, they have an appointment for Wayne to be seen at Riley Children's Hospital, 3 hours away at the University Medical Center in Indianapolis, for a recurring cyst located behind his left ear. Plans are being made for a driver to take Mary, Elmer, Wayne, Aaron, Annie, and two of Mary's sisters to Indianapolis for the appointment. Because it is on the way, they plan to stop in Fort Wayne to see an Amish healer who gives nutritional advice and does "treatments." Aaron, Annie, and Elmer have been there before, and the other women are considering having treatments, too. Many Amish and non-Amish go there and tell others how much better they feel after the treatments.

They know their medical expenses seem minor in comparison to the family who last week lost their barn in a fire and to the young couple whose 10-year-old child had brain surgery after a fall from the hay loft. Elmer gave money to help with the expenses of the child and will go to the barn raising to help rebuild the barn. Mary's sisters will help to cook for the barn raising, but Mary will not help this time because of the need to care for her newborn.

The state health department is concerned about the low immunization rates in the Amish communities. One community health nurse who works in the area where Elmer and Mary live has volunteered to talk with Elmer, who is on the Amish School Board, to learn about how the health department could work more closely with the Amish and also learn more about what the people know about immunizations. The county health commissioner thinks this is a waste of time and what they need to do is let the Amish know that they are creating a health hazard by neglecting or refusing to immunize their children.

## STUDY QUESTIONS

1. Develop three open-ended questions or statements you would use in learning from Mary and Elmer what health and caring mean to them and to the Amish culture.

2. List four or five areas of perinatal care that you would want to discuss with Mary.

3. Why do you think Mary placed the baby on a pillow as she was leaving the doctor's office?

4. If you were the nurse to whom Mrs. Miller confided her interest in taking the baby to the folk healer, how would you learn more about their simultaneous use of folk and professional health services?

5. List three items to discuss with the Millers to prepare them for their consultation at the Medical Center.

6. If you were preparing the reference for consultation, what would you mention about the Millers that would help to promote culturally congruent care at the medical center?

7. Imagine yourself participating in a meeting with state and local health department officials and several local physicians and nurses to develop a plan to increase the immunization rates in the counties with large Amish populations. What would you suggest as ways to accomplish this goal?

8. Discuss two reasons many Old Order Amish choose not to carry health insurance.

9. Name three health problems with genetic linkages that are prevalent in some Amish communities.

10. How might health-care providers use the Amish values of the three-generational family and their visiting patterns in promoting health in the Amish community?

11. List three Amish values to consider in prenatal education classes.

12. Develop a nutritional guide for Amish women who are interested in losing weight. Consider Amish values, daily lifeways, and food production and preparation patterns.

13. List three ways in which Amish express caring.

## References

Allen, F. (1989, September 20). Country doctor: How a physician solved riddle of rare disease in children of Amish. *Wall Street Journal*, pp. 1, A16.

Armstrong, P. & Feldman, S. (1986). *A midwife's story*. New York: Arbor House.

Bender, H. S. & Smith, C. H. (Eds.). (1956). *The Mennonite encyclopedia* (Vols. 1–4). Scottdale, PA: Mennonite Publishing House.

Boehm, F. E. A prayer for the dying. (1995, March 2). *The Atlanta Journal-Constitution*, p. 15.

Bowman, H. S. & Procopio, J. (1963). Hereditary non-sperocytic hemolytic anemia of the pyruviate kinase deficient type. *Annals of Internal Medicine, 58,* 561–591.

Detera-Wadleigh, S. D., et al. (1987). Close linkage of C harvey ras-1 and insulin gene to affective disorder is ruled out in three North American pedigrees. *Nature, 325,* 806–808.

Egeland, J.A. (1967). Belief and behavior as related to illness: A community case study of the Old Order Amish (Doctoral dissertation, Yale University). *American Doctoral Dissertation,* 1996–1967, p. 250.

Enninger, W. & Wandt, K-H. (1982). Pennsylvania German in the context of an Old Order Amish settlement. *Yearbook of German-American Studies 17,* 123–143.

Ericksen, J. A., Ericksen, E. P., Hostetler, J. A., & Huntington, G. E. (1979). Fertility patterns and trends among the Old Order Amish. *Population Studies, 33*(2), 255–275.

Ericksen, J. A. & Klein, G. L. (1981). Women's roles and family production among the Old Order Amish. *Rural Sociology, 46*(2), 282–296.

Fuchs, J. A., et al. (1990). Health risk factors among Amish: Results of a survey. *Health Education Quarterly, 17*(2), 197–211.

Ginns, E. D., et al. (1992). Update on the search for DNA markers linked to manic-depressive illness in the Old Order Amish. *Journal of Psychiatric Research, 26*(4), 305–308.

Haag, C. (1982). *A Pennsylvania-German reader and grammar.* University Park, PA: Pennsylvania State University Press.

Hall, E. T. (1976). *Beyond culture.* Garden City, NJ: Anchor Press.

Heikes, J. (1985). *Differences among the Old Order Amish of Wayne County, Ohio, and their use of health care services.* Unpublished master's thesis, Ohio State University, Columbus, OH.

Hodgkinson, S., et al. (1987). Molecular genetic evidence for heterogeneity in manic depression. *Nature, 325,* 805–806.

Hostetler, J. A. (1993). *Amish society,* (4th ed.). Baltimore, MD: John Hopkins University Press.

Hostetler, J. A. & Huntington, G. E. (1992). *Amish children: Education in the family, school, and community* (2nd ed.). Dallas: Harcourt Brace Jovanovich College Publishers.

Huffines, M. L., (1994). Amish languages. In J. R. Dow, W. Enninger, & J. Raith (Eds.), *Internal and external perspectives on Amish and Mennonite life 4: Old and new world Anabaptist studies on the language, culture, society and health of Amish and Mennonites* (pp. 21–32). Essen, Germany: University of Essen.

Huntington, G. E. (1987, November). *Cultural interaction during times of crises: Permeable boundaries and Amish cultural success.* Paper presented at annual meeting of the American Anthropological Association, Chicago.

Huntington, G. E. (1988). The Amish family. In C. Mindel & R. Haberstein (Eds.), *Ethnic families in America,* (3rd ed.) (pp. 367–399). New York: Elsevier.

Huntington, G. E. (1993). Health care. In D. B. Kraybill (Ed.), *The Amish and the state.* Baltimore, MD: The Johns Hopkins University Press.

Jones, M. W. (1990). A study of trauma in an Amish community. *Journal of Trauma, 30*(7), 899–902.

Kaiser, G. H. (1986). *Dr. Frau: A woman doctor among the Amish.* Intercourse, PA: Good Books.

Kelsoe, J. R., Ginns, E. D., Egeland, J. A., et al. (1989). Re-evaluation of the linkage relationship between chromosome 11p loci and the gene for bipolar affective disorder in the Old Order Amish. *Nature, 342,* 338–342.

Kelsoe, J. R., Kristobjanarson, H., Bergesch, P., et al. (1993). A genetic linkage study of bipolar disorder and 13 markers on chromosome 11 including the D2 dopamine receptor, *Neuropsychopharmocology, 9*(4), 293–307.

Ketterling, R. P., Bottema, C. D., Koberl, D. D., Setsuko Ii, & Sommer, S. S. (1991). T$^{296}$M, a common mutation causing mild hemophilia B in the Amish and others: Founder effect, variability in factor IX activity assays, and rapid carrier detection. *Human Genetics, 87,* 333–337.

Kraybill, D. R. (1989). *The riddle of Amish culture.* Baltimore, MD: The Johns Hopkins University Press.

Kraybill, D. R. (1993). *The Amish and the state.* Baltimore, MD: The Johns Hopkins University Press.

Kraybill, D. R. & Olshan, M. A. (1994). *The Amish struggle with modernity.* Hanover, NH: University Press of New England.

Law, A., Richard III, C. W., Cottingham, R. W. Jr., Lathrop, M. G., Cox, D. R., & Myers, R. M. (1992). Genetic linkage analysis of bipolar affective disorder in an Old Order Amish pedigree. *Human Genetics, 88,* 562–568.

Lucas, C. A., O'Shea, R. M., Zielezny, M. A., Freudenheim, J. L., & Wold, J. F. (1991). Rural medicine and the closed society. *New York State Journal of Medicine, 91*(2), 49–52.

Martin, P. H., Davis, L., & Askew, D. (1965). High incidence of phenylketonuria in an isolated Indiana community. *Journal of the Indiana State Medical Association, 56,* 997–999.

McKusick, V. A. (1978). *Medical genetics studies of the Amish: Selected papers assembled with commentary.* Baltimore, MD: The Johns Hopkins University Press.

McKusick, V. A., Egeland, J. A., Eldridge, D., & Krusen, E. E. (1964). Dwarfism in the Amish I. The Ellis-van Creveld syndrome. *Bulletin of the Johns Hopkins Hospital, 115,* 306–330.

McKusick, V. A., Eldridge, R., Hostetler, J. A., Ruanquit, U., & Egeland, J. A. (1965). Dwarfism in the Amish II. Cartilage hair hypoplasia. *Bulletin of the Johns Hopkins Hospital, 116,* 285–326.

Meyers, T. J. (1983). *Stress and the Amish community in transition.* Unpublished doctoral dissertation, Boston University.

Meyers, T. J. (1993). Education and schooling. In D. Kraybill (Ed.), *The Amish and the state* (pp. 87–106). Baltimore, MD: The Johns Hopkins University Press.

Meyers, T. J. (1994a). Lunch pails and factories. In D. R. Kraybill & M. A. Olshan (Eds.), *The Amish struggle with modernity* (pp. 165–181). Hanover, NH: University Press of New England.

Meyers, T. J. (1994b). The Old Order Amish: To remain or to leave. *Mennonite Quarterly Review, 68,* 378–395.

Morton, D. H., Bennett, M. J., Seargeant, L. E., Nichter, C. A., & Kelly, R.I. (1991). Glutaric aciduria type I: A common cause of episodic encephalopathy and spastic paralysis in the Amish of Lancaster County, Pennsylvania. *American Journal of Medical Genetics, 41,* 89–95.

Nolt, S. (1992). *A history of the Amish.* Intercourse, PA: Good Books.

Olshan, M. A. (1991). The opening of Amish society: Cottage industry as a trojan horse. *Human Organization, 50*(4), 378–384.

Olshan, M. A. (1993). The national Amish steering committee. In D. B. Kraybill, *The Amish and the state,* (pp. 67–84). Baltimore: The Johns Hopkins University Press.

Pauls, D. L., Morton, L. A., & Egeland, J. A. (1992). Risks of affective illness among first-degree relatives of bipolar and Old Order Amish probands. *Archives of General Psychiatry, 49,* 703–708.

Ratnoff, O. D. (1958). Hereditary defects in clotting mechanisms. *Advances in Internal Medicine, 9,* 107–179.

Tripp-Reimer, T. & Schrock, M. (1982). Residential patterns of ethnic aged: Implications for transcultural nursing. In C. Uhl, & J. Uhl (Eds.), *Proceedings of the Seventh Annual Transcultural Nursing Conference* (pp. 144–153). Salt Lake City: University of Utah, Transcultural Nursing Society.

Tripp-Reimer, T., Sorofman, B., Lauer, G.,

Martin, M., & Afifi, L. (1988). *Journal of Cross-Cultural Gerontology, 3* 185–195.

Troyer, H. (1994). Medical considerations of the Amish. In J. R. Dow, W. Enninger, & J. Raith (Eds.), *Internal and external perspectives on Amish and Mennonite life 4: Old and new world Anabaptist studies on the language, culture, society and health of the Amish and Mennonites* (pp. 68–87). Essen, Germany: University of Essen.

Wenger, A. F. (1980, October). *Acceptability of perinatal services among the Amish.* Paper presented at a March of Dimes Symposium, Future Directions in Perinatal Care, Baltimore, MD.

Wenger, A. F. Z. (1988). The phenomenon of care in a high context culture: The Old Order Amish (Doctoral dissertation, Wayne State University, 1988), *Dissertation Abstracts International,* 50/02B.

Wenger, A. F. Z. (1991a). Culture-specific care and the Old Order Amish. *Imprint, 38*(2), 81–82, 84, 87, 93.

Wenger, A. F. Z. (1991b). The culture care theory and the Old Order Amish. In M.M. Leininger (Ed.), *Cultural care diversity and universality: A theory of nursing* (pp. 147–178). New York: National League for Nursing.

Wenger, A. F. Z. (1991c). The role of context in culture-specific care. In P. L. Chinn (Ed.), *Anthology of caring* (pp. 95–110). New York: National League for Nursing.

Wenger, A. F. Z. (1994). Health and healthcare decision-making: The Old Order Amish. In J. R. Dow, W. Enninger, & J. Raith (Eds.), *Internal and external perspectives on Amish and Mennonite life 4: Old and New World Anabaptists studies on the language, culture, society and health of the Amish and Mennonites* (pp. 88–110). Essen, Germany: University of Essen.

Wenger, A. F. Z. (1995). Cultural context, health and healthcare decision-making. *Journal of Transcultural Nursing. 7*(1), 3–14.

Wenger, A. F. Z. & Wenger, M. R. (1988). Community and family care patterns of the Old Order Amish. In M. Leininger, *Care: Discovery and uses in clinical and community nursing* (pp. 39–54). Detroit: Wayne State University Press.

Wenger, M. R. (1970). *A Swiss German dialect study: Three linguistic islands in midwestern USA.* Ann Arbor, MI: University Microfilms.

What is in a language? (1986, February). *Family Life,* p. 12.

Wolkomir, R., & Wolkomir, J. (1991, July). The doctor who conquered a killer, *Readers Digest, 139,* 161–166.

Yoder, D. (1972). Folk medicine (pp. 191–215). In R. M. Dorson (Ed.), *Folklore and life.* Chicago: University of Chicago Press.

# Appalachians

*Larry D. Purnell and Mona Counts*

---

• Key terms to become familiar with in this chapter are:

| | |
|---|---|
| Appalachian Regional Commission | Home |
| Asafetida bag | Insider |
| Being | Low blood |
| Doing | Outsider |
| Fatalism | "Sit a spell" |
| High blood | |

## OVERVIEW, INHABITED LOCALITIES, AND TOPOGRAPHY

### Overview

Appalachians have only recently been identified as a specific cultural group. The name *Appalachia* is derived from the Apalache Indians who inhabited much of the area known today as the Appalachian Mountain Region of the United States. DeSoto gave the region its name when he got lost in the Appalachian Mountains in 1569 (McNeil, 1989). The term *Appalachian* is used in this chapter to describe the people born in the region and their descendants who live in or near the Appalachian Mountain range. Appalachians generally characterize themselves according to their family name and by their county of origin. People living in this area have been called "our contemporary ancestors" (Cunningham, 1987), "mountain people" (Hitch, 1989), "yesterday's people" (Miles, 1975), "the invisible minority" (Obermiller & Malong, 1994A; Wenger, 1987), "the neglected minority" (Simon, 1987; Tripp-Reimer & Freidl, 1977), and "Elizabethans" (Wilson, 1987).

During the 1960s through the 1980s, much was written about Appalachia, but no consensus exists as to what characteristics properly belong to the culture, or even whether such a culture exists (Marger & Obermiller, 1987). Many authors have represented the people of Appalachia in negative terms, and some writings have generalized characteristics of small groups to Appalachians in general. These generalizations and negativism are not representative of the people or culture as a whole. During the 1970s, sociocultural studies of the people of Appalachian heritage living outside the region implied that they have a unique set of values and beliefs. Such studies resulted in the view that Appalachians could be considered a distinct ethnic group (Obermiller & Philliber, 1987), and the term "urban Appalachian" replaced the term "Appalachian migrant" (Cunningham, 1987). In 1970, the Appalachian Identity Center, operated by people from Appalachia, was established in Cincinnati, Ohio, to provide support and play an advocacy role for migrants from rural Appalachia. In 1979, the Appalachian Urban Council came into existence to increase the availability of university and community resources to Appalachians (Wenger, 1987).

Despite the variations among groups within this large geographic region, there are similarities in beliefs and practices of individuals and families who are descendants of the people who first settled this area from the 17th through 19th centuries. Therefore, health-care providers must look not only at the dominant values but also the variant characteristics of this group (Tripp-Reimer, 1982) and use them as a guide when providing health-care services. Intraethnic variations such as socioeconomic status, religion, education, gender, military status, rural versus urban residence, age, and generation require that each person be assessed individually rather than being stereotyped.

The Appalachian region is federally defined according to the *Appalachian Regional Commission* (ARC) and comprises 397 counties in 13 states—Georgia, Alabama, Mississippi, Virginia, West Virginia, North Carolina, South Carolina, Kentucky, Tennessee, Ohio, Maryland, New York, and Pennsylvania. In addition, the region is divided into Southern Appalachia, Central Appalachia, and Northern Appalachia. West Virginia is the only state entirely within Appalachia. The vast majority of the Appalachian region is rugged, mountainous terrain that is partially responsible for its residents' values and traditions. The reality of Appalachian existence is a deep-seated work ethic, low cost of living, and high quality of life. Yet the perception is a "cabin in the woods, with a tireless car sitting in the yard" (Casto, 1993, p. 34). Appalachians are loyal, caring, family-oriented, religious, hardy, independent, honest, patriotic, and resourceful (Marger & Obermiller, 1987).

In some areas of Appalachia, insufficient roads, public bus transportation systems, rail transportation systems, and airports prevent easy access. One county in the center of Appalachia has the largest land mass of any county east of the Mississippi and has no public transportation. No Standard Metropolitan Statistical Area exists in the entire state of West Virginia. Difficulty in accessing the area is partially responsible for continued geographic and sociocultural isolation. Even though the Appalachian region includes several large cities, a significant number of people live in settlements of less than 2500 with rugged roads that separate people and, thus, help to preserve their identity (Cunningham, 1987).

Readers interested in additional sources about the nonhealth-related cultural beliefs of Appalachian people are referred to books such as *She Walks These Hills*, *The Hangman's Beautiful Daughter*, *Bimbos of the Death Sun*, *If Ever I Return*, *Pretty Peggy-O*, *Sick of Shadows*, *Macpherson's Lament*, *The Dollmaker*, and the *Foxfire* series. In addition, the movie *Deerhunter* and the television series *Christy* depict Appalachian mountain culture.

## Heritage and Residence

Most Appalachians trace their heritage to Scotland, Ireland, Wales, England, Germany, and France (Neely, 1987). Most native Appalachians identify a family link with Native-Americans who populated the area before them. Historically, the population has been predominantly white, with only 3.2 percent of the population of black descent (Marger & Obermiller, 1987). Within the last 30 years, an increase has occurred in other ethnically and culturally diverse populations moving into the Appalachian region.

## Reasons for Migration and Associated Economic Factors

Initially, people migrated to Appalachia for religious freedom to practice their beliefs (Tripp-Reimer, 1982). They wanted to have space for themselves and away from each other. When people migrate from Appalachia into larger urban settings, the migration pattern is a regional one, where individuals from one area primarily migrate to the same areas as their relatives and friends (Wenger, 1987). This regional migration pattern provides a supportive network of family and friends that is important for the culture of Appalachians and serves as a network for obtaining employment in new locations (Borman & Obermiller, 1994). The limited opportunities for employment often require the wage earner to leave the family at home while working elsewhere, returning home as frequently as resources allow. The Appalachian concept of "home" is associated with the land and the family, not a physical structure. The average Appalachian moves no farther than 30 miles from the family of origin (Counts, 1994). During the decades of the 1940s through the 1960s, 7 million people migrated in and out of the Appalachian region (Brown & Hillary, 1963). Since 1950, 3.5 million people have migrated to northern cities where they "live city" and "feel country" (Obermiller & Malong, 1994A). Today, significant migration in and out of the region continues, but the great migration is over and the number of people migrating into the area approximates the number of people migrating out (Philliber, 1987), resulting in the relative stabilization of the Appalachian population at approximately 24 million (Obermiller & Oldendick, 1987; Simon, 1987). During the 1960s, the ARC appropriated funds for building roads to attract industry and provided loans for residents to start their own businesses. Since that time, there has been a greater propensity for migration (peaking in the 1950s) from the mountains to urban areas (DeStafano, 1994). Unemployment continues to be above the national average, with some Appalachian rural areas having rates as high as 37 to 50 percent (Russell & Rocha, 1993).

Migration patterns reflect the economic conditions found in Appalachia and some of the Appalachian values of home, connections to the land, and importance of the family. Working-age persons move to "make their living" and return to the area to "retire." Because of these patterns, Appalachia has the highest existing aging population and the highest returning aging population of any region. The pattern of returning home to retire has given rise to challenges for health-care delivery with the aging population. A Johns Hopkins physician, Dr. Henry Taylor, who works and lives in Central Appalachia, is quoted as saying, "We are five years ahead of the rest of America in the proportion of aging people; we can develop the models for care."

The Appalachian region has a large population living in poverty and working in low-paying jobs. In fact, many areas in Appalachia are poorer today than they were three and four decades ago. This increase in poverty can be attributed to changing industrial patterns and the decrease in coal mining and timbering in the area (Flaskerud, 1984).

The original economic base of Appalachia consisted of extractive industries that were headquartered outside the area. The depletion of natural resources and changes in the utilization of resources has led to the current poor economic base. The increase in poverty may also be partially attributed to increasing standards in society, a heightened awareness regarding poverty in our society, and the overall rate of poverty in the United States, which now approaches 15.1 percent of the population (*U.S. Statistical Abstracts*, 1995).

## Educational Status and Occupations

The original immigrants to this area were highly educated on arrival, but limited formal education resulted in isolation of later generations from mainstream society (Jones, 1983). This led to a disparity in educational and health-care facilities despite the value placed on education. Knowledge of the larger society and what could be made available to Appalachians was greatly depressed due to limited educational stimulus during the early part of this century (Wheeler, 1994). Educational disparities have resulted in a dichotomous population of persons who are either poorly educated or extremely well-educated.

Continued education beyond elementary levels is not considered important by some because it is perceived not to be needed to earn a living. Many parents do not value the importance of continuing formal education for their children because it was not necessary for them in their traditional occupations (Obermiller & Malong, 1994A). In addition, many Appalachian parents do not want their children influenced by mainstream American values (Hooker, 1987). Parents who value education encourage their children to seek quality education at the best institutions possible. However, those who return to the area highly educated are often unable to secure suitable employment.

Today in Appalachia IQ scores of children are higher by 10 points at all ages than in previous decades. In a study of Tennessee mountain children, the greatest improvement in IQ test performance occurred in children between the ages of 6 and 15 years, with the increase in IQ gain being the largest in students who had access to larger schools. However, in those instances where formal education was stopped, the average child who had an IQ of 94.7 at age 6 years experienced a drop to 73.5 by the age of 16 years. This drop is attributed to the decreased educational stimuli in the rural environment (Wheeler, 1994).

Fewer children drop out of school today than in previous decades (Obermiller & Malong, 1994A). The high-school dropout rate for Appalachian youths in 1980 was 27 percent, and in 1989, the dropout rate decreased to 17 percent (Penn, Borman, & Hoeweler, 1994), which is still higher than that evidenced in other cultural or ethnic groups in the area. Edwards, Lenz, and East-Odom (1993) reported a high school dropout rate of 36 percent. Because of the high cultural value placed on cars and trucks, several states within the Appalachian region have laws that tie driving privileges to completion of schooling, which has influenced dropout rates significantly. No change has occurred in graduation rates from college; they remain at 36 percent as compared with 45 percent for their non-Appalachian counterparts (Penn, Borman, & Hoeweler, 1994). Throughout the region, the ARC sponsors programs such as Linking Education with Economic Development and Partnering with Parents for Successful Early Childhood Educational Project to increase educational performance at all levels (Hoffman, 1993). Factors such as improved mobility, access to better schools with qualified teachers, increased employment opportunities in some regions, and utilization of technology with access to the information highway are responsible for improved socioeconomic conditions and better performance on standard IQ tests. Educational levels of individuals within the Appalachian region vary (Maloney & Borman, 1987), and thus it is essential for the health-care provider to assess the educational status of individuals when providing health teaching. Educational materials and explanations must be presented at a level consistent with the client's capabilities and within each client's cultural framework and beliefs.

Original immigrants lived off the land, with subsistence farming providing the necessities for living. From the 1800s until the 1970s, mining was a major occupation for families for generations. With a decrease in the use of coal for factories and homes, unemployment increased. Predominant occupations in the region today are family subsistence farming, mining, timbering, textile manufacturing, furniture making, pottery making, crafts, automobile manufacturing (Obermiller & Malong, 1994B), fabricated materials, glass manufacturing, industrial machinery, and defense-related manufacturing (Hawthorne, 1994). Since the 1960s, an increased number of service industries and factories have moved into the area. Many of the industries that locate in the Appalachian region contribute to an increased risk for respiratory diseases (Obermiller & Smith, 1994). The recent surge in access to technology and the Internet has created new employment opportunities in high-technology industry for one segment of the population.

Appalachian whites are three times more likely to be of a lower socioeconomic status than non-Appalachian whites (Philliber & Obermiller, 1987). Most Appalachians work in semiskilled or unskilled jobs and lag behind others in educational and occupational attainment (Wenger, 1987). To improve employment opportunities, the ARC appropriated monies to establish hospitality training programs to prepare individuals for careers as janitors, maids, and waitresses, and for positions in tourist industries (Miles, 1975). These types of programs have caused a backlash because they encourage individuals to enter lower-paying occupations. Technical and community colleges in the Appalachian region have both day and evening classes to prepare individuals to seek steady employment in higher-paying occupations.

Being knowledgeable about the work backgrounds of Appalachians is essential for health screening and promotion to prevent, detect, and treat occupational illnesses. Health-care personnel must also examine personal beliefs, attitudes, and past experiences that may negatively affect care when working with clients who come from different socioeconomic or educational backgrounds.

# COMMUNICATIONS

## Dominant Language and Dialects

The dominant language of the Appalachian region is English, with many words antedating to sixteenth-century Saxon and Gaelic (Miles, 1975). Some insular groups in Appalachia speak Elizabethan English, which gives the area the appellation Elizabethan America (Wilson, 1989). Elizabethan English has its own distinctiveness and syntax that can cause communication difficulties with practitioners who are not familiar with the dialect. Some examples of variations in pronunciation for words are *allus* for "always," and *fit* for "fight." Word meanings that may be different include *poke* or *sack* for "paper bag," and *sass* for "vegetables." The Appalachian region is also noted for its use of strong preterits (Wilson, 1989) such as *clum* for "climbed," *drug* for "dragged," and *swelled* for "swollen." Plurals for monosyllabic words are formed like Chaucerian English, which adds *es* to the word. Examples include the following: "post" becomes *postes,* "beast" becomes *beastes,* "nest" becomes *nestes,* and "ghost" becomes *ghostes.* Many people, especially in the nonacademic environment, drop the *g* on words ending in *ing.* For example, "writing" becomes *writin,* "reading" becomes *readin,* and "spelling" becomes *spellin.* In addition, vowels may be pronounced with a diphthong that can cause difficulty to one unfamiliar with this dialect, which includes such variations in pronunciation as *poosh* for "push," *boosh* for "bush," warsh for "wash," *hiegen* for "hygiene," *deef* for "deaf," *welks* for "welts," *whar* for "where," *hit* for "it," *hurd* for "heard," and *your'n* for "your" (DeStafano, 1994). However, when the word is written, the meaning is apparent. Comparatives and superlatives are formed by adding a final *er* or *est,* making the word "bad" become *badder* and "preaching" become *preachin'est* (Wilson, 1989).

If the health-care practitioner is unfamiliar with the exact meaning of a word, it is best to ask the client to elaborate on the meaning. Otherwise, miscommunication can occur and result in an incorrect diagnosis. The health-care practitioner may want to have the person write the words (if the person has writing skills) to help prevent any error in communication.

## Cultural Communications Patterns

Appalachians practice the ethic of neutrality, which helps shape communication styles, worldview, and other aspects of the Appalachian culture. According to Barnett, et al. (1994), four dominant themes that affect communication patterns in the Appalachian culture are (1) avoiding aggression and assertiveness, (2) not interfering with others' lives, (3) avoiding dominance over others, and (4) avoiding arguments and seeking agreement.

Because Appalachians tend to accept others and do not want to judge others, they may use fewer adjectives and adverbs when speaking and writing. Thus, many

Appalachians may be less precise in describing emotions, be more concrete in conversations, and answer questions in a more direct manner (Simon, 1987). The health-care provider may need to use more open-ended questions when obtaining health information and eliciting opinions and beliefs about health-care practices.

Appalachians are private people who want to offend no one and may not easily trust or share their thoughts and feelings with *outsiders* (foreigners) (Flaskerud, 1980; Hitch, 1987; Lewis, Messner, & McDowell, 1985; Miles, 1975; Tripp-Reimer, 1982). They are likely to say what they think the listener wants to hear rather than what the listener should hear (Wigginton, 1971). In addition, many Appalachians dislike authority figures and institutions that attempt to control behavior. Individualism and self-reliant behavior are idealized; thus, personalism and individualism are admired, and people are accepted on the basis of their personal achievements and qualities and their family lineage.

Appalachians' perceptions of family and self influence many aspects of their communication style. The family is more than genetic relationships and has been described by some as the brothers, sisters, aunts, uncles, parents, grandparents, in-laws, and out-laws. The entire concept of self is "we." This perception of continuity transcends the concept of self as "I." The use of the pronoun we throughout speech patterns recognizes the concept of self. "We can make it," "We will survive," "We will be there" all may only refer to the person speaking; yet the pronoun we is used in place of I.

The interactions in an Appalachian community are illustrated by this story of a key informant from the Genesis project of Counts (1985 through 1994). Miss Ruth, a 94-year-old native Appalachian, was interviewed in the house in which she was born. She had had her appendix removed in the living room of this same house by a traveling nurse. After returning from a trip to Africa (she had a doctorate and liked to travel but always returned home), Miss Ruth described the concept of "neighboring" as a double-edged sword. The positive side is that when you are sick, everyone comes around to take care of you; however, on the negative side, when you try to do something quietly, everyone knows about it.

Appalachians may be sensitive to direct questions about personal issues. Sensitive topics are best approached with indirect questions and suggestions because individuals are often very sensitive to hints of criticism (Tripp-Reimer, 1982; Heath, 1983). Traditionally, Appalachians are taught to deny anger and not complain (Flaskerud, 1980). Information should be gathered in the context of broader relationships with respect for the ethic of equality, which implies more horizontal than hierarchical relationships, allowing for cordiality to precede information sharing. Starting with sensitive issues may invite ineffectiveness (Barnett, et al., 1994); thus, the health-care provider may need to "sit a spell" and "chat" before getting down to the business of collecting health information. To establish trust, the health-care provider must show interest in the client's family and other personal matters, drop hints instead of give orders, and solicit the client's opinions and advice. This increases self-worth and self-esteem and helps to establish the trust that is needed for effective working relationships. Health-care providers who are outsiders must be more attuned to these cultural patterns. An understanding of the relationships among Appalachian people and authority figures that have resulted from historical inequities assists in the health providers' acceptance of these differences.

Because Appalachians like personal space, they are more likely to stand at a distance when talking with people in both social and health-care situations. This physical distancing has its origins in religious persecution endured by this group in the earlier part of the century and has been perpetuated by isolationism, which encourages family members to become the main contact for individuals (Flaskerud, 1980).

Some Appalachians may perceive direct eye contact, especially from strangers, as aggression or hostility (Hooker, 1987). Because direct eye contact is considered impolite, they may avoid it when communicating their needs to outsider health-care providers (Flaskerud, 1980).

To communicate effectively with Appalachian clients, nonverbal behavior must be assessed within the contextual framework of the culture. Many Appalachians are comfortable with silence, and when talking with health-care providers who are outsiders, they are likely to speak without emotion, facial expression, or gestures (Flaskerud, 1980). Health-care providers unfamiliar with the culture may interpret these nonverbal communication patterns as not caring.

## Temporal Relationships

The traditional Appalachian culture is "being"-oriented as compared with "doing"-oriented. Individuals are usually more relaxed, are more in tune with body rhythms than time or clocks, and enjoy spontaneous activity (Lewis, Messner, & McDowell, 1985; Simon, 1987; Tripp-Reimer, 1982). For many engulfed in poverty and isolation due to the harsh terrain, the trend is to live for today, relying on tradition for things that they cannot control. This outlook on life is common with present-oriented temporal relationships where some higher power is in charge of life and its outcomes (Simon, 1987; Tripp-Reimer, 1982). As the area becomes more inundated with communication systems such as televisions, satellite dishes, and the information highway, temporal relationships are becoming more futuristic.

One may come early or late for an appointment and still expect to be seen. If individuals are not seen because they are late for an appointment and are asked to reschedule, they may not return because they may feel rejected by the health-care provider (Lewis, Messner, & McDowell, 1985). Many Appalachians are hesitant to make appointments because "somethin better might come up."

## Format for Names

Although the format for names in Appalachia follows the standard given name, or family name, individuals address nonfamily members by their last name. A common practice of respect for the elderly is to call persons by their first names with the title Miss or Mr., for example, Miss Lillian or Mr. Bill. Miss Lillian may or may not be married. There is also a need to link with both families of origin. Many times Appalachians refer to a female as *she was a __*. This links the families and enhances the feeling of continuity.

Health-care providers working with Appalachian families must adopt an attitude of respect and flexibility and demonstrate a willingness to listen. These behaviors demonstrate interest and help to bridge barriers imposed by the health-care providers' own personal ideologies and cultural values.

## FAMILY ROLES AND ORGANIZATION

### Head of Household and Gender Roles

The traditional Appalachian household is patriarchal (Flaskerud, 1980; Miles, 1975; McCoy & McCoy, 1987; Tripp-Reimer, 1982), with many families becoming more egalitarian in belief but not in practice (McCoy & McCoy, 1987). For many Appalachians, "a rift is set between the sexes at babyhood and it widens with the passing of years" (Miles, 1975, p. xxii). In previous decades, primarily because of family self-sufficiency and independence, gender roles were more clearly defined. However, for many families, women still take care of the house and assume responsibility for childrearing (Obermiller & Smith, 1994). Women are seen as the providers of emotional strength; older women are responsible for the preservation of the culture (Miles, 1975), have a lot of clout in health-care matters, and are usually the ones responsible for preparing herbal remedies and folk medicines. Men do work that requires manual strength and brings money home. When necessity requires, men, women, and children work side by side to make a living. A gradually changing gender role identification is heightened in urban settings.

Fewer women of Appalachian descent living in urban areas work outside the home and register to vote than do non-Appalachian women (McCoy & McCoy, 1994). In the urban setting, women's roles are disrupted more than men's roles. Eighty-two percent of Appalachian men do not believe women should work outside the home unless economic conditions necessitate this, nor should women have authority over men. Unmarried women are less confined in gender roles (McCoy & McCoy, 1994). Analysis of decision making in Appalachian households demonstrates that matriarchal decision making is perceived as the man's choice. In reality, females, especially older women and grandmothers, actually make the decisions, yet the men folk think they decide. With the advent of better access to education and improved roads throughout the Appalachian region, more women are working outside the home, thus creating an environment where gender roles may become less well-defined. In a survey of health-care professionals who participated in a cultural diversity conference in Chillicothe, Ohio, in June, 1994, many believed that their culture is progressing toward a more egalitarian household, especially if the female in the household makes more money than her male counterpart.

Appalachian women marry early, usually by the age of 20 years and men by the age of 28 years (McNeil, 1989), and Appalachian families are larger than non-Appalachian families in the rest of the United States. Several studies suggest that many do not formally marry to avoid loss of income from welfare sources.

## Prescriptive, Restrictive, and Taboo Behaviors for Children and Adolescents

Children are important to the Appalachian culture. Large families are common and children are accepted regardless of what they do (Helton, Barnes, & Borman, 1994). Publicly, parents impose strict conformity for fear of community censure and parental feelings of inferiority (Flaskerud, 1980). Permissive behavior at home is unacceptable, and hands-on physical punishment to a degree that some perceive as abuse is common.

For Appalachian children having problems with school performance, the most effective approach for increasing performance is individualized attention rather than group support or attention (Penn, Borman, & Hoeweler, 1994). To be effective with changing negative behavior, it is necessary to emphasize positive points.

As children progress into their teens, mischievous behavior is accepted but not condoned. Continuing formal education may not be stressed because many teens are expected to get a job to help support the family. Children are seen as being important, and to many, having a child, even at an early age, means fulfillment (Hansen & Resick, 1990). Motherhood increases the woman's status in the church and community (Horton, 1984). It is not uncommon for teenagers to marry by the age of 15 years, and some as early as 13 years (Fisher & Page, 1987; Borman & Steglin, 1994). Aid to Families with Dependent Children (commonly known as AFDC) reimbursement strategies encourage such behaviors in economically deprived areas. Children, single or married, may return to their parents' home, where they are readily accepted, whenever the need arises.

Many teens in Appalachia may be in a cultural dilemma with exposure to other beliefs outside the home and family. Health-care providers can assist adolescents and family members in working through these cultural differences by helping them to resolve personal conflicts in ways that convey respect for the family's culture; by discussing personal parenting practices; and by providing information about disease, illness, and treatments in culturally congruent ways.

## Family Roles and Priorities

Appalachian families take great pride in being independent and doing things for themselves. Even though economics may permit others to do some tasks, great pride is taken in being able to do for oneself. For many, family priorities include men getting a job to make a living and women bearing children (Horton, 1984). Because the nuclear and extended family are traditionally important (Crissman, 1987; Halperin, 1994; Hooker, 1987; McCoy & McCoy, 1994; Tripp-Reimer, 1982;) in the Appalachian culture, family members frequently live in close proximity. Relatives are frequently sought for advice on childrearing and most other aspects of life.

Elders are respected and honored in the Appalachian family. Grandparents frequently care for grandchildren, especially if both parents work. This child care is readily accepted and is an expectation in large extended families (Lewis, Messner, & McDowell, 1985). Elders usually live close to or with their children when they are no longer able to care for themselves. The physical structure of the home is designed to assist aging parents in maintaining function. Many adult children do not consider nursing home placement because, to many, it is the equivalent of a death sentence (Halperin, 1994). Migration of children out of the home area can cause a particular dilemma for the elderly (Rowles, 1983). Many elderly are forced to relocate outside their home area to be with their children. A dilemma occurs because they have an equally strong Appalachian value of attachment to place and family (Chovan & Chovan, 1985; LaFargue, 1980).

One's obligation to extended family outweighs the obligations to school or work (Halperin, 1994; McCoy & McCoy, 1994). The nuclear family feels a personal responsibility for nieces and nephews and readily takes in relatives when the need arises. This extended family is important regardless of the socioeconomic level (Hooker, 1987).

Crissman's study (1987) explored the family structural changes that occur with urban migration and found that the extended family remains dominant among rural Appalachians but that the nuclear family is dominant with urban Appalachians. This strong sense of family, where the family distrusts outsiders and values privacy, is responsible for some Appalachians' not getting involved in community activities or joining group activities (Mccoy & Mccoy, 1994).

The Appalachian family network can be a rich resource for the health-care provider when health teaching and assistance with personalized care is needed. For programs to be effective with Appalachians, support must begin with the family, specifically the grandmothers and immediate neighborhood activities (Penn, Borman, & Hoeweler, 1994). The health-care provider must respect each person as an individual and be nonbureaucratic in nature. The family rather than the individual must be considered as the basic treatment unit.

Social status is gained from having the respect of family and friends. Formal education and position do not gain one respect, which has to be earned by proving that one is a good person and "living right." Living right is based on the principles of the ethic of neutrality (Tripp-Reimer & Freidl, 1977; Wigginton, 1971; Wigginton & Bennett, 1984; Wigginton & Bennett, 1986). Having a job, regardless of what the work might be, is as important as having a prestigious position. Families are very proud of their family members and let the entire community know about their accomplishments. The health-care provider must respect Appalachian values even when they conflict with their own.

## Alternative Lifestyles

Alternative lifestyles are usually readily accepted in the Appalachian culture. Single and divorced parents are readily accepted into the extended family. Same-sex couples and families living together are accepted but rarely discussed. Such acceptance is congruent with the ethic of neutrality, the Appalachian need for privacy and not interfering with other's lives, avoiding arguments, and seeking agreement, even though agreement is not spoken.

## WORKFORCE ISSUES

### Culture in the Workplace

Because many Appalachians value family, reporting to work may take a backseat when a family member is ill or other family obligations are pressing. Liberal leave policies for funerals and family emergencies are essential for a positive work environment among traditional Appalachians. Because personal space is important, many Appalachians use a greater distance when communicating in the workplace. This practice should not interfere with positive working relationships when both parties understand each other's cultural behaviors. Appalachians prefer to work in a harmonious environment that fosters cooperation and agreement in decision making (Tripp-Reimer & Freidl, 1977). For many, the preferred work pattern is to work for a while, take time off, and then return to work. Work patterns may change for Appalachians, but the reality for Appalachians is a deep-seated work ethic (Castro, 1993). Professionals from other countries may have difficulty establishing rapport in the workplace because of outsidedness.

Appalachian individuals wish to maintain independent lifeways. Although on one hand they want progress, they also wish to remain isolated from the mainstream. More traditional groups may be slower to assimilate values of middle-class society into their work habits.

### Issues Related to Autonomy

The Appalachian ethic of neutrality and values of individualism with a strong people orientation may pose a dichotomous perception at work for outsiders who may not be familiar with Appalachian lifeways. However, when conflicts occur, mutual collaboration for seeking agreement is consistent with their ethic of neutrality. In addition, because many Appalachians align themselves more closely with horizontal rather than hierarchical relationships, they are sometimes reluctant to take on management roles. When Appalachians do accept management roles, they take great pride in their work and in the organization as a whole.

Most middle-class Americans gain self-actualization through work and personal involvement with doing. Appalachians seek fulfillment through kinship and neighborhood activities of being. To foster positive and mutually satisfying working relationships, organizations should capitalize on the individual strengths such as independence, sensitivity, and loyalty that are recognized in the Appalachian culture. Many Appalachians prefer to work at their own pace, devising their own work rules and methods to get the job done. Some factories and health-care facilities in the region who hire managers and administrators from outside the region provide educational seminars about the Appalachians' worldview, work culture, and lifeways to foster cultural sensitivity.

Once outsiders learn the Appalachian dialect and their ears become accustomed to the accent, the language barrier is minimized. Word meanings may differ, but this usually does not present a major problem. Because the Appalachian dialect tends to be more concrete than that of middle-class Americans (Simon, 1987), exposure to this dialect is necessary so that misunderstandings do not occur. Negative interpretations of Appalachian behaviors by non-Appalachian professionals can be detrimental to health-care working relationships (Tripp-Reimer, 1982).

## BIOCULTURAL ECOLOGY

### Skin Color and Biologic Variations

Since its first settlement, the Appalachian region has had a predominantly white population with little variation over time. Some individuals can trace their heritage to a mixture of white ancestry and Cherokee or Apalache Native-American Indian. A few blacks, a distinct minority of 3.2 percent, may identify themselves as Appalachian (Marger & Obermiller, 1994). The influence of Native-Americans can be seen in skin color.

### Diseases and Health Conditions

Many Appalachians live in cities with serious degradation and are affected disproportionately by environmental problems stemming from industrial pollution (Obermiller & Smith, 1994). The predominant occupations of farming, textile manufacturing, mining, furniture making, and timber industries place residents at an increased risk for respiratory diseases such as black lung, emphysema, and tuberculosis. People living in some rural areas that lack electricity, running water, and plumbing have an increased susceptibility to parasitic conditions. Other health conditions such as hypochromic anemia, otitis media, cardiovascular diseases, female obesity, and non-insulin-dependent diabetes mellitus are 400 to 600 percent greater than the national norm (Brown & Obermiller, 1994). Children are at greater risk for sudden infant death syndrome, congenital malformations, and infections (Obermiller & Rappold, 1994; Spurlock, Moser, & Flynn, 1989). Cancer, suicide, and accidents are 150 to 400 percent greater in Appalachia than the national average (Edwards, Lenz, and East-Odom, 1993). The risk of heart attack, stroke, accidental injury, and emotional and mental illness are 150 to 400 percent greater in the Appalachian population as compared with non-Appalachians (Brown & Obermiller, 1994; Obermiller & Rappold, 1994). Educational information presented in a nonjudgmental manner can have a significant impact on the improvement of the health status of Appalachian clients. The presentation of health and educational material needs to be linked with improvement in function to be taken seriously.

### Variations in Drug Metabolism

The literature reports no studies specific to the pharmacodynamics of drug interactions among Appalachians. Given the diverse gene pool of many residents, the health-care professional needs to observe each individual for adverse drug interactions.

## HIGH-RISK BEHAVIORS

Appalachians, as compared with non-Appalachians, are less concerned about their overall health and risks associated with smoking (Obermiller & Oldendick, 1994). The use of smokeless tobacco is the highest in the country. Underage use of alcohol is the most widespread abusive activity among teens (Penn, Borman, & Hoeweler, 1994). Dietary practices and lifestyle account for the higher risk of heart attack, stroke, mental illness, and accidental injury among this population. There continues to be a low rate of exercise and a diet high in fats and refined sugars (Edwards, Lenz, and East-Odom, 1993). The Appalachian definition of health encompasses three levels: body, mind, and spirit. This definition precludes viewing disease as a problem unless it interferes with one's functioning. Consequently, many conditions are denied or ignored until they progress to the point of decreasing function. Nutrition practices are covered more extensively under the section on nutrition.

## Health-care Practices

A ten-step pattern of health-seeking behaviors has been identified among Appalachians. The steps are as follows:

1. At the onset of symptoms, the "typical" Appalachians implement self-care practices that are usually learned from mothers.

2. When the symptoms persist, they call their mother, if available.

3. If mother is unavailable, they call the female in their kin network who is perceived as knowledgeable regarding health. If a nurse is available, they may seek the nurse's advice.

4. If relief is not achieved, they use over-the-counter (OTC) medicine they have seen on television that most closely matches their symptoms.

5. When that is ineffective, they use some of "Mable's medicine" (she lives down the road, had similar symptoms, and did not finish her medicine).

6. Next, they ask the local pharmacist for a recommendation; this marks the first professional encounter if no nurse was available earlier. (Of course, they usually do not tell the pharmacist that they tried Mable's medicine.) The pharmacist strongly suggests they see a health-care provider; however, on their insistence, the pharmacist recommends another OTC medication, which typical Appalachians try.

7. When no relief is achieved, they seek a local health-care provider who may or may not speak understandable English. The provider treats them to the best of his or her ability.

8. If the condition does not resolve, the local health-care provider refers them to a specialist in the area.

9. The specialist treats the condition to his or her best ability.

10. If unsuccessful, the specialist refers them to the closest tertiary medical center.

These ten steps may not always follow the same sequence as presented here; some steps may be skipped, and not all steps are always completed. Moreover, the time frame around these ten steps may be several years. Often by the time typical Appalachians are referred for definitive treatment, compensatory reserves have been depleted and they die at large medical centers. The story is then passed on in the "holler." So-and-So went to _____ and died. This pattern leads to a significant mistrust of large medical centers and a reluctance to use these facilities effectively.

Health-care providers can have a significant impact on improving a client's health-seeking behaviors by providing information early in this pattern. Nurses especially can help to reverse this pattern because they are viewed as knowledgeable, nonjudgmental, and respectful of Appalachian lifestyles.

# NUTRITION

## Meaning of Food

As with most ethnic and cultural groups, food has meaning beyond providing nutritional sustenance. To many Appalachians, wealth means having plenty of food for family, friends, and social gatherings (Wigginton, 1971; Wigginton, 1981; Wigginton & Bennett, 1986).

## Common Foods and Food Rituals

Many Appalachians, especially those living in rural areas, eat wild game (Wigginton, 1979), which includes muskrat, groundhog, rabbit, squirrel, duck, and venison. Wild game traditionally has a lower fat content than meat raised for commercial purposes. However, consistent with traditional practices from previous decades, most parts of both wild and domesticated animals are eaten. High-cholesterol–containing organ meats such as tongue, liver, heart, lungs (called lights), and brains are considered delicacies. In addition, bone marrow is used to make sauces, and stomach, intestines (chitlins or chitterlings), pigs' feet, tail, and ribs are also commonly eaten (Wigginton, 1979). Low-fat game meat is usually breaded and fried, negating the overall gains from these low-fat meat sources.

Food preparation practices may increase dietary risk factors for cardiac disease because many recipes contain lard and meats are preserved with salt. Other foods common in particular regions of Appalachia that may be unfamiliar to nonnative Appalachians are sweet potato pie; molasses candy; apple beer; gooseberry pie; pumpkin cake; and pickled beans, fruit, corn, beets, and cabbage, all of which are high in sodium (Gillespie, 1982). Frying foods with bacon grease or lard is a common practice. Fried green tomatoes, biscuits, and thick gravies are favorites.

Appalachians celebrate not only Thanksgiving, Christmas, and other national and religious holidays with food, but many other occasions as well. In rural areas, people celebrate with food when game and livestock are slaughtered because this is usually an extended family or community affair. The value of self-reliance is enhanced during the "cannin" season when foodstuffs are preserved. "Cannin" becomes a social or family occasion and is an excellent avenue for health teaching if the health-care provider is willing to participate and learn. Additional celebrations with food occur during times of death and grieving, when friends and participants bring dishes specifically prepared for the occasion.

## Dietary Practices for Health Promotion

Many Appalachians believe that good nutrition has an effect on one's health. In one study with rural Appalachians, young mothers were asked what it meant to eat well for good health. They referred to "taking fluids" and "eating right," but they were unable to describe healthy eating patterns any further. In a study by Hansen and Resick (1990), the respondents had no real knowledge of healthy nutrition for primary prevention.

Many believe that the sooner a baby can take food other than milk, the healthier it will be. Babies from the first month are fed grease, sugar, and coffee to promote hardiness (Miles, 1975). The Women, Infants, and Children program, commonly known as WIC, has done much to change some of these practices. Health-care providers have a rich opportunity to provide primary education in healthy eating practices. Factual information that describes health risks with early feeding of solid foods may help prevent later nutritional allergies in children.

The severity of hypertension in one community was decreased significantly when a health-care provider participated in the "cannin" of beans and showed the residents that the beans would remain crisp with a "tige of vinegar" rather than a "pile of salt." It is essential for the health-care provider to assess each person's specific food practices and preparation to provide effective dietary counseling for health promotion and wellness. Health-care providers in clinics and school settings have the opportunity to have a positive impact on the nutritional status of individuals and families. School breakfast and lunch programs, Meals on Wheels, and church-sponsored meal plans are some of the ways in which health-care providers can encourage and support families in attaining better nutrition practices.

## Nutritional Deficiencies and Food Limitations

Many rural and urban Appalachian children replace meals with snacks. The most common snacks are candy, salty foods, desserts, and carbonated beverages (Ezell, Skinner, & Penfield, 1985). Another survey reported that 34 percent of adolescents skip breakfast and 27 percent either skip lunch entirely or eat snack foods (Ezell, Skinner, & Penfield, 1985). Both of these studies revealed that the Appalachian diet is deficient in vitamin A, iron, and calcium.

There are no specific food limitations or enzyme deficiencies among Appalachians. With subsistence farming and commercial farms from nearby areas, all foods for a healthy diet are readily available during the growing season. Limitations may come from lack of readily accessible grocery stores and lack of financial ability to purchase nutritious foods.

## PREGNANCY AND CHILDBEARING PRACTICES

### Fertility Practices and Views toward Pregnancy

Contraceptive practices of Appalachians follow the general pattern of the U.S. population (Hochstrasser, Garkovich, & Modern, 1986). Methods include birth control pills, prophylactics, and tubal ligation; abortion is an individual choice. A popular belief among many is that taking laxatives facilitates an abortion. However, in practice, a disproportionate number of teenage pregnancies continues to occur at a younger age among Appalachians as compared with non-Appalachians (Hansen & Resick, 1990).

Fertility practices and sexual activity, both sensitive topics for many teenagers, are areas in which outsiders unknown to the family may be more effective than health-care practitioners who are known to the family. To be effective, counseling by the health-care provider must be accomplished within the cultural belief patterns of this group and must be approached in a nonhierarchical manner, preferably with a health-care provider of the same gender.

## Prescriptive, Restrictive, and Taboo Practices in the Childbearing Family

The literature reports no specific research or studies related to prescriptive, restrictive, or taboo practices during pregnancy. Pregnant women subscribe to the belief that to have a healthy baby, they need to eat well and take care of themselves (Horton, 1984). Other beliefs include that boys are carried higher and the belly appears pointy, whereas girls are carried low; picture taking can cause a stillbirth; reaching over one's head can cause the cord to strangle the baby; wearing an opal ring during pregnancy may harm the baby; being frightened by a snake or eating strawberries or citrus fruit can cause birthmarks; and if the mother experiences a tragedy, a congenital anomaly may occur. Childbearing is a family affair. The birthing mother is expected to accept childbirth as a short, intense, natural process that must be endured (Horton, 1984) and that will bring her closer to the earth.

The literature reports no specific studies on beliefs related to postpartum practices. When a new baby is born, relatives and extended family members gather to assist the new mother with household chores until she is able to complete them herself. Some newborns wear a band around the abdomen to prevent umbilical hernias and an *asafetida bag* around the neck to prevent or ward off contagious disease.

The health-care professional providing pregnancy counseling to the Appalachian family needs to demonstrate an openness to discuss cultural differences. Misinformation or incorrect information might be harmful to the pregnant mother or infant.

# DEATH RITUALS

## Death Rituals and Expectations

When a death is expected, family and friends may stay through the night and prepare food for the event. Because death is such an important occasion in Appalachia, many factories give workers 3 days' funeral leave for deaths of extended family members (Obermiller & Oldendick, 1994). After a death, extended family and friends may spend the night with the deceased's immediate family to prevent loneliness (Wigginton, 1973).

Deaths in Ohio are frequently published in West Virginia newspapers with a notice that the individual will be returned to the mountains for burial. Funeral services serve an important social function and are usually simple in Appalachia. This is a time when extended family and friends come together for services that can last for 3 hours. The length of time for a service varies according to the age of the deceased (Wigginton, 1975; Dorgan, 1989). The service for an elderly person is usually longer than that for a younger person. The body is displayed for hours, either in the home or at the church, so that all those who wish to can view the body. At the end of the service, all who wish to can view the body again, with the closest relative being the last to view the body. Many Appalachian families go to specific funeral homes that specialize in services more personal to the Appalachian culture, and the Appalachian urban areas have funeral homes that specialize in long-distant transport for burial. These funeral homes are familiar with Appalachian customs and meet their culturally specific requirements (Obermiller & Rappold, 1994).

The deceased is usually buried in his or her best clothes. Some persons have a custom-made set of clothes in which to be buried and may even design their own funeral services (Obermiller & Rappold, 1994). A common practice is to bury the deceased with personal possessions. At the funeral home, the person's favorite chair, a picture of the deceased, or other personal items may be displayed. After the funeral services are completed, elaborate meals are served either in the home or at the church. Services are accompanied by singing before, during, and after the service. Cemeteries throughout Appalachia show frequent visitations and give a sense of place and relationship to the land. Plots are carefully tended with displays of flowers, wreaths, and flags. Other beliefs regarding burial practices include placing graveyards on hillsides for fear that graves may be flooded out in low-lying areas. If the body is exhumed and reburied, it is believed that the person may not go to heaven (Lewis, Messner, & McDowell, 1985).

## Responses to Death and Grief

Clergy help families through the grieving process by providing counseling and support to family members. Appalachians are particularly good at working through the grieving process (Obermiller & Rappold, 1994). Flowers are more important than donations to a charity. Cremation is an acceptable practice, and what to do with the ashes is a personal decision (Wigginton & Bennett, 1986).

## SPIRITUALITY

### Religious Practices and Use of Prayer

The original inhabitants in Appalachia were mostly Protestant and Episcopalian. Central organization was difficult in the wilderness; thus, people individualized their chosen church structure. Today the predominant religions in the Appalachian region are Baptist, Methodist, Presbyterian, Holiness, Pentecostal, Episcopalian, and a few Roman Catholic and Jehovah's Witness. Fifty different religious groups in Appalachia call themselves Baptists (Dorgan, 1989). These sects are quite diverse, with important central beliefs. Most of these sects have a strong belief in autonomy at the local level. As a result, many divisions have occurred within and among churches to accommodate more personal beliefs and philosophies. Regardless of the denomination, the vast majority of churches in the region stress fundamentalism in religious practices and use the King James version of the bible (Dorgan, 1987; Wigginton & Bennett, 1977; Wigginton, 1984).

Many small churches have lay preachers instead of trained ministers. Most believe that to be a preacher, a person must have a divine calling, not something one consciously chooses, and that a person needs to have been moved to this calling. Thus, a minister may or may not be a preacher. Many of the Baptist faiths believe that baptism must be done in a river, pond, or lake so that the body can be submerged. Another practice, feet washing, where men wash men's feet and women wash women's feet, demonstrates humbleness. Many fundamentalist churches segregate women and children on one side of the church and men on the other side. Some denominations believe in divine healing, and the region is full of examples to testify to its effectiveness (Dorgan, 1989; Wigginton, 1979).

Services in many churches can be an interesting experience for outsiders unfamiliar with the specific religious services. Revival meetings are common practice along with two or more weekly services. Revival meetings tend to be lively (Dorgan, 1989), allowing persons to shout out when the spirit moves them to do so. Other denominations speak in tongues and believe in visions. Stringed music is played in many churches (Dorgan, 1989).

Some freewill churches, for example, Holiness Church (Hitch, 1989), preach against attending movies, ball games, and social functions where dancing occurs. Other sects believe in poisonous snake handling (rare), wherein the snake will not bite those who have faith. Each year, a few people get snake bites and usually heal themselves, but a few deaths occur each year after snake handling (Dorgan, 1989; Wigginton & Bennett, 1986).

Ingesting strychnine in small doses is used by some during religious services to increase sensory stimuli. This practice can precipitate convulsions if ingested in large enough amounts. Fire handling is still practiced by some groups, again with the belief that the hot coals will not burn those who have the faith (Dorgan, 1989; Schwarz, 1991; Wigginton & Bennett, 1984).

Prayer for many Appalachians is a primary source of strength. Prayer is personally designed around specific church and religious beliefs and practices, which vary widely throughout the region and between and among churches of similar faith (Gillespie, 1983). More religiously devoted persons pray daily whether or not they attend church formally. The religious beliefs are of a more spiritual nature and not tied to the tenets of any singular faith. They are part of the harmony of the mountains and being at one with life. Churches in many parts of Appalachia serve as the social centers of the community.

The health-care practitioner who is aware of clients' religious practices and spirituality needs are in a better position to promote culturally competent health care and to incorporate nonharmful practices into clients' care plans. The practitioner must indicate an appreciation and respect for the dignity and spiritual beliefs of Appalachians without expressing negative comments about differing religious beliefs and practices.

## Meaning of Life and Sources of Strength

Meaning in life comes from the family and "living right," which is defined by each person and usually means living right with God and in the beliefs of a chosen church (Dorgan, 1987; Wigginton & Bennett, 1984). Religion tends to be less focused on institutional rituals and ceremonies and consists more of personalized beliefs in God, Christ, and church (McCoy & McCoy, 1994). Because of the sometimes harsh lifestyle in the mountainous region, religious beliefs and faith make life worth living in a grim situation. The church provides a way of coping with the hurts, pains, and disappointments of a sometimes hostile environment and becomes a source for celebration (Dorgan, 1989).

Common themes that give Appalachians strength are family, traditionalism, personalism, self-reliance, religiosity, a worldview of being, and not having undue concern about things that man cannot control, such as nature and the future. Appalachians believe that rewards come in another life (Flaskerud, 1980), where God repays one for kind deeds on earth.

## Spiritual Beliefs and Health-care Practices

Within the context of *fatalism,* the belief that what happens to one is largely a result of God's will (Wigginton, 1979), Appalachians may not seek health care until symptoms of illness are well advanced. This practice is described more thoroughly under High-Risk Behaviors earlier in this chapter.

## HEALTH-CARE PRACTICES
### Beliefs that Influence Health-care Practices

Beliefs that influence health-care practices for many Appalachians are derived from such concepts as family, fatalism, traditionalism, self-reliance, and individualism (Counts & Boyle, 1987; Dillard, 1983; Jones, 1975; Helton, Barnes, & Borman, 1994). Even though many Appalachians believe that much of health is due to God's will, the concept of self-reliance fosters good health practices through self-care (Obermiller & Oldendick, 1994). Many may not see formal biomedical health-care practitioners until self-medicating and folk remedies have been exhausted. Appalachians, as compared with non-Appalachians, are less likely to use the emergency room or to have private physicians (Obermiller & Handy, 1994). For many, when they do seek formal health care, the condition is in a severe form, takes longer to treat, and has a less favorable outcome. The ten steps in the pattern of health care (see High-Risk Behaviors) illustrate this influence. Appalachians have an increased length of hoc pitalization, increased use of sick time, and are absent from school more than non-Appalachians (Obermiller & Oldendick, 1994). Health information on the Appalachian client should be gathered in the context of broader family relationships and cordiality that precedes information sharing (Barnett, et al., 1994). The health-care provider must consider the family rather than the individual as the basic unit for treatment (Heath, 1983). Because direct approaches are frowned upon, health-care providers need to approach sensitive topics indirectly. Many Appalachians expect the health-care provider to establish an advocacy role and to understand and accept their cultural differences; thus, it is best to involve professionals from the same backgrounds if they are available (Heath, 1983; Obermiller & Smith, 1994; Tripp-Reimer, 1982).

Obermiller and Oldendick (1994) surveyed a large sample of Northern Appalachians and asked what they thought was responsible for good health. Sixty-four percent stated that good health is due to self-care; 39 percent, family relationships; 36 percent, heredity; 26 percent, luck; 22 percent, God's will; and 6 percent, physicians. Seventy percent of those in the study believed that death is predetermined. Myerberg, et al. (1995), in their West Virginia study of risk-related interventions, were able to decrease infant mortality rates by 21.4 percent when services were affordable, available, accessible, and acceptable to the client. Approaching the client's beliefs and health responses in a nonjudgmental manner avoids defensiveness and enhances respect for the health-care provider. Effective health-care education can be accomplished by recognizing and encouraging positive self-care activities.

## Responsibility for Health Care

When Appalachians enter the biomedical health-care arena, many feel powerless in regard to their own health, abdicate responsibility for their own care, expect that the physician will take over their care completely (Chovan & Chovan, 1988), have high expectations and unrealistic dependence on the health-care system, and abandon self-reliance activities (Counts & Boyle, 1987). In addition, emergency rooms and formal health-care organizations are impersonal, sometimes drastic, and frequently ineffective (Heath, 1993; Obermiller & Oldendick, 1994).

Bureaucratic forms foster a fear and suspicion of health-care providers, which can lead to confusion, distrust, and negative stereotyping by both parties (Heath, 1983). When physicians are sought in outlying rural areas, they make their fee payment schedules more flexible, they dispense drugs, and they give injections in their offices. For many, a "being" orientation blocks prevention and enhances a crisis orientation (Chovan & Chovan, (1987). One method to enhance utilization of health services is to give one-on-one attention (Chovan & Chovan, 1987).

A major health concern for many Appalachians is the state of the **blood**, which is described as being thick or thin, good or bad, and **high** or **low**; these conditions can be regulated through diet (Tripp-Reimer & Freidl, 1977). Venereal disease and Rh-negative blood fall into the category of bad blood. Sour foods can also cause bad blood. Appalachian men report a greater number of backaches, and women report a greater number of headaches than the rest of society (Horton, 1984).

The Appalachian region has the highest rate of cervical cancer in the United States (Fisher & Page, 1988). When a program was initiated to offer Pap smears in one high-risk community, the most common reason that women consented to having the examination was one of convenience. If the Pap smear was not done on the first visit and clients were given a return appointment, they were less likely to return to have the test. Women under the age of 30 years were more likely to have a Pap smear done than older women (Fisher & Page, 1988). The primary focus on health for many

Appalachians is self-care. Self-care is primarily perceived as an individual responsibility (Counts & Boyle, 1987), and care is focused within the family rather than within the community (Hansen & Resick, 1990). Because many Appalachians value the ability to respond to and cope with events of daily life, many home remedies, treatments, and active consultation with kin and family members are sought before seeking outside help (Counts & Boyle, 1987).

Care within the medical system is used when the condition is perceived as serious, does not respond to self-care treatment, or has a high potential for death. Furthermore, because self-reliance activities and nature are predominant over people, many believe that it is best to let nature heal (Counts & Boyle, 1987). The health-care provider should give explanations and instructions within the context of the Appalachian culture to make them more acceptable to the client and family.

When elderly Appalachians go to a physician, many expect help immediately. A physician dispensing the medicine in the office is seen as being helpful. If the physician gives a prescription to the person, this may be interpreted as rejection (Lewis, Messner, & McDowell, 1985).

## Folk Practices

The strong belief in folk medicine is a traditional part of the Appalachian culture. Using herbal medicines, poultices, and teas is common practice among persons of all socioeconomic levels (Bushey, 1992). Table 5–1 presents a reference guide for the health-care practitioner with the major ingredients and conditions for which the folk treatments are used, so that these treatments can be adjusted to accommodate prescription therapies or education regarding folk treatments. Information in this table has been derived from the *Foxfire* series, the authors' backgrounds and experiences, and health-care professionals at a cultural diversity conference in northern Appalachia. Specific amounts are not given. In many cases the amounts vary from person to person, according to the geographic region, and among families. Local names are given rather than scientific names because this is how the residents gather them. Many folk and traditional practices were learned from the Cherokee and Apalache Indians living in the region and have been passed down from generation to generation (Wigginton & Bennett, 1986). Although many of these home remedies are not harmful, some may have a deleterious effect when used to the exclusion of, or in combination with, prescription medications, as should already be evident from the ten-step pattern health-seeking behaviors among Appalachians presented in the section Health-care Practices.

Because ingredients in some of these herbal medicines can have serious side effects, especially if taken in large quantities, the health-care provider must become familiar with folk medicines used by Appalachians as part of the client assessment. The health-care provider must ascertain if the person intends to use folk medicines simultaneously with prescription medications and treatment regimens so that they can be incorporated into the plan of care or dialogue undertaken to prevent adverse treatments.

## Barriers to Health Care

Barriers to health care for Appalachians include the rugged terrain, the economic conditions in the region, lack of access to health-care facilities, and a shortage of health-care providers (Edwards, Lenz, & East-Odom, 1993; Tripp-Reimer & Freidl, 1977). In the mid-1970s, the Appalachian region had 34 percent fewer physicians and 20 percent fewer nurses than other areas of the United States (Tripp-Reimer & Freidl, 1977; Chovan & Chovan, 1985). Because the physician shortage in Appalachia

## Table 5–1 • Health Conditions and Appalachian Folk Medicine Practices

| Health Condition | Folk Medicine Practices |
| --- | --- |
| Arthritis | Make tea from boiling the roots of ginseng. Drink the tea or rub it on the arthritic joint. |
| | Mix roots of ginseng and goldenseal in liquor and drink it. Ginseng is used heavily by many Koreans and was exported to Korea in the 18th and 19th centuries. |
| | Eat large amounts of raw fruits and vegetables. |
| | Carry a buckeye around in your pocket. |
| | Drink tea from the stems of the barbell plant. |
| | Drink a mixture of honey, vinegar, and moonshine (or other liquor). |
| | Drink tea made from alfalfa seeds or leaves. |
| | Drink tea made from rhubarb and whiskey. |
| | Place a magnet over the joint to draw the arthritis out of the joint. |
| Asthma | Drink tea from the bark of wild yellow plum trees, mullein leaves, and alum. Take every 12 hr. |
| | Combine gin and heartwood of a pine tree. Take twice a day. |
| | Suck salty water up your nose. |
| | Smoke or sniff rabbit tobacco. |
| | Swallow a handful of spiderwebs. |
| | Smoke strong tobacco until you choke. |
| | Drink a mixture of honey, lemon juice, and whiskey. |
| | Inhale smoke from ginseng leaves. |
| Bedbugs/chiggers | Apply kerosene liberally to all parts of the body. *Caution:* Kerosene can cause significant irritation to sensitive skin, especially when exposed to sunlight. |
| Bleeding | Place a spiderweb across the wound. This is also used in rural Scotland. |
| | Put kerosene oil on the cut. |
| | Place soot from the fireplace into a cut. Be sure to wash out the soot after bleeding is stopped or the area will scar. |
| | Apply a mixture of honey and turpentine on the bleeding wound. |
| | Apply a mixture of soot and lard on the wound. |
| | Place a cigarette paper over the wound. |
| | Put pine resin over the cut. |
| | Place kerosene oil on the wound. *Caution:* If used in large doses, kerosene will burn the skin. |
| High Blood Pressure (not to be mistaken for high blood) | Drink sasparilla tea. |
| | Drink a half cup of vinegar. |
| Blood Builders | Drink tea from the bark of a wild cherry tree. |
| | Combine cherry bark, yellowroot, and whiskey. Take twice each day. |
| | Eat fried pokeweed leaves. |
| Blood purifiers | Drink tea from burdock root. |
| | Drink tea from spice wood. |
| Blood tonic | Take a teaspoonful of honey and a tiny amount of sulfur. |
| | Take a teaspoon of molasses and a tiny amount of sulfur. |
| | Drink tea made from bloodroot. |
| | Soak nails in a can of water until they become rusty. Drink the rusty water. |
| Boils or Sores | Apply a poultice of walnut leaves or the green hulls with salt. |
| | Apply a poultice of the houseleek plant. |

Table 5–1 • **Health Conditions and Appalachian Folk Medicine Practices** (*Continued*)

| Health Condition | Folk Medicine Practices |
| --- | --- |
| | Apply a poultice of rotten apples. |
| | Apply a poultice of beeswax, mutton tallow, sweet oil, oil of amber, oil of spike, and resin. |
| | Apply a poultice of kerosene, turpentine, Vaseline, and lye soap. |
| | Apply a poultice of heart leaves, lard, and turpentine. |
| | Apply a poultice of bread and milk. |
| | Apply a poultice of slippery elm and pork fat. |
| | Apply a poultice of flaxseed meal. |
| | Apply a poultice of beef tallow, brown sugar, salt, and turpentine. |
| Burns | Apply a poultice of baking soda and water. |
| | Place castor oil on the burn. |
| | Apply a poultice of egg white and castor oil. |
| | Place a potato on the burn. |
| | Wrap the burn in a gauze and keep moist with salt water. |
| | Place linseed oil on the burn. |
| | Apply a poultice of lard and flour. |
| | Put axle grease on the burn. This is also a practice with some Germans in Minnesota. |
| Chapped hands and lips | Apply lard, grease, or tallow from pork or mutton. |
| Chest congestion | Apply poultice to the chest made of kerosene, turpentine, and lard. Make sure the poultice is not applied directly to the chest but rather on top of a cloth. |
| | Apply mutton tallow directly to the chest. |
| | Apply a warm poultice of onions and grease. |
| | Rub pine tar on the chest. |
| | Chew leaves and stems of peppermint. |
| | Drink a combination of ginger and sugar in hot water. |
| | Make a mixture of rock candy and whiskey. Take several teaspoons several times each day. |
| | Drink tea made from ginger, honey, and whiskey. |
| | Drink tea made from pine needles. |
| | Put goose grease on your chest. |
| | Drink red pepper tea. |
| | Eat roasted onions. |
| | Drink brine from pickles or kraut. |
| | Make tea from boneset, rosemary, and goldenrod. |
| | Make tea from the butterfly weed. |
| Colic | Make tea from calamus root and catnip. (Calamus is a suspected carcinogen.) |
| | Tie an asafetida bag around the neck. |
| | Drink baking soda and water. |
| | Chew and swallow the juice of camel root. |
| | Massage stomach with warm castor oil. |
| | Drink ginseng tea. |
| Constipation | Take two tablespoons of turpentine. |
| | Combine castor oil and mayapple roots. |
| | Take castor oil or Epsom Salts. |
| Croup | Have child wear a bib containing pine pitch and tallow. |
| | Apply cloth to the chest saturated with groundhog fat, turpentine, and lamp oil. |
| | Drink juice from a roasted onion. |
| | Apply to the back a poultice made from mutton tallow and beeswax. |

**Table 5–1 • Health Conditions and Appalachian Folk Medicine Practices** (*Continued*)

| Health Condition | Folk Medicine Practices |
| --- | --- |
| | Eat a spoonful of sugar with a drop of turpentine.<br>Eat honey with lemon or vinegar.<br>Eat onion juice and honey. |
| Diarrhea | Drink water from boiling the lady-slipper plant.<br>Place soot in a glass of water, let the soot settle to the bottom of the glass, and drink the water.<br>Drink tea made from blackberry roots.<br>Drink tea from red oak bark.<br>Drink blackberry or strawberry juice.<br>Drink tea made from strawberry or blackberry leaves.<br>Drink tea made out of willow leaves.<br>Drink the juice from the bark of a white oak tree or a persimmon tree. |
| Earache | Place lukewarm salt water in the ear.<br>Put castor oil or sweet oil in the ear.<br>Put sewing machine oil in the ear.<br>Place a few drops of urine in the ear.<br>Place cabbage juice in the ear.<br>Blow smoke from tobacco in the ear.<br>Place a Vicks-soaked cotton ball in the ear. |
| Eye ailments | Place a few drops of castor oil in the eye.<br>Drop warm salty water in the eye. |
| Fever | Drink tea made from rabbit tobacco or snakeroot.<br>Drink tea made from the butterfly weed, wild horsemint, or feverweed.<br>Mash garlic bulbs and place in a bag tied around the pulse points.<br>Drink water from wild ginger. |
| Headache | Drink tea made of lady's slipper plants.<br>Tie warm fried potatoes around your head.<br>Take Epsom salts.<br>Tie ginseng roots around your head.<br>Place crushed onions on your head.<br>Rub camphor and whiskey on your head. |
| Heart trouble | Drink tea made from heartleaf leaves or bleeding heart.<br>Eat garlic. |
| Kidney trouble | Drink tea made from peach leaves or mullein roots.<br>Drink tea made from corn silk or arbutus leaves. |
| Liver trouble | Drink tea made from lion's tongue leaves.<br>Drink tea made from the roots of the spinet plant. |
| Poison Ivy | Urinate on the affected area.<br>Take a bath in salt water and then apply Vaseline.<br>Wash the area with bleach.<br>Wash the area with the juice of the milkweed plant.<br>Apply a poultice of gunpowder and buttermilk.<br>Apply baking soda to wet skin. |
| Sore throat | Gargle with sap from a red oak tree.<br>Eat honey and molasses.<br>Eat honey and onions.<br>Drink honey and whiskey.<br>Tie a poultice of lard or cream with turpentine and Vicks to your neck.<br>Apply a poultice of cottonseed to your throat.<br>Swab your throat with turpentine. |

Table 5–1 • **Health Conditions and Appalachian Folk Medicine Practices** (*Continued*)

| Health Condition | Folk Medicine Practices |
| --- | --- |
| Worms | Drop turpentine on a spoonful of sugar or honey. Drink tea made from the root of snakeroot. Drink tea made from the roots of red sassafras. |
| Warts | Apply milkweed juice. |

has been greater than the nurse shortage, nurses have historically delivered the bulk of primary care (Lenz & Edwards, 1982). Today, the area is still underserved by all types of health-care practitioners because of its geographic isolation and the underuse of health resources (Hansen & Resick, 1990). Even though the ARC has sponsored road-building campaigns in the mountainous regions of Appalachia since 1965, transportation problems continue to exist in parts of the region (Fig. 5–1). A disproportionate number of Appalachians, especially those who are self-employed, unemployed, or underemployed do not have prepurchased health insurance. Health-care facilities are closing in some areas owing to decreasing employment opportunities, necessitating individuals to relocate, and therefore, making it more difficult for those people remaining to obtain needed services (Edwards, Lenz, & East-Odom, 1993).

## Cultural Responses to Health and Illnesses

Appalachians generally take care of their own. Their view is to accept the person as a "whole individual"; thus, the mentally deficient and handicapped are readily accepted and not turned out (Lewis, Messner, & McDowell, 1985). The mentally handicapped are not crazy but rather have "bad nerves"; they are "quite turned" or "odd turned" (Lewis, Messner, & McDowell, 1985).

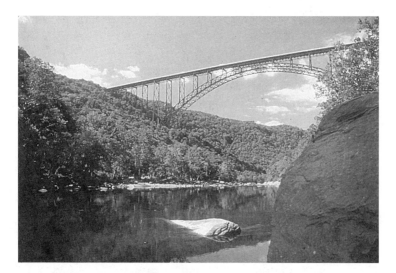

**Figure 5–1.** Before the construction of the New River Gorge bridge, many people were isolated from health care. (Courtesy of West Virginia Division of Tourism and Parks.)

Although non-Appalachian health professionals recommend psychiatric treatment for behaviors labeled as "lazy," "mean," "immoral," "criminal," or "psychic" by Appalachian mental health professionals, Appalachian mental health professionals recommend punishment by either the social group or the legal system or tolerance of these behaviors (Flaskerud, 1980). When unemployment increases and individuals go on welfare or receive food stamps, the use of mental health facilities shows an associated increase (Banziger & Foos, 1983; Banziger, Smith, & Foos, 1982).

Traditional Appalachians believe that disability is a natural and an inevitable part of the aging process (Hansen & Resick, 1990; Horton, 1984). Their culture of being discourages the use of rehabilitation as an option (Obermiller & Rappold, 1994).

Irvine's study (1989) of clients with diabetes mellitus found that less than 20 percent of clients stayed on their diets, foot care was sporadic, exercise was too infrequent to be effective, and blood and urine testing were rarely done. Only 36 percent of individuals in the study had any previous health teaching regarding their disease. Those clients who were compliant tended to be older persons who were in better perceived health and had more education. Also, those clients with more severe diabetes maintained better adherence to health-care prescriptions. To establish trust and rapport when working with the Appalachian client with a chronic disease, the health-care provider must avoid assumptions regarding health beliefs and provide health maintenance interventions within the scope of cultural customs and beliefs.

Individual responses to pain cannot be classified among Appalachians. The Appalachian background is too varied and no studies regarding cultural beliefs about pain could be found in the literature. For many Appalachians, pain is something that is to be endured and accepted stoically (Miles, 1975). However, when a person does become ill or has pain, personal space collapses inward and the person expects to be waited on and cared for by others. A belief among many is that if one places a knife or ax under the bed or mattress of a person in pain, the knife will help cut the pain. This practice occurs with childbearing and other conditions that cause pain (Wigginton, 1975). The author is aware of an Appalachian woman who requested to have a knife or ax placed under the bed or mattress postoperatively to help cut (or decrease) the pain associated with surgery. The author offered a small pocket knife or butter knife to place under the bed. Both were unacceptable; the pocket knife was too small and the butter knife was too dull to be of any use. A sharp meat-cutting knife from the dietary department was deemed appropriate because it was both large enough and sharp enough to help cut the pain.

## Blood Transfusion and Organ Donation

Appalachians generally do not have any specific rules or taboos about receiving blood, donating organs, or undergoing organ transplantation (Wigginton, 1973; Wigginton, 1984). These decisions are largely one's own, but advice is usually sought from family and friends.

## HEALTH-CARE PRACTITIONERS

## Traditional Versus Biomedical Practitioners

For decades, both lay and trained nurses have provided significant amounts of health care, including obstetrics, in this mountainous region. Granny and trained midwives have provided obstetric services throughout the history of the region. Folk practitioners are primarily older women but may be men (Lenz & Edwards, 1983).

The Frontier Nursing Service, started in 1927 by Mary Breckenridge, is a notable example of nurses taking the initiative to provide health care in Appalachia (Severence, 1992), and one of the oldest and most well-known nurse-run clinics in the United States. It was started in one of the most rural areas of Appalachia in response to a lack of physicians and the high birth and mortality rates among children in the area (Ruffing-Rahal, 1991; Severence, 1992). Lay-midwives had been practicing in Appalachia for decades, but the Frontier Nursing Service introduced formally trained nurse-midwives. By all subjective and objective evaluations, the service has been successful. Since the formation of this service, other nurse-organized and nurse-managed clinics that provide primary care to women and children include the Mountain City Extended Hours Health Center, operated by the College of Nursing of East Tennessee State University (Edwards, Lenz, & East-Odom, 1993); the ambulatory nurse practitioner health-care center with a Veterans Administration Hospital in West Virginia (Lewis, Messner, & McDowell, 1985); and a family practice center in Boone, North Carolina, developed in 1986 (Fisher & Page, 1987). With changing laws and decreasing barriers for independent practice by nurse practitioners, independent nurse practitioner–managed primary care clinics are becoming quite successful. Their success is attributed to programming based on the provision of culturally congruent care respectful of Appalachian lifeways and the employment of local people whenever possible.

Many Appalachians prefer to go to *insider* health-care professionals, especially in the more rural areas, because the system of payment for services is accepted on a sliding scale and even an exchange of goods for health services exists in some communities. One nurse practitioner in private practice states that the only time she locks her car is when the zucchini are "in." If she does not, when she gets in her car after a clinic session, she has no room to drive because of all the "presents" of the large vegetable.

Locally respected Appalachians are engaged to facilitate acceptance of outside programs and of the staff who participate at the grassroots level in planning and initiating the programs. For Appalachian clients to become more accepting of biomedical care, it is important for health-care providers to approach persons in an unhurried manner consistent with their relaxed lifestyle, to engage clients in decision making and care planning, and to use locally trained support staff whenever possible.

## Status of Health-care Providers

Most herbal and folk practitioners are highly respected for their treatments, mostly because they are well-known to their people and trusted by those in need of health care. Physicians and other health-care professionals are frequently seen as outsiders to the Appalachian population and, therefore, are mistrusted (Hansen & Resick, 1990; Simon, 1985). This initial mistrust is rooted in outsider behaviors that exploited the Appalachian people and took their land for timbering and coal mining in earlier generations (Simon, 1985). Trust for outsiders is gained slowly (Chovan & Chovan, 1987). Once the person gets to know and trust the health-care provider, the provider is given much respect.

Many of the physicians who practice in the remote areas of Appalachia are from foreign countries and are distrusted, not for gender or profession, but for hierarchical relationships, communication styles, and outsidedness. Appalachians prefer home-based nurses, health-care and social workers. To obtain full cooperation, the health-care provider needs to ask clients what they consider to be the problem before devising a plan of care; otherwise, the clients may resent the health-care provider (Helton, Barnes, & Borman, 1994). It is equally important to decrease language barriers by decoding the jargon of the health-care environment.

---

**CASE STUDY**

William Kapp, aged 55 years, and his wife Gloria, aged 37 years, have recently moved from an isolated rural area of Northern Appalachia to Denver, Colorado, because of Gloria's failing health. Mrs. Kapp has had pulmonary tuberculosis for several years. They decided to move to New Mexico because they heard that the climate was better for Mrs. Kapp's pulmonary condition. For an unknown reason, they stayed in Denver where William obtained employment making machine parts.

The Kapp's oldest daughter, Ruth, aged 20 years, Ruth's husband Roy, aged 24 years, and their daughter Rebecca, aged 17 months, moved with them so that Ruth could help care for her ailing mother. After 2 months, Roy returned to Northern Appalachia because he was unable to find work in Denver. Ruth is 3 months' pregnant.

Because Mrs. Kapp has been feeling "more poorly" in the last few days, she has come to the clinic and is accompanied by her husband William, her daughter Ruth, and her granddaughter, Rebecca. On admission, Gloria is expectorating greenish sputum, which her husband estimates to be about a teacup-full each day. Gloria is 5'5" tall and weighs 92 pounds. Her temperature is 101.4°F, her pulse is regular at 96 beats per minute, and her respirations are 30 per minute and labored. Her skin is dry and scaly with poor turgor.

While the physician is examining Mrs. Kapp, the nurse is taking additional historical and demographic data from Mr. Kapp and Ruth. The nurse finds that Ruth has had no prenatal care and that her first child Rebecca was delivered at home with the assistance of a neighbor. Rebecca is pale, suffers from frequent bouts of diarrhea and colicky symptoms. Mr. Kapp declines to offer information regarding his health status and states that he takes care of himself.

This is the first time that Mrs. Kapp has seen a health-care provider since their relocation. Mr. Kapp has been treating his wife with a blood tonic he makes from soaking nails in water, a poultice he makes from turpentine and lard, which he applies to her chest each morning, and a cough medicine that he makes from rock candy, whiskey, and honey, of which he has her take a tablespoon four times a day. He feels that this has been more beneficial than the prescription medication given to them before they relocated.

The child Rebecca has been taking a cup of ginseng tea for her colicky symptoms each night, and a cup of red bark tea each morning for her diarrhea.

Ruth's only complaint is the "sick headache" that she gets three to four times a week. She takes ginseng tea and Epsom salts for the headache.

Mrs. Kapp is discharged with prescriptions for isoniazid, rifampin, and an antibiotic and with instructions to return in 1 week for follow-up based on the results of blood tests, chest radiograph, and sputum cultures. She is also told to return to the clinic or emergency department if her symptoms worsen before then. The nurse gives Ruth directions for making appointments with the prenatal clinic for herself and the pediatric well-child clinic for Rebecca.

---

**STUDY QUESTIONS**

1. Describe the migration patterns of Appalachians over the last 50 years.

2. Discuss issues related to autonomy in the workforce for Appalachians.

3. Identify high-risk behaviors common in the Appalachian region.

4. Describe barriers to health care for people living in Appalachia.

5. What might the nurse or physician do to encourage Mrs. Kapp to be compliant with her prescription regimen?

6. What would your advice be regarding each of the home remedies that Mrs. Kapp is taking? Would you encourage or discourage her from continuing them?

7. What might the nurse have done to help ensure that Ruth would make the appointments for herself and her daughter?

8. What advice would you give Ruth regarding the home remedies that she and her daughter are currently taking? Would you encourage or discourage their use?

9. Do you think that Mrs. Kapp will return for her appointment next week? Why? What would you do if she does not return for her appointment?

10. Do you think that Ruth will make and keep appointments for herself and her daughter?

11. What would you do to encourage Mr. Kapp to consent to a health assessment?

12. What additional services could you suggest to assist the Kapp family at this time?

13. What additional follow-up do you consider essential for the Kapp family?

14. What advice would you give Ruth regarding her daughter's frequent bouts of diarrhea?

## References

Banziger, G., Smith, R. K., & Foos, D. (1982). Economic indicators of mental health service utilization in rural Appalachia. *American Journal of Community Psychology, 10*(6), 669–687.

Banziger, G. & Foos, D. (1983). The relationship of personal financial status to the utilization of community mental health centers in rural Appalachia. *American Journal of Community Psychology, 11*(5), 543–552.

Barnett, D., Bauer, A., Baker, B., Ehrhardt, K. E., & Stoller, S. (1994). A case for naturalistic assessment and intervention in an urban Appalachian community. In K. M. Borman & P. J. Obermiller (Eds.), *From mountain to metropolis: Appalachian migrants in American cities* (pp. 94–104). Westport, CT: Greenwood Publishing Group.

Borman, K. M. & Obermiller, P. J. (1994). *From mountain to metropolis: Appalachian migrants in American cities.* Westport, CT: Greenwood Publishing Group.

Borman, K. M. & Steglin, D. (1994). Social change and urban Appalachian children: Youth at risk. In K. M. Borman & P. J. Obermiller (Eds.), *From mountain to metropolis: Appalachian migrants in American cities* (pp. 167–180). Westport, CT: Greenwood Publishing Group.

Brown, J. S. & Hilary, G. A. (1963). The great migration: 1940–1960. In T. R. Ford (Ed.), *The Southern Appalachian region: A survey* (pp. 119–223). Lexington: University of Kentucky.

Brown, K. M. & Obermiller, P. J. (1994). The health status of children living in urban Appalachian neighborhoods. In K. M. Borman & P. J. Obermiller (Eds.), *From mountain to metropolis: Appalachian migrants in American cities* (pp. 70–82). Westport, CT: Greenwood Publishing Group.

Casto, J. E. (1993). Ohio learns the power of a positive image. *Appalachia, 26*(3), 32–36.

Chovan, M. J. & Chovan, W. (1985). Stressful events and coping responses among older adults in two sociocultural groups. *Journal of Psychology, 119*(3), 253–260.

Counts, M. M. & Boyle, J. S. (1987). Nursing, health, and policy within a community context. *Advances in Nursing Science, 9*(3), 12–23.

Crissman, J. K. (1987). The impact of the urban milieu on the Appalachian family. In P. J.

Obermiller & W. W. Philliber (Eds.), *Too few tomorrows: Urban Appalachians in the 1980's* (pp.81–88). Boone, NC: Appalachian Consortium Press.

Cunningham, R. (1987). *Apples on the flood: The Southern mountain experience.* Knoxville: The University of Tennessee Press.

DeStafano, J. S. (1994). Readin, writin, and route 23: A road to economic but not educational success. In K. M. Borman & P. J. Obermiller (Eds.), *From mountain to metropolis: Appalachian migrants in American cities* (pp. 12–24). Westport, CT: Greenwood Publishing Group.

Dorgan, H. (1987). *Giving glory to God in Appalachia: Worship practices of six Baptist subdenominations.* Knoxville: University of Tennessee Press.

Dorgan, H. (1989). *The old regular Baptist of central Appalachia: Brothers and sisters in hope.* Knoxville: University of Tennessee Press.

Edwards, J. B., Lenz, C. L., & East-Odom, J. C. (1993). Nurse-managed primary care: Serving a rural Appalachian population. *Family and Community Health, 16*(2), 50–56.

Fisher, S., & Page, A. L. (1987). Women and preventive health care: An exploratory study of the use of pap smears in a potentially high-risk Appalachian population. *Women's Health, 11*(3/4), 83–99.

Flaskerud, J. H. (1980). Perceptions of problematic behavior by Appalachians, mental health professionals and lay non-Appalachians. *Nursing Research, 29*(3), 140–149.

Gillespie, P. F. (1982). *Foxfire 7.* Garden City, NY: Anchor Press.

Halperin, R. H. (1994). Appalachians in cities: Issues and challenges for research. In K. M. Borman & P. J. Obermiller (Eds.), *From mountain to metropolis: Appalachian migrants in American cities* (pp. 181–198). Westport, CT: Greenwood Publishing Group.

Hansen, M. M. & Resick, L. K. (1990). Health beliefs, health care, and rural appalachian subcultures from an ethnographic perspective. *Family and Community Health, 13*(1), 1–10.

Hawthorne, A. (1994). Enhancing manufacturing competitiveness. *Appalachia, 26*(1), 26–36.

Heath, S. B. (1983). *Ways and words: Language, life, and work in communities and classrooms.* Cambridge: Cambridge University Press.

Helton, L. R., Barnes, E. C., & Borman, K. M. (1994). Urban Appalachia and professional intervention: A model for education and social service providers. In K. M. Borman & P. J. Obermiller (Eds.), *From mountain to metropolis: Appalachian migrants in American cities* (pp. 106–120). Westport, CT: Greenwood Publishing Group.

Hitch, M. A. (1989). Life in a blue ridge hollow. In W. K. McNeil (Ed.), *Appalachian images in folk and popular culture* (pp. 243–254). London: U. M. I. Press.

Hochstrasser, G. G., Garkovich, D., & Modern, L. (1986). Contraceptive practices in rural appalachia. *American Journal of Public Health, 85*(9), 1004–1008.

Hoffman, C. (1993). Excellence in education. *Appalachia, 26*(1), 4–11.

Hooker, W. (1987). The contribution of culture: Implications for the nursing process. In R. B. Murray and M. M. Huelskoetter (Eds.), *Psychiatric Mental Health Nursing* (pp. 237–256). East Norwalk, CT: Appleton & Lange.

Horton, C. F. (1984). Women have headaches, men have backaches: Patterns of illness in an Appalachian community. *Social Science Medicine, 19*(6), 647–654.

Irvine, A. A. (1989). Self care behaviors in a rural population with diabetes. *Patient Education and Counseling, 13,* 3–13.

LaFargue, J. P. (1980). A survival strategy: Kinship networks. *American Journal of Nursing, 80*(9), 1636–1640.

Lenz, C. L., & Edwards, J. E. (1982). Nurse-managed primary care: Tapping the rural community power base. *Journal of Nursing Administration, 22*(9), 57–61.

Lewis, S., Messner, R., & McDowell, W. A. (1985). An unchanging culture. *Journal of Gerontological Nursing, 11*(8), 22–26.

Maloney, M. E. & Borman, K. M. (1987). Effects of schools and schooling upon Appalachian children in Cincinnati. In P. J. Obermiller & W. W. Philliber (Eds.), *Too few tomorrows: Urban Appalachians in the 1980's* (pp. 89–98). Boone, NC: Appalachian Consortium Press.

Marger, M. N. & Obermiller, P. J. (1987). Urban Appalachians and Canadian maritime migrants: Comparative study of emergent ethnicity. In P. J. Obermiller & W. W. Philliber (Eds.), *Too few tomorrows: Urban Appalachians in the 1980's* (pp. 23–34). Boone, NC: Appalachian Consortium Press.

McCoy, C. B. & McCoy, H. V. (1987). Appalachian youth in cultural transition. In P. J. Obermiller & W. W. Philliber (Eds.), *Too few tomorrows: Urban Appalachians in the 1980's* (pp. 99–110). Boone, NC: Appalachian Consortium Press.

McNeil, W. K., (1989). *Appalachian images in folk and popular culture.* Ann Arbor: U. M. I. Press.

Miles, E. B. (1975). *The spirit of the mountains.* Knoxville: The University of Tennessee Press.

Myerberg, D., et al. (1995). Reducing postneonatal in West Virginia: A statewide intervention program targeting risk identification at and after birth. *American Journal of Public Health, 85,*(5), 631–637.

Neely, S. K. (1987). The ethnic entrepreneurer in the urban Appalachian community. In P. J. Obermiller & W. W. Philliber (Eds.), *Too few tomorrows: Urban Appalachians in the 1980's* (pp. 43–48). Boone, NC: Appalachian Consortium Press.

Obermiller, P. J. & Handy, W. (1994). Health education strategies for urban Blacks and Appalachians. In K. Borman & P. J. Obermiller (Eds.), *From mountain to metropolis: Appalachian migrants in American cities,* (pp. 61–71). Westport, CT: Greenwood Publishing Group.

Obermiller, P. J. (1987). Labeling urban Appalachians. In P. J. Obermiller & W. W. Philliber (Eds.), *Too few tomorrows: Urban Appalachians in the 1980's* (pp. 35–42). Boone, NC: Appalachian Consortium Press.

Obermiller, P. J. & Malong, M. E. (1994a). Living city, feeling country: The current status and future prospects of urban Appalachians. In K. M. Borman & P. J. Obermiller (Eds.), *From mountain to metropolis: Appalachian migrants in American cities* (pp. 3–12). Westport, CT: Greenwood Publishing Group.

Obermiller, P. J. & Malong, M. E. (1994b). Looking for Appalachians in Pittsburg: Seeking deliverance, finding the deer hunter. In K. M. Borman & P. J. Obermiller (Eds.), *From mountain to metropolis: Appalachian migrants in American cities* (pp. 13–25). Westport, CT: Greenwood Publishing Group.

Obermiller, P. J. & Oldendick, R. W. (1994). Urban Appalachian health concerns. In K. M. Borman & P. J. Obermiller (Eds.), *From Mountain to metropolis: Appalachian migrants in American cities* (pp. 51–60). Westport, CT: Greenwood Publishing Group.

Obermiller, P. J. & Oldendick, R. W. (1987). Moving on: Recent patterns of Appalachian migration. In P. J. Obermiller & W. W. Philliber (Eds.), *Too few tomorrows: Urban Appalachians in the 1980's* (pp. 51–62). Boone, NC: Appalachian Consortium Press.

Obermiller, P. J. & Oldendick, R. W. (1987). Two studies of Appalachian civic involvement. In P. J. Obermiller & W. W. Philliber (Eds.), *Too few tomorrows: Urban Appalachians in the 1980's,* (pp. 69–80). Boone, NC: Appalachian Consortium Press.

Obermiller, P. J. & Philliber, W. W. (1987). *Too few tomorrows: Urban Appalachians in the 1980's.* Boone, NC: Appalachian Consortium Press.

Obermiller, P. J. & Rappold, R. (1994). The sense of place and culture among urban Appalachians: A study in post-death migration. In K. M. Borman & P. J. Obermiller (Eds.), *From mountain to metropolis: Appalachian migrants in American cities*, (pp. 25–33). Westport, CT: Greenwood Publishing Group.

Obermiller, P. J. & Smith, A. (1994). Concerning contamination: Attitudes on environmental issues among urban minority groups. In K. M. Borman & P. J. Obermiller (Eds.), *From mountain to metropolis: Appalachian migrants in American cities* (pp. 83–92). Westport, CT: Greenwood Publishing Group.

Penn, E. M., Borman, K. M., & Hoeweler, F. (1994). Echoes from the hill: Urban Appalachian youths and educational reform. In K. M. Borman & P. J. Obermiller (Eds.), *From mountain to metropolis: Appalachian migrants in American cities* (pp. 121–140). Westport, CT: Greenwood Publishing Group.

Philliber, W. W. (1987). The changing composition of Appalachian migration. In P. J. Obermiller & W. W. Philliber (Eds.), *Too few tomorrows: Urban Appalachians in the 1980's* (pp. 51–62). Boone, NC: Appalachian Consortium Press.

Philliber, W. W. & Obermiller, P. J. (1987). Appalachians in midwestern cities: Regionalism as a basis of ethnic group formation. In P. J. Obermiller & W. W. Philliber (Eds.), *Too few tomorrows: Urban Appalachians in the 1980's* (pp. 19–22). Boone, NC: Appalachian Consortium Press.

Rowles, G. D. (1983). Between worlds: A relocation dilemma for the Appalachian elderly. *International Journal of Aging and Human Development, 17*(4), 301–314.

Ruffing-Rahal, M. A. (1991). Ethnographic traits in the writing of Mary Breckenridge. *Journal of Advanced Nursing, 16,* 614–620.

Russell, J. & Rocha, C. (1993). Appropriations clear house. *Journal of the Appalachian Regional Commission, 26*(3), 2–3.

Schwarz, B. E. (1991). Ordeal by serpents, fire, and strychnine: A study of some provocative psychosomatic phenomena. In W. K. McNeil (Ed.), *Appalachian images in folk and popular culture,* (pp. 285–306). London: U. M. I. Press.

Severence, D. (1992). Appalachian health care: Candles in the darkness. *Frontier Nursing Service Quarterly Bulletin, 67*(3), 22–29.

Simon, J. M. (1987). The care of the elderly in Appalachia. *Journal of Gerontological Nursing, 13*(7), 32–35.

Tripp-Reimer, T. (1982). Barriers to health care: Variations in interpretation of Appalachian client behavior by Appalachian and non-Appalachian professionals. *Western Journal of Nursing Research, 4*(2), 179–191.

Tripp-Reimer, T. & Freidl, M. C. (1977). Appalachians: A neglected minority. *Nursing Clinics of North America, 12*(1), 41–54.

*U.S. Statistical Abstracts* (1995). Washington, DC: Bureau of the Census.

Wenger, T. E. (1987). Too few tomorrows. In P. J. Obermiller & W. W. Philliber (Eds.), *Too few tomorrows: Urban Appalachians in the 1980's* (pp. 3–12). Boone, NC: Appalachian Consortium Press.

Wigginton, E. (1971). *Foxfire Book.* Garden City, NY: Anchor Press/Doubleday.

Wigginton, E. (1973). *Foxfire 2.* Garden City, NY: Anchor Press/Doubleday.

Wigginton, E. (1975). *Foxfire 3.* Garden City, NY: Anchor Press.

Wigginton, E. (1977). *Foxfire 4.* Garden City, NY: Anchor Press/Doubleday.

Wigginton, E. (1979). *Foxfire 5.* Garden City, NY: Anchor Press.

Wigginton, E. (1981). *Foxfire 6.* New York: Doubleday.

Wigginton, E. & Bennett, M. (1984). *Foxfire 8.* New York: Doubleday.

Wigginton, E. & Bennett, M. (1986). *Foxfire 9.* New York: Doubleday.

Wilson, C. M. (1989). Elizabethan America. In W. K. McNeil (Ed.), *Appalachian images in folk and popular culture* (pp. 205–216). London: U. M. I. Press.

# Arab-Americans

*Patricia AbuGharbieh*

• Key terms to become familiar with in this chapter are:

| | |
|---|---|
| Allah | Inshallah |
| Arabic | Islam |
| *Dayah* | *Jinn* |
| Ethnic identity | Maalesh |
| Familism | Mosque |
| *Hadith* | *Mukrah* |
| *Halal* | Muslim |
| *Haram* | Prophet Muhammad |
| *Hijab* | *Qur'an* (Koran) |
| Imam | Ramadan |
| | Sheikh |

## OVERVIEW, INHABITED LOCALITIES, AND TOPOGRAPHY

### Overview

Arabs trace their ancestry and traditions to the nomadic desert tribes of the Arabian Peninsula. They share a common language, **Arabic,** and the majority are united by **Islam,** a major world religion that originated in seventh-century Arabia. Despite these common bonds, even Arab residents of a single Arab country are characterized by diversity in thought, attitude, and behavior. Country of origin, degree of development and westernization, rural versus urban upbringing, education, social class, and religion shape the Arab, influencing thoughts, attitudes, and behaviors. Indeed, a poor tradition-bound farmer from rural Yemen may appear to have little in common with a Western-educated professional from cosmopolitan Beirut. Additional factors such as refugee status, time since arrival, **ethnic identity,** disparity between cultures, employment status, social support, and English language skills influence the immigration experience and the Arab-American's adjustment to life in America (Lipson & Meleis, 1985).

The diversity among Arabs makes presenting a representative account of Arab-Americans a formidable task. Three related difficulties include author bias, personal experiences with certain subgroups of Arabs, and paucity of literature describing

Arab-Americans. Zogby (1990) attributed this scarcity to the Arab-American community's "invisibility." Early immigrants, predominantly Christians from present-day Lebanon and Syria, valued assimilation and were rather easily absorbed into mainstream America. Similarly, as an unofficial minority, Arab-Americans "disappear" in national studies because they are included in "white" population figures. Therefore, to portray Arab-Americans as fully as possible, literature describing Arabs is used to supplement research completed by groups studying Arab-Americans residing in Michigan and the San Francisco Bay area of California. An underlying assumption is that the attitudes and behaviors of first-generation immigrants are somewhat similar to those of their Arab world counterparts.

Islamic doctrines and practices are emphasized because most post-1965 Arab-American immigrants are **Muslims** (El-Badry, 1994). Religion, whether official Islam or a local folk variant, is an integral part of everyday Arab life. Moreover, because Arabism and Islam are so intrinsically interwoven and because Islam incorporates elements of Christianity, Arabs, whether Christian or Muslim, share many basic traditions and beliefs. Consequently, knowledge of Islam is critical to understanding the Arab-American client's cultural frame of reference and for providing care and health teaching that accommodate and show respect for the specific religious beliefs and practices of Arab Muslim clients.

## Heritage and Residence

Arab-Americans are defined as immigrants from the Arabic-speaking world: northern African countries of Morocco, Algeria, Tunisia, Libya, Sudan, and Egypt, and the western Asian countries of Lebanon, occupied Palestine, Syria, Jordan, Iraq, Kuwait, Bahrain, Qatar, United Arab Emirates, Saudi Arabia, Oman, and Yemen. The Arab-American Institute (1994) estimates that there are 3 million Arab-Americans. Arab immigration has been described as occurring in two waves (Zogby, 1990), which are distinct with respect to immigrants' characteristics. First-wave immigrants and their descendants typically reside in urban centers of the northeast: New York; Washington, D.C.; Boston, Massachusetts; Bergen-Passaic, New Jersey; Pittsburgh and Philadelphia, Pennsylvania; and Nassau-Suffolk counties, New York. Second-wave Arab-American immigrants have settled in cities in the Midwest and West; they outnumber U.S.-born Arab-Americans in Illinois (Chicago) and California. Detroit-Dearborn, Michigan, is the largest and perhaps most visible Arab-American community (Zogby, 1990). Houston, Texas, and Cleveland, Ohio, are also among the top 10 cities for Arab-Americans (El-Badry, 1994).

## Reasons for Migration and Associated Economic Factors

First-wave immigrants came to the United States between 1890 and 1940 seeking economic opportunity and perhaps the financial means to return home and buy land or set up shop in their ancestral village. While the majority of these first Arab-Americans engaged in pack peddling, others worked in the textile, steel, and auto industries (Vincent-Barwood, 1986). About half of today's Arab-Americans are descendants of these Lebanese and Syrian Christian immigrants.

Second-wave immigrants entered the United States after World War II, increasing dramatically after passage of the Immigration Act of 1965. Unlike the more economically motivated Lebanese-Syrian Christians, most second-wave immigrants are refugees from nations beset with war and political instability—chiefly occupied Palestine, Jordan, Iraq, Yemen, Lebanon, and Syria. Included in this group are a large number of professionals and individuals seeking educational degrees who subsequently remained in the United States. The majority are Muslims with a political consciousness and sense of ethnic identity unknown to first-wave immigrants (Zogby, 1990).

## Educational Status and Occupations

Because Arabs favor professional occupations, education as a prerequisite to white-collar work is valued. Not surprisingly, both U.S.- and foreign-born Arab-Americans are more educated than the average American (Zogby, 1990). Their educational accomplishments are particularly impressive because, just fifty years ago, education for most Arab youths meant attendance at a Koranic school. Reading and reciting **Qur'an,** under the instruction of a religious **sheikh** or elder, was often the only education many received (Nydell, 1987). Perhaps because of this instruction, rote learning by repetition, recitation in chorus, and memorization are favored methods of instruction in Arab educational institutions. Similarly, theory tends to receive more emphasis than practical application.

Literacy rates among women in the Arab world vary from approximately 30 percent in Egypt and Iraq to almost 70 percent in Lebanon and Jordan, where women often earn university degrees (Kurian, 1992). For example, 45 percent of the graduates from the University of Jordan between 1965 and 1987 were women (University of Jordan, 1988). Significantly, many illiterate individuals have memorized the *Qur'an.*

In comparison with Americans, Arab-Americans are more likely to be self-employed and much more likely to be in managerial and professional specialty occupations (Zogby, 1990). Nearly 25 percent are involved in retail trade. Conversely, Arab-Americans are less likely to be involved in farming, forestry, fishing, precision production, crafts, or work as operators and fabricators.

Despite the affluence of Arab-Americans as a group, their poverty rate is substantially higher than the U.S. national average because of the differences between U.S.- and foreign-born Arab-Americans. Whereas U.S.-born Arab-Americans tend to be employed and prosperous, foreign-born Arab-Americans are more likely to be unemployed and poor, with one in five immigrant households having an income of $5000 or less (*Note:* 1979 income figures). Zogby's (1990) demographic profile is based on individuals who completed the 1980 census long form, declared Arabic ancestry, and provided 1979 income data.

## COMMUNICATIONS

### Dominant Language and Dialects

Arabic is the official language of the Arab world. Modern Standard Arabic or classical Arabic is a universal form of Arabic used for all writing and formal situations ranging from radio newscasts to lectures. Dialectal or colloquial Arabic, of which each community has a typical variety, is used for everyday spoken communication. Arabs often mix Modern Standard Arabic and colloquial Arabic according to the complexity of the subject and the formality of the occasion. The presence of numerous dialects with differences in accent, inflection, and vocabulary may interfere with communication, particularly in a field such as psychiatry where shades of meaning are significant (Racy, 1977).

The Arab's speech is likely to be characterized by repetition, exaggeration, and gesturing, particularly when involved in spirited discussions. Arabs may shout when angry or excited and punctuate remarks with oaths to stress their sincerity. Westerners witnessing such impassioned communication may assume an argument is taking place; however, Arabs are not usually as angry as they appear. To Arabs, displays of emotion connote deep and sincere concern for the outcome of a discussion (Nydell, 1987).

English is a common second language in Egypt, Jordan, Lebanon, Yemen, Bahrain, and Kuwait (Nydell, 1987). Despite this, and the finding that 83.7 percent of Arab-born U.S. census respondents report speaking English "well" (Zogby, 1990), there is ample evidence that language and communication pose formidable problems in American health-care settings. For example, Lipson, et al.'s (1987) medical record review revealed a large number of clients whose English was poor. Even English-speaking Arab-Americans report difficulty expressing their needs and understanding health-care providers (Laffrey, et al., 1989; Young, et al., 1987). Similarly, Arab-American clients rank Arabic-speaking health providers as a most important service (Laffrey, et al., 1989).

Health-care providers have cited numerous interpersonal and communication problems, including presentation of confusing diagnostic pictures (Lipson, et al., 1987; Sullivan, 1993), failed appointments, clients' agreement but subsequent non-compliance, reluctance to disclose personal health information, docile patients with demanding and overanxious relatives (Lipson, et al., 1987), passivity in the physician's presence (Meleis & Jonsen, 1983), unwillingness to engage in self-care (Laffrey, et al., 1989), and a tendency to exaggerate when describing complaints (Dubovsky, 1983; Sullivan, 1993). Similarly, Meleis and Jonsen (1983) described an Egyptian family's negative reactions to personal questions, requests for written informed consent, and frank discussions of diagnosis and prognosis.

## Cultural Communication Patterns

Arabs have been described as highly contexted (Hall, 1979), with more communication contained in the context of the situation than the words spoken. Arabs value privacy and resist disclosure of personal information to strangers. Conversely, among friends and relatives, Arabs express feelings freely. These patterns of communication become more comprehensible when interpreted within the Arab's cultural frame of reference. Many personal needs may be anticipated without the individual having to verbalize them because of close family relationships (Laffrey, et al., 1989). The family may rely more on unspoken expectations and nonverbal cues than overt verbal exchange (Budman, Lipson, & Meleis, 1992).

Arabs need to become familiar with personal interactions and get to know someone, developing feelings for the person, before thoughts can be shared. Because meaning may be attached to compliments, as well as indifference, manner and tone are as important as what is said. Arabs are sensitive to the courtesy and respect they are accorded, and good manners are a salient factor in evaluating a person's character (Nydell, 1987). Therefore greetings, inquiries about well-being, pleasantries, and a cup of tea precede business. Conversants stand close together, maintain steady eye contact, and touch (only between members of the same sex) the other's hand or shoulder. Sitting and standing properly is critical; to do otherwise is taken as a lack of respect. Within the context of personal relationships, verbal agreements are considered binding. Keeping promises is considered a matter of honor.

Substantial efforts are directed at maintaining pleasant relationships and preserving dignity and honor. Hostility in response to perceived wrongdoing is warded off by an attitude of *maalesh*, "never mind, it doesn't matter." Individuals are protected from bad news for as long as possible and then informed as gently as possible. When disputes arise, Arabs hint at their disagreement or simply fail to follow through. Alternatively, an intermediary, someone with influence, may be used to intervene in disputes or present requests to the top man. Mediation saves face if a conflict is not settled in one's favor and reassures the petitioner that maximum influence has been employed (Nydell, 1987).

Guidelines for communicating with Arab-Americans include the following:

1. Employ an approach that combines expertise with warmth. Minimize status differences as Arab-Americans report feeling uncomfortable and self-conscious in the presence of authority figures. Pay special attention to the person's feelings. Arab-Americans perceive themselves as sensitive, with the potential for being easily hurt, belittled, and slighted (Reizian & Meleis, 1987).

2. Take time to get acquainted before delving into business. If sincere interest in the Arab-American's home country and adjustment to American life is expressed, the Arab-American is likely to enjoy relating such information, much of which is essential to assessing risk for traumatic immigration experience (see "Barriers to Health Care" below) and understanding the person's cultural frame of reference. Sharing a cup of tea does much to give an initial visit a positive beginning (Lipson & Meleis, 1983).

3. Nurses may need to clarify role responsibilities regarding history taking, performing physical examinations, and providing health information for newer immigrants. Arabs are accustomed to nurses' functioning as medical assistants and housekeepers (see Status of Health-care Providers).

4. Perform focused rather than comprehensive assessments. Explain the relationship of the information needed for physical complaints.

5. Interpret family members' communication patterns within a cultural context. Recognize that a spokesperson(s) may answer questions directed to the client and that the family's role is to relate the client's complaints with greater vehemence than the client (Reizian & Meleis, 1986). Family members can also be expected to act as the client's advocates; they may attempt to resolve problems by taking appeals "to the top" or by seeking the help of an influential intermediary.

6. Convey hope and optimism. The concept of "false hope" is not meaningful to Arabs because they regard God's power to cure as infinite. The amount and type of information given should be carefully considered.

## Temporal Relationships

Arabs believe in predestination, that is, that the events of one's life have been prerecorded. Accordingly, individuals should work hard to make the best of life while acknowledging that God has ultimate control over all that happens. Consequently, plans and intentions are qualified with the phrase ***inshallah***, "if God wills," and blessings and misfortunes are attributed to God rather than to the actions of individuals.

Throughout the Arab world, there is a nonchalance about time and deadlines; the pace of life is more leisurely than in the West. Social events and appointments tend not to have a fixed beginning or end. Although certain individuals may arrive on time for appointments, the tendency is to be somewhat late.

## Format for Names

Etiquette requires shaking hands on arrival and departure. However, when an Arab man is introduced to an Arab woman, the man waits for the woman to extend her hand. Titles are important and are used in combination with the person's first name (e.g., Mr. Khalil or Dr. Ali). Some may prefer to be addressed as mother (Um) or father (Abu) of the eldest son (e.g., Abu Khalil, or "father of Khalil").

# FAMILY ROLES AND RESPONSIBILITIES

## Head of Household and Gender Roles

Arab families are characterized by a strong patriarchal tradition and a hierarchical structure. Women are subordinate to men, and young people are subordinate to older people. Consequently, within his immediate family, the man is the head of the family and his influence is overt. In public, a wife's interactions with her husband are formal and respectful. However, behind the scenes, she typically wields tremendous influence, particularly in matters pertaining to the home and children. A wife may sometimes be required to hide her power from her husband and children to preserve the husband's view of himself as head of the family (Budman, Lipson, & Meleis, 1992).

Within the larger extended family, the senior male figure assumes the role of decision maker. The family matriarch attains status in advancing years, particularly if she is the mother of many sons (Racy, 1977). The bond between mothers and sons is typically strong, and most men make every effort to obey their mother's wishes, and even her whims (Nydell, 1987).

Gender roles are clearly defined and regarded as a complementary division of labor. Men are breadwinners, protectors, and decision makers, whereas women are responsible for the care and education of children and for maintenance of a successful marriage by tending to their husbands' needs.

Although women in more westernized Arab countries such as Lebanon, Syria, Jordan, and Egypt often have professional careers, with some joining in calls for women's liberation, family and marriage remain primary commitments for the majority. In fact, many women express a genuine respect for the traditional way of life, which "offers dignity, protection, and an easier way of life" (Barakat, 1985, p. 70). For example, many Muslim women view the **hijab,** "covering the body except for one's face and hands," as offering them protection in situations where the sexes mix, because it is a recognized symbol of Muslim identity and good moral character.

Ironically, many Americans associate the *hijab* with oppression rather than protection. Similarly, the authority structure and division of labor within Arab families are often misinterpreted, fueling common stereotypes of the overtly dominant Arab male and the passive and oppressed Arab woman. Health-care professionals should recognize and maintain the positive cultural meanings of care by Arab males, specifically their role responsibilities with respect to surveillance, protection, and maintenance of the family, rather than narrowly stereotyping Arab males as controlling (Luna, 1994).

## Prescriptive, Restrictive, and Taboo Behaviors for Children and Adolescents

In the traditional Arab family, the roles of the father and mother as they relate to the children are quite distinct. Typically, the father is the disciplinarian, whereas the mother is an ally and mediator, an unfailing source of love and kindness. Although some fathers feel that it is advantageous to maintain a degree of fear, family relationships are usually characterized by affection and sentimentality. Children are dearly loved, indulged, and included in all family activities.

Among Arabs, raising children so they reflect well on the family is an extremely important responsibility. A child's character and successes (or failures) in life are attributed to upbringing and parental influence. Because of the emphasis on **familism** rather than individualism within the Arab culture, affiliative behavior is favored at the expense of differentiating behavior (El-Islam, 1982). Correspondingly, childrearing methods are oriented toward accommodation, conformity, and cooperation. Children are taught to do things because "that is how it is done," and to avoid actions because "nobody does that—what would people say!" (Nydell, 1987, p. 82). Regard for public opinion and maintenance of family honor are important reasons for modifying behavior.

Childrearing patterns also include strong disapproval of aggression toward parents and authority, fostering of sibling rivalry as a means of achieving character, and early differentiation of sex role in terms of sex-specific tasks, play, and dress (Racy, 1977). The "good child" is obedient, respectful of adults, quiet, clever, and mannerly.

Methods of discipline include physical punishment and shaming. Children are made to feel ashamed because others have seen them misbehave rather than to experience guilt arising from self-criticism and inward regret.

While adolescence in the West is centered on acquiring a personal identity and completing the separation process from family, Arab adolescents are expected to remain enmeshed in the family system. Family interests and opinions often influence career and marriage decisions. Arab adolescents are pressed to succeed academically, in part because of the connections between professional careers and social status. Conversely, behavior that would bring family dishonor, such as academic failure, sexual activity, illicit drug use, and juvenile delinquency, is avoided. For girls in particular, chastity and decency are required. While adolescence in Arab countries is described as less turbulent than in the West (Racy, 1977), cultural differences related to childrearing often cause significant family conflict for Arab-American families. Arab-American parents cite multiple concerns related to conflicting values regarding dating, summer jobs, methods of discipline, and sex education (Laffrey, et al., 1989).

## Family Roles and Priorities

The family is the central socioeconomic unit in Arab society. Family members cooperate to secure livelihood, rear children, and maintain standing and influence within the community. Family members live nearby, sometimes intermarry (first cousins), and expect a great deal from one another regardless of practicality or ability to help. Loyalty to one's family takes precedence over personal needs. Maintenance of family honor is paramount.

Within the hierarchical family structure, older family members are accorded great respect. Children, sons in particular, are held responsible for supporting elderly parents. Similarly, caring for aging parents is a religious duty for Muslims. Therefore, regardless of the sacrifices involved, the elderly parents are almost always cared for within the home. Senile dementia is viewed as a normal developmental stage not requiring intervention (Racy, 1977).

Responsibility for family members rests with the older men of the family. In the absence of the father, brothers are responsible for unmarried sisters. In the event of death, the husband's family provides for his widow and children. In general, family leaders are expected to use influence and render special services and favors to kinsmen.

Although educational accomplishments (doctoral degrees), certain occupations (medicine, engineering, law), and acquired wealth contribute to social status, family origin is the primary determinant. Certain character traits such as piety, generosity, hospitality, and good manners may also enhance social standing (Nydell, 1987).

## Alternative Lifestyles

The vast majority of adults marry. Although the Islamic right to marry up to four wives is sometimes exercised, particularly if the first wife is chronically ill or infertile, most marriages are monogamous and for life. Whereas homosexuality occurs in all cultures to some extent, it is stigmatized among Arab cultures; fearing family disgrace and ostracism, gays and lesbians remain closeted.

## WORKFORCE ISSUES

### Culture in the Workplace

Cultural differences that may impact work life include beliefs regarding family, gender roles, one's ability to control life events, maintaining pleasant personal relationships, guarding dignity and honor, and the importance placed on maintaining one's reputation. Arabs and Americans may also differ in attitudes toward time, instructional methods, and patterns of thinking, and amount of emphasis placed on objectivity. However, because many second-wave professionals were educated in the United States and thereby socialized to some extent, differences are probably more characteristic of less educated, first-generation Arab-Americans.

Stress is a common denominator in recent studies of first generation immigrants. Sources of stress include separation from family members, difficulty adjusting to American life, marital tension, and intergenerational conflict, specifically coping with adolescents socialized in American values through school activities (Laffrey, et al., 1989). Although discrimination is not mentioned as a specific stressor, Arab-Americans are keenly aware of the misperceptions Americans hold about Arabs, such as notions that Arabs are inferior, backward, sinister, and violent. Arab-American Muslims are additionally burdened by the American public's ignorance of mainstream Islam and stereotyping of Muslims as fanatics, extremists, and martyrdom-seeking terrorists.

Indeed, Muslim Arab-Americans face a variety of challenges as they practice their faith in a secular American society. For example, Islamic and American civil law differ on matters such as marriage, divorce, banking, and inheritance. Individuals who wish to attend Friday prayer services and observe religious holidays frequently encounter job-related conflicts. Children are often torn between fulfilling Islamic obligations regarding prayer, dietary restrictions and dress, and hiding their religious identity so as to fit into the American public school culture.

### Issues Related to Autonomy

Whereas American workplaces tend to be dominated by deadlines, profit margins, and maintaining one's competitive edge, a more relaxed, cordial, and relationship-oriented atmosphere prevails in the Arab world. Friendship and business are mixed over cups of sweet tea to the extent that it is unclear where socializing ends and work begins. Managers promote optimal performance by using personal influence and persuasion, and performance evaluations are based on personality and social behavior as well as job skills. Not surprisingly, Arabs often find the American work atmosphere cold and impersonal; they often note Americans who omit greetings (Nydell, 1987).

Significant differences also exist in workplace norms. In the United States, position is usually earned, laws are applied equally, work takes precedence over family, honesty is an absolute value, facts and logic prevail, and direct and critical appraisal is regarded as valuable feedback. In the Arab world, position is often attained through one's family and connections, rules are bent, family obligations take precedence over the demands of the job, lying is sometimes appropriate, subjective perceptions often dictate actions, and criticism is often taken personally as an affront to dignity and family honor (Nydell, 1987). In Arab offices, supervisors and managers are expected to praise their employees to assure them that their work is noticed and appreciated. Whereas such direct praise may be somewhat embarrassing for Americans, Arabs expect and want praise when they feel they have earned it (Nydell, 1987).

# BIOCULTURAL ECOLOGY

## Skin Color and Biologic Variations

Although Arabs are uniformly perceived as swarthy, and while many do, in fact, have dark or olive skin, they may also have blonde or auburn hair, blue eyes, and fair complexions. Because color changes are more difficult to assess in dark-skinned persons, pallor and cyanosis are best detected by examination of the oral mucosa and conjunctiva.

## Diseases and Health Conditions

The major public health concerns in the Arab world include trauma related to motor vehicle accidents, maternal-child health, and control of communicable diseases. The incidence of infectious diseases such as tuberculosis, malaria, trachoma, typhus, hepatitis, typhoid fever, dysentery, and parasitic infestations varies between urban and rural areas and from country to country. For example, disease risks are relatively low in modern urban centers of the Arab world but quite high in the countryside where animals such as goats and sheep virtually share living quarters, open privies are commonplace, and running water is not available. Schistosomiasis (also called bilharzia), infecting about one-fifth of Egyptians, has been called Egypt's number one health problem. Its prevalence is related to an entrenched social habit of using the Nile River for washing, drinking, and urinating (Gammal, 1988). Similarly, outbreaks of cholera and meningitis are continuous concerns in Saudi Arabia during the Muslim pilgrimage season. In Jordan, where contagious diseases have declined sharply, emphasis has shifted to preventing accidental death and controlling noncommunicable diseases such as cancer and heart disease. Correspondingly, seat belt use, smoking habits, and pesticide residues in locally grown produce are major issues. Campaigns directed at improving children's health include hepatitis B vaccinations and dental health programs. Table 6–1 illustrates the range of health conditions existing in the major homelands of second-wave Arab-American immigrants.

Glucose-6-phosphate dehydrogenase (G-6-PD) deficiency, sickle cell anemia, and the thalassemias are extremely common in the Eastern Mediterranean region, probably because carriers enjoy an increased resistance to malaria (Hamamy & Alwan, 1994; Robinson & Linden, 1993). High consanguinity rates—roughly 30 percent of marriages in Iraq, Jordan, Kuwait, and Saudi Arabia are between first cousins—and the trend of bearing children up to menopause also contributes to the prevalence of genetically determined disorders in Arab countries (Hamamy & Alwan, 1994).

With modernization and increased life expectancy, multifactorial disorders—hypertension, diabetes, coronary heart disease—have also emerged as major problems in Eastern Mediterranean countries (Hamamy & Alwan, 1994). In many countries, cardiovascular disease is a major cause of death. In Lebanon, the increased frequency of familial hypercholesterolemia (Braunwald, et al., 1987) is a contributing factor. Individuals of Arabic ancestry are also more likely to inherit familial Mediterranean fever, a disorder characterized by recurrent episodes of fever, peritonitis, or pleuritis alone or in some combination.

The extent to which these conditions affect the health of Arab-Americans is unknown because morbidity and mortality statistics for Arab-Americans are unavailable. However, research suggests that Arab-Americans are similar to the U.S. population as a whole with respect to health conditions (Young, et al., 1987) and physical complaints (Lipson, Reizian, & Meleis, 1987). However, the Arab Wayne County Behavioral Risk Factor Survey (BRFS) (1994), a telephone survey including Arabs (N = 388) residing in the Detroit area, identified cardiovascular disease as one of two particular risks based on high prevalence rates for cigarette smoking, high cholesterol

## Table 6–1 • Health Status Indicators for Major Homelands of Second-Wave Arab-Americans

| Country | Syria | Jordan | Lebanon | Iraq | Yemen* | | Egypt |
| --- | --- | --- | --- | --- | --- | --- | --- |
| | | | | | North | South | |
| Life Expectancy (Male/female) | 68/70 | 68/71 | 66/70 | 66/68 | 48/49 | 50/54 | 60/61 |
| Infant mortality | 38/1000 | 55/1000 | 49/1000 | 67/1000 | 129/1000 | 110/1000 | 90/1000 |
| Fertility rate (Births per woman) | 6.7 | 6.2 | 3.7 | 7.3 | 7.6 | 7.0 | 4.7 |
| Access to safe water | 76% | 96% | 93% | 87% | 42% | 54% | 73% |
| Major health problems | Trachoma Gastrointestinal and parasitic disease | Trachoma Intestinal and parasitic disease | Eye Infections TB Polio Heart disease accounts for ⅓ of reported deaths | Trachoma TB Parasitic diseases Dysentery Typhus Malaria Nutritional deficiencies Decline in the quality of health care with Gulf War | Trachoma TB Dysentery Typhus Malaria Typhoid Hepatitis Measles Whooping Cough Poor hygiene and sewage disposal practices, inadequate diet, and scarcity of health-care personnel | | Trachoma Tuberculosis Dysentery Hookworm Typhus Schistosomiasis |

*Source:* Data compiled from Kurian (1992). Life expectancy, infant mortality, and fertility statistics are 1990 figures. Population with access to safe water data is the "latest" available.

* Statistics obtained before the unification of North and South Yemen.

diets, obesity, and sedentary lifestyles. Although the prevalence of hypertension was lower in the Arab community than in the rest of Wayne County, Arab respondents were less likely to report having their blood pressure checked. In fact, lower rates for appropriate testing and screening, such as cholesterol testing and uterine and breast cancer screening, were considered the second area of major risk for this group of Arab-Americans.

## Variations in Drug Metabolism

Information describing drug disposition and sensitivity in Arabs is limited. One to 1.4 percent of Arabs are known to be poor metabolizers of debrisoquine and substances similarly metabolized: antiarrhythmics, antidepressants, beta-blockers, neuroleptics, and opioid agents. Consequently, a small number of Arab-Americans may experience elevated blood levels and adverse effects when customary dosages of antidepressants are prescribed. Conversely, typical codeine dosages may prove inadequate because poor metabolizers cannot metabolize codeine to morphine (Levy, 1993) to promote optimal analgesic effect.

## HIGH-RISK BEHAVIORS

Despite Islamic beliefs discouraging tobacco use, smoking remains deeply ingrained in Arab culture. For many Arabs, offering cigarettes is a sign of hospitality. Consistent with their cultural heritage, Arab-Americans are characterized by higher smoking rates and lower quitting rates than their national counterparts (Rice & Kulwicki, 1992; Wayne County Health Department, 1994). Middle-aged men (53.3 percent) and women (42.2 percent) and older women (49.1 percent) are most likely to smoke. Young women (18.7 percent) are least likely to be cigarette smokers (Wayne County Health Department, 1994).

Islamic prohibitions do appear to influence patterns of alcohol consumption and attitudes toward drug use (Wayne County Health Department, 1994). Ninety percent of the Arab BRFS respondents reported that they abstain from drinking alcohol. None reported heavy drinking, with a limited number reporting binge drinking (2.2 percent) and driving under the influence of alcohol (1.4 percent). All respondents believed that occasional use of cocaine entails "great" risk with most saying the same about occasional use of marijuana.

Although the actual risk for, and incidence of, human immunodeficiency virus infection and acquired immunodeficiency syndrome (AIDS) among Arab-Americans is unknown, 4 percent (N = 411) of the Arab-American respondents surveyed by Kulwicki and Cass (1994) reported that they were at high-risk for AIDS. In addition, the sample demonstrated less knowledge about primary routes of transmission and more misconceptions regarding unlikely modes of transmission than other populations surveyed. The Arab Wayne County BRFS (1994) confirmed these findings noting respondents' great reluctance to interact with people with AIDS.

## Health-care Practices

According to the Arab Wayne County BRFS (1994), Arab-Americans' risk in terms of safety is mixed. Factors enhancing safety include low rates of gun ownership and high recognition of the risks associated with having guns in the house. Conversely, lower rates of fire escape planning and seat belt usage for adults and older children (car seats are used), as well as higher rates of physical assaults, threaten their safety. Although passivity regarding health has been linked to the attitude known as *in-*

*shallah,* if God wills (Dubovsky, 1983), Islamic teachings stress an activist approach to maintaining one's health as well as an acceptance of God's will.

In the majority of health areas surveyed through the Arab Wayne Country BRFS (1994), education and income were important determinants of risk for persons of Arab descent. For example, lower levels of household income and education were associated with less positive perceptions of health, lack of knowledge about certain health issues, less accessibility to health care, and higher prevalence rates for chronic diseases such as diabetes and hypertension.

## NUTRITION

### Meaning of Food

Sharing meals with family and friends is a favorite pastime. Offering food is also a way of expressing love and friendship, hospitality, and generosity (Fig. 6–1). For the Arab woman whose primary roles are caring for her husband and children, the preparation and presentation of an elaborate midday meal is taken as an indication of her love and caring. Similarly, in entertaining friends, the types and quantity of food served, often several entrees, is a measure of one's hospitality and esteem for one's guests. Honor and reputation are based on the manner in which guests are received. In return, family members and guests express appreciation by eating heartily.

### Common Foods and Food Rituals

Although cooking and national dishes vary from country to country and seasoning from family to family, Arabic cooking shares many general characteristics. Familiar spices and herbs such as cinnamon, allspice, cloves, ginger, cumin, mint, parsley, bay leaves, garlic, and onions are used frequently. Skewer cooking and slow simmering are typical modes of preparation. All countries have rice and wheat dishes,

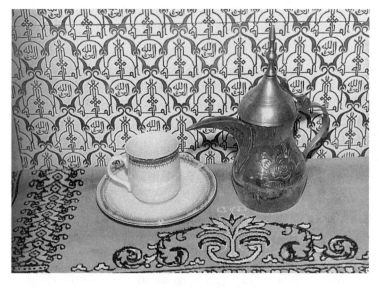

**Figure 6–1.** Generosity and hospitality are traits highly valued in the Arab culture. Offering hot, cardamon-flavored coffee is an important duty of the host. (Photograph by Nabil AbuGharbieh.)

stuffed vegetables, nut-filled pastries, and fritters soaked in syrup. Dishes are garnished with raisins, pine nuts, pistachios, and almonds.

Favorite fruits and vegetables include dates, figs, apricots, guava, mango, melon, papaya, bananas, citrus, carrots, tomatoes, cucumbers, parsley, mint, spinach, and grape leaves. Lamb and chicken are the most popular meats and poultry. Muslims are prohibited from eating pork and pork products (for example, lard). Similarly, because the consumption of blood is forbidden, Muslims are required to cook meats and poultry until well done. Bread accompanies every meal and is viewed as a gift from God. In many respects, the traditional Arab diet is representative of the U.S. Department of Agriculture's food pyramid. Bread is a mainstay, grains and legumes are often substituted for meats, fresh fruit and juices are especially popular, and olive oil is widely used. In addition, because foods are prepared "from scratch," consumption of preservatives and additives is limited.

Lunch is the main meal in Arab households. Encouraging guests to eat is the host's duty. Guests often begin with a ritual refusal and then succumb to the host's insistence. Food is eaten with the right hand because it is regarded as clean. Beverages may not be served until after the meal because some Arabs consider it unhealthy to eat and drink at the same time. Similar concerns may exist regarding mixing hot and cold foods.

Health-care providers should also be knowledgeable about **Ramadan**, the Muslim month of fasting. The fast, which is meant to remind Muslims of their dependence on God and the poor who experience involuntary fasting, involves abstinence from eating, drinking (including water), smoking, and marital intercourse during daylight hours. Although the sick are not required to fast, many pious Muslims insist on fasting while hospitalized, necessitating adjustments in meal times and medications, including medications given by nonoral routes. In outpatient settings, health-care providers need to be alert to potential "noncompliance." Patients may omit or adjust the timing of medications. Of particular concern are medications requiring constant blood levels, adequate hydration, or both (for example, antibiotics that may crystallize in the kidneys). Providers may need to provide appointment times after sunset during Ramadan for individuals requiring injections (for example, allergy shots).

## Dietary Practices for Health Promotion

Arabs associate good health with eating properly, consuming nutritious foods, and fasting to cure disease. For some, concerns about amounts and balance among food types (hot, cold, dry, moist) may be traced to the **Prophet Muhammad** who taught that "the stomach is the house of every disease, and abstinence is the head of every remedy" (Al-Akili, 1994, p. 7). Within this framework, illness is related to excessive eating, eating before a previously eaten meal is digested, eating nutritionally deficient food, mixing opposing types of foods, and consuming elaborately prepared foods. Conversely, abstinence allows the body to expel disease.

The condition of the alimentary tract has priority over all other body systems in Arabs' perception of health (Meleis & La Fever, 1984). Gastrointestinal complaints are often the reason Arab-Americans seek care (Lipson, et al., 1987; Reizian and Meleis, 1987; Young, et al., 1987). Obesity is a problem for older Arab-American women (Lipson, et al., 1987), the majority of whom report trying to lose weight by reducing caloric intake (Wayne County Health Department, 1994).

## Nutritional Deficiencies and Food Limitations

In Arab countries, diet is influenced by income, government subsidies for certain foods (for example, bread, sugar, oil), and seasonal availability. Arab-Americans most at risk for nutritional deficiencies include newly arrived immigrants from Yemen and Iraq (Kurian, 1992) and Arab-American households below the poverty level.

Poverty and preferential feeding of males may contribute to nutritional deficiencies in girls (Issacs, 1989; West, 1987). Lactose intolerance sometimes occurs in this population. However, the practice of eating yogurt and cheese, rather than drinking milk, probably limits symptoms in sensitive persons.

Many of the most common foods are available in American markets. Some Muslims may refuse to eat meat that is not *halal*, or slaughtered in an Islamic manner. *Halal* meat can be obtained in Arabic grocery stores and through Islamic centers or **mosques.**

Islamic prohibitions against the consumption of alcohol and pork have implications for American health-care providers. Conscientious Muslims are often wary of eating outside the home and may ask multiple questions about ingredients used in meal preparation: Are the beans vegetarian? Was wine used in the meat sauce, or lard in the pastry crust? Muslims are equally concerned about the ingredients and origins of mouthwashes, toothpastes, and medicines (for example, alcohol-based syrups and elixirs), and insulins and capsules (gelatin coating) derived from pig. However, if no substitutes are available, Muslims are permitted to use these preparations.

## PREGNANCY AND CHILDBEARING PRACTICES

### Fertility Practices and Views toward Pregnancy

Fertility rates in the countries from which most Arab-Americans emigrated (see Table 6–1) range from 3.7 in Lebanon to 7.6 in North Yemen (Kurian, 1992), with an average rate of 5.98. Fertility practices of Arabs are influenced by traditional Bedouin values supporting tribal dominance, popular beliefs that "God decides family size" and "God provides," and Islamic rulings regarding birth control, treatment of infertility, and abortion.

High fertility rates are favored. Procreation is regarded as the purpose of marriage and the means of enhancing family strength. Accordingly, Islamic jurists have ruled that the use of "reversible" forms of birth control such as *mukrah*, are "undesirable but not forbidden." They should be employed only in certain situations, listed in decreasing order of legitimacy, such as threat to the mother's life, too frequent childbearing, risk of transmitting genetic disease, and financial hardship. Moreover, irreversible forms of birth control such as vasectomy and tubal ligation are *haram*, "absolutely unlawful." Muslims regard abortion as *haram* except when the mother's health is compromised by pregnancy-induced disease or her life is threatened (Ebrahim, 1989). Therefore, unwanted pregnancies are dealt with by hoping one miscarries "by an act of God" or by covertly arranging for an abortion.

Among Jordanian husbands, religion and the fatalistic belief that "God decides family size" were most often given as reasons why contraceptives were not used. Contraceptives were used by 27 percent of the husbands, typically urbanites of high socioeconomic status. Although the IUD and the "pill" were most widely favored, 4.9 percent of females used sterilization despite religious prohibitions (The Hashemite Kingdom of Jordan, 1985). A review of the medical records of Arab-Americans revealed much the same pattern: few requests for birth control despite large family size with two women accepting tubal ligations (Lipson, et al., 1987).

Indeed, among Arab women, in particular, fertility may be more of a concern than contraception because sterility in a woman could lead to rejection and divorce. Islam condones treatment for infertility, as **Allah** provides progeny as well as a cure for every disease. However, approved methods for treating infertility are limited to artificial insemination using the husband's sperm and in vitro fertilization involving the fertilization of the wife's ovum by the husband's sperm. All other techniques are seen as involving an element of adulterous union that could undermine the institution of marriage (Ebramin, 1989).

## Prescriptive, Restrictive, and Taboo Practices in the Childbearing Family

Because of the emphasis on fertility and the bearing of sons, pregnancy usually occurs early in Arab marriages. The pregnant woman is indulged and her cravings satisfied, lest she develop a birthmark in the shape of the particular food she craves. Because of the preference for males, the sex of the child can be a stressor for mothers without sons. Friends and family often note how the mother is "carrying" the baby as an indicator of the baby's sex (that is, high for a girl and low for a boy). Practices that may adversely influence fetal growth include the consumption of large quantities of olive oil (Cline, et al., 1986), and failure to stop smoking or to limit caffeine. Inadequate weight gain in some mothers may be attributed to the practice of giving the "best food" to one's spouse and children (Cline, et al., 1986). Although pregnant women are excused from fasting during Ramadan, some Muslim women may be determined to fast and thus suffer potential consequences for glucose metabolism and hydration.

Labor and delivery are women's affairs. In Arab countries, home delivery with the assistance of *dayahs*, midwives, or neighbors is common because of limited access to hospitals, "shyness," and financial constraints. Iraqi refugees residing in Detroit have maintained the pattern of home birth (Young, et al., 1987). During labor, women openly express pain through facial expressions, verbalizations, and body movements. They do not ordinarily accept breathing and relaxation techniques, and few desire anesthesia because of the fear and myth surrounding epidural and spinal anesthesia (Meleis and Sorrell, 1981).

Care for the infant includes wrapping the stomach at birth, or as soon thereafter as possible, to prevent cold or wind from entering the baby's body (Luna, 1994). The call to prayer is recited in the Muslim newborn's ear. Male circumcision is almost a universal practice, and for Muslims, it is a religious requirement.

Folk beliefs influence bathing and breast-feeding. Arab mothers may be reluctant to bathe postpartum because of the beliefs that air gets into the mother and causes illness (Luna, 1994) and because of the belief that washing the breasts "thins the milk" (Cline, et al., 1986). Breast-feeding is often delayed until the second or third day after birth because of beliefs that the mother requires rest, that nursing at birth causes "colic" pain for the mother, and that "colostrum makes the baby dumb" (Cline, et al., 1986). Postpartum care also includes special foods such as lentil soup to increase milk production and tea to flush and cleanse the body.

Statistics describing the pregnancy and birth experiences of Michigan mothers, including 2755 Arab-Americans (Office of the State Registrar and Division of Health Statistics, Michigan Department of Public Health, 1993), depict the experiences of Arab-American mothers and infants as fairly comparable to their white counterparts with respect to variables such as adequacy of prenatal care, maternal complications, infant mortality, and birth complications. In addition, fewer Arab-American mothers smoke, drink alcohol, or gain too little weight.

Although these statewide statistics are quite favorable, it is important to mention that earlier studies revealed an alarming rate of infant mortality among Arab-American mothers in Dearborn, Michigan, a particularly disadvantaged community of new immigrants with high rates of unemployment. Factors contributing to poor pregnancy outcomes include poverty; lower level of education; inability to communicate in English; personal, family, and cultural stressors; cigarette smoking; and early or closely spaced pregnancies. Fear of being ridiculed by American health-care providers and a limited number of bilingual providers limit access to health-care information (Kulwicki, 1989).

## DEATH RITUALS

### Death Rituals and Expectations

Although Arabs insist on maintaining hope regardless of prognosis, death is accepted as God's will. According to Muslim beliefs, death is foreordained and worldly life is but a preparation for eternal life:

> Every soul will taste of death. And ye will be paid on the Day of Resurrection only that which ye have fairly earned. Whoso is removed from the Fire and is made to enter Paradise, he indeed is triumphant. The life of this world is but comfort of illusion. (Surah III, v. 185, p.70)

Muslims are not to struggle with the sort of "if only . . . then . . ." hindsight common to Americans. Accidents occur so that death finds a means (Wikan, 1988). Muslim death rituals include turning the patient's bed to face the Holy City of Mecca and reading from the Qur'an, particularly verses stressing hope and acceptance.

After death, the deceased is washed three times by a Muslim of the same sex. The body is then wrapped, preferably in white material, and buried as soon as possible in a brick or cement-lined grave facing Mecca. Prayers for the deceased are recited at home, at the mosque, or at the cemetery. Women do not ordinarily attend the burial unless the deceased is a close relative or husband. Instead, they gather at the deceased's home and read the *Qur'an*. Cremation is not practiced.

Family members do not generally approve of autopsy because of respect for the dead and feelings that the body should not be mutilated. Islam allows forensic autopsy and autopsy for the sake of medical research and instruction (Darsh, n.d.).

### Responses to Death and Grief

The recognition of death as inevitable is reinforced by Islamic guidelines limiting expressions of grief and periods of mourning (Darsh, n.d.). Family members are asked to endure with patience and good faith in Allah what befalls them of death. While friends and relatives are to restrict mourning to 3 days, a wife may mourn for 4 months and 10 days. Although weeping is allowed, beating the cheeks or tearing garments is prohibited.

However, in some Arab Muslim communities, popular beliefs more than Islamic teachings may shape responses to loss. For example, Wikan (1988) described intense, heart-rending grieving and endless reminiscing over the deceased as characteristic of the poor in Cairo. Because of beliefs that humans are required to do whatever is necessary to make the best of life and that expression of emotion is necessary for health, these poor Egyptians see no contradiction between submitting to God's will and fully expressing what they regard as detrimental emotion.

## SPIRITUALITY

### Religious Practices and Use of Prayer

The majority of Arabs are Muslims. Prominent Christian groups include the Copts in Egypt, the Chaldeans in Iraq, and the Maronites in Lebanon. Despite their distinctive practices and liturgies, Christians and Muslims share certain beliefs because of

Islam's origin in Judaism and Christianity. Muslims and Christians believe in the same God and many of the same Prophets, the Day of Judgment, Satan, heaven, hell, and an afterlife. One major difference is that Islam has no priesthood. Islamic scholars or religious *sheikhs,* the most learned individuals in an Islamic community, assume the role of **imam**, or "leader of the prayer." The imam also performs marriage ceremonies, funeral prayers, and acts as a spiritual counselor or reference on Islamic teachings. Obtaining the opinion of the local imam may be a helpful intervention for Arab-American Muslims struggling with health-care decisions.

Observance of religious practices varies among Muslims. Patai (1958) makes a distinction between official Islam, as practiced by the educated, and popular beliefs and practices that influence the religious life of the "untutored folk." In addition, as with any other religion, there are nominal as well as practicing Muslims. However, because Islam is the state religion of most Arab countries, and in Islam, there is no separation of church and state, a certain degree of religious participation is obligatory.

To illustrate, consider a few examples of Islam's impact on Jordanian life. Because of Islamic law, abortion is investigated as a crime and foster parenting is encouraged, whereas adoption is forbidden. The infertility treatments available are those approved by Islamic jurists. *Shariah,* Islamic law courts, rule on matters such as marriage, divorce, guardianship, and inheritance. Classes on Islam and prayer rooms are part of public schools. School and work schedules revolve around Islamic holidays and the weekly prayer. During Ramadan, restaurants remain closed during daylight hours, and work days are shortened to facilitate fasting. Because Muslims gather for communal prayer on Friday afternoons, the workweek runs from Saturday through Thursday. Finally, because of Islamic tradition that adherents of other monotheistic religions be accorded tolerance and protection, Jordan's Christians have separate religious courts and schools, and non-Muslims attending public schools are not required to participate in religious activities.

## Meaning of Life and Individual Sources of Strength

For Muslims, adherents of the world's largest religion, Islam, religious faith means "submission to Allah." Life centers on worshipping Allah and preparing for one's afterlife by fulfilling religious duties as described in the holy *Qur'an* and the **hadith**. The five major duties or pillars of Islam are: (1) declaration of faith, (2) prayer five times daily, (3) almsgiving, (4) fast during Ramadan, and 5) completion of a pilgrimage to Mecca.

Despite the dominance of familism in Arab life, religious faith is often regarded as more important. Whether Muslim or Christian, Arabs identify strongly with their respective religious group and religious affiliation is as much a part of their identity as family name. God and His power is acknowledged in everyday life.

## Spiritual Beliefs and Health-care Practices

Many Muslims believe in combining spiritual medicine, performance of daily prayers, and reading or listening to *Qur'an,* with conventional medical treatment. The devout patient may request that his or her chair or bed be turned to face Mecca and that a basin of water be provided for ritual washing or ablution before praying. Providing for cleanliness is particularly important because the Muslim's prayer is not acceptable unless the body, clothing, and place of prayer are clean.

Islamic teachings urge Muslims to eat wholesome food; abstain from pork, alcohol, and illicit drugs; practice moderation in all activities; be conscious of hygiene; and face adversity with faith in Allah's mercy and compassion, hope, and acceptance.

Muslims are also advised to care for the needs of the community by visiting and assisting the sick and providing for needy Muslims.

Illness is often regarded as punishment for one's sins. Correspondingly, by providing cures, Allah manifests mercy and compassion and supplies a vehicle for repentance and gratitude (Al-Akili, 1994). Others emphasize that sickness not be viewed as punishment but as a trial or ordeal that brings about expiation of sins and that may strengthen character (Ebrahim, 1989). Common responses to illness include patience and endurance of suffering because it has a purpose known only to Allah, unfailing hope that even "irreversible" conditions might be cured "if it be Allah's will," and acceptance of one's fate. Euthanasia and suicide are forbidden.

## HEALTH-CARE PRACTICES

## Health-seeking Beliefs and Practices

Good health is conceptualized as the ability to fulfill one's roles. Diseases are attributed to a variety of factors such as inadequate diet, hot and cold shifts, exposure of one's stomach during sleep, emotional or spiritual distress, and envy or the evil eye. Arabs are expected to express and acknowledge their ailments when ill. Muslims often mention that the Prophet urged physicians to perform research and the ill to seek treatment because "Allah has not created a disease without providing a cure for it," except for the problem of old age (Ebrahim, 1989, p.5).

Despite beliefs that one should care for health and seek treatment when ill, Arab women are often reluctant to seek care. Because of the cultural emphasis placed on modesty, some women express shyness about disrobing for examination. Similarly, some families object to female family members being examined by male physicians. Fear that a diagnosed illness such as cancer or psychiatric illness may influence marriageability of the woman and her female relatives may contribute to delays in seeking medical care. For example, in Egypt, breast cancer is often far advanced at diagnosis (Ali & Khalil, 1991). Among Jordanian women, the majority sought care when the tumor was 5 cm or more (Shahin, 1989). Similarly, health-care visits for gynecologic problems or pregnancy were rare among Detroit-area Iraqi refugees (Young, et al., 1987).

Evidence also suggests that the cultural preference for boys influences the health care that low-income parents provide for female children. In poor communities in Jordan, boys were better nourished, more likely to be immunized, and more apt to receive prompt medical attention for illnesses (West, 1987). Delay in seeking treatment was noted by a local health-care provider who diagnosed "failure to thrive" in a young Iraqi female infant when her refugee parents sought medical attention for a feverish male sibling.

While Arab-Americans readily seek care for actual symptoms, preventive care is not generally sought. Among two groups of Arab-Americans, there was not one health-care visit for physical examination (Lipson, et al., 1987; Young, et al., 1987). Similarly, pediatric clinics are used primarily for illness and injury rather than for well-child visits (Lipson, et al., 1987). Laffrey, et al. (1989) attributed these patterns to Arabs' present orientation and reluctance to plan and to the meaning Arab-Americans attach to preventive care. Whereas American health-care providers focus on screening and managing risks and complications, Arab-Americans value information that aids in coping with stress, illness, or treatment protocols. Arab-Americans' failure to use preventive care services may be related to other factors such as insurance coverage, the availability of female physicians who accept Medicaid patients, and the novelty of the concept of preventive care for immigrants from developing countries.

## Responsibility for Health Care

Dichotomous views regarding individual responsibility and one's control over life's events often cause misunderstanding between Arab-Americans and health-care providers (AbuGharbieh, 1993). For example, individualism and an activist approach to life are the underpinnings of the American health-care system. Accordingly, practices such as informed consent, self-care, advanced directives, risk management, and preventive care are valued. Patients are expected to use information seeking and problem solving in preference to faith in God, patience, and acceptance of one's fate as primary coping mechanisms. Similarly, American health-care providers expect that the patient's hope be "realistic" in accordance with medical science.

However, in the Arab culture, quite the opposite values—familism and fatalism—influence health care and responses to illness. For Arabs, the family is the context within which health care is delivered (Lipson, et al., 1987). Rather than engage in self-care and decision making, clients often allow family members to oversee care. Family members indulge the individual and assume the ill person's responsibilities. Although the patient may seem overdependent and the family over protective by American standards, family members' vigilance and "demanding behavior" should be interpreted as a measure of concern. For Muslims, care is a religious obligation associated with individual and collective meanings of honor (Luna, 1994). Individuals are seen as expressing care through the performance of gender-specific role responsibilities as delineated in the *Qur'an.*

Although most American health-care professionals consider full disclosure an ethical obligation, most Arab physicians do not believe that it is necessary for a client to know a serious diagnosis or full details of a surgical procedure. In fact, communicating a grave diagnosis is often viewed as cruel and tactless because it deprives clients of hope. Similarly, preoperative instructions are thought to cause needless anxiety, hypochondriasis, and complications. Apart from the educated, most clients are not interested in actively participating in decision making (AbuGharbieh, 1993). They expect physicians, because of their expertise, to select treatments. The client's role is to cooperate. As authority figures, accorded great respect in Arab society, physicians are seldom challenged or questioned. When treatment is successful, the physician's skill is recognized; adverse outcomes are attributed to God's will (Sullivan, 1993) unless there is evidence of blatant malpractice. As corroborated by Ali and Khalil (1991), faith (submission to God), the support of others, and compliance with the medical regimen are the most commonly employed coping strategies.

Not all Arabs may be familiar with the American concept of health insurance. Traditionally, insurance is provided by the family unit through its communal resources. Certain Arab countries, such as Saudi Arabia and Kuwait, provide free medical care, whereas in other countries, many citizens are government employees entitled to low-cost care in government-sector facilities. Private physicians and hospitals are preferred because of beliefs that the private sector offers the best care.

Because many medications requiring a prescription in the United States are available over the counter in Arab countries, Arabs are accustomed to seeking medical advice from pharmacists. In comparison with their Wayne County counterparts, Arab-Americans in the Wayne County BRFS (1994) were less like to take prescription medications and more likely to use medications as directed.

## Folk Practices

Although Islam disapproves of superstition, witchcraft, and magic, concerns about the powers of jealous people, the evil eye, and certain supernatural agents such as the devil and *jinn* are part of the religion. Those who envy the wealth, success, or

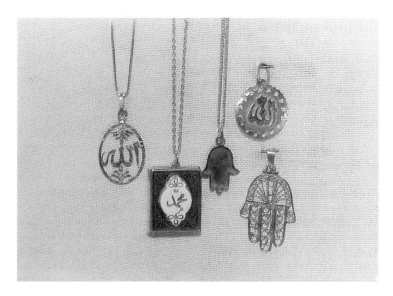

**Figure 6–2.** Jewelry reflects the integration of Islam and art. In the necklace *(far left)* is the word "Allah." "Mohammad" is inscribed on the *Qur'an (second from left)*. At the right are amulets, which are believed to offer the wearer protection from evil. (Photograph by Nabil AbuGharbieh.)

beauty of others are believed to cause adversity by a gaze, which transmits malignant radiating energy and upsets the victim's natural balance (Al-Akili, 1994). Newborns are believed to be particularly susceptible to the evil eye (Luna, 1994; Meleis & Sorrell, 1981), and expressions of congratulations may be interpreted as envy. Protection from the evil eye is afforded by wearing amulets, such as blue beads or figures involving the number five, reciting the *Qur'an,* or invoking the name of Allah (Fig. 6–2). Persons suspecting themselves of possessing the evil eye are to pray "Lord, bless what he has" (Al-Akili, 1994, p. 128).

Unacceptable wishes, feelings, and acts may be assigned to the devil, enabling people to doubt or to disavow them as the devil's ideas, instead of their own (El-Islam, 1982). Similarly, unreasonable, bizarre, and unpredictable behavior may be attributed to possession by an evil *jinn*. The Arabic word for insanity, *jenun* is derived from *jinn*.

Traditional Islamic medicine is based on the theory of four humors and the spiritual and physical remedies prescribed by the Prophet. Because illness is viewed as an imbalance between the humors—black bile, blood, phlegm, and yellow bile—and the primary attributes of dryness, heat, cold, and moisture, therapy involves treating with the disease's opposite: hot disease–cold remedy. Although methods such as cupping, cautery, and phlebotomy may be employed, treating with special prayers or simple foods such as dates, honey, salt, and olive oil is preferred (Al-Akili, 1994). Saudi Arabian patients use cautery in combination with modern medical technology (Sullivan, 1993).

## Barriers to Health Care

At particular risk for both increased risk exposure and inadequate access are newly arrived, unskilled refugees from poorer, less developed parts of the Arab world. Factors such as refugee status, recent arrival, incongruence between cultures (potentially greater for Muslims, rural Arabs, or both), financial concerns, and poor master of English add to the trauma of immigration (Lipson & Meleis, 1985), affecting both health status and responses to health problems. Moreover, these immigrants are less likely to receive adequate health care because of cultural and language barriers, lack of transportation, limited health insurance, poverty, a lack of awareness of existing services, and poor coordination of services (Kulwicki, 1989).

Although insurance noncoverage affects a significant number of Arab Wayne County BRFS (1994) respondents, other studies suggest that Arab-Americans regard other barriers and services as more significant. Recent refugees from Iraq rated doctor and refugee communication and transportation as the most significant obstacles to health care (Young, et al. 1987), whereas another group of Arab-Americans rated services such as health education programs, Arabic-speaking health providers, and appropriate referral (Laffrey, et al., 1989) as more important than health insurance and financial assistance.

## Cultural Responses to Health and Illness

Arabs regard pain as unpleasant and something to be controlled (Reizian & Meleis, 1986). Because of their confidence in Western medicine, Arabs anticipate immediate postoperative relief. This expectation, in combination with a belief in conserving energy for recovery, often contributes to a reluctance to comply with typical post-operative routines such as frequent ambulation. Although expressive, emotional, and vocal responses to pain are usually reserved for the immediate family, under certain circumstances, such as childbirth and illnesses accompanied by spasms, Arabs express pain more freely (Reizian & Meleis, 1986). The tendency of Arabs to be more expressive with their family and more restrained in the presence of health professionals may lead to conflicting perceptions regarding the adequacy of pain relief. Whereas the nurse may assess pain relief as adequate, family members may demand that their relative receive additional analgesia.

The attitude that mental illness is a major social stigma is particularly pervasive (Budman, Lipson, & Meleis, 1992). Psychiatric symptoms may be denied, attributed to "bad nerves" or supernatural beings, or explained as a consequence of physical trauma, emotional trauma, or both (Racy, 1977). Underrecognition may occur because of the somatic orientation of Arab patients and physicians, patients' tolerance of emotional suffering, and relatives' tolerance of behavioral disturbances (El-Islam, 1982). Indeed, home management with automatic but crucial adjustments within the family may abort or control symptoms until remission occurs (Racy, 1977). For example, female family members manage postpartum depression by assuming care of the newborn, telling the mother she needs more help or more rest. Islamic legal prohibitions further confound attempts to estimate the incidence of problems such as alcoholism and suicide, resulting in underreporting of these conditions because of a potential for severe social stigma.

When persons suffering from mental distress seek medical care, they are likely to present with a variety of vague complaints, such as abdominal pain, lassitude, anorexia, and shortness of breath. Patients often expect and may insist on somatic treatment, at least "vitamins and tonics" (El-Islam, 1982). When mental illness is accepted as a diagnosis, somatic treatments rather than psychotherapy are preferred (Racy, 1977). Hospitalization is resisted because such placement is viewed as abandonment (Budman, Lipson, & Meleis, 1992). Although Arab-Americans report family and marital stress (Laffrey, et al., 1989) and multiple mental health symptoms (Young, et al., 1987), Arab-Americans do not seek psychiatric services (Young, et al., 1987) or accept psychiatric referrals when suggested (Lipson, et al., 1987).

Reiter, Mar'i, and Rosenberg (1986) and Yousef (1993) described the Arab public's attitude toward the disabled as generally negative and expectations with respect to education and rehabilitation are low. Yousef (1993) related misconceptions about mental retardation to the dearth of Arab literature and the public's lack of experience with the disabled. Because of social stigma, the disabled are often kept from public view. Similarly, although there is a trend toward educating some children with mild mental retardation in regular schools, special education programs are generally institutionally based.

Indeed, Reiter, Mar'i, and Rosenberg (1986) discovered that parents, those most intimately involved with the developmentally disabled, their parents, held rather positive attitudes. Among Israeli Arab parents, Muslims, the less educated, and residents of smaller villages expressed more tolerant views than Christians, the educated, and residents of larger villages with mixed populations. Reiter, Mar'i, and Rosenberg linked the less positive attitudes of the latter groups to the process of modernization, which effects a drive toward status and a weakening of family structures and traditions. Traditions include regarding the handicapped as coming from God, accepting the disabled person's dependency, and providing care within the home.

Dependency is accepted. Family members assume the ill person's responsibilities. The ill person is cared for and indulged. From an American frame of reference, the patient may seem overdependent and the family overprotective.

## Blood Transfusion and Organ Donation

Although blood transfusions and organ transplants are widely accepted, Islamic jurists have established certain restrictions regarding the harvesting of organs (Darsh, n.d.). While there is no objection to living-related or living-unrelated donation, provided the permission of the donor is freely given, taking organs from an individual assuming death is inevitable is not allowed because the time of death is known only to Allah. After death occurs, organs may be harvested with the prior permission of the deceased or relatives of the deceased. In Jordan as well as in Saudi Arabia (Nicholls, 1989), the first locally harvested cadaveric grafts were transplanted in the late 1980s.

## HEALTH-CARE PRACTITIONERS

## Traditional Versus Biomedical Care

Although Arab-Americans combine traditional and Western biomedical care practices, they favor intrusive treatments, regarding them as more effective (Meleis, 1981). Intramuscular injections are preferred over pills, and intravenous over intramuscular treatments. In comparison with radiation and chemotherapy, excision of a cancer is more often associated with "cure" (Dodd, et al., 1985). Similarly, Arabs do not readily accept psychotherapy and occupational therapy as treatments of psychiatric conditions (Meleis & La Fever, 1984).

Gender, and to a lesser extent, age are considerations in matching Arab patients and health-care providers. In Arab societies, unrelated males and females are not accustomed to interacting. Shyness in women is appreciated, and Muslim men may ignore women out of politeness. Health-care settings, client units, and sometimes waiting rooms are segregated by sex. Male nurses never care for female patients.

Given this background, many Arab-Americans may find interacting with a health-care professional of the opposite sex quite embarrassing and stressful. Discomfort may be expressed by refusals to discuss personal information and by a reluctance to disrobe for physical assessments and hygiene. Western male physicians (Dubovsky, 1983; Sullivan, 1993) often express the concern that illnesses that are usually easily diagnosed with a history and physical examination alone (for example, thyroid disorders) may be missed, and that veiling of the face prevents observation of facial expression, precluding intimate disclosure. In addition, Arab women may be unaccustomed to a thorough physician examination. As an Egyptian physician explained, Arab male physicians often limit physical examination to "touching the stethoscope to the chest." Thus, a thorough examination may be misperceived as making indecent advances and, in Arab society, violating a woman's honor is a grave offense; therefore, client and provider should be matched by sex. Female providers for female clients; for males, a male or an older (that is, mother figure) female staff member.

## Status of Health-care Providers

Among Arab-Americans, older male physicians are viewed as most trustworthy (Lipson & Meleis, 1985). At times of crisis Arab Americans find consultation with the senior-ranking physician or department chair particularly reassuring.

Although medicine is perhaps the most respected profession in Arab societies, nursing is viewed as menial work that also conflicts with societal norms proscribing certain female behavior. In this conservative culture, where contact between unrelated males and females is often discouraged, nursing is considered particularly undesirable as an occupation requiring close contact between the sexes and work during evening and night hours (AbuGharbieh, 1993). American nurses are regarded more favorably because of their Western education, expertise, and performance of roles ascribed solely to Arab physicians (for example, physical examination).

Perhaps because Arab physicians tend to be older males and Arab nurses, young females, the status and roles of physicians and nurses mirror the hierarchical family structure of Arab society. Physicians require that nurses "know their place" and leave the interpretation of data, decision making, and disclosure of information to them. Nurses conform to the role expectations of physicians and the public and function as medical assistants and housekeepers rather than as critical thinkers and health educators. In Jordan, physicians represent nursing on national committees despite the availability of doctorally prepared Jordanian nurses (AbuGharbieh & Suliman, 1992). Some may interpret this as evidence that physicians have protective dominion over nurses just as men have over women.

---

### CASE STUDY

Mrs. Ayesha Said is a 39-year-old Muslim housewife and mother of six who immigrated to the United States from a rural town in southern Iraq 2 years ago. Her mother-in-law and her husband, Mr. Ahmed Said, accompanied her to the United States as participants in a post–Gulf War resettlement program, after spending some time in a Saudi Arabian refugee camp. Their relocation was coordinated by a local international institute that provided an array of services for finding employment and establishing a household, enrolling children in the public schools, and applying for federal aid programs.

Mr. Ahmed, who completed the equivalent of high school, works in a local plastics factory. He speaks some English. He plans to attend an English language class held at the factory for its many Iraqi employees. Mrs. Ayesha, who has very little formal schooling, spends her day cooking and caring for her children and spouse with the assistance of her mother-in-law. She leaves their home, a three-bedroom upper flat in a poor area of the city, only when she accompanies her husband shopping or they attend gatherings at the local Islamic center. These events are quite enjoyable because the majority of those using the center are also recently arrived Iraqi immigrants. She also socializes with other Iraqi women by telephone. Except for interactions with the American personnel at the institute, Mr. Ahmed and Mrs. Ayesha Said remain quite isolated from American society. They have discussed moving to Detroit because of its large Arab community.

Four of the Said family's children attend public elementary schools, participating in the English as a Second Language (commonly known as ESL) program. Mr. Ahmed and Mrs. Ayesha are dismayed by their children's rapid acculturation. Although holidays such as Halloween, Christmas, Valentine's Day, and Easter, are contrary to Islam, their children plead to participate in these school-related activities. Their eldest child, a seventh-grade girl, wants to discard the *hijab* and join in coed swimming and physical education classes.

Mrs. Ayesha is being admitted to the surgical unit after a modified radical mastectomy. According to the physician's notes, she discovered a "lump that didn't go away" about 6 months ago while breast-feeding her youngest child. She delayed seeking care, hoping that *inshallah*, the lump would vanish. Access to care was also limited by Mrs. Ayesha's preference for a female physician and financial constraints, that is, finding a female surgeon willing to treat a patient with limited financial means. Her past medical history includes measles, dental problems, and headaches and a reproductive history of seven pregnancies. One child, born prematurely, died soon after birth.

As you enter the room, you see Mrs. Ayesha dozing. Her husband, mother-in-law, and a translator are at the bedside.

## STUDY QUESTIONS

1. Describe Arab-Americans with respect to religion, education, occupation, income, and English language skills. Compare the Said family with Arab-Americans as a group.

2. Assess the Said family's risk for experiencing a stressful immigration by relating factors and personal characteristics discussed by Lipson and Meleis (1985).

3. Describe the steps you would take to develop rapport with Mrs. Ayesha and her family during your initial encounter. Include nonverbal behavior and social etiquette, as well as statements or questions that might block communication.

4. Identify interventions that you would employ to accommodate Mrs. Ayesha's "shyness" and modesty.

5. You notice that although Mrs. Ayesha is alert, her husband and sometimes her mother-in-law reply to your questions. Interpret this behavior within a cultural context.

6. Although Mrs. Ayesha is normothermic and states her pain is "little," Mr. Ahmed insists that his wife be covered with several additional blankets and receive an injection for pain. When you attempt to reassure him of his wife's satisfactory recovery, noting as evidence of her stable condition that you plan to "get her up" that evening, he demands to see the physician. Interpret his behavior within a cultural context.

7. Discuss Arab food preferences as well as the dietary restrictions of practicing Muslims. If you filled out Mrs. Ayesha's menu, what would you order?

8. When you give Mrs. Ayesha and her family members discharge instructions, what teaching methods would be most effective? What content regarding

recovery from a mastectomy might most Arab-Americans consider "too personal"?

9. Identify typical coping strategies of Arabs. What could you do to facilitate Mrs. Ayesha's use of these strategies?

10. Discuss predestination as it influences the Arab-American's responses to death and bereavement.

11. Discuss Islamic rulings regarding the following health matters: contraception, abortion, infertility treatment, autopsy, and organ donation and transplant.

12. Describe the Arab-American's culturally based role expectations for nurses and physicians. In what ways do the role responsibilities of Arab and American nurses differ?

13. What illness and conditions is the Arab-American unlikely to disclose because of Islamic prohibitions or an attached stigma?

14. Compile a health profile (strengths versus areas of concern) of Arab-Americans by comparing beliefs, values, behaviors, and practices favoring health and those negatively influencing health.

## References

AbuGharbieh, P. & Suliman, W. (1992). Changing the image of nursing in Jordan through effective role negotiation. *International Nursing Review, 39*(5) (Issue 305), 149–152, 144.

AbuGharbieh, P. (1993). Culture shock. Cultural norms influencing nursing in Jordan. *Nursing & Health Care, 14*(10), 534–540.

Ali, N. & Khalil, H. (1991). Identification of stressors, level of stress, coping strategies, and coping effectiveness among Egyptian mastectomy patients. *Cancer Nursing, 14*(5), 232–239.

Al-Akili, M. (1993). *Natural healing with the medicine of the prophet.* Philadelphia, PA: Pearl Publishing House.

Arab American Institute. (1994). *Arab Americans: Making a difference.* [Brochure]. Kasem, C: Author.

Barakat, H. (1985). The Arab family and the challenge of social transformation. In E. Fernea (Ed.), *Women and the family in the Middle East. New voices of change* (pp. 27–48). Austin, TX: University of Texas Press.

Braunwald, L., Isselbacher, K., Petersdorf, R., Wilson, J., Martin, J. & Fauci, A. (Eds.). (1987). *Harrison's principles of internal medicine* (11th ed.) (pp. 288, 764–765). New York: McGraw-Hill.

Budman, C., Lipson, J., & Meleis, A. (1992). The cultural consultant in mental health care: The case of an Arab adolescent. *American Journal of Orthopsychiatry, 62*(3), 359–370.

Cline, S., Abuirmeileh, N., Roberts, A., et al. (1986). *Woman's life cycle. Fundamentals of health education* (pp. 48–77). Yarmouk, Jordan: Yarmouk University.

Darsh, S. (n.d.). *Islamic health rules.* Jeddah, Saudi Arabia: Abul Qasim Bookstore.

Dodd, M., Ahmed, N., Lindsey, A., & Piper, B. (1985). Attitudes of patients living in Egypt about cancer and its treatment. *Cancer Nursing, 8*(5), 278–284.

Dubovsky, S. (1983). Psychiatry in Saudi Arabia. *American Journal of Psychiatry, 140*(11),1455–1459.

Ebrahim, A. (1989). *Abortion, birth control & surrogate parenting. An Islamic perspective.* Indianapolis, IN: American Trust Publications.

El-Badry, S. (January, 1994). The Arab-American market. *American Demographics,* 22–31.

El-Islam, M. (1982). Arabic cultural psychiatry. *Transcultural Psychiatric Research Review, 19,* 5–24.

El-Islam, M. (1994). Cultural aspects of morbid fears in Qatari women. *Social Psychiatry Psychiatric Epidemiology, 29,* 137–140.

Gammal, S. (1988, December 31). Egypt battles tradition in fight against Nile-borne disease. *Jordan Times,* p. 5.

Hall, E. (1979, August). Learning the Arabs' silent language. *Psychology Today,* pp. 45–54.

Hamamy, H. & Alwan, A. (1994). Hereditary disorders in the Eastern Mediterranean Region. *Bulletin of the World Health Organization, 72*(1), 145–154.

The Hashemite Kingdom Jordan, Department of Statistics. (1985). *Jordan's husbands' fertility survey.* Amman, Jordan: The Hashemite Kingdom of Jordan, Department of Statistics in collaboration with Division of Reproductive Health, Centers for Disease Control, Atlanta, GA.

Issacs, P. (1989). Growth parameters and blood values in Arabic children. *Pediatric Nursing, 15*(6), 579–585.

Kulwicki, A. (1989, October). Infant mortality among Arab Americans in Michigan is cause for concern. *Michigan Nurse,* 12–13.

Kulwicki, A. & Cass, P. (1994). An assessment of Arab American knowledge, attitudes, and beliefs about AIDS. *IMAGE: Journal of Nursing Scholarship, 26*(1), 13–17.

Kurian, G. (Ed.). (1992). *Encyclopedia of the Third World.* New York: Facts on File.

Laffrey, S., Meleis, A., Lipson, J., Solomon, M., & Omidian, P. (1989). Assessing Arab-American health care needs. *Social Science & Medicine, 29*(7), 877–883.

Levy, R. (1993). Ethnic and racial differences in response to medicines: Preserving individualized therapy in managed pharmaceutical programmes. *Pharmaceutical Medicine, 7,* 139–165.

Lipson, J. & Meleis, A. (1983). Issues in health care of Middle Eastern patients. *The Western Journal of Medicine, 139*(6), 854–861.

Lipson, J. & Meleis, A. (1985). Culturally appropriate care: The case of immigrants. *Topics in Clinical Nursing, 7*(3), 48–56.

Lipson, J., Reizian, A., & Meleis, A. (1987). Arab-American patients: A medical record review. *Social Science & Medicine, 24*(2), 101–107.

Luna, L. (1989). Transcultural nursing care of Arab Muslims. *Journal of Transcultural Nursing, 1*(1), 22–26.

Luna, L. (1994). Care and cultural context of Lebanese Muslim immigrants: Using Leininger's theory. *Journal of Transcultural Nursing, 5*(2), 12–20.

*The meaning of the glorious Qur'an.* (1977). (Pickthall, M., text and trans.) Mecca, Saudi Arabia: Muslim World League.

Meleis, A. (1981, June). The Arab American in the health care system. *American Journal of Nursing, 8*(6), 1180–1183.

Meleis, A. & La Fever, C. (1984). The Arab American and psychiatric care. *Perspectives in Psychiatric Care, 22,* 72–86.

Meleis, A. & Jonsen, A. (1983). Ethical crises and cultural differences. *The Western Journal of Medicine 138,*(6), 889–893.

Meleis, A., Lipson, J., & Paul, S. (1992). Ethnicity and health among five Middle Eastern immigrant groups. *Nursing Research, 41*(2), 98–103.

Meleis A. & Sorrell, L. (1981). Arab American women and their birth experiences. *Maternal-Child Nursing, 6,* 171–176.

Nicholls, P. (1989, August). Transplanted to Saudi Arabia. *American Journal of Nursing, 89*(8), 1048–1050.

Nydell, M. (1987). *Understanding Arabs. A guide for Westerners.* Yarmouth, ME: Intercultural Press.

Office of the State Registrar and Division of Health Statistics, Director of Statistical Services, MDPH, Lansing, MI, 1993.

Patai, R. (1958). *The kingdom of Jordan.* Princeton, NJ: Princeton University Press.

Racy, J. (1977). Psychiatry and the Arab East. In L. Brown & N. Itzkowitz (Eds.), *Psychological dimensions of Near Eastern studies* (pp. 279–329). Princeton, NJ: The Darwin Press.

Reiter, S., Mar'i, S., & Rosenberg, Y. (1986). Parental attitudes toward the developmentally disabled among Arab communities in Israel: A cross-cultural study. *International Journal of Rehabilitation Research,9*(4), 335–362.

Reizian, A. & Meleis, A. (1986). Arab-Americans' perceptions of and responses to pain. *Critical Care Nurse, 6*(6),30–37.

Reizian, A. & Meleis, A. (1987). Symptoms reported by Arab-American patients on the Cornell Medical Index (CMI). *Western Journal of Nursing Research, 9*(3), 368–384.

Rice, V. & Kulwicki, A. (1992). Cigarette use among Arab Americans in the Detroit metropolitan area. *Public Health Reports, 107*(5), 589–594.

Robinson, A. & Linden, M. (1993). *Clinical Genetics Handbook* (2nd ed.) Boston: Blackwell Scientific.

Shahin, M. (1989, August 31–September 1). Breast cancer in Jordan—A question of increasing awareness. *Jordan Times.*

Sullivan, S. (1993) The patient behind the veil: Medical culture shock in Saudi Arabia. *Canadian Medical Association Journal, 148*(3), 444–446.

University of Jordan, Planning & Statistical Department. (1988). *Statistical yearbook.* Amman, Jordan: The University of Jordan.

Vincent-Barwood, A. (1986). The Arab immigrants. *Aramco World Magazine, 37*(5), 10–13,15.

Wayne County Health Department. (1994). *Arab community in Wayne County, Michigan: Behavior risk factor survey.* East Lansing, MI: Michigan State University, Institute for Public Policy and Social Research.

West, M. (1987, April 29). Surveys indicate girls face discrimination in provision of nutrition and health care. *Jordan Times.*

Wikan, U. (1988). Bereavement and loss in two Muslim communities: Egypt and Bali compared. *Social Science and Medicine, 27,* 451–460.

Young, R., Bukoff, A., Waller, J., Jr., & Blount, S. (1987). Health status, health problems and practices among refugees from the Middle East, Eastern Europe and Southeast Asia. *International Migration Review, 21*(3), 760–782.

Yousef, J. (1993). Education of children with mental retardation in Arab countries. *Mental Retardation 31*(2), 117–121.

Zogby, John. (1990). *Arab America today. A demographic profile of Arab Americans.* Washington, DC: Arab American Institute.

# Chinese-Americans

*Linda K. Matocha*

---

• Key terms to become familiar with in this chapter are:

| | |
|---|---|
| *Dan wei* | *Pu tong hua* |
| *Dao* | *Qi* |
| *Guan xi* | *Shen* |
| Han | *Xue* |
| *Jing* | Yang |
| *Jing luo* | Yin |
| *Jing ye* | *Zang fu* |
| *Mai* | *Zhong guo* |

## OVERVIEW, INHABITED LOCALITIES, AND TOPOGRAPHY

## Overview

Although some Western health-care providers categorize all Asians into the same group, each group is very different. Cultural values differ among Chinese according to location within their country of origin, such as north versus south, east versus west, rural versus urban, and interior versus port cities. Chinese immigrants to Western countries are even more varied, with a mixture of traditional and Western values and beliefs. These differences must be acknowledged and appreciated.

Most of the Chinese are considered **Han** (91.96 percent), with the remaining a mixture of 56 different nationalities, religions, and ethnic groups. Because of the complexity of their values, it is impossible to develop specific cultural interventions appropriate for all Chinese clients. Therefore, the information included in this chapter should serve simply as a guide or beginning for understanding Chinese persons, not as a definitive profile.

Children born to Chinese in Western countries tend to adopt Western culture easily. Their parents and grandparents tend to maintain their traditional Chinese culture in varying degrees. Chinese who live in the "Chinatowns" of America maintain many of their cultural and social beliefs and values and insist that the health-care provider respect these values and beliefs with their prescribed interventions.

## Heritage and Residence

The Chinese culture is one of the oldest recorded and includes dynasties from 2200 B.C. (the Xia) to the current People's Republic of China. The Chinese consider their country and their civilization as the center of the world. The Chinese name for their country is **Zhong guo,** which literally means "middle kingdom" or "center of the earth." Many of the current values and beliefs of the Chinese remain grounded in the tradition of their history. Confucian (Confucius 551–479 B.C.) ideals continue to play an important part in the values and beliefs of Chinese. These ideals emphasize the importance of accountability to family and neighbors and reinforce the idea that all relationships embody power and rule.

During early Communist rule, an attempt was made to break down the values grounded in Confucianism and substitute values consistent with equal social responsibility. This was initially achieved, and rank in society was no longer seen as important. During the People's Revolution, feudal rank frequently meant loss of social importance, physical punishment, imprisonment, and even death. Later, during the Cultural Revolution the young were responsible for the deaths of many previously esteemed elderly and educated Chinese.

Today, many of the Confucian values have reasserted themselves in Chinese society. Families, elderly, and highly educated persons are again viewed as important. Research completed by the Chinese Culture Connection (a group of Chinese sociologists) lists 40 values of importance in modern China, including filial piety, industry, patriotism, order of relationships by status and observance of this order, tolerance of others, loyalty to superiors, respect for rites and social rituals, knowledge, benevolent authority, thrift, patience, courtesy, and respect for tradition (Hu & Grove, 1991).

Because more Chinese are living in Western societies, it is important that healthcare providers understand the historical and cultural changes that influence their values. Rawl (1992) noted that 7.3 million Asians and Pacific Islanders live in the United States. Every year the quota for the immigration of Chinese has been filled with more than 40,600 arriving from mainland China, Taiwan, and Hong Kong. More Asian-Americans are immigrating to the United States than any other ethnic group (Chin, 1991). The larger communities of Chinese are located in cities, mostly in the Western part of the United States, with small groupings of Chinese inhabitants evident in almost all communities. The largest Chinese community in the United States is located in New York City, with over 300,000 residents (Halporn, 1992), and the second largest is centered in San Francisco.

The Ministry of Public Health (1992) states that the population of China is 1.13 billion people (1990 census) with 80 percent of Chinese living in rural communities. The country is over 9.6 million square kilometers (3.7 million square miles) with 23 provinces, 5 regions, including Tibet, Hong Kong, and Taiwan, and 3 municipalities. Each province, region, and municipality functions independently in many ways. The Chinese consider each region as part of greater China and predict that the day will come when all of China is reunited. Tibet has already been reassimilated, and Hong Kong is returning to Chinese control in 1997.

## Reasons for Migration and Associated Economic Factors

The largest numbers of Chinese immigrated to the United States at three points in history: in the 1800s, 1950s, and recent years (Campbell & Chang, 1981). Among Chinese immigrants to America are those who came for education or business reasons. Although these Chinese may be considered visitors, they are an integral part of American society.

Chinese immigration was initially based on economic needs (Halporn, 1992).

Over 100,000 male peasants from Guangdong and Fujian China came to the United States without their families to make their fortune on the transcontinental railroad, starting in 1833, and during the Gold Rush of 1849 (Halporn, 1992). Many believed that they could make money in the United States to help their families and later return to China. Unfortunately, most found that opportunities were limited to hard labor and other vocations that were not desired by European-Americans. Because of their cultural diversity and their unusual physical features, it was difficult for them to assimilate into American society. They looked different, and unlike other European cultures, they could not simply change their names to try to blend with others. Racial violence and prejudice against them were common, and the courts could not punish the violators because the Chinese had few rights because they could not become American citizens. Compared with other ethnic groups, their immigration numbers were small until 1952 when the McCarran-Walters Bill relaxed immigration laws and permitted more Chinese to enter America.

For their safety and the maintenance of their cultural values, most Chinese settled in closed communities that have become the Chinatowns of today. Even as late as 1924, they were excluded by immigration laws. In fact, at times more Chinese left the United States than immigrated (Marden & Meyer, 1973). In 1965 Public Law 89-232 removed immigration barriers and made it possible for Asians to immigrate more easily (Chang, 1981).

## Educational Status and Occupations

Education is compulsory in China, and most children receive the equivalent of a ninth-grade education (Chin, 1988). Middle school students must complete a state examination to determine their eligibility to enter a general high school, to go to a preparatory high school before entering technical school or college, or to begin their lives as workers. Those who complete either the general or preparatory high school experience compete academically to continue their education at college and university levels. The system is complex and not presented here in its entirety; thus, further study of the educational system is encouraged.

A university education is valued above all; however, few have the opportunity to achieve this life goal because places in better educational institutions are limited. Because competition for top universities is keen, many families select less valued universities to ensure that their child is accepted into a university rather than slated for a technical school education. Many young adults come to Western countries to attend universities because a foreign education is considered prestigious in China.

In the West, the educational levels of Chinese are divided between the highly educated and the poorly educated (Liu, 1991). This dichotomy results in health-care providers categorizing their clients in a similar manner. Unfortunately, more often they assume that the clients have a poor education because the Chinese have not always been successful in attaining positions of power or high economic levels (Sue & Sue, 1992). Many people believe that Chinese occupations are limited to restaurants, service employment, and the garment industry.

Because of the competitive educational system in China where only the brightest students go to a university, Chinese immigrants with a college education are often very intelligent. Student immigrants are expected to return to China when their education is completed. However, many do not return and elect to remain in Western countries. This places a severe drain on one of China's most important resources, their young scholars. As a result, it has become increasingly difficult for Chinese students to come to the West to study.

Another group of Chinese immigrants are professionals from Hong Kong who are moving to Canada, the United States, and other Western countries to avoid the repatriation in 1997. These immigrants usually have family connections or close friends in Western countries who are highly educated and skilled.

A third group of immigrants consists of uneducated individuals with diverse manual labor skills. Finding employment opportunities for these Chinese may be more difficult. They often settle with family members who are not skilled or highly educated. This arrangement drains family resources for many years until they obtain financial security, learn the language, and become acculturated in other ways.

## COMMUNICATIONS

### Dominant Language and Dialects

The official language of China is Mandarin (***pu tong hua***, which is spoken by about 70 percent of the population, primarily in north China), but there are many distinct dialects (10 major ones), including Cantonese, Fujianese, Shanghainese, Toishanese, and Hunanese (Kaplan, Sobin, & deKeijzer, 1990). For example, *pu tong hua* is spoken in Beijing, the capital of China in the north, and Shanghainese is spoken in Shanghai. The two cities are only 1462 kilometers apart, but because the dialects are so different, the two groups cannot understand one another verbally. Even though people from one part of China cannot understand those from other regions, the written language is the same throughout the country. The written language consists of over 50,000 characters (about 5000 common ones); thus, most children are at least 10 to 12 years old before they can read the newspaper.

Although many times Chinese sound loud when talking with other Chinese, they generally speak in a moderate to low voice. Talking loudly may be interpreted by the Chinese person as anger. Americans are considered loud to most Chinese, and thus, the health-care provider must be cautious about tones when interacting with Chinese-Americans so that intentions are not misinterpreted.

When possible, the provider should use the Chinese language to communicate (Table 7–1 for some common phrases), being careful to avoid jargon and to use the simplest terms. Many times verbs can be omitted because the Chinese language has only a limited number of verbs. The Chinese appreciate any attempt to use their language. They do not mind mistakes and will correct you when they believe that it does not cause the conversants to lose face.

Negative queries are difficult for Chinese to understand. For example, do not say, "You know how to do that, don't you?" Instead say, "Do you know how to do that?" It is easier for them to understand instructions placed in a specific order, such as "One, at nine o'clock every morning get the medicine bottle; two, take two tablets out of the bottle; three, get your hot water; four, swallow the pills with the water." Do not use complex sentences with "ands" and "buts." The Chinese have difficulty deciding what to respond to first when the speaker uses compound or complex sentences.

When asked whether they understand what was just said, the Chinese invariably answer yes, even when they do not understand. Such an admission causes loss of face; thus, it is better to have the person repeat your instructions.

### Cultural Communication Patterns

Chinese have a reputation of not openly displaying their emotions. Although this may be true among strangers, among family and friends they are open and demonstrative. The Chinese share information freely with health-care providers once a trusting relationship has developed. This is not always easy because Western health-care providers may not have the patience or time to develop such relationships. In situations where the Chinese perceive that health-care practitioners or other persons of authority may lose face or be embarrassed, they may choose not to be totally truthful.

## Table 7–1 • **Frequently Used Words and Phrases**

| English Word or Phrase | Chinese Pinyin | Phonetic Pronunciation |
|---|---|---|
| Hello | *Nǐ hǎo* | Nee how (note tones to be used*) |
| Goodbye | *Zài jiàn* | Dzai jee en |
| How are you? | *Nǐ hǎo mā* | Nee how mah |
| Please | *Qing* | Ching |
| Thank you | *Xīe xie* | Shee eh shee eh |
| I don't understand | *Wǒ bù dǒng* | Wah boo doong |
| Yes | *Shì de or dui* | Shur da or doee (no real yes or no comparable saying—this means I agree or okay) |
| No | *Bú shì de or bu hǎo* | Boo shur or boo how |
| My name is | *Wǒ jiào* | Wah djeeow |
| Very good | *Hen hǎo* | Hun hao |
| Hurt | *Téng* | Tung |
| I, you, he/she/it | *Wǒ, nǐ, tā* | Wah, nee, tah |
| Hot | *Rè* | Ruh |
| Cold | *Leng* | Lung |
| Happy | *Gāo xìngu* | Gow shing |
| Where | *Na li* | Na lee |
| Not have | *Mei you* | May yo |
| Doctor | *Yi shēng* | Yee shung |
| Nurse | *Hù shì* | Who shur |

*Note: Each *pu tong hua* Chinese word is pronounced with five different tones:
1. First tone is high and even across the word ( ˉ ).
2. Second tone starts low and goes high ( ´ ).
3. Third tone starts neutral, goes low, and then goes high ( ˇ ).
4. Fourth tone curt and goes low ( ` ).
5. Fifth tone is neutral and pronounced very lightly.

Touching between health-care providers and Chinese clients should be kept to a minimum. Most Chinese maintain a formal distance with each other, which is a form of respect. Many are uncomfortable with face-to-face communications, especially when there is direct eye contact. Because they prefer to sit next to others, the health-care practitioner may need to rearrange seating to promote positive communication. When touching is necessary, the practitioner should provide explanations to Chinese clients.

Facial expressions are used extensively among family and friends. The Chinese love to joke and laugh. They use and appreciate smiles when talking with others. However, if the situation is formal, smiles may be limited. Other body movements are used when communicating with family and friends or when they are angry. In formal business situations or greeting persons of high rank, their use of body movements may be limited. It is best to watch them for cues of expression.

## Temporal Relationships

The Chinese concept of time is cyclical and identified with the changing of seasons and the cycle of birth, life, and death. Chinese, therefore, tend to integrate the idea of time into life rather than to try to master it as do most Western societies. The

Chinese way of thinking is very similar; they think in terms of relationships. Rather than breaking thinking into linear thoughts and Western logic, the Chinese conceptualize and use concrete examples. This enables them to mobilize quickly toward a common goal. They look for similarities among events and objects in their daily lives.

Health-care providers may observe two opposing views of time among Chinese-Americans. The first view is one of "Chinese time," whereby lateness for appointments is to be expected. A more recent view emphasizes the importance of punctuality. Because tardiness is a sign of disrespect, those who subscribe to this view arrive on time and expect others to do the same. To Westerners who plan their calendars weeks and even months in advance, this can be frustrating. Therefore, health-care providers should be prepared for both concepts of time.

## Format for Names

The health-care provider should be polite and formal and address Chinese clients by their whole name or by their family name and title. The Chinese method of introduction, whether by name card or verbally, is different from that of Western countries. For example, the family name is stated first and then the given name. Calling persons by any name except their family name is rude unless they are close friends or relatives. If a person's family name is Li and the given name is Ruiming, then the proper form of address is Li Ruiming. Men are addressed by their family name, such as *Ma*, and a title such as *Ma xian sheng* (Mister Ma) or *lao Ma* (old, respected Ma) or *xiao Ma* (young Ma). Titles are important to a Chinese person, so when possible identify the person's title and use it.

Women in China do not use their husband's name after marriage. Therefore, unless the woman is from Hong Kong or Taiwan or has lived in a Western country for a long time, do not assume that her name is the same as her husband's. Her family name comes first, followed by her other names and finally by her title.

Many Chinese take an English name as an additional given name because many Westerners cannot accurately pronounce Chinese names. Their English name is correct to use in many settings. It is better to address them by Miss Millie or Mr. Jonathan than simply by their English name. Even though they have adopted an English name, many Chinese believe that to use only the first name is improper. Some Chinese may give permission to use only the English name. In addition, some Chinese switch the order of their names to be the same as Westerners, with their family name last. Because this practice can be confusing, the health-care provider should ask the person how they wish to be addressed.

## FAMILY ROLES AND ORGANIZATIONS

### Head of Household and Gender Roles

Kinship traditionally has been organized around the male lines. Fathers, sons, and uncles are the important, recognized relationships between and among families in politics and in business. Each family maintains a recognized head who has great authority and assumes all major responsibilities of the family.

Another traditional practice in many Chinese families in rural areas is the submissive role of the daughter-in-law to the mother-in-law. Many times the mother-in-law is demanding and hostile to the daughter-in-law and may treat her worse than the servants. Such relationships continue to influence Chinese families today (Fairbank, 1983) to some extent.

The Chinese view of women is perpetuated to ensure male dominance in a society that has existed for centuries. Men still remain in control of the country largely because people's ideas remain stereotypical of men and women (Butterfield, 1990).

However, in recent years, Communism has attempted to change that perception. In 1949, women were given recognition by the Communist Party, which stated that women "hold up half the sky," and are legally equal to men. In China today, over 90 percent of the women work (Chin, 1988), and many hold professional positions or are prestigious leaders.

Even though legally women are considered equal, they are frequently forced to accept positions of more menial labor. The traditional gender roles of women are changing, but a sense remains that the woman's responsibility is to maintain a happy and efficient home life, especially in rural China. In recent times, some Chinese men are beginning to include housework, cooking, and cleaning as their responsibilities when their spouses work. Most Chinese believe that the family is most important, and thus, each family member assumes changes in roles to achieve this harmony.

Teenage pregnancy is not common among the Chinese but is increasing among Chinese-Americans (Butterfield, 1990). Young men and women enter the workforce immediately after high school. Many continue to live with their parents and contribute to the family even after marriage (in their 20s) and the birth of a child (in their 30s).

Boys and girls play together when they are young, but as they get older, this is not encouraged because their roles and the corresponding expectations predetermined by Chinese society discourages doing things together. Both sexes study hard. Boys are more active and take pride in their bodies being fit. Girls are not nearly as interested in fitness as boys (Chin, 1988) and often enjoy reading, art, and music.

## Prescriptive, Restrictive, and Taboo Behaviors for Children and Adolescents

Children are highly valued in China, especially now that China's one-child rule is in effect. Families often wait many years before they can afford a child. After the child is born, many family resources are lavished on the child. Families may only be able to afford to live with relatives in a two-room apartment, but if the family believes that the child benefits by having a piano, then the family finds the resources to provide that piano. Children are well dressed and kept clean and well fed.

In China, the child is protected from birth, and independence is not fostered. The entire family makes decisions for the child even into young adulthood (Bond, 1991; Hu & Grove, 1991; Lin & Fu, 1990). Children usually depend on the family for everything. Few teens earn money because they are expected to study hard and to help the family with daily chores rather than to seek employment.

Children feel a lot of pressure to succeed to help improve the future of the family and the country. Their common goal is to score well on the national examinations when they reach age 18 years. Most value studying over play and peer relationships. They recognize that they are constantly evaluated on having healthy bodies and minds and achieving excellent marks in school.

In rural communities, male children are more valued than female children because they continue the family line and provide labor. In urban areas, female children are valued as highly as male children. Children in China are taught to curb their expression of feelings because the person who does not stand out is successful. The young in China today frequently think that their parents are too cautious. The children are becoming even more outspoken as they read more and watch more television and movies (Chin, 1988).

Children in elementary school through young adults in universities take courses in Marxist politics and learn not to question the doctrine of the country. If they do question politics, they may be interrogated and ridiculed for their radical thoughts. Nationalism is important to Chinese children, and they want to help their country continue to be the center of the world.

Children are expected to help their parents in the home. Many times in the cities when children get home from school before their parents, they are expected to do their homework immediately and then do their household chores. They exhibit their independence not so much by expressing their individual views but rather by performing chores on their own.

Lin and Fu (1990) studied 138 children (44 Chinese, 46 Chinese-American, and 48 white American) in kindergarten through second grade and found that both the Chinese and Chinese-American parents expected increased achievement and parental control over their children. One surprising finding was the high expectation for independence in Chinese and Chinese-American children. Researchers postulated that perhaps the measurement used was actually measuring another trait; thus, more research needs to be done to confirm this finding.

Adolescents are expected to determine who they are and where they want to end up in life. They maintain their respect for elders even when they disagree with them (Sue & Sue, 1992). They may argue with their parents and teachers but not for long. They have learned that it seldom does any good. Teens value a strong and happy family life and seldom do things that jeopardize that unanimity. Adolescents question affairs of life and make great efforts to see at least two sides of every issue. They enjoy exploring different views with their peers and try to explore them with their parents.

## Family Roles and Priorities

The Chinese perception of family is through the concept of relationships. Each person identifies himself or herself in relation to others in the family (Chin, 1988). The individual is not lost, just defined differently from individuals in Western cultures. Personal independence is not valued; rather, Confucian teachings state that true value is in the relationships a person has with others, especially the family.

Older children who experienced the Cultural Revolution may feel some discomfort with their traditional parents. During the Cultural Revolution, the young informed on their elders and their peers who did not espouse the doctrine of the time. Most of those who were reported were sent to "re-education camps" where they did hard labor and were "taught the correct way to think." As a result, many families have been permanently separated.

Extended families are important to the Chinese and work as units to get ahead. Many times children live with their grandparents or aunts and uncles so individual family members can obtain a better education or reduce financial burdens. Relatives are expected to help each other through connections (**guan xi**), which are used by Chinese society in a manner similar to the use of money in other cultures. Such connections are perceived as obligations and are placed in a mental bank with deposits and withdrawals. These commitments may remain in the "bank" for years or generations until they are used to get jobs, housing, business contacts, gifts, medical care, or anything that demands a payback.

Filial loyalty to family is extended to other Chinese. When Chinese immigrants are in need of additional assistance, the health-care provider may be able to call on local Chinese organizations to obtain help for the client.

Elderly persons in China are venerated just as they were in earlier years. Leaders in the Chinese government are elderly and remain in power until their 70s, 80s, and even older. Traditional Chinese view elderly persons as being very wise. This wisdom replaces physical strength (Butterfield, 1990). Communism has not changed this view. Chinese children are expected to care for their parents, and in China, this is mandated through law.

Younger Chinese who adopt Western ideas and values may find that the expectations of their elders are too demanding. Even though younger Chinese-Americans do not live with their elders, they maintain respect and visit them more frequently than Americans (Ying, 1994). The elderly Chinese mother is viewed as central to family feelings, and the elderly father retains his role as leader. As generations live in areas removed from China, families become more Westernized, and family relationships need to be assessed on an individual family basis.

An extended family pattern is common and has existed for over 2000 years. The traditional marriage still remains nuclear. Historically in China, marriage was used to strengthen positions of families in society.

Kinship relationships are based on the concept of loyalty, and the young experience pressure to improve the family's standing. Many parents give up items of daily living to provide more for their children, thereby increasing opportunities for the them to get ahead.

Maintaining face is very important to the Chinese and is accomplished by adhering to the rules of society. Because power and control are important to Chinese society, rank is very important. True equality is not something that exists in the Chinese mind; their history has demonstrated that equality cannot exist. If more than one person is in power, then consensus is important. If the actual person in power is not present at decision-making meetings, barriers are raised and any decisions made are negated unless the person in power agrees. Even after negotiations have been concluded and contracts signed, the Chinese continue to negotiate.

Even more important than recognized social status and corresponding values and beliefs is the Chinese concept of privacy. The Chinese words for privacy have a negative connotation and mean something underhanded, secret, and furtive. People grow up in crowded conditions, they live and work in small areas, and their value of support for the group does not make privacy highly valued. The Chinese may ask many personal questions about salary, life at home, age, and children. Refusal to answer personal questions is accepted as long as it is done with care and feeling. The one subject that is taboo is sex and anything related to sex. Privacy is also limited by territorial boundaries. Waiting in an orderly line may not be the Chinese way of doing things. The Chinese may enter rooms without knocking or invade privacy by not allowing a person to be alone. The need to be alone is viewed as "not good" to the Chinese, and they may not understand when a Westerner wants to be alone. A mutual understanding of these beliefs is necessary for harmonious working relationships.

## Alternative Lifestyles

Alternative lifestyles are not common and not encouraged by Chinese society. The Chinese do not condone same-sex relationships, and in many provinces, they are illegal and punishable by death. The goals of every man and woman are supposed to be marriage and the procreation of one child. Chinese women and men generally do not marry before the ages of 25 and 28 years because the government discourages earlier marriages (Butterfield, 1990). There are few one-parent families unless a death has occurred. Divorce is legal but not encouraged.

## WORKFORCE ISSUES

### Culture in the Workplace

China is becoming more westernized with high technology and increased knowledge. Communism is responsible for establishing the **dan wei**, local Chinese work units that are responsible for jobs, homes, health, enforcing governmental regulations, and problem solving for families. Recent immigrants may know that the workplace is different in the United States, but they still may expect their employers to provide the necessities of living such as housing.

Chinese-American workers have the appearance of being slow. They are not lazy; they simply believe that working slowly is just as good as working quickly. In China, the government assures them a job; therefore, ambition is not valued. In fact, to be noticed for working faster and harder may not be in a person's best interest. Rather, it may cause others to complain or be envious. The Chinese adapt readily to the Western workforce, but the employer needs to be aware of these differences in work-related habits and values.

The Chinese acculturate by learning as much as possible about their new culture. They observe people from the culture and listen closely for nuances in language and interpersonal connections. They frequently call on other Chinese to teach them how to fit in more quickly. Chinese are supportive of one another in new cultures and help each other find resources and learn to live effectively and efficiently in the new culture. They also watch television and go to movies to learn about Western ways of life. They read about the new culture in magazines, books, and newspapers. They love to travel, and when an opportunity arises to see different aspects of the new culture, they do not hesitate to do so.

## Issues Related to Autonomy

Historically, the Chinese have been autonomous. They had to exhibit this characteristic to survive difficult times. However, their autonomy is limited and is based on functioning for the good of the group. When a new situation arises that requires independent decision making, many times the Chinese know what should be done but do not take action until the leader or superior gives permission.

The Western workforce expects independence, and certain Chinese groups may need to be taught that true autonomy is necessary to advance. Chinese immigrants may need assertiveness training. The health-care provider should be aware, however, that the training may not be successful because it is foreign to Chinese cultural values. It is best to try to demonstrate alternatives; it will remain up to persons to determine if assertiveness can be a part of their life. After acculturation has taken place, Chinese-Americans do not differ significantly in assertiveness (Sue, Sue, & Ino, 1990).

Language is a barrier for the Chinese person seeking assimilation into a Western workforce. Western languages and Chinese have many differences, among them sentence structure and the use of intonation. The Chinese do not have verbs that denote tense like Western languages. The ordering of the words in a sentence is basically the same, with the subject first and then the verb, but the Chinese place their descriptive words in different orders. Intonation in Chinese is in the words themselves rather than in the sentence. The Chinese who have taken English lessons can usually read and write English competently, but they may have difficulty in understanding and speaking it. The health-care provider should write instructions rather than verbalize them.

## BIOCULTURAL ECOLOGY

### Skin Color and Other Biologic Variations

The skin color of Chinese is varied. Many have skin color similar to Westerners with pink undertones. Others have a yellow tone, and still others are very dark. Mongolian spots, dark bluish spots over the lower back and buttocks, are present in about 80 percent of infants. Bilirubin levels are usually higher in Chinese newborns, with the highest levels occurring the fifth or sixth day after birth (Giger, Davidhizar, & Wieczorek, 1993; Overfield, 1985).

The Chinese are distinctively of Mongolian race, but their Asian characteristics have many variants. The country is very large and includes people from many different backgrounds, including Mongols and Tibetans. Generally, men and women are shorter than Westerners, but some Chinese are over 6 feet tall. Differences in bone structure are evidenced in the ulnar bone, which is longer than the radius. Hip measurements are significantly smaller. Females are 4.14 cm smaller and males 7.6 cm smaller than Westerners (Quick Reference, 1994). Not only is overall bone length shorter, but bone density is less. Chinese have a high hard palate, which may cause problems when wearing Western dentures. Hair color is generally black and straight, but some do have naturally curly hair. Most Chinese men do not have much facial hair. The Rh-negative blood group is rare, and twins are not common in Chinese families (Giger, et al., 1993) but are greatly valued, especially since the emergence of China's one-child law.

## Diseases and Health Conditions

Many Chinese who come to the United States settle in large cities like San Francisco and New York. Thus, the Chinese are at risk for the same problems and diseases experienced by other inner-city populations. For example, crowding in large cities often results in poor sanitation, and increases the incidence of infectious diseases, air pollution, and violence.

Another major problem for Chinese is their lack of understanding of the Western health-care system. In China, the government is primarily responsible for providing basic health care in a multilevel system. Native Chinese who are accustomed to the neighborhood work units called *dan wei,* which answer their questions and provide health-care services, may have trouble locating the appropriate level or source of health care in the United States. The language barrier further complicates their ability to use the American health-care system and increases the health risks of Chinese clients. The tendency of many health-care providers to treat everyone who looks Asian alike can make their situation even more problematic, because each ethnic group is different and should be treated differently.

The three major causes of death in China are the same as in the United States: heart disease, other circulatory diseases, and cancers (Lawson & Lin, 1994; Ryan, 1992b). Life expectancy for the Chinese is 67 years for males and 71 years for females. This is similar to life expectancy in the United States and has increased from 35 to 70 years in the last 30 years (Lawson & Lin, 1994). Disease incidence has decreased as well, but major problems still exist in rural China, where perinatal deaths and deaths from infectious diseases remain high (Lawson & Lin, 1994). Tobacco use is a major problem and results in an increased incidence of lung disease. Health-care providers must screen newer immigrants from China for these health-related conditions and provide interventions in a culturally congruent manner.

$\alpha$-Thalassemia, a genetic disease, affects Chinese people in one of two ways. One form is evidenced by a smaller but increased number of red blood cells and does not usually affect one's health status; the other form is evidenced as anemia followed by an early death (Burns, 1983; Gaspard, 1994). A sex-linked genetic disease common in the Chinese is glucose-6-phosphate dehydrogenase deficiency (G-6-PD), an enzyme deficiency affecting the person's red blood cells resulting in anemia (Burns, 1983; Gaspard, 1994). Finally, the Chinese have an increased incidence of lactose intolerance, resulting in diarrhea, indigestion, and bloating when milk and milk products are consumed (Burns, 1983; Porth, 1994).

An increased incidence of hepatitis B and tuberculosis is evidenced by many Chinese immigrants (Chin, 1991). Poor living conditions and overcrowding in China enhance the development of these diseases, which persist after immigrants settle in other countries.

Studies by the Office of Minority Health Resource Center in Washington, D.C., have found that Chinese-American women have a 20 percent higher rate of pancreatic cancer (1994b) and higher rates of suicide after the age of 45 years (1994d), and all Chinese have higher death rates due to diabetes (1994c). The incidence of different types of cancer, including cervical, liver, lung, stomach, multiple myeloma, esophageal, pancreatic and nasopharyngeal cancers, is higher among Chinese-Americans (Office of Minority Health Resource Center, 1994a; Olsen & Frank-Stromborg, 1993). Overall, the incidence of disease in this population has not been studied sufficiently, and continuing research is desperately needed.

## Variations in Drug Metabolism and Interactions

Multiple studies outlining problems with drug metabolism and sensitivity have been conducted among Chinese. Results suggest a poor metabolism of mephenytoin (for example, diazepam) in 15 to 20 percent of Chinese; sensitivity to beta-blockers, such as propranolol, as evidenced by a decrease in the overall blood levels accompanied by a seemingly more profound response; atropine sensitivity as evidenced by an increased heart rate; and increased responses to antidepressants and neuroleptics given at lower doses. Analgesics have been found to cause increased gastrointestinal side effects, despite a decreased sensitivity to them. In addition, the Chinese have an increased sensitivity to the effects of alcohol (Levy, 1993).

Delineating specific variations in drug metabolism among the Chinese is difficult, because various studies tend to group them in aggregate as Asians. Much more research needs to be completed to determine variations between Westerners and Asians as well as among Asians (Fong & Mokuau, 1994).

## HIGH-RISK BEHAVIORS

High-risk behaviors are difficult to determine with accuracy among Chinese in the United States because most of the data group Chinese into an aggregate called Asian-Americans (Chin, 1991). Even in this grouping, the representation of Asian-Americans usually does not exceed 5 percent of the population. More than half (50 to 67 percent) are newer immigrants (Chin, 1991; Sue & Sue, 1992), requiring additional help assimilating into the healthcare system.

Smoking is a high-risk behavior for many Chinese men and careless teenagers (Yang & Lawson, 1991). Most Chinese women do not smoke, but recently the numbers for women are increasing, especially after immigration to the United States. Travelers in China see more cigarette vendors in the streets than any other type of vendor. The decrease in smoking in the United States resulted in cigarette manufacturers' identifying China as a good market in which to sell their product (Chin, 1991). Even though alcohol consumption among Chinese has been high at times, the level is currently low (Weatherspoon, Danko, & Johnson, 1994). Despite these findings, the use of alcohol contributes to a high incidence of vehicular accidents and related trauma (Lawson & Lin, 1994).

## Health-care Practices

Younger Chinese usually do not hesitate to seek health-care providers when necessary. They generally practice Western medicine unless they feel that it does not work for them; then they use traditional Chinese medicine. Elderly persons may try traditional Chinese medicine first and only seek Western medicine when the traditional medicine does not seem to work. This results in sicker elderly persons seeking care from Western health-care providers. Even after seeking Western medical care, elderly Chinese may continue to practice traditional Chinese medicine in some form. Health-care providers need to understand this practice and include it in their care. A trusting relationship between provider and client is necessary for the Chinese to share all aspects of health care with the practitioner.

# NUTRITION

## Meaning of Food

Food habits are important to the Chinese, who offer food to their guests at any time of the day or night. Most celebrations with family and business events center on food. Foods at meals have a specific order, with the focus on a balance for a healthy body. The importance of food is demonstrated daily in its use to promote good health and to combat disease and injury. Traditional Chinese medicine frequently uses food and food derivatives to cure diseases and increase the strength of the weak and elderly persons.

## Common Foods and Food Rituals

The typical Chinese diet is difficult to describe. Each region in China has its own traditional diet. Peanuts and soy beans are popular, and common grains include wheat, sorghum, and maize (Worcester, 1983). The Chinese eat steamed and fried rice noodles called *bun*. Rice is usually steamed but can be fried with eggs, vegetables, and meats. Many Chinese eat beans or noodles instead of rice. Chinese noodles are usually eaten with a broth base and include vegetables and meats. Meat choices include pork (the most common), chicken, beef, duck, shrimp, fish, scallops, and mussels. Tofu, an excellent source of protein, is a staple of the Chinese diet. It is prepared in many different ways, from fried to boiled, or cold like ice cream. Bean products are another source of protein, and many of the desserts or sweets in Chinese diets are prepared with red beans.

Before-dinner toasts are made to family and business colleagues. The toasts may be interspersed with speeches, or the speeches may be incorporated in the toasts. Cold appetizers may be on the table and often include peanuts and fruits in season. Chopsticks, a chopstick holder, a small plate, and a glass(es) are part of the table setting. If the foods are messy, like Beijing duck, then a finger towel may be available. Frequently a Westerner can ask for forks and spoons. The Chinese have ceramic or porcelain spoons and use them routinely for soup. Knives are unnecessary because the food is usually served in bite-sized pieces. Chopsticks may be difficult for some at first, but the Chinese are good-natured and are pleased by any attempt to use them. Chopsticks should never be stuck in the food upright because that is considered bad luck. Westerners soon learn that slurping, burping, and other noises are not only ignored but appreciated. The Chinese are very relaxed at meals and commonly rest their elbows on the table.

Drinks with dinner include tea, soft drinks, juice, or beer. Foreign-born Chinese do not like ice in their drinks. They believe that it is damaging to their body and shocks the body systems out of balance. On the other hand, hot drinks are enjoyed and believed to be safe for the body. This "goodness" of hot drinks may stem from tradition, when the only safe drink came from boiled water. All food is put in the center of the table. It may come all at one time, but usually multiple courses are served. The host either serves the most important guests or signals everyone to start.

## Dietary Practices for Health Promotion

Fruits and vegetables may be peeled or eaten raw. Some fruits and vegetables commonly eaten raw by Westerners are usually cooked by the Chinese. Unpeeled raw fruits and vegetables are sources of contamination due to unsanitary conditions in China. The Chinese enjoy their vegetables lightly stir-fried in oil. Salt, oil, and oil products are important parts of the Chinese diet.

The health-care provider needs to provide special instructions regarding risk factors associated with diets high in fats and salt. For example, the Chinese may need education regarding the use of salty fish and condiments, which increase the risks for nasopharyngeal, esophageal, and stomach cancers.

## Nutritional Deficiencies and Food Limitations

The Chinese diet is generally vegetarian, although meat is often served. Little information is available about dietary deficiencies in the Chinese diet. The life span of the Chinese is long enough to suggest that severe dietary deficiencies are not common as long as food is available. Periodically, some deficiencies such as rickets and goiters have occurred. The Chinese government added iodine into water supplies, and fish rich in iron is encouraged to enhance the diets of people with goiters. Native Chinese generally do not drink milk or eat milk products because of a genetic tendency for lactose intolerance. Their healthy selection of green vegetables limits the incidence of calcium deficits. The health-care provider may need to screen newer immigrants for these deficiencies and assist them in planning an adequate diet.

Most Chinese do not eat desserts high in sugar content. Their desserts are usually peeled or sliced fruits or desserts made of bean and bean curd. The higher death rate from diabetes in Western countries may be due to a change from the typical Chinese diet with few sweets to a Western diet with many sweets.

## PREGNANCY AND CHILDBEARING PRACTICES

### Fertility Practices and Views toward Pregnancy

China is attempting to slow the rate of population growth by enforcing a one-child law. If a family does decide to have another child, they are expected to wait at least 5 years. Three children are not allowed by the law.

The most popular form of birth control is the intrauterine device. About 50 percent of the Chinese use it (Butterfield, 1990). Sterilization is common, and oral contraception is available. Contraception is free in China. Abortion is fairly common, but statistics are hard to find. Most Chinese families see pregnancy as positive, and many wait a long time to have the first and sometimes only child. If a woman does become pregnant before the couple is ready to start a family, she may have an abortion. When the pregnancy is desired, the nuclear and extended family rejoices in the new family member. Overall, pregnancy is seen as women's business although the Chinese male is beginning to demonstrate an active interest in pregnancy and the welfare of the mother and baby. Health-care practitioners need to understand this traditional view. Because Chinese women are very modest, many women insist on a female midwife or physician. Some agree to use a male physician only when an emergency arises.

### Prescriptive, Restrictive, and Taboo Practices in the Childbearing Family

Pregnant women usually add more meat to their diets because their blood needs to be stronger for the fetus. Many women increase the amount of organ meat in their diets, and even during times of severe food shortages, the Chinese government has tried to ensure that pregnant women receive adequate nutrition. These tradition are reflected in the Chinese family living in the Western world.

Other dietary restrictions and prescriptions may be practiced by the pregnant woman. Shellfish may be avoided during the first trimester because it causes allergies (Campbell & Chang, 1981). Some mothers may be unwilling take iron because they believe that it makes the delivery more difficult (Bobak & Jensen, 1993).

The Chinese government is proud of the fact that since the People's Revolution, infant mortality has been significantly reduced (Ministry of Public Health, 1992). This has been accomplished by providing a three-level system of care for the pregnant woman in rural and urban populations. Over 90 percent of childbirths are done under sterile conditions either by a physician or a midwife. This has reduced the maternal mortality rate significantly (Ministry of Public Health, 1992). Therefore, most Chinese who have immigrated to Western countries are knowledgeable about modern sterile deliveries.

In China, a woman stays in the hospital for 5 to 7 days after delivery to help recover her strength and body balance. Traditional postpartum care includes 1 month of recovery, with the mother eating foods that decrease the yin (cold) energy (Campbell & Chang, 1981). The Chinese government supports this 1-month recuperation period through labor laws that entitle the mother from 56 days to 6 months of maternity leave with full pay (Ministry of Public Health, 1992). Women who return to work are allowed time off for breast-feeding, and in many cases, factories provide a special lounge for the women to breast-feed. Families who come to Western societies expect the same importance to be placed on motherhood and may be surprised to find that many Western countries do not provide similar benefits.

Prescriptive and restrictive practices are used by many Chinese women during the postpartum period. Fruits and vegetables are avoided because they are considered "cold" foods. Mothers eat five to six meals a day including rice, soups, and seven to eight eggs. Rice wine is encouraged to increase the strength of the mother, but mothers need to be cautioned that it may also increase the bleeding time. Many mothers do not expose themselves to the cold air and do not go outside or bathe because the cold air can enter the body (Campbell & Chang, 1981). Women wear many layers of clothes even in the summer to keep the air away from their bodies.

## DEATH RITUALS

### Death Rituals and Expectations

The Chinese tradition in death and bereavement is centered on ancestor worship. Ancestor worship is frequently misunderstood; it is not a religion, but rather a form of paying respect. Many Chinese believe that their spirits can never rest unless living descendants provide care of the grave and worship their memory of the deceased. These practices were so important to the Chinese that early Chinese pioneers to the West had statements written into their work contract that their ashes or bones be returned to China (Halporn, 1992).

The belief that the Chinese greet death with stoicism and fatalism is a myth. In fact, the Chinese fear death, avoid references to it, and teach their children this avoidance (Chang, 1981; Huang, 1992). The number four is considered unlucky by many Chinese because it sounds like the word for death, and people avoid using it in their lives (similar to the bad luck associated with the number 13 by many Western societies). Wei C. Huang (1992) writes:

> At a very young age, a child is taught to be very careful with words that are remotely associated with the "misfortune" of death. The word "death" and its synonyms are strictly forbidden on happy occasions, especially during holidays. People's uneasiness about death often is reflected in their emphasis on longevity and ev-

erlasting life. . . . In daily life, the character "Long Life" appears on almost everything: jewelry, clothing, furniture, and so forth. It would be a terrible mistake to give a clock as a gift, simply because the pronunciation of the word "clock" is the same as that of the word "ending." Recently, many people in Taiwan decided to avoid using the number "four" because the number has a similar pronunciation to the word "death." (p. 1)

The purchase of insurance may be avoided because of a fear that it is inviting death. The color white is associated with death and is considered bad luck. Black is also a bad luck color. Red is the ultimate good luck color.

Many Chinese believe in ghosts, and the fear of death is extended to the fear of ghosts. Some ghosts are good and some are bad, but all have great power. Communism discourages this thinking and sees it as a hindrance to future growth and development of the society, but the ever-pragmatic Chinese believe it is better not to invite trouble with ghosts just in case they might exist (Ryan, 1992a).

The dead may be viewed in the hospital or in the family home. Extended family members and friends come together to mourn. Honor is given to the dead by placing around the coffin objects that signify the life of the dead such as food, spirit money, and other articles made of paper. In China, cremation is preferred by the state because of a lack of wood for coffins and a lack of space for burial. The ashes are placed in an urn and then in vaults. As cities grow, even the space for vaults is limited. In rural areas, many families prefer traditional burial and have family burial plots. Preference is to bury an intact body in a coffin.

## Responses to Death and Grief

The Chinese react to death in various ways. Most are more accepting of death than are Westerners. Death is viewed as a part of the natural cycle of life, and most believe that something good happens to them after they die. These beliefs foster the impression that Chinese are stoic. In fact they feel emotions similar to those of Westerners; they just do not overtly express those emotions to strangers (Chen, 1992). A person does not have to go to work but instead can use this mourning time for remembering the dead and planning for the future. Bereavement time in the larger cities is 1 day to 1 week, depending on the policy of the government agency and the relationship of family members to the dead (Ryan, 1992a). Mourners are recognized by black arm bands and white strips of cloth tied around their heads.

## SPIRITUALITY

### Religious Practices and Use of Prayer

Most Chinese consider religion to be a form of superstition, but in some parts of China, religion is becoming more popular. The main formal religions in China are Buddhism, Catholicism, Protestantism, Taoism, and Islam (Woo, 1990). Formal religious services as a practice are minimal. However, the ideals and values of the different religions are practiced alone rather than with people coming together to participate in a formal religious service. An understanding of this concept is essential when the health-care provider attempts to obtain chaplaincy services for Chinese clients.

Prayer is generally a source of comfort and improved life. Some Chinese do not acknowledge a religion such as Buddhism, but if they go to a shrine they burn incense and offer prayers.

## Meaning of Life and Individual Sources of Strength

The Chinese view life in terms of cycles and interrelationships, believing that life gets its meaning from the context in which it is lived. Life cannot be broken into simple parts and examined because the parts are interrelated. When the Chinese attempt to explain life and what it means, they speak about what happened to them, what happened to others, and the importance and interrelatedness of those events. They speak not only of the importance of the current phenomena but also about the importance of what occurred many years, maybe even centuries, before their lives. They live and believe in a true systems framework.

"Life forces" are sources of strength to the Chinese. These forces come from within the individual, the environment, the past and future of the individual, and society. Chinese use these forces when they need strength. If one usual source of strength is unsuccessful, they try another. The individual may use many different techniques, such as meditation, exercise, massage, and prayer. Drugs, herbs, food, good air, and artistic expression may also be used. Good-luck charms are cherished, and traditional and nontraditional medicines are used.

The family is usually one source of strength. Individuals draw on family resources and are expected to give back resources to strengthen the family. Resources may be financial, emotional, physical, mental, or spiritual. Calling on ancestors to provide strength as a resource requires giving back to the ancestors when necessary.

The larger society is also used for support and neighbors help each other. The government is expected to provide the means for improving life, and people resist if the government attempts to take away resources. The individual is also expected to give back to the government. The interconnectedness of life provides a source of strength for individuals from before birth to death and beyond.

## Spiritual Beliefs and Health-care Practices

Health-care practices of the Chinese reflect their cyclical explanation of life, in which everything is connected to health. The health-care provider needs to understand this multidimensional manner of thinking and believing. Assessments, goal setting, interventions, and evaluations may be different for the Chinese client. The context of client problems is the emphasis, and the physical, mental, and spiritual aspects of the person's life are the foci.

## HEALTH-CARE PRACTICES

### Health-seeking Beliefs and Practices

Health care in China is provided for most citizens. Every work unit and neighborhood has its own clinic and hospital. Traditional Chinese medicine shops abound (Fig. 7–1). Even department stores and supermarkets have Western medicines and traditional Chinese medicines and herbs.

While many Chinese have made the transition to Western medicine, others maintain their roots in traditional Chinese medicine, and still others practice both types of medicine (Unschuld, 1985). The Chinese are similar to other nationalities in seeking the most effective cure available. However, the Chinese frequently do not tell health-care providers about other forms of treatment because they are conscious of saving face. They believe that if they inform one health-care provider about another, then each of the providers loses face. Members of the health-care team need to de-

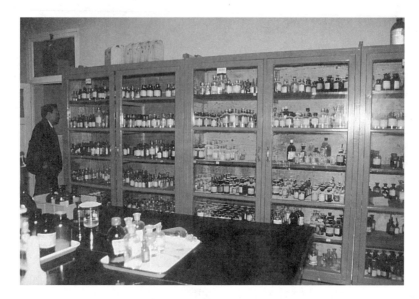

**Figure 7–1.** A traditional Chinese medicine shop. Many Chinese practice traditional Chinese medicine, either alone or in conjunction with Western medicine.

velop a trusting relationship with the Chinese client so that all information is disclosed. The health-care provider must impress on the client the importance of disclosing all treatments because many treatments have antagonistic effects.

The focus of health care has not changed over the centuries and includes having a healthy body, a healthy mind, and a healthy spirit. Preventive health-care practices are a major focus of China today. An additional focus is placed on infectious diseases such as schistosomiasis, tuberculosis, childhood diseases, and malaria; cancer; heart diseases; and maternal-infant care. Reported human immunodeficiency virus remains at low levels in China. The reason may be the stigma associated with sexually transmitted diseases and drug use in the society (Chinese Fail to Seek, 1992).

## Responsibility for Health Care

The Chinese self-medicate when they think that they know what is wrong or they have been successfully treated by medicine or herbs in the past. They share their knowledge about treatments and their medicine with friends and family members. Health-care providers need to recognize that sharing medications is an accepted practice among the Chinese. Thus, health-care providers should inquire about this practice when making assessments, setting goals, and evaluating the results of treatments. A trusting relationship between members of the health-care team and the client and family is necessary to enhance the disclosure of all treatments.

The Chinese culture uses two health-care systems. One is grounded in Western medical care, and the other is anchored in traditional Chinese medicine. The educational preparation of physicians, nurses, and pharmacists is similar to Western health-care education. Ancillary workers have responsibility in the health-care system, and midwifery practice is widely accepted by the Chinese. Physicians in Chinese medicine are trained in universities, and traditional Chinese pharmacies remain an integral part of health care.

# Folk Practices

Traditional Chinese medicine is practiced widely, with concrete reasons for the preparation of medicine, the taking of medicine, and expected outcomes. Western medicine needs to be explained to the Chinese in equally concrete terms.

Traditional Chinese medicine has many facets, including the five basic substances (**Qi**, the energy, **Xue**, the blood, **Jing**, the essence, **Shen**, the spirit, and **Jing ye**, the body fluids); the pulses and vessels for the flow of energetic forces (**Mai**); the energy pathways (*Jing*); the channels and collaterals, including the 14 Meridians for acupuncture, moxibustion, and massage (**Jing Luo**); the organ systems (**Zang Fu**); and the tissues of the bones, tendons, flesh, blood vessels, and skin (Ross, 1985). The scope of traditional Chinese medicine is vast and should be studied with more care by professionals who provide health-care for Chinese clients.

The Chinese believe that health and a happy life can be maintained if the two forces, the **yang** and **yin**, are balanced. This balance is called the **Dao**. Heaven is the yang, earth the yin; man the yang, woman the yin; the sun the yang, and the moon the yin; the hollow organs (bladder, intestines, stomach, gallbladder, and *San jiao* or triple burner), head, face, back, and lateral parts of the body the yang; and the solid viscera (heart, lung, liver, spleen, kidney, and pericardium), abdomen, the chest, and the inner parts of the body the yin. The yin is cold and the yang is hot. Health-care providers need to be aware that the functions of life and the interplay of these functions, rather than the structures, are important to the Chinese.

Central to traditional medicine is the concept of the *Qi*. It is considered the vital force of life and includes air, breath, or wind and is present in all living organisms. Some of the *Qi* is inherited, and other parts come from the environment, such as in food. The *Qi* circulates through the 14 meridians and organs of the body to give the body nourishment. The channels of flow are also responsible for elimination of the bad *Qi*. All channels (the meridians and organs) are interconnected. The results resemble a system where a change in one part of the system results in change in other parts, and one part of the system can assist other parts in total functioning.

Diagnosis is made through close inspection of the outward appearance of the body, the vitality of the person, the color of the person, the appearance of the tongue, and the person's senses. The practitioner uses listening, smelling, and questioning. Palpation is used by feeling the 12 pulses and different parts of the body. Treatments are based on the imbalances that occur. Many are directly related to the obvious problem, but many more are related through the interconnectedness of the body systems. Many of the treatments not only "cure" the problem but are also used to "strengthen" the entire human being. Traditional Chinese medicine cannot be learned quickly because of the interplay of symptoms and diagnoses. It takes many years for practitioners to become adept in all phases of diagnosis and treatment.

Acupuncture and moxibustion are used in many of the treatments (Gu & Zhang, 1992). Acupuncture is the insertion of needles into precise points along the channel system of flow of the *Qi* called the 14 meridians. (The system has over 400 points.) Many of the same points can be used in applying pressure and massage to achieve relief from imbalances in the system. The same systems approach is used to produce localized anesthesia.

Moxibustion is the application of heat from different sources to various points. For example, one source, such as garlic, is placed on the distal end of the needle after it is inserted through the skin, and the garlic is set on fire. Sometimes the substance is burned directly over the point without a needle insertion. Localized erythema occurs with the heat from the burning substance, and the medicine is absorbed through the skin. Cupping is another common practice. A heated cup or glass jar is put on the skin creating a vacuum, which causes the skin to be drawn into the cup. The heat that is generated is used to treat joint pain.

T'ai chi, practiced by many Chinese, has its roots in the 12th century. This type of exercise is suitable for all age groups, even the very old. Da Liu (1972) stated, "It relaxes the mind as well as the body. It helps digestion, quiets the nervous system, benefits the heart and blood circulation, makes joints loose, and refreshes the skin" (p. 1). T'ai chi involves different forms of exercise, and some can be used for self-defense. The major focus of the movements is mind and body control. The concepts of yin and yang are included in the movements, with a yin movement following a yang movement. Total concentration and controlled breathing are necessary to enable the smoothness and rhythmic quality of movement. The movements resemble a slow-motion battle, with the participant both attacking and retreating. Movements are practiced at least twice a day to bring the internal body, the external body, and the environment into balance.

Herbal therapy is integral to traditional Chinese medicine. It is even more difficult to learn than diagnosis, acupuncture, and moxibustion. Herbs fall into four categories of energy (cold, hot, warm and cool), five categories of taste (sour, bitter, sweet, pungent, and salty), and a neutral category (Jewell, 1983). Different methods are used to administer the herbs, including drinking and eating, applying topically, and wearing on the body. Each treatment is specific to the underlying problem or a desire to increase strength and resistance.

## Barriers to Health Care

Chinese clients face many of the same barriers to health care faced by Westerners; however, there are some special concerns. Tan (1992) summarized these as follows:

1. The Chinese have more difficulties facing diagnoses of cancer because families are the main source of support for patients, and many family members are still in China.

2. The Chinese pay less attention to the need for purchasing medical insurance, so any serious illness leads to heavy financial burdens on the family.

3. Once the client responds to initial treatment, the family tends to stop treatment and the client is lost to follow-up or becomes noncompliant.

4. Chinese families may be reluctant to allow postmortem examinations because of their fear of being "cut up."

5. The most difficult barrier is frequently the reluctance to disclose the diagnosis to the patient or the family.

In times of sickness many Chinese are reluctant to enter the hospital because many Chinese associate hospitals with death (Kraut, 1990). The family is expected to care for the person, which can be done more easily in the home, and most patients would rather stay at home with families. Many try traditional Chinese medicine at home and only enter the hospital if that has failed or they become seriously ill. The routines of hospitals are not understood, they interfere with daily activities, and the food does not satisfy the person's taste. Hot water, warm rooms, and putting on warm clothing is seen as good for the health. These ideas are opposite from what they can expect in Western hospitals. Even when a Chinese interpreter can be found, the dialect or correct form of the language may not be the same as the patient's.

Lack of knowledge and communication problems multiply when the Chinese attempt to apply for financial assistance. The rules and regulations placed on public agencies and assistance programs such as Medicaid and Medicare block effective use, and applying for insurance and collecting claims can be equally problematic.

# Cultural Responses to Health and Illness

Chinese express their pain in ways similar to those of Americans, but their description of pain differs. A study by Moore (1990) includes not only the expression of pain but also common treatments used by Chinese. The Chinese tend to describe their pain in terms of more diverse body symptoms, whereas Westerners tend to describe pain locally. The Western description includes words like stabbing and localized, whereas the Chinese describe pain as dull and more diffuse. They tend to use explanations of pain from the traditional Chinese influence of imbalances in the yang and yin combined with location and cause. The study determined that the Chinese cope with pain by using externally applied methods, such as oils and massage. They also use warmth, sleeping on the area of pain, relaxation, and aspirin.

The balance between the yang and yin is used to explain mental as well as physical illness and health. This belief, coupled with the influence of Russian theorists such as Pavlov, influence the Chinese view of mental illness. Mental illness results more from metabolic imbalances and organic problems. The effect of social situations on a person's mental well being (such as stress and crises) is considered to be inconsequential, but rather physical imbalances from genetics are the important factors. Because a stigma is associated with having a family member who is mentally ill, many families initially seek the help of a folk healer. Bentelspacher, Chitran, and Rahman (1994) found that many use a combination of traditional and Western medicine. Many mentally ill clients are treated as outpatients and remain in the home.

Although Chinese do not readily seek assistance for emotional and nervous disorders, a study of 143 Chinese-Americans found that younger, lower socioeconomic, and married Chinese with better language ability seek help more frequently (Ying & Miller, 1992). The researchers recommended that new immigrants be taught that help is available when needed for mental disorders within the mental health–care system.

Chinese in larger cities are becoming more supportive of the disabled, but for the most part, support services are rare. Since the focus has been on improving the overall economic growth of the country, the needs of the disabled have not had priority. The son of Deng Xiaoping was crippled in the Cultural Revolution and has been active in making the country more aware of the needs of the disabled. In the summer of 1994, games for the physically disabled were held in Beijing, China. Because most city households have televisions, the televised games increased the awareness of the Chinese people about the abilities of the disabled. Overall, the Chinese still view mental and physical disabilities as a part of life that should be hidden.

The expression of the sick role depends on the level of education of the client. More educated persons who have been exposed to Western ideals and culture are more likely to assume a sick role similar to that of Westerners. However, the highly educated and acculturated may exhibit some of the traditional roles associated with illness. Each client needs to be assessed individually for responses to illness and for expectations of care. Foo (1992) provided extensive insight into the sick role of the Chinese. Traditionally, the Chinese ill person is viewed as being passive and accepting of illness. They do not get as angry as the typical Westerner at the inconvenience or unfairness of an illness. To the Chinese, illness is expected as a part of the life cycle. However, they do try to avoid danger and to live as healthy a life as possible. To the Chinese, all of life is interconnected; therefore, they will seek explanations and connections for illness and injury in all aspects of life. Their explanations to health-care providers may not make sense, but the health-care provider should try to determine those connections so the connections can be incorporated into treatment regimens. The Chinese believe that because the illness or injury is caused from an imbalance, there should be a medicine or treatment that can restore the balance. If the medicine or treatment does not seem to do this, then they may refuse to use it.

Native Chinese and Chinese-Americans like treatments that are comfortable and do not hurt. Treatments that hurt are physically stressful and drain their energy.

Health-care providers who have been ill themselves can appreciate this way of thinking, because sometimes the cure seems worse than the illness. Explanations that are consistent with the Chinese way of thinking about treatments will be more successful.

The Chinese depend on their families and sometimes on their friends to help them while they are sick. These people provide much of the direct care; health-care providers are expected to manage the care. The family may seem to take over the life of the sick person, and the sick person is very passive in allowing them the control. One or two primary people assume this responsibility, usually a spouse. Health-care providers need to include the family members in the plan of care and, in many instances, in the actual delivery of care.

## Blood Transfusions and Organ Donation

Modern-day Chinese accept blood transfusions, organ donations, and organ transplants as long as they are safe and effective. Blood transfusions in China are not always safe because of the high incidence of hepatitis B; therefore, health-care providers often select other types of treatments. No overall ethnic or religious practices prohibit the use of blood transfusions, organ donations, or organ transplants. Of course, some persons may have religious or personal reasons to deny their use.

# HEALTH-CARE PRACTITIONERS

## Traditional Versus Biomedical Practitioners

As discussed previously, self-medication and self-diagnosis are common among the Chinese, and many times they will not seek help from health-care practitioners until they have tried their own medications, herbs, and other treatments. They may discuss their problems with family members and close friends, who help them diagnose their problem and even obtain treatments. Sharing of medicines and herbal treatments are common.

The Chinese respect their bodies but may not seem modest. Their bathrooms usually have no doors, and they frequently go to communal showers. However, they are very modest when it comes to touch. They feel uncomfortable touching their own bodies, which may be problematic when they need to use touch to provide their own health care (for example, breast self-examinations) (Lovejoy, et al., 1989). Persons of the same sex may use touch if they are close friends or family. Men and women do not touch each other, and even couples who have been married for a long time do not show physical affection in public. Chinese women feel uncomfortable when being touched by health-care providers, and most seek a woman health-care provider (Rawl, 1992).

## Status of Health-care Providers

Traditional Chinese medicine practitioners are shown great respect by the Chinese. In many instances, they are shown equal, if not more, respect than Western practitioners. The Chinese may distrust Western practitioners because of the pain and invasiveness of their treatments. The hierarchy among Chinese health-care providers is similar to that of the Chinese society. Older health-care providers receive respect from the younger providers. Men usually receive more respect than women, but that is beginning to change. Physicians receive the highest respect, followed closely by nurses with a university education. Other nurses with limited education are next in the hierarchy, followed by ancillary personnel. Liu (1991) provides an extensive historical view of the evolution of nursing in China.

Health-care practitioners are usually given the same respect as elders in the family (Louie, 1985). They are recognized by Chinese children as being authority figures. Physicians and nurses are viewed as persons who can be trusted with the health of a family member. Nurses are generally perceived as caring individuals (Morales & Jiang, 1993), but many times they do not provide much direct care for patients. The family is expected to oversee the direct care, while the physician makes the decisions about the type of treatment. Adult Chinese also respond to practitioners in the same way, but if they disagree with the health-care provider, they may not follow instructions. Moreover, they may not verbally confront the health-care provider because they fear that either they or the provider will suffer a loss of face.

## CASE STUDY

An elderly Asian-looking man is admitted to the emergency room with chest pain, difficulty breathing, diaphoresis, vomiting, pale, cold clammy skin, and apprehension. He is accompanied by three people speaking a mixture of English and a foreign language to one another. The nurse tries to speak English with the man, but he cannot understand anything said. Accompanying the elderly man are two women (one elderly and very upset and one younger who stands back from the other three people) and one younger man. The younger man states that the elderly man, whose name is Li Ying Bin, is his father, the elderly woman his mother, and the younger woman his wife. The son serves as the translator. Li Ying Bin comes from a small village close to Beijing, he is 68 years old, and he has been suffering with minor chest pain and trouble breathing for 2 days. He is placed in the cardiac room and the assessment is continued.

Mr. Li is on vacation visiting his son and daughter-in-law in the city. His son and daughter-in-law have only been married 1 year, but the son has lived in the West for 7 years. Mr. Li's daughter-in-law looks Chinese but was born in the United States. She does not speak very many words of Chinese.

Further physical assessment reveals that Mr. Li has a history of "heart problems," but the son does not know much about them. Mr. Li had been to the hospital in Beijing but did not like the care he received there and returned home as soon as possible. He goes to the local clinic periodically when the pain increases, and the health-care provider in China uses traditional Chinese medicine herbs and acupuncture. In the past, those treatments relieved his symptoms.

Medications are ordered to relieve pain, and Mr. Li undergoes diagnostic procedures to determine his cardiac status. They reveal that he did sustain massive heart damage. Routine interventions are ordered including heart medications, anticoagulants, oxygen, intravenous fluids, bedrest, and close monitoring. His condition is stabilized, and he is sent to the cardiac intensive care unit.

In the cardiac unit, the nurse finds Mrs. Li covering up Mr. Li until he sweats, and she argues with the nurse every time Mr. Li is supposed to dangle his legs. She complains that he is too cold and brings in hot herbal beverages for him to drink. She does not follow the nurse's and physician's orders for dietary restrictions, and she begins to hide her treatments from the staff. Her son and daughter-in-law try to explain to her that this is not good, but she continues the traditional Chinese medicine treatments.

Mr. Li is a very quiet patient. He lies in bed and never calls for help. He frequently seems to be meditating and exercising his arms. When he does talk to his son, he speaks of the airplane ride and the problems of being so high. He believes that may have caused his current heart problem. Mr. Li also wonders if Western food could be bad for his system. Mr. Li's condition gradually deteriorates over the next few days. Nurses and physicians attempt to tell the family about his condition and possible death, but the family will not talk with them about it. Mr. Li dies on the fifth day.

## STUDY QUESTIONS

1. What were the main reasons the Chinese immigrated to the United States initially? How were they treated by Americans? What impact has that had on the way the Chinese are viewed by Westerners today?

2. If you were to go to China on a business trip, how would you design your name card so that the Chinese would not be confused?

3. If you wished to have a meeting with a Chinese delegation of health-care providers, would you expect them to be on time? Why?

4. If the meeting included a meal with Chinese food, what kinds of food would you expect to be served? How would it be presented? If something is served that you do not like, would you eat it anyway?

5. Compare and contrast the Chinese meaning of life and way of thinking with the Western meaning and way of life.

6. What are the common health risks for the development of chronic obstructive pulmonary disease among Chinese people?

7. What are some of the reasons that Mr. Li waited so long to enter the hospital?

8. Mr. Li did not complain of chest pain in the cardiac intensive care unit. Is this a common behavior? Why?

9. True or False. The Chinese family will expect health-care providers at the hospital to provide most of the care for Mr. Li.

10. Why must the physician be careful with the amounts of medication ordered?

11. Mrs. Li is curt, demanding, and disagreeable toward her daughter-in-law. Why does she act this way?

12. Explain why Mr. Li blames the airplane ride and the Western food for his heart attack. Why does he meditate and do exercises?

13. Is Mr. Li's stoicism during dying surprising? Why do the family members refuse to discuss his health and possible death?

14. What is the preferred method of body disposal for Chinese?

15. Describe common mourning rituals for the Chinese.

16. Describe bereavement in a Chinese family.

17. Describe a common view of death among Chinese.

# References

Bentelspacher, C. E., Chitran, S., & Rahman, M. A. (1994, May). Coping and adaptation patterns among Chinese, Indian, and Malay families caring for mentally ill relative. *The Journal of Contemporary Human Services, 4*(5), 287–294.

Bond, M. H. (1991). *Beyond the Chinese face: Insights from psychology.* Hong Kong: Oxford University Press.

Burns, G. W. (1983). *The science of genetics: An introduction to heredity* (5th ed.). New York: Macmillan.

Butterfield, F. (1990). *China: Alive in the bitter sea* (rev. ed.). New York: Random House.

Campbell, T. & Chang, B. C. (1981). Health care of the Chinese in America. In G. Henderson & M. Primeaux (Eds.), *Transcultural health care* (pp. 162–171). Menlo Park, CA: Addison-Wesley.

Chang, B. (1981). Asian-American patient care. In G. Henderson & M. Primeaux (Eds.), *Transcultural health care* (pp. 255–278). Menlo Park, CA: Addison-Wesley.

Chen, C. (1992). Bereavement in Chinese-Americans. In C. L. Chen, W. C. Lowe, D. Ryan, A. H. Kutscher, R. Halporn, & H. Wang (Eds.), *Chinese Americans in loss and separation* (pp. 58–76). New York: Foundation of Thanatology.

Chin, A. (1988). *Children of China: Voices from recent years.* New York: Alfred A. Knopf.

Chin, J. L. (1991). Health care issues for Asian-Americans. *Journal of Multi-cultural Community Health, 1*(2), 17–22.

Chinese fail to seek help for HIV. (1992), *Nursing Times, 88*(21), 8.

Da Lui . (1972). *T'ai chi and i ching: A choreography of body and mind.* New York: Harper & Row.

Fairbank, J.K. (1983). *The United States and China* (4th ed.). Cambridge, MA: Harvard University Press.

Fong, R. & Mokuau, N. (1994). Not simply "Asian Americans": Periodical literature review on Asians and Pacific Islanders. *Social Work, 39*(3), 298–305.

Foo, S. (1992). Coping with major stroke and death: A neurologist's observation of first generation Chinese immigrants. In C. L. Chen, W.C. Lowe, D. Ryan, A.H. Kutscher, R. Halporn, & H. Wang (Eds.), *Chinese Americans in loss and separation* (pp. 38–40). New York: Foundation of Thanatology.

Gaspard, K. J. (1994). The red blood cell and alterations in oxygen transport. In C. M. Porth (Ed.), *Pathophysiology: Concepts of altered states* (4th ed., pp. 323–339). Philadelphia: J. B. Lippincott

Giger, J. N., Davidhizar, R.E., & Wieczorek, S.C. (1993). Culture and ethnicity. In I. M. Bobak & M. D. Jensen (Eds.), *Maternity and gynecologic care: The nurse and the family* (pp. 43–69). St. Louis: Mosby.

Gu, J. & Zhang, L. (1992). Acupuncture and moxibustion in primary health care in rural China. *World Health Forum, 13*(1), 51.

Halporn, R. (1992). Introduction. In C. L. Chen, W.C. Lowe, D. Ryan, A. H. Kutscher, R. Halporn, & H. Wang (Eds.), *Chinese Americans in loss and separation* (pp. v–xii). New York: Foundation of Thanatology.

Hu, W. & Grove, C.L. (1991). *Encountering the Chinese.* Yarmouth, MN: Intercultural Press.

Huang, W. (1992). Attitudes toward death: Chinese perspectives from the past. In C. L. Chen, W. C. Lowe, D. Ryan, A. H. Kutscher, R. Halporn, & H. Wang (Eds.), *Chinese Americans in loss and separation* (pp. 1–5). New York: Foundation of Thanatology.

Jewell, J. A. (1983). Traditional therapies II: Chinese materia medica. In S. M. Hillier & J. A. Jewell (Eds.), *Health care and traditional medicine in China, 1809–1982* (pp. 267–305). London: Routledge & Kegan Paul.

Kaplan, F. M., Sobin, J. M., & deKeijzer, A. J. (1990). *The China guide book* (11th ed.). New York: Harper & Row.

Kraut, A. M. (1990). Healers and strangers: Immigrant attitudes toward the physician in America—A relationship in historical perspective. *JAMA, 263*(13), 1807–1811.

Levy, R. A. (1993). Ethnic and racial differences is response to medicines: Preserving individualized therapy in managed pharmaceutical programmes. *Pharmaceutical Medicine, 7,* 139–165.

Lawson, J.S. & Lin, V. (1994), Health status differentials in the People's Republic of China. *American Journal of Public Health, 84*(5), 737–741.

Lin, C.C. & Fu, V.R. (1990). A comparison of child-rearing practices among Chinese, Immigrant Chinese, and Caucasian-American parents. *Child Development, 61,* 429–433.

Liu, C. (1991). From *san gu po* to caring scholar: The Chinese nurse in perspective. *International Journal of Nursing Studies, 28*(4), 315–324.

Louie, L.B. (1985). Providing health care to Chinese clients. *Topics in Clinical Nursing, 7*(3), 118–125.

Lovejoy, N.C., Jenkins, C., Wu, T., Shankland, S., & Wilson, C. (1989). Developing a breast cancer screening program for Chinese-American women. *Oncology Nursing Forum, 16*(2), 181–187.

Marden, C.F. & Meyer, G. (1973). *Minorities in American society.* New York: D. van Nostrand.

Ministry of Public Health, People's Republic of China. (1992). *A brief introduction to China's medical and health services.* Beijing, People's Republic of China.: Author.

Moore, R. (1990). Ethnographic assessment of pain coping perceptions. *Psychosomatic Medicine, 52,* 171–181.

Morales, E.T. & Jiang, S. L. (1993), Applicability of Orem's conceptual framework: A cross-cultural point of view. *Journal of Advanced Nursing, 18,* 737–741.

Office of Minority Health Resource Center. (1994a). Cancers of cervix, stomach, esophagus run high for some. *Closing the gap: Cancer and minorities,* (p. 1.) Washington DC: Author.

Office of Minority Health Resource Center. (1994b). *Closing the gap: Health and minorities in the U.S.* (p. 1). Washington, DC: Author.

Office of Minority Health Resource Center. (1994c). High diabetes rates linked to diet. *Closing the gap: Diabetes and minorities* (p. 1.) Washington, DC: Author.

Office of Minority Health Resource Center. (1994d). Older Chinese women at high risk for suicide. *Closing the gap: Homicide, suicide, unintentional injuries, and minorities* (p. 1). Washington, DC: Author.

Olsen, S.J. & Frank-Stromberg, M. (1993). Cancer prevention and early detection in ethnically diverse populations. *Seminars in Oncology Nursing, 9*(3), 198–209.

Porth, C. M. (1994). *Pathophysiology.* Philadelphia: J. B. Lippincott.

Quick reference to cultural assessment. (1994). St. Louis: Mosby.

Rawl, S. M. (1992). Perspectives on nursing care of Chinese Americans. *Journal of Holistic Nursing, 10*(1), 6–17.

Ross, J. (1985). *Zang Fu: The organ systems of traditional Chinese medicine* (2nd ed.). London: Churchill Livingstone.

Ryan, D. (1992a). Death customs in urban China today. In C. L. Chen, W.C. Lowe, D. Ryan, A. H. Kutscher, R. Halporn, & H. Wang (Eds.), *Chinese Americans in loss and separation* (pp. 6–13). New York: Foundation of Thanatology.

Ryan, D. (1992b). Health care in Daian, China today. In C. L. Chen, W. C. Lowe, D. Ryan, A. H. Kutscher, R. Halporn, & H. Wang (Eds.), *Chinese Americans in loss and separation* (pp.

15–21). New York: Foundation of Thanatology.

Sue, D. & Sue, D. W. (1992). Counseling strategies for Chinese Americans. In C. C. Lee & B. L. Richardson (Eds.), *Multicultural issues in counseling: New approaches to diversity* (pp. 79–90). Alexandria, VA: American Association for Counseling and Development.

Sue, D., Sue, D.M., & Ino, S. (1990). Assertiveness and social anxiety in Chinese-American women. *The Journal of Psychology, 124*(2), 155–163.

Tan, C. M. (1992). Treating life-threatening illness in children. In C. L. Chen, W. C. Lowe, D. Ryan, A. H. Kutscher, R. Halporn, & H. Wang (Eds.), *Chinese Americans in loss and separation* (pp. 26–33). New York: Foundation of Thanatology.

Unschuld, P. U. (1985). *Medicine in China: A history of ideas.* Berkeley, CA: University of California Press.

Weatherspoon, A. J., Danko, G. P., & Johnson, R. C. (1994, March). Alcohol consumption and use norms among Chinese Americans and Korean Americans. *Journal of Studies on Alcohol,* pp. 203–206.

Worcester, N. (1983). Diet and nutrition in the People's Republic of China. In S. M. Hillier & J. A. Jewell (Eds.), *Health care and traditional medicine in China, 1809–1982* (pp. 408–425). London: Routledge & Kegan Paul.

Yang, P. & Lawson, J. S. (1991), Health care for a thousand million. *World Health Forum, 12,* 151–155.

Ying, Y. (1994). Chinese American adult's relationship with their parents. *The Journal of Social Psychiatry, 40*(1), 35–45.

Ying, Y. & Miller, L. S. (1992). Help-seeking behavior and attitude of Chinese Americans regarding psychological problems. *American Journal of Community Psychology, 20*(4), 549–556.

# Cuban-Americans

*Divina Grossman*

---

• Key terms to become familiar with in this chapter are:

| | |
|---|---|
| *barrenillos* | Machismo |
| botanica | *Marielitos* |
| *Choteo* | *Orisha* |
| *Compadrazgo* | *Personalismo* |
| *Decaimientos* | Santeria |
| *Decensos* | *Santero* |
| *Ebo* | *Simpatia* |
| Honor | *Verguenza* |

## OVERVIEW, INHABITED LOCALITIES, AND TOPOGRAPHY
### Overview

Although Cuban-Americans are the smallest Hispanic group, they are the largest ethnic group in the metropolitan Miami, Florida, area and have been credited with the socioeconomic transformation of that city. Miami has become established as the dominant center of Cuban settlement, with the second-largest population of Cubans in the world next to Havana (Grenier & Stepick, 1992).

Before the Cuban migration, Miami was a city of transplanted northerners and was mostly favored by tourists and retirees. On their arrival, the Cubans created businesses and rejuvenated the economy, leading some to speak of the "Great Cuban Miracle." In 1987, Cubans owned more than 30,000 small businesses in Miami, with aggregate revenues of $3.8 billion. In 1989, the average Cuban family's income approximated that of a native-born family (Portes & Stepick, 1993).

The experience of Cubans in their homeland and in the United States is distinct from that of other Hispanic groups. The history and culture of Cuba and the Cuban people have been heavily influenced by Spain, the United States, the Soviet Union, and, through the slave trade in Cuba's sugar industry, by West African influences such as the Yoruba (Szapocznik & Hernandez, 1988).

Cuba was under Spanish control from 1511 to 1898, making it one of Spain's last colonies in the New World. The stranglehold on the sugar industry by Spanish *peninsulares* (individuals born in Spain), who were opposed by the growing class of *criollo* landowners (individuals of Spanish ancestry born in Cuba) and the *independentista* movement, created political turmoil and social imbalances that gave rise to the Cuban national character. The mistrust of government reinforced a strong personalistic tradition, a sense of national identity evolving from family and interpersonal relationships (Szapocznik & Hernandez, 1988).

As compared with other immigrant groups, Cubans were welcomed by the U.S. government, provided with support (for example, the Cuban Refugee Program begun by the Kennedy administration), and met with relatively little prejudice (Portes & Zhou, 1994). Cubans engaged in a wide range of entrepreneurial activity, both in sales and services, within the shelter of the Cuban community. Consequently, newer Cuban immigrants found networks of support and were somewhat protected from the difficulties associated with a competitive labor market. Like Eastern European Jews on New York's Lower East Side and Japanese immigrants in California, Cubans in Miami formed a true ethnic enclave (Grenier & Stepick, 1992).

Cubans in the United States are a strong presence not only economically but also politically. Their predominant political stance is characterized by an exile ideology, a preoccupation with events in Cuba, and a militant opposition to the regime of Fidel Castro. Overwhelmingly, Cuban-Americans tend to be conservative, Republican, and anticommunist. They have demonstrated high voter turnout and tend to vote in blocks during local and national elections (Boswell, 1991; Grenier & Stepick, 1992).

Cubans have managed to adjust to mainstream American culture while remaining close to their Cuban roots, a process that Szapocznik, et al. (1980) termed *biculturation*. The work of Gomez (1990) suggests that among Cuban-Americans, biculturation was positively related to psychological well-being, self-esteem, and to a lesser degree, job satisfaction. The bicultural individual and family are able to interact successfully with the host culture while retaining the skills and abilities to interact with their culture of origin (Szapocznik, Kurtines, & Fernandez, 1980). This may be attributed in part to the existence of Cuban ethnic enclaves. Thus, many Cubans tend to possess a strong ethnic identity, speak Spanish at home and in their daily activities, and adhere to traditional Cuban values and practices.

## Heritage and Residence

Cuba, the largest island in the Caribbean, lies between the coast of Florida and the Yucatan Peninsula of Mexico. To the west of Cuba is the Gulf of Mexico, and to the east are the islands of Hispaniola and Puerto Rico. Cuba is about 600 miles long and 50 miles wide. Racially, Cubans are 51 percent mulatto, 36 percent white, 11 percent black, and 1 percent Chinese (Mendez, 1994).

Cubans have a rich historical heritage. Spain launched its conquest of Mexico from Cuba in 1519. During the Spanish colonial period from 1511 to 1898, Spanish boats stopped in Havana on their way to Mexico and Central America. In the 19th century, the Monroe Doctrine led to a special relationship between Cuba and the United States. Cuba was controlled by a U.S. military government from 1898 to 1902. From 1902 to 1959, Cuba became politically independent as a capitalist state. In 1959, the revolution under Fidel Castro tried to free Cuba of U.S. influence. Castro subsequently established a socialist government, which still controls the country today (Boswell & Curtis, 1983; Mendez, 1994).

Of the 22,354,000 Hispanic people in the United States, about 1,044,000 are of Cuban origin. Of these, 735,000 reside in the South, 184,000 in the Northeast, 88,000 in the West, and 37,000 in the Midwest. The highest concentration of Cuban-Americans is in Florida where, according to the U.S. Department of Commerce, Bureau of the Census (1990), 674,052 Cubans live. Metropolitan centers with large Cuban ethnic enclaves include Miami, Florida; Union City, New Jersey; and West New York, New Jersey.

## Reasons for Migration and Associated Economic Factors

About 1 million Cubans immigrated to the United States between 1959 and 1980. The majority arrived on the U.S. mainland after the 1959 revolution that brought Fidel Castro to power and forever changed the social, economic, and political landscape of Cuba. Although the American government has defined the exodus as a political rather than an economic migration, a combination of these factors provided the motivation for migration. The desire for personal freedom, the hope of refuge and political exile, and the promise of economic opportunities have been the main determinants of Cuban immigration.

Portes and Bach (1985) described the six stages of Cuban immigration to the United States as follows:

First stage: includes departures from January 1959 to October 1962. When Fidel Castro overthrew the government of Fulgencio Batista in January 1959, approximately 250,000 landowners, industrialists, professionals, and merchants left on commercial flights from Havana to the United States.

Second stage: includes departures from November 1962 to September 1965. The confrontation between Cuba and the United States over Russian missiles in Cuba ended all direct flights from Cuba to the United States. At this time, about 56,000 people left on small boats and rafts because no direct transportation was available.

Third stage: includes departures from October 1965 to April 1973. Cuba and the United States reached an understanding in which an airlift was allowed from Varadero Beach to Miami. These "freedom flights" or "family reunification flights" yielded about 297,000 people.

Fourth stage: includes departures from May 1973 to September 1978. The Cuban government unilaterally ended the airlift. Travel to Spain, Mexico, and Jamaica became the only means of leaving Cuba. About 39,000 people arrived in the United States this way on commercial flights.

Fifth stage: includes departures from October 1978 to March 1980. Fidel Castro allowed political prisoners from Cuban jails to leave with their families. About 10,000 people arrived in this manner on airplane flights, boats, and rafts.

Sixth stage: includes departures from April to September 1980. The Cuban government again allowed a massive boatlift from the Mariel Harbor to Key West, Florida. Approximately 125,000 people arrived, including persons with criminal records, homosexuals, deaf-mutes, lepers, and patients from mental institutions. About 5000, or 4 percent, of these were hard-core criminals, causing an increase in the levels of violent crime in the metropolitan Miami and New York areas.

Since December 1960, the Cuban Refugee Program under the Department of Health, Education, and Welfare has been responsible for coordinating the processing and resettlement of Cubans in the United States. Between 1962 and 1971, the federal government spent over $730 million to support Cuban immigrant assistance programs, which covered relocation costs, housing subsidies, job training, medical care, low-cost college loans, food distribution, and cash allotment (Boswell & Curtis, 1984; Olson & Olson, 1995; Portes & Bach, 1985).

In the two decades of Cuban immigration, significant change has been observed in the waves of immigrants from the elite classes of the first stage, called the "Golden Exiles," to the *Marielitos* of the sixth stage. Although the waves were diverse in composition, the earliest immigrants were of higher educational achievement and economic status in Cuba, whereas the later group was more representative of the Cuban population. The motivation for immigration also changed from the desire to escape political and religious persecution in the earlier waves to the hope for economic improvement in the later waves (Boswell & Curtis, 1983).

## Educational Status and Occupations

The level of educational attainment of Cuban-Americans is higher than that of other Hispanic groups and approximates that of the white non-Hispanic American population (Ginzberg, 1991). Cubans under 35 years of age also have the highest school enrollment rates of any population in the United States, including non-Hispanic whites. Even at the preschool level (children aged 3 and 4) about 42 percent of Cuban children are enrolled in school (Perez, 1984).

In comparison with other Hispanic groups, Cubans exhibit a higher proportion of self-employed persons. Relatively high proportions of Cubans are found in these industrial categories: wholesale and retail trade, banking and credit agencies, insurance, real estate, and finance. Relative lower proportions of Cubans are employed in the extractive industries, public administration, and the manufacture of durable goods (Perez, 1984). By occupations, higher proportions of Cubans than other Hispanic groups and the total U.S. population (57 percent versus 38 percent and 56 percent, respectively) are found in nonclerical white-collar occupations such as executive, administrative, and managerial; professional and technical; and sales (Ginsberg, 1991). Cuban-Americans report the highest income of all three Hispanic groups and are more likely to report dual-income families (Smart & Smart, 1992). In 1987, the unemployment rate among Cubans was 5.5 percent—the lowest of any ethnic group in the U.S.—as compared with 7 percent for the rest of the country (Olson & Olson, 1995).

## COMMUNICATION

### Dominant Language and Dialects

Language is often used as an index of assimilation of an immigrant group into the dominant culture. Virtually all first-generation Cubans in the United States speak Spanish as their first language. A survey by Diaz (1980) found that the vast majority of Cuban immigrants speak only Spanish at home, with slightly over 50 percent speaking only Spanish at work. In contrast, more than 50 percent who attend school speak English exclusively and less than 20 percent of those speak mostly Spanish. For all age groups, Cubans with a higher level of education are more likely to speak English at home.

A study by the National Commission for Employment Policy (1982) revealed that only 18 percent of Cuban-born Americans consider English to be their dominant language, as compared with 30 percent for the Mexican and Puerto Rican populations. Because Cubans live and transact business in Spanish-speaking ethnic enclaves, they have little need or motivation to learn English (Boswell & Curtis, 1983).

The large number and variety of Spanish-language media, including newspapers, magazines, and radio programs, also reflect Cuban immigrants' preference for Spanish over English. Research by Diaz (1980) indicated that about 60 percent of Cubans listen mostly to Spanish-language programs and over 55 percent read mainly newspapers in Spanish. Taking a stroll through Little Havana in Miami or Little Havana North along New Jersey's Union City—West New York corridor, the preference for Spanish is once again reflected in billboard and poster advertisements. There signs announcing *joyeria* (jewelry store), *carniceria* (butcher shop) *muebleria* (furniture store), *farmacia* (drug store), or *zapateria* (shoe store) are quite commonplace (Boswell, 1991).

The inability to speak English has been identified as one of the most important problems faced by first-generation Cuban immigrants. According to a study by Portes and Clark (1980), three years later, learning English was still identified as the foremost problem, with economic difficulties moving to second place and transportation to third place.

As compared with their first-generation predecessors, second generation Cubans speak Spanish but frequently in a functional, elementary way. They may speak Spanish exclusively at home but may converse with friends or peers in "Spanglish," a mixture of Spanish and English. The smooth transition from Spanish to English and vice versa in the same sentence may be observed, as in the expressions *Vamos de shopping* or *Tenga un nice day* (Boswell & Curtis, 1983). In addition, Cubans in the United States have incorporated into their everyday Spanish many English words such as *futbol, rosbif, coctel, sueter, frigidaire, and bridge* (Fernandez, 1977). For Cuban-Americans, Spanglish becomes a pattern of life that reflects both their Cuban and American heritage.

## Cultural Communication Patterns

Like other Hispanic groups, Cubans value **simpatia** and **personalismo** in their interactions with others. *Simpatia* refers to the need for smooth interpersonal relationships and is characterized by courtesy, respect, and the absence of harsh criticism or confrontation. *Personalismo* pertains to an emphasis on intimate interpersonal relationships as more important than impersonal bureaucratic relationships. **Choteo**, a lighthearted attitude with teasing, bantering, and exaggerating, may be observed often in the way Cubans communicate with one another (Bernal, 1994; Queralt, 1984).

Conversations among Cubans are characterized by animated facial expressions, direct eye contact, and hand gestures and gesticulations. Voices tend to be loud and the rate of speech faster than what may be observed with non-Cuban groups. Linguistically, the use of the second person form *usted* to address older persons and authority figures has fallen into disuse, replaced by the familiar form *tu* (Sandoval, 1979). The use of *tu* in interpersonal situations serves to reduce distance and promotes *personalismo* (Bernal, 1994). Touching in the form of handshakes or hugs is acceptable among family, friends, and acquaintances. In the health-care setting, clients and family members may hug or kiss the health-care provider to express gratitude and appreciation.

Cubans feel a sense of "specialness" about themselves and their culture that may be conveyed in communication with others. This sense of specialness arises from pride in their unique culture, a fusion of European and African, the geopolitical importance of Cuba in relation to powerful countries in history, and the exceptional success they have achieved in adapting to their new environment. The sense of specialness, combined with the fast rate and loud volume of speech, may sometimes be interpreted as arrogance or grandiosity in a non-Cuban cultural context (Bernal, 1994).

## Temporal Relationships

Cubans tend to be present-oriented as compared with future-oriented European-Americans. A greater emphasis is laid on current issues and problems rather than on projections into the future. In the clinical setting, health-care providers must realize that Cuban clients tend to be motivated to seek help in response to crisis situations. Hence, visits to the health-care provider for resolution of a crisis must be used as opportunities for teaching and promotion of personal growth (Szapocznik, et al., 1978; Queralt, 1984).

*Hora cubana* (Cuban time) refers to a flexible time period that stretches about 1 to 2 hours beyond the designated clock time. A Cuban understands that when a party starts at 8 P.M., the socially acceptable time to arrive is between 9 and 10 P.M. However, families who have acculturated to American values may adhere to a more rigid clock time. When setting up appointments for clinic visits, the health-care provider must determine the client's level of acculturation with respect to time and make arrangements for flexible scheduling if necessary.

## Format for Names

As in other Latin American societies, Cubans use two surnames representing the mother's and father's sides of the family. To illustrate: A woman may carry the name Regina Morales Colon, indicating that her patriarchal surname is Morales and her matriarchal surname Colon. When a Cuban woman marries, she adds *de* and her husband's name after her father's surname and drops her mother's surname. In the previous example, if Regina marries Mr. Ordonez, her name will be Regina Morales de Ordonez (Boswell & Curtis, 1983).

When addressing Cuban clients, especially elderly ones, the health-care provider should use the formal rather than the familiar form unless told otherwise. In the previous example, the appropriate appellation would be Senora Morales, or Mrs. Morales, instead of Regina.

## FAMILY ROLES AND ORGANIZATION

### Head of Household and Gender Roles

Among Cubans, the family is the most important social unit (Bernal, 1994). The traditional Cuban family structure is patriarchal, characterized by a dominant and aggressive male and passive, dependent female (Queralt, 1984). Fox (1979) found that the concepts of *la casa* (the home) and *la calle* (the street) underscore the distinction between the roles of men and women. *La casa* is considered the province of the woman, and *la calle* the domain of the man. *La calle* includes everything outside the home, which is considered a proper testing ground for masculinity but dangerous and inappropriate for women (Fox, 1979).

Traditionally, Cuban wives are expected to stay at home, manage the household, and care for the children. Husbands are expected to work, provide, and make major decisions for the family. Richmond's (1980) work on Cuban family structure demonstrated that Cuban husbands tended to help very little with household chores, but those whose wives worked tended to help more. In the same study, Cuban wives who contributed to the family income were more likely to receive help from their husbands with household chores and acquired greater decision-making power than women who did not work (Richmond, 1980).

Cultural values acquired through four centuries of Spanish domination influence the behavior of Cuban men and women toward each other. The concept of **honor** is described as personal goodness or virtue, which can be lost or diminished by an immoral or unworthy act. Honor is maintained mainly by fulfilling family obligations and by treating others with *respeto* (respect). **Verguenza**, a consciousness of public opinion and the judgment of the entire community, is considered to be more important for women than men. **Machismo** dictates that men display physical strength, bravery, and virility (Fox, 1979).

Fox (1979) reported that the qualities Cuban men found most admirable in women were *puntuales a sus esposos*, *obediente*, and *atienda bien a sus esposos*, all indicating submissive and passive qualities. In women, being *moral* (virtuous), *aseada* (clean), and *decente* are desirable qualities. A double standard is often applied to male and female behavior (Fox, 1979). For example, it may be socially acceptable for men, but not for women, to engage in extramarital affairs. On the other hand, chaperoning is expected for single, respectable women who go out on dates (Boswell & Curtis, 1983).

Since the massive migration from Cuba to the United States in 1959, the traditional Cuban family has undergone transition to a less male-dominated, less segregated, and more egalitarian structure. Cuban women who arrived in the United States were frequently the first in the family to locate jobs and contribute to the survival of the family. According to Gallagher (1980), Cuban immigrant women were more receptive to life in the United States, more flexible, and were more readily hired for jobs than men. Eventually, as their contributions to the family's economic well-being increased, women's power to make decisions was enhanced. Cuban-American women have the highest rate of labor participation when compared with other groups of women in the Unites States (Suarez, 1993). Thus, contemporary Cuban families from the 1980s to the present may demonstrate greater gender equality in decision making for the family (Szapocznik & Hernandez, 1988). Although customs are changing, the gender role distinctions are still greater among Cuban-Americans than European-Americans in the United States (Queralt, 1984).

## Prescriptive, Restrictive, and Taboo Practices for Children and Adolescents

Cuban parents tend to pamper and overprotect their children, showering them with love and attention (Queralt, 1984). Fox (1979) reported that in Cuban families, the expectation is that children study, respect their parents, and follow *el buen camino* (the straight and narrow). Children are encouraged to acquire knowledge and learning *porque eso no te lo puede quitar nadie* (because no one can take that away from you) (Bernal, 1994).

Gender differences are evident in differing expectations of boys and girls. A boy is expected to learn a trade or prepare himself for work, whereas a girl is expected "to keep herself honorable while single" and to prepare herself for marriage. Boys are enjoined to stay away from vices. Girls are instructed to avoid the opposite sex and not to go out without "ample protection" (Fox, 1979).

When a Cuban daughter reaches the age of 15 years, a *quince,* or 15th birthday party, is typically held to celebrate this rite of passage. Socially, the *quince* is indicative of the young woman's readiness for courting by a *novio* (boyfriend). In Cuba, the *quince* was celebrated with plenty of good food, music, and dancing with family and friends. In Miami's Cuban enclave, the *quince* is a major social event. Parents may save up for years to prepare for a daughter's *quince,* which has today evolved into a large, extravagant party (Mendez, 1994).

Evidence suggests that younger and second-generation Cubans are acculturating faster than older and first-generation Cubans (Bernal, 1994). Cuban adolescents may undergo an identity crisis, not knowing whether they are fully Cuban or American. During this time, they may reject traditional cultural values, and parents may feel threatened that their authority is being challenged. The opposing values and demands of their Cuban heritage and American society create a potential for tension and conflict between Cuban adolescents and their parents. Some examples are the Cuban practice of chaperoning unmarried couples when they go dating. The custom has persisted of protecting young unmarried daughters and expecting them to live at home with the family until they marry (Boswell & Curtis, 1983).

## Family Roles and Priorities

Cubans have tightly knit nuclear families that allow for inclusion of relatives and *padrinos* (godparents). *La familia* (the family) is the most important source of emotional and physical support for its members (Caudle, 1993). Multigenerational house-holds are common, with grandparents often being part of the nuclear family.

In comparison with other ethnic or cultural groups, Cubans have the lowest proportion of families with children. Cubans also have the highest proportion of persons aged 65 years and older who live with their relatives. The high proportion of elderly persons living with family members has led to the typical three-generation Cuban family (Perez, 1984). The percentage of elderly women living with a relative is 68 percent for Cubans as compared with 38 percent for whites (Jackson, 1980). Mintzer, et al. (1992) reported that Cuban elderly women with Alzheimer's disease resided primarily with their daughter-caregivers, whereas white American women with the disease lived in institutional settings.

In Cuban families, lineal or hierarchical relationships are the norm, with hus-bands expecting obedience from their wives and parents from their children (Sza-pocznik & Hernandez, 1988). As is typical of many Latin American societies, Cubans tend to rely more on family and personal relationships rather than on the government or organizations (Boswell & Curtis, 1983).

A system of personal relationships known as **compadrazgo** is also typical. A set of godparents or *compadres* is selected for each child who is baptized and confirmed. *Compadres* tend to be close friends or relatives of the child's natural parents and may be counted on for moral or financial assistance. *Compadres* are usually consid-ered part of the Cuban family whether or not a true blood relationship exists (Boswell & Curtis, 1983).

As Cubans undergo biculturation, the traditional closely knit family may be dis-rupted. Intergenerational differences may occur, with highly Americanized children feeling alienated from their parents. A large proportion of Cubans who are now be-tween the ages of 40 and 60 years will be elderly persons by the beginning of the 21st century. Thus, the number of Cubans over the age of 65 years can be expected to double (Perez, 1994).

## Alternative Lifestyles

There is a high proportion of divorced women among Cuban-Americans as compared with other Hispanic and non-Hispanic groups in the United States. In spite of this, Cubans have the highest rate of children under 18 years living with both parents, a low percentage of families headed by women with no husbands present, and the lowest rate of mothers and children living within a larger family. One explanation for these patterns may be that divorced Cuban women return to their parents' home but, because of a low reproductive rate, do not tend to be accompanied by children (Perez, 1994).

In dealing with some Cuban-Americans, health-care providers may hear the term *Marielito* used in a derogatory manner to refer to the estimated 4 percent of the 125,000 Cubans who arrived during the Mariel boatlift. Because some of the *Marie-litos* were hard-core criminals released from Cuba's jails, the increased levels of crime in metropolitan Miami and New York have been attributed in part to their arrival. Although only a small minority of them were criminals, unfortunately the negative attitudes toward them have been extended to Cuban-Americans as a group. The Mar-ielitos were predominantly single, black, working-class Cuban males, in contrast with the professional and managerial workers of earlier waves of migration (Boswell & Curtis, 1984). They experienced many difficulties in adjusting to life in the United States, had lower median incomes, and were more likely to be unemployed and receiving public assistance than earlier Cuban immigrants (Olson & Olson, 1995).

Little or no data are available on the occurrence of homosexuality among Cuban-Americans, although the gay lifestyle would be contradictory to the prevailing ma-chismo orientation of Cuban culture. Same-sex couples living together may be alien-ated from their families, especially among first-generation Cubans who adhere closely to traditional gender roles and family values. Given the stigma associated with homosexuality in this culture, a matter-of-fact, nonjudgmental approach must be used by health-care workers when questioning Cuban clients regarding sexual orientation or sexual practices.

# WORKFORCE ISSUES

## Culture in the Workplace

As stated previously, Cubans have enjoyed tremendous economic success in the United States. According to 1989 Bureau of the Census figures, 62 percent of Cubans have completed a high school education, a higher percentage than for other Hispanic groups. The relatively high educational achievement is reflected in the proportion of Cuban-Americans (57 percent) who are employed in professional and technical jobs, the two highest occupational categories. Cuban families also have proportionately more persons participating in the labor force and earning a higher median income than Mexican or Puerto Rican families (Suarez, 1993).

Cuban-Americans exhibit strong entrepreneurial abilities, and many own their own businesses. These businesses tend to be concentrated in construction, transportation, textiles, wholesale, and retail trades. Cuban-American businesses have the highest annual gross receipts when compared with those of other recent immigrant groups (Olson & Olson, 1995). The existence of several Cuban ethnic enclaves with a familiar language and culture has created numerous employment opportunities for recent Cuban immigrants.

Blank and Slipp (1994) discussed some of the workplace concerns of Hispanics, including Cubans. A major complaint is that regardless of different cultural heritages, Hispanics tend to be lumped together as a group. Although they share the same language with other Hispanic groups, Cubans prefer to be identified with their specific group and take pride in their heritage.

In a study of Cuban immigrants, Martinez (1984) found that one of the most frequently encountered workplace difficulties was in the area of interpersonal relationships. Cubans tend to be lineal in their relationships, recognizing supervisors or superiors as authority figures and treating them with respect and deference. In mainstream American culture, collegial relationships where workers can exercise initiative, question the supervisor, and participate in decision making may make Cubans uncomfortable. Cubans value a structure characterized by *personalismo*, an orientation toward people, as being more important than concepts or ideas. For Cubans, strong personal relationships at work are considered an extension of family relationships. Cuban workers may function best in a working environment that is warm, friendly, and fosters *personalismo*. Because of the emphasis on the job or task in the American workplace, many Cubans view this workplace as being too individualistic, businesslike, and detached.

A frequent source of tension in the workplace is the tendency of Cubans to speak Spanish with other Cuban or Hispanic coworkers. Speaking the same language allows them to form a common bond, relieve anxieties at work, and feel comfortable with one another. In Blank and Slipp's (1994) study, one Cuban supervisor asserted, "Others should know that we tend to go back and forth in language—Spanish when we're talking personally and English when it's professional."

## Issues Related to Autonomy

Diaz (1980) reported that the percentage of Cuban-Americans who spoke Spanish exclusively at work was 34 percent in Miami and 39 percent in Union City, New Jersey. A small proportion spoke only English at work—23 percent in Miami and 17 percent in New Jersey. The existence of a Cuban ethnic enclave and the high labor force participation among Cuban-Americans suggest that proficiency in English was not a requisite for employment for the majority of individuals in this group (Boswell & Curtis, 1983). Nevertheless, for Cuban-Americans as a whole, the slow progress of linguistic assimilation has created a political backlash from European-Americans and African-Americans, who fear further latinization of their community. In 1980, overwhelming support in Miami for an antibilingualism ordinance stating that "the expenditure of county funds for the purpose of utilizing any language other than English, or promoting any culture other than that of the United States, is prohibited" is cited as a manifestation of the anti-Cuban sentiment (Portes & Stepick, 1993). To some degree, the language barrier may have also insulated Cuban-Americans from the dominant culture, retarded acculturation, and fostered some interethnic tensions (Grenier & Stepick, 1992).

## BIOCULTURAL ECOLOGY

### Skin Color and Other Biologic Variations

The Cuban population in the United States contains a high concentration of whites, higher than the proportion found in Cuba and in the total U.S. population. In the 1990s, more than 80 percent of Cuban-Americans are white and only 5 percent are black (Olson & Olson, 1995). During the period of Spanish colonization, the Arawak Indians in Cuba were almost completely annihilated and replaced with African slaves. Unlike Mexicans, therefore, Cubans lack an Indian ancestry (Queralt, 1984; Williamson, 1992).

Because of their predominantly European ancestry, Cubans in the United States have skin, hair, and eye colors that vary from light to dark. A smaller minority who are of African-Cuban extraction are dark-skinned and may have physical features similar to African-Americans.

### Diseases and Health Conditions

Data from the Hispanic Health and Nutrition Survey (HHANES) indicate that 29 percent of Cuban-American males and 34 percent of Cuban-American females are overweight, as compared with 25 percent and 37 percent of Puerto Rican males and females, and 30 percent and 39 percent of Mexican-American males and females (National Center for Health Statistics, 1989; Council on Scientific Affairs, 1991). The same study found that 16 percent of Cuban-Americans aged 45 to 74 years had diabetes mellitus, as compared with 26 percent of Puerto Ricans and 24 percent of Mexican-Americans (Council on Scientific Affairs, 1991).

Among Cuban-Americans in Dade County, Florida, approximately 23 percent of the males and 16 percent of the females were hypertensive—rates that are significantly lower than those for whites and blacks nationally. Cuban-American hypertensive men were more likely to be on medication than Puerto Rican and Mexican hypertensive men. With the hypertension threshold designated as 160/95 and the control threshold considered to be 140/90, the proportion of men with controlled hypertension was 26 percent for Cuban-Americans, as compared with 23 percent for Mexicans and 12 percent for Puerto Ricans (Pappas, Gergen, & Carroll, 1990). The Cuban population in Miami was found to have an inordinately high rate of nonalcoholic cirrhosis, but attempts to link this trend with the hepatitis B surface antigen have not proved successful (Diaz, 1980).

The HHANES Survey revealed that the prevalence of self-reported bronchitis was lower among Cuban-Americans (1.7 percent) and Mexican-Americans (1.7 percent) than among Puerto Ricans (2.9 percent). The prevalence of chronic bronchitis was two times greater among smokers than nonsmokers among Cubans and Puerto Ricans but less for Mexican-Americans (Bang, Gergen, & Carroll, 1990).

In the HHANES Survey, Cubans had a significantly higher prevalence of total tooth loss than both Mexican-Americans and Puerto Ricans. In adults, Cuban-Americans had the highest mean number of filled teeth of the three Hispanic subgroups. Also, the prevalence of gingival inflammation and periodontitis in Cuban- Americans is higher than that in the white non-Hispanic population (Ismail & Szpunar, 1990). The Cuban diet, which is high in sugar and starches, may explain the high prevalence of these conditions among Cuban-Americans.

## Variations in Drug Metabolism

Although some studies have reported differences in drug metabolism among Hispanics, little or no data is available specific to Cuban-Americans.

## HIGH-RISK BEHAVIORS

The HHANES Survey found that Hispanic men were twice as likely to smoke as Hispanic women, with a prevalence rate of 42 percent for Cuban-American men. The prevalence rate of smoking among Cuban women was 24 percent, as compared with 30 percent among Puerto Ricans and 24 percent among Mexicans. All three Hispanic groups showed higher smoking rates than the non-Hispanic white population in the National Health Interview Survey (Sandoval, 1994). The prevalence of smoking among Cuban-American women in their 30s was higher than the national average, and they smoked significantly more cigarettes than Puerto Rican and Mexican-American women in the same age group (Pletsch, 1991).

The HHANES Survey also revealed that drinking alcohol was significantly more common among Cuban males than females, and among younger versus older Cuban groups, a pattern that was similar to that in Mexicans and Puerto Ricans. Among middle-aged and older Cuban males, who tend to be relatively well educated and have higher income, control of intoxication is important, as compared with the younger, more recent Cuban immigrants. Among Cuban women, the proportion of life-long abstainers increased significantly from the younger to the older groups (Black & Markides, 1994).

Violent deaths account for high mortality rates among adolescents and young adults of Cuban, Mexican-American, and Puerto Rican origin. Cuban and Puerto Rican suicide rates also exceed those of the white non-Hispanic population (Council on Scientific Affairs, 1991).

## Health-care Practices

An obstacle to good nutritional practice is the Cuban cultural perspective of the "healthy body." A healthy and beautiful Cuban infant is one that is fat. Even among adults, a little heaviness is considered attractive. *Que gordo estas!* (How fat you are!) is considered a compliment. The traditional Cuban diet, high in calories, starches, and saturated fats, predisposes to the development of obesity (Feinsilver, 1993).

As shown in the HHANES Survey, about one-third of Cuban males and females are overweight (National Center for Health Statistics, 1989). Lopez (1993) found that unmarried Cuban-American women who had little recreational activity tended to have a higher mean weight. In addition, in contrast to Mexican-American and Puerto Rican women, body fatness in Cuban-American women was not significantly associated with income (Lopez & Masse, 1993).

In Cuba, health care is viewed as a basic human right and occupies a prominent place in the Cuban government's domestic and foreign policies. Polyclinics in communities are the basic unit of health care. Physician-nurse teams attend clients in these polyclinics as well as in the home, school, day-care center, and workplace (Feinsilver, 1993). In the United States, Cubans exhibit high levels of preventive health behavior, as evidenced by routine physical examinations within the last 2 years. The utilization of preventive services was usually associated with accessibility, which in turn was significantly influenced by education, annual income, and age. (Solis, et al., 1990).

## NUTRITION

### Meaning of Food

Food has a powerful social meaning among Cuban-Americans, allowing families to reaffirm kinship ties, promote a sense of community, and perpetuate their customs and heritage (Boswell & Curtis, 1983). To grasp this fully, one needs only to observe multigenerational families assembled for dinner on a Saturday or Sunday evening in a Cuban restaurant in Miami's Little Havana or Cuban friends sharing a cup of cafe cubano and pastelitos at a stand-up sidewalk counter. In Miami alone, the demand for Cuban food and food products has resulted in the establishment of about 400 Latin restaurants, mostly Cuban, and some 700 *bodegas,* or grocery stores.

### Common Foods and Food Rituals

Cuban foods reflect the environmental influences of Cuba's tropical climate and agriculture, the historical influences of Spanish colonial rule, the African slave trade, and the Arawak Indians' cultivation methods. Figure 8–1 depicts the food guide pyramid for Cubans. Typical staple foods are root crops like yams, yuca, malanga, and boniato; plantains; and grains. Traditional Spanish dishes like *arroz con pollo* and *paella* are frequently served. Many dishes are prepared with olive oil, garlic, tomato sauce, vinegar, wine, lime juice, called *sofrito,* and spices. Meat is usually marinated in lemon, lime, sour orange, or grapefruit juice before cooking (Boswell & Curtis, 1983).

The main course in Cuban meals is meat, usually pork or chicken. Some popular entrees are roast pork (*lechon*), fried pork chunks (*masas de puero*), sirloin steak (*palomilla*), shredded beef (*ropa vieja*), pot roast (*boliche*), and roasted chicken (*pollo asado*). A roasted suckling pig is traditionally served on Christmas Eve and New Year's Day, and during other festive celebrations. Black beans are prepared with a sauce containing fat, pork, and other spices. Ripe plantains (*platanos maduros*) or green plantains *(platanos verdes)* are served fried. Fried green plantains (*tostones* or *mariquita*) may also be smashed between a brown paper bag and the fist (*un cartucho y el puno*), giving them the familiar name *platanos y punetazo*. Desserts are rich and very sweet, such as custard (*flan*), egg pudding (*natilla*), rice pudding (*arroz con leche*), coconut pudding (*pudin de coco*), or bread pudding (*pudin de pan*) (Boswell & Curtis, 1983).

Beverages may include sugar cane juice (*guarapo*), iced coconut milk (*coco frio*), milk shakes (*batidos*), Cuban soft drinks such as Iron Beer or Materva, sangria, or beer. The strong and bittersweet coffee called *cafe cubano* is a standard drink after meals and throughout the day, whether at home, in restaurants, or in other social situations. In the United States, Cubans may drink the *cafe cubano* as *cortadito* or with a dash of milk to cut the strength and bittersweet taste (Boswell & Curtis, 1983). A traditional Cuban meal includes a generous helping of white rice with black beans or black bean soup, fried plantains, roasted pork or fried chicken, a tuber such as malanga or yuca, followed by dessert and espresso. Thus, the typical diet is high in

# The Food Guide Pyramid
### for
### *Cubans*

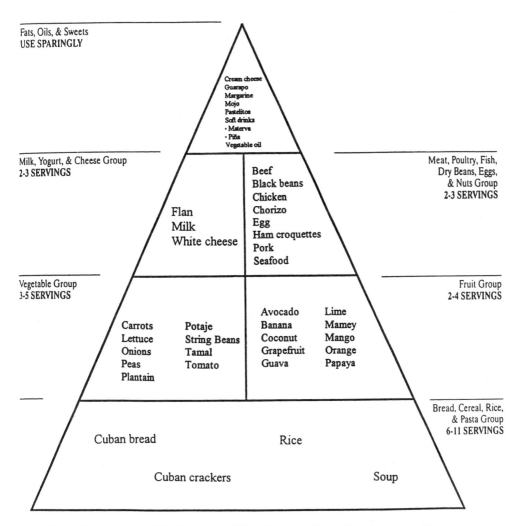

Fats, Oils, & Sweets
USE SPARINGLY

Cream cheese
Guarapo
Margarine
Mojo
Pastelitos
Soft drinks
• Materva
• Piña
Vegetable oil

Milk, Yogurt, & Cheese Group
2-3 SERVINGS

Meat, Poultry, Fish,
Dry Beans, Eggs,
& Nuts Group
2-3 SERVINGS

Flan
Milk
White cheese

Beef
Black beans
Chicken
Chorizo
Egg
Ham croquettes
Pork
Seafood

Vegetable Group
3-5 SERVINGS

Fruit Group
2-4 SERVINGS

Carrots
Lettuce
Onions
Peas
Plantain

Potaje
String Beans
Tamal
Tomato

Avocado
Banana
Coconut
Grapefruit
Guava

Lime
Mamey
Mango
Orange
Papaya

Bread, Cereal, Rice,
& Pasta Group
6-11 SERVINGS

Cuban bread

Rice

Cuban crackers

Soup

**Figure 8–1.** The Food Guide Pyramid for Cubans. (From Rodriguez, A: Hispanic Americans in Florida: An Overview of Their Food Habits, 1995.)

calories, starches, and saturated fats. As in Spain and other Hispanic countries, a leisurely noon meal (*almuerzo)* and a late evening dinner, sometimes as late as 10 or 11 p.m., (*comida)* are customary (Boswell & Curtis, 1983; Feinsilver, 1993).

## Nutritional Deficiencies and Food Limitations

As seen in Figure 8–1, the major food groups are well represented in the Cuban diet; however, leafy green vegetables may be lacking in the average Cuban meal. Therefore, in assessing the nutritional adequacy of a Cuban client's diet, the health-care provider must ensure that there is sufficient fiber content.

## PREGNANCY AND CHILDBEARING PRACTICES

### Fertility Practices and Views toward Pregnancy

The fertility rate of Cuban women is 49.8 per 1000 live births, as compared with 106 for Mexican-Americans and 86 for Puerto Ricans (Smith & Weinman, 1995). The low rate of reproduction, which is consistent in every maternal age group, has been attributed to three factors:

1. Cuban-American women have a high rate of labor force participation.

2. Before the revolution, Cuba had the lowest birth rate in Latin America.

3. Cuba's current reproductive rate is among the lowest in the developing world (Perez, 1984).

In an analysis of HHANES data, Stroup-Benham and Trevino (1991) found that Cuban-American women were twice less likely to use oral contraceptives (8 percent) than Mexican-American women (16 percent). Among Cuban-American females who were considered at risk for pregnancy, only 9 percent took oral contraceptives, as compared with 11 percent among Puerto Ricans and 20 percent among Mexican-Americans.

In the same study, hysterectomies, oophorectomies, and tubal ligations were found to be less common among Cuban-American women than among either Mexican-American or Puerto Rican women. Based on these data, Cuban-American women appear to be at greatest risk for unintended pregnancies. Paradoxically, they have the lowest birth rate among the three groups of Hispanic women (Stroup-Benham & Trevino, 1991). A possible explanation for this inconsistency may be the high divorce rate and the high labor force participation rate among Cuban-American females.

The rate of prenatal care among Cuban mothers is 85 percent, as compared with 80 percent in white non-Hispanics, 59 percent in Mexican-Americans, and 65 percent in Puerto Ricans (U.S. Department of Health and Human Services, 1993). The prevalence of preterm births (infants born before 37 weeks of gestation) was found to be the lowest (13 percent) among Cuban-American women, followed by Mexican-American (14 percent) and Puerto Rican women (15%), as compared with 11 percent for non-Hispanic white women (Mendoza, et al., 1991).

In the Linked Birth and Infant Death data sets of 1983 and 1984, the neonatal mortality risk (the risk of death in infants less than 28 days after birth) was 1.0 among Cuban-Americans and Mexican-Americans as compared with 2.3 among Puerto Rican Islanders and 1.5 among continental Puerto Ricans. The postneonatal mortality risk, the risk of death in infants between 28 to 364 days of life, was highest among Puerto Ricans (1.2) and lowest among Cuban-Americans (0.6) (Becerra, et al., 1991).

Many Cuban folk beliefs and practices surround pregnancy. For example, some Cuban women believe that they have to eat for two during the pregnancy and end up gaining excessive weight. Some believe that morning sickness is cured by eating coffee grounds, that eating a lot of fruit ensures a baby with a smooth complexion, and that wearing necklaces during pregnancy causes the umbilical cord to be wrapped around the baby's neck (Brewer, 1995).

Among Cuban-Americans, childbirth is a time for celebration. Family members and friends congregate in the hospital, awaiting the delivery of the baby. Although traditionally it was not acceptable for Cuban men to attend the birth of their children, the younger and more acculturated Cuban fathers tend to be present to support their wives during labor. In the postpartum period, it is believed that ambulation, exposure to cold, and bare feet places the mother at risk for infection. Because of this, family members and relatives often care for the mother and baby for about 4 weeks post-partum (Brewer, 1995).

## Prescriptive, Restrictive, and Taboo Practices in the Childbearing Family

Thomas and DeSantis (1995) found that the majority of Cuban women (77 percent) who migrated to the United States in the 1980s considered breast-feeding better than bottle feeding, but only 40 percent chose to breast-feed one or more of their infants. In the same study, Cuban mothers weaned infants from the breast and introduced solid foods at a median age of 3 months. Weaning from the bottle occurred in Cuban infants at a median age of 4 years, as compared with 1 year of age recommended in the medical literature.

Thomas and DeSantis (1995) related the early introduction of solid foods and prolonged bottle feeding of Cuban children to the traditional Cuban beliefs that "a fat child is a healthy child" and that breast-feeding may contribute to a deformity or asymmetry of the breasts. In the same study, 97 percent of Cuban mothers indicated that they administer vitamin preparations to promote healthy development of their children. Cuban mothers also used advice about child health given by their spouses, mothers, mothers-in-law, and clerks and pharmacists who sold them over-the-counter drugs (Thomas & DeSantis, 1995).

## DEATH RITUALS

### Death Rituals and Expectations

In death as in life, the support of the extended family network is important. Whether in the hospital or at home, the dying person is typically attended by a large gathering of relatives and friends. In Catholic families, individual and group prayers are held for the dying to provide a peaceful passage to the hereafter. Religious artifacts such as rosary beads, crucifixes, *estampitas* (little statues of saints) are placed in the dying person's room.

Depending on the dying person's religious beliefs, a Catholic priest, Protestant minister, a rabbi, or a **santero** may be summoned to the deathbed to perform appropriate death rites. For adherents of **santeria,** death rites may include animal sacrifice, chants, and ceremonial gestures. Health-care providers need to be open-minded and responsive to both the physical and psychosocial needs of the dying and the bereaved and, regardless of religious beliefs, accord them the utmost respect and privacy.

After a person's death, candles are lighted to illuminate the path of the spirit to the afterlife. A funeral wake, or *velorio,* is usually held at a funeral parlor, where friends and relatives gather to support the bereaved family. The wake lasts for 2 to 3 days until the funeral. Burial in a cemetery is the common practice for Cuban Catholics, although others may resort to cremation.

### Responses to Death and Grief

Bereavement is expressed openly among Cuban-Americans, with loud crying and other physical manifestations of grief considered socially acceptable. Death is an occasion for far-away relatives to visit and commiserate with the bereaved family. Women from the immediate family usually dress in black during the period of mourning. Visitors make offerings of candles and floral wreaths (*coronas*), provide assistance with household chores, and attend to visitors or funeral arrangements. Cuban-Americans customarily remember and honor the deceased on their birthdays or death anniversaries by lighting candles, offering prayers or masses, bringing flowers to the grave, or gathering with family members at the grave site.

## SPIRITUALITY

### Religious Practices and Use of Prayer

Approximately 85 percent of Cuban-Americans are Roman Catholics, with the remaining 15 percent being Protestants, Jews, and believers in the African-Cuban cult of *santeria*. The Roman Catholic Church has been an important source of support, especially for first-generation Cuban immigrants. A number of predominantly Cuban parishes with Cuban clergy are located in Florida and New Jersey where large Cuban populations reside. In South Florida, about 1 in 5 Cuban Catholics regularly attends mass (Jorge, Suchlicki, & Leyva de Varona, 1991). The Catholic Church has exerted an important influence on Cuban families by providing educational opportunities at Catholic schools. Many Cuban parents, especially the upper middle class, prefer to have their children educated in private Catholic schools.

The difference between Roman Catholicism as practiced by Cubans and as practiced by mainstream Catholics is its personalistic instead of institutional nature. The religious practice of Cuban Catholics is characterized by devotion and intimate, confiding relationships with the Virgin Mary, Jesus, and the saints (Boswell & Curtis, 1984).

Some families may have shrines dedicated to *La Caridad del Cobre* (the patron saint of Cuba) or other saints at the entrance to their homes, in their yards, or in commercial establishments. The three favorite saints that are enshrined are Santa Barbara, San Lazaro, and *La Caridad del Cobre*. Inside the home, crucifixes and pictures or statues depicting images of saints may be found. When someone is ill, small pictures of saints called *estampitas* may be placed under the pillow or at the sick person's bedside.

Significant religious holidays for Cuban families include Christmas, *Los Tres Reyes Magos* (Three Kings Day), and the festivals of the *La Caridad del Cobre* and Santa Barbara (Boswell & Curtis, 1984). The Cuban community usually celebrates the feast of *La Caridad del Cobre* (September 8) by transporting the statue of the patron saint on a boat to a specific location, where a Mass is held in her honor. Cuban families also celebrate Christmas Eve (*Noche Buena*), when a traditional Cuban meal is served. The pork is typically cooked all day in a wooden box lined in metal (*una caja china*) and set in the backyard. The pig is placed at the bottom of the box and the charcoal on top. The pork is served with black beans and rice, yuca, and *turones* (Spanish dessert). The evening is concluded with the family attending midnight mass (*Misa de Gallo*).

*Santeria,* or *Regla de Ocha,* is a 300-year-old African-Cuban religious system that combines Roman Catholic elements with ancient Yoruba tribal beliefs and practices. Santeria originated among the Yoruba people of Nigeria, who brought their beliefs with them when they arrived in the New World as slaves. As a condition of their entry into the West Indies, slaves were required to be baptized as Roman Catholics (Murphy, 1988). In the process of adaptation to their new non-African environment, the slaves altered their beliefs to incorporate those of their predominantly Catholic masters. Thus, Santeria became the product of a syncretism between "the gods of the slaves and the Catholic saints of their masters" (Sandoval, 1979, p. 138).

Santeria evolved from two main cultural antecedents: the worship of **Orisha** among the Yoruba tribe of Nigeria and the cult of saints from the Roman Catholicism of Spain. Through their exposure to the Catholic religion, the slaves came to associate their African gods, called *orishas,* with the Roman Catholic saints, or *santos.* The worship of orishas and its associated beliefs, rituals, incantations, magic, and spirit possession are central to Santeria.

Table 8–1 displays the seven African powers or main *orishas* (Martinez & Wetli, 1982). As shown, for example, the Yoruba deity of fire and thunder called *Chango* became identified with Santa Barbara, who was the patron saint of the Spanish artillery and who appeared in Catholic lithographs in red, the color of the *orisha* (Sandoval, 1979). *Chango,* the most popular god in Santeria, controls thunder, violent storms, lightning, and fire. The six other *orishas,* the Catholic saints with whom they are identified, and their corresponding functions and powers are also shown in Table 8–1.

When persons decide to practice Santeria, their *orishas* become known to them and must be worshipped throughout their lives. Followers of Santeria believe in the magical and medicinal properties of flowers, herbs, weeds, twigs, and leaves. Sweet herbs such as *manzanilla, verbena,* and *mejorana* are used for attracting good luck, love, money, and prosperity. Bitter herbs such as *apasote, zarzaparilla,* and *yerba bruja* are used to banish evil and negative energies (Gonzales-Whippler, 1982).

Adherents of Santeria also believe in the power of consecrated objects such as

### Table 8–1 • Seven African Powers or Main Orishas

| Orisha | Christian Saint | Function/Power | Punishment | Propitiation |
|---|---|---|---|---|
| *Eleggua* | Holy Child of Atocha | Guardian of entrances, roads, and paths; Trickster | | Blood of goats; black rooster; smoked fish; smoked junia; yams, sugar cane |
| *Obatala* | Our Lady of Mercy | Father of all human beings, gives advice, is source of energy, wisdom, purity, and peace | Blindness, paralysis, and birth deformities | White pigeons, white canaries; female goat; plums; yam puree |
| *Chango* | Saint Barbara | Warrior diety that controls thunder and violent storms, lightning and fire | Death, suicide by fire | Roosters, goats, lambs; apples, and bananas |
| *Oshun* | Our Lady of Charity | Diety that controls money and love, makes marriages, protects genitals | Abdominal distress, social and domestic strife | Female goat, white chickens, sheep; honey |
| *Yemaya* | Our Lady of Regla | Primary mother of the santos, protects womanhood, owns seas | Respiratory distress | Ducks, lambs, female goats; watermelons; black-eyed peas |
| *Babaluaye* | Saint Lazarus | Patron of the sick, especially diseases of the skin | Leprosy, gangrene, skin diseases | Spotted rooster; snakes; cigars; pennies; glasses of water |
| *Ogun* | Saint Peter | Warrior deity, owns all metals and weapons | Violent death (such as an automobile accident) | Blood and feathers; young bulls, roosters; steel knife; railroad tracks |

*Source:* Adapted from Martinez, R., & Wetli, C. (1982). Santeria: A magicoreligious system of Afro-Cuban origin. *American Journal of Social Psychiatry, 2*(3), p 34, with permission.

stones (*otanes*) in which the *orishas* reside. Necklaces, bracelets, and charms may be given by *santeros* to their clients to protect them from evil and to strengthen their well-being. The *orishas* must be propitiated for the person to avoid punishment, as seen in Table 8–1. For example, white pigeons and plums must be offered to the god Obatala to avoid the punishments of blindness, paralysis, and birth deformities (Martinez & Wetli, 1982).

Sacrifice, or **ebo** (pronounced egbo or igbo), is a central ritual in Santeria. The main purpose of *ebo* is to establish communication between the spirits and human beings. The initiation of a *santero* involves the sacrifice of a four-legged animal and a series of rites lasting over 7 days (Brandon, 1990). Transition through major life events such as birth, death, and marriage require ritual sacrifice to appease the gods and solicit their support.

Sacrificial objects in Santeria include plants, foods, and animals. Plants and foods include plantains, malanga, yam, okra, flour, gourds, and ground black-eyed peas wrapped in plantain leaves. Animals used for sacrifice, such as hens, birds, lambs, or goats, are killed by wringing the head or severing the carotid arteries with a knife. The animal's blood is offered as a type of communion with the deities (Brandon, 1990). In 1993, the Supreme Court struck down antianimal sacrifice laws in Hialeah, Florida, and recognized the right of a Santeria sanctuary, the Church of Chango Eyife, to offer animal sacrifice as a religious sacrament (Gonzalez, 1995).

Santeria is viewed as a link to the past and is used among Cubans and other Hispanic groups to cope with physical and emotional problems. When someone is sick, that person's physical complaints may be diagnosed and treated by a physician, but the *santero* may be summoned to assist in balancing and neutralizing the various aspects of the illness. Santeria is actively practiced by middle-class Cubans in Miami, Florida, and in areas of New York, New Jersey, and California where Cubans reside (Sandoval, 1979).

In eliciting a complete history from the client, health-care providers must include information regarding the type of religion being practiced, if any. Clients' religious beliefs and practices must be viewed in an open, sincere, and nonjudgmental manner. In the hospital setting, maintenance of privacy is important if clients and families need to perform certain rituals or prayers. A visit from a priest, rabbi, or *santero* may provide a sense of psychological support and spiritual well-being. At times, santeros have been known to make sacrificial offerings at the client's hospital bedside. As long as standards of safety and sanitation are maintained, families must be allowed space and privacy to be able to engage in specific religious ceremonies.

## Meaning of Life and Individual Sources of Strength

As in other Latin American communities, the family is the most important source of strength, identity, and emotional security. Cubans usually rely on a network of family members and relatives for assistance in times of need. The sense of specialness Cubans feel, stemming from pride in their culture and their remarkable success in adapting to their new country, is likewise a source of self-esteem and self-identity. For many Cubans, deeply held religious beliefs have provided guidance and strength during the long and difficult process of migration and adaptation and continue to play an important role in their day-to-day lives.

## Spiritual Beliefs and Health-care Practices

Research indicates that Cubans tend to be fatalistic, feeling that they lack control over circumstances influencing their lives (Szapocznik, et al., 1978). The belief in a higher power is evident in a variety of practices Cubans may engage in for the purpose of maintaining health and well-being or curing illness, such as using magical herbs, special prayers or chants, ritual cleansing, and sacrificial offerings.

When Cuban clients consult a health-care provider, in all likelihood they have already tried some folk remedies advised by older women in their family or obtained from a botanica. The majority of folk remedies are harmless and do not interfere with biomedical treatment (Pachter, 1994). In most cases, clients may be allowed to continue using these remedies, such as herbal teas.

Health-care providers should be alert to the frequent practice of sharing prescription medications in families and among relatives. A family member who found an antibiotic effective in curing an ailment may share the medication with another relative suffering from the same symptoms. The health history must always include assessment of past or present medication use, whether traditional, over the counter, or prescription. Appropriate explanations must be given regarding the actions and adverse effects of drugs and the reasons why they cannot be shared with other family members.

# HEALTH-CARE PRACTICES

## Health-seeking Beliefs and Practices

As in other Latin American societies, Cubans rely on the family as the primary source of health advice. Typically, the older women in the family are sought out for information such as traditional home remedies for common ailments. Herbal teas or mixtures may be concocted to relieve mild or moderate symptoms. Concurrently or alternatively, a *santero* may be consulted or a trip to the botanica may be warranted to obtain treatment.

Socialized into a strong health ideology and successful primary care system in Cuba, Cubans are able to use biomedical services as a primary or secondary source of care. Cuba has a regionalized, hierarchically organized national health system that provides universal coverage and standardization of services. An innovative family practice program assigns physicians and nurses to city blocks and remote communities to promote physical fitness, detect risk factors for disease, and cure disease (Feinsilver, 1993). In the United States, many Cuban clinics that have sprung up have evolved into health maintenance organizations (HMOs).

## Responsibility for Health Care

Of the three Hispanic groups, Cuban-Americans with the most education and the highest incomes are the most likely to have private insurance (Council on Scientific Affairs, 1991). The Current Population Survey (U.S. Department of Commerce, Bureau of the Census, 1989a) estimated that the rate of uninsured was 20 percent for Cuban-Americans, as compared with 37 percent for Mexican-Americans, 16 percent for Puerto Ricans, and 10 percent for non-Hispanic whites. In addition, Cuban-Americans averaged more visits to a physician (6.2 visits) than Mexican-Americans (3.7 visits) and white non-Hispanics (4.8 visits) (Trevino, et al., 1991).

Research indicates that the utilization of preventive services by Cuban-Americans was determined more by access to care than by acculturation. Among Cuban-Americans without health insurance, 40 percent reported not having visited a physician for more than 1 year (Trevino, et al., 1991). Moreover, among Cuban-Americans, access to care was positively associated with education, annual income, and age (Solis, et al., 1990).

## Folk Practices

Cubans may use traditional medicinal plants in the form of teas, potions, salves, or poultices. In Cuban communities like Little Havana in Miami, stores called **botanicas** (Fig. 8–2) sell a variety of herbs, ointments, oils, powders, incenses, and religious figurines to relieve maladies, bring luck, drive away evil spirits, or break curses. In addition, Santeria necklaces and animals used for ritual sacrifice are available at botanicas (Lantigua, 1995; Scott, 1981).

Herbal teas that may be used to treat common ailments include (Estape, 1995):

*Cosimiento de anis* (anise): to relieve stomachaches, flatulence, and baby colic; also to calm nerves

*Cosimiento de limon con miel de abeja* (lemon and honey): to relieve cough and respiratory congestion

*Cosimiento de apasote* (pumpkin seed): to treat gastrointestinal worms

*Cosimiento de canela* (cinnamon): to relieve cough, respiratory congestion, and menstrual cramps

*Cosimiento de manzanilla* (chamomile): to relieve stomachaches

*Cosimiento de naranja agria* (sour orange): to relieve cough and respiratory congestion

*Cosimiento de savila* (aloe vera): to relieve stomachaches

*Cosimiento de tilo* (linden leaves): to calm nerves

*Cosimiento de yerba buena* (spearmint leaves): to relieve stomachaches and calm nerves

Fruits and vegetables, abundant in the natural tropical environment of Cuba, that may be used include:

*Chayote* (vegetable): to calm nerves

*Sanaoria* (carrots): to help problems with vision

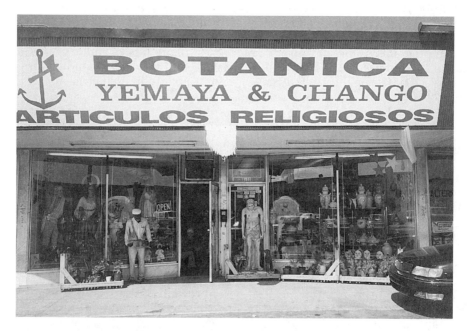

**Figure 8–2.** In Cuban communities, *botanicas* such as this one sell herbs, ointments, oils, powders, incenses, and religious figurines to relieve maladies, bring luck, or drive away evil spirits.

*Toronja y ajo* (grapefruit and garlic): to lower blood pressure

*Papaya y toronja, y pina* (papaya, grapefruit, and pineapple): to eliminate gastrointestinal parasites

*Remolacha* (beets): to treat influenza and anemia

*Cascara de mandarina* (fruit): to relieve cough

Other home remedies that may be used include:

*Agua con sal* (salt water): to relieve sore throat

*Agua de coco* (coconut water): to relieve kidney problems and infections

*Agua raja* (turpentine): applied to sore muscles and joints to relieve pain

*Bicarbonato*, limon y agua (baking soda, lemon, and water): to relieve stomach
upset or heartburn

*Cebo de carnero* (fat of lamb): applied directly on the skin to treat contusions and
swelling

*Mantequilla* (butter): applied directly on burns to soothe pain

*Clara de huevos* (egg white): applied directly over scalp to promote hair growth

Cuban families may use an *azabache, la manito de coral,* or *ojitos de Santa Lucia*
for various protective purposes. The *azabache* is a black stone placed on infants and
children as a bracelet or pin to protect them from the "evil eye." *La manito de coral,*
symbolic of the hand of God protecting a person, may also be worn as a necklace or
bracelet. *Los ojitos de Santa Lucia,* or the eyes of Saint Lucy, may be hung on a
bracelet or necklace for prevention of blindness and protection from the evil eye.

## Barriers to Health Care

Poverty may be a barrier to health care for only 14 percent of Cuban families, as
compared with 65 percent of Puerto Ricans, 47 percent of Mexicans, and 10 percent
of non-Hispanic whites in the United States (Juarbe, 1995). In a study of Cuban households, Diaz (1980) examined difficulties encountered in the utilization of health-care
services. Nearly half of those who used public clinics and public hospitals reported
at least one or more types of difficulties. These included language, time lag, red tape,
and transportation. For those who used private clinics and private health practitioners, the difficulties were cost of services, inconvenient hours, language, and red
tape.

Moreover, Cuban families that used hospitals, both public and private, named
language as a major difficulty in using health services. Thus, hospitals may not be as
accommodating to the bilingual needs of Cuban clients as other types of health-care
providers (Diaz, 1980).

## Cultural Responses to Health and Illness

Because of multiple losses they experienced in leaving their homeland and the difficulties associated with adaptation to a new culture and environment, Cuban immigrants may suffer from loneliness, depression, anger, anxiety, insecurity, and
health problems (Queralt, 1984). In evaluating Cuban families, Bernal (1994) suggested that health-care providers assess the following:

1. *Migration phase associated with the family.* It is important to know how long the
   family has lived in the United States and the reasons for migration. Information
   about political and social pressures that prompted the move should be elicited.
   Because family members acculturate at different rates, the level of acculturation
   should also be determined.

2. *Degree of connectedness to the culture of origin.* Conflicts in value orientations must be identified when assessing Cuban families. For example, the varying expectations between mainstream American and Cuban cultures with respect to dependence and independence may give rise to tension and conflict.

3. *Differentiation between the stresses of migration and differences in cultural values and family developmental conflicts.* In a clinical situation, the health-care provider must be able to recognize whether the client's response is due to migration-related problems, value orientation conflicts, or dysfunctional family development.

Among Cuban-Americans, dependency is a culturally acceptable sick role. Sick family members are showered with attention and support. Frequently, a hospitalized Cuban client will have a room full of flower arrangements and visitors. Favorite dishes may be brought to the hospital from home. The extended family network is relied on to assume temporarily the household chores and other tasks usually performed by the sick person. Family members are consulted and typically participate in decision making relative to the client's treatment.

Cuban-Americans tend to seek help in response to crisis situations (Delgado, 1981). The experience of pain constitutes a signal of a physical disturbance that would warrant consultation with a traditional or biomedical healer. Similar to other Hispanic clients, Cuban-Americans tend to be expressive of their pain and discomfort. Verbal complaints, moaning, crying, and groaning are culturally appropriate ways of dealing with pain. The expression of pain itself may serve a pain-relieving function and may not necessarily signify a need for administration of pain medication.

African-Cubans may seek biomedical care for organic diseases but consult a *santero* for spiritual or emotional crises. Conditions such as **decensos** (fainting spells) or **barrenillos** (obsessions) may be treated solely by a *santero* or simultaneously with a physician. As pointed out by Sandoval (1979), the trance state achieved through Santeria enables the Cuban client to act out emotional problems in a manner that is nonthreatening to the person's self-esteem.

## Blood Transfusion and Organ Donation

Receiving blood transfusions and organ donations are usually acceptable for Cubans. This is probably due to their experience with the sophisticated, high-technology medical care system in Cuba.

## HEALTH-CARE PRACTITIONERS

### Traditional Versus Biomedical Care

As with many other cultural groups, Cubans use both traditional and biomedical care. Initially, folk remedies may be used at home to treat an ailment or illness. If the condition persists, folklore practitioners such as *santeros* and biomedical practitioners may be used either simultaneously or successively. When seeing a Cuban client, the health-care provider must always ask about the use of folk remedies and consultations with folk practitioners to prevent conflicting therapeutic regimens.

Although Santeria was associated with the lower, uneducated classes in Cuba, it has emerged as a viable and dynamic religious and health system among middle-class Cubans in the United States. The *santero* may prescribe treatment or perform the appropriate rituals or ceremonies to enable ill persons to recover. The *santero* may invoke various types of supernatural deities to intervene in their lives and make them well. Often, even if a physician is being consulted, clients may believe that the *santero* is needed to rally supernatural forces toward their recuperation (Sandoval, 1979).

Some health problems that *santeros* may treat are **decaimientos** (conditions related to tired blood), *descensos,* or *barrenillos. Santeros* believe that illness arises from a person's failure to comply with the desire of an *orisha* (saint). The ceremonies, sacrifices, and rituals performed by the *santero* are meant to placate the anger of the *orisha.* Unlike most health-care agencies, which are open for only 8 or 9 hours a day, santeria cult houses are open to help their adherents about 18 hours a day (Sandoval, 1979).

Many Cubans consult a family physician for primary care. Before the revolution, Cuba had an organized government-supported health program that provided medical care to the majority of citizens. Since the 1959 revolution, the Cuban government has articulated a fundamental principle that health care is a right of all and a fundamental responsibility of the state. Thus, a national health-care system provides universal coverage, equitable geographic distribution of health-care facilities, and standardization of health services (Feinsilver, 1993). Cuba has been a leader in the establishment of prepayment health plans and has had them in operation since the 1880s (Gallagher, 1980).

In a survey of Cuban households, Diaz (1980) found that the majority of Cuban families in Miami, Florida (57 percent), and in Union City, New Jersey (88 percent), used the private health practitioner as a source of medical care. The most frequent reasons presented for utilizing this type of care were as follows: (1) advice of friends and relatives, (2) high quality of service, and (3) specific type of service.

Cuban families in Miami, Florida, gained access to primary health-care services predominantly through private health practitioners and private clinics, whereas in Union City, New Jersey, the main sources of health care were private health practitioners. An extensive network of privately owned and operated health clinics exist in Dade County, mainly located in Miami's Cuban ethnic enclaves, Little Havana and Hialeah. The private health clinics are believed to be popular among the Cubans because they provide services that are culturally sensitive to Cuban needs, such as emphasis on the family, use of the Spanish language, focus on preventive health-care behaviors, and low cost (Diaz, 1980).

In contrast to the high utilization rate of private clinics, very small proportions of Cuban families in Miami and Union City used public clinics for primary health-care services. Moreover, only 1 percent of Cuban households in both cities reported using a *santero* for health-care services, a surprisingly low proportion given the popular belief that the practice of Santeria is more widespread. In contrast, 7 percent of the Miami respondents and 23 percent of the Union City respondents indicated they would approach a *santero* if needed. Diaz suspected some degree of underreporting in this survey because of the sensitive nature of the question; therefore, the true figures may actually be higher.

## Status of Health-care Providers

Although Hispanics, including Cubans, will soon exceed 10 percent of the U.S. population, they are seriously underrepresented in the health occupations. Only 1 percent of registered nurses; 2 to 3 percent of dentists, pharmacists, and therapists; and 5 percent of physicians are of Hispanic origin (Ginzberg, 1991; Rojas, 1994). In Florida, although 12 percent of the population is Hispanic, only 5 percent of nursing students and 2 percent of nursing faculty are Hispanic (Grossman, et al., 1995). More effort needs to be directed toward increasing the number of Hispanic students in health professional schools as well as enhancing programs and resources to assist in successful retention and completion.

## CASE STUDY

Mrs. Demetilla Hernandez is a 63-year-old Cuban woman who seeks consultation at the Liberty HMO Clinic because of weakness, lethargy, and fatigue that she has experienced in the last 2 months. A week ago, while cooking dinner at her daughter Mariana's house, she momentarily lost her balance and slipped on the kitchen floor. Although Mrs. Hernandez sustained only a mild bruise on her leg, her daughter Mariana insisted on taking her to the clinic for a check-up because of her persistent symptoms.

Mrs. Hernandez, widowed 4 years ago when her husband died of a heart attack, lives with her daughter Mariana, aged 40 years. Mariana is divorced and has three children: Luis, 15; Carolina, 10; and Sofia, 7. Since moving into Mariana's house, Mrs. Hernandez has been managing the household while Mariana is at work. Mrs. Hernandez prepares the family's meals, attends to the children when they come home from school, and performs light housekeeping chores. Mariana is employed full time as a supervisor at the local telephone company. The family, originally from Cuba, has been living in Miami for 12 years. Carolina and Sofia were born in Miami, but Luis came from Cuba with his parents when he was 3 years old. Mrs. Hernandez, who does not speak English, converses with her daughter and grandchildren in Spanish. Although the children and their mother occasionally speak English among themselves, the family's language at home is Spanish.

At the Liberty HMO Clinic, Mrs. Hernandez was diagnosed with essential hypertension and noninsulin-dependent diabetes mellitus. The physician prescribed an oral hypoglycemic drug and advised Mrs. Hernandez to exercise daily and to limit her food intake to 1500 calories a day. Mrs. Hernandez was concerned because she usually prepares traditional Cuban meals at home and was not sure whether she could tolerate being on a diet. Besides, she explained to Mariana, she thought the dishes she prepares are very "healthy." Proof of that, she stated, is that her three grandchildren are plump and nice-looking. Mrs. Hernandez told her daughter that instead of buying the prescribed medicine, perhaps she should go to the botanica and obtain some herbs that would help lower her blood sugar.

## STUDY QUESTIONS

1. As a health-care provider, what are the typical Cuban communication patterns you need to be aware of in dealing with Mrs. Hernandez?

2. Describe the traditional Cuban food patterns. How would you assist Mrs. Hernandez in developing a plan for a 1500-calorie diet and regular exercise?

3. Would you encourage Mrs. Hernandez to go to the botanica to purchase some herbs? How would you approach her desire to use herbs instead of the prescribed oral hypoglycemic agent?

4. Discuss some common folklore practices that Cuban families may use to maintain health or cure common ailments.

5. Explain how time orientation may influence Mrs. Hernandez' compliance with follow-up clinic visits.

6. Formulate three important goals in teaching Mrs. Hernandez and her family about health care.

7. Identify the typical family and value structure among Cuban-Americans.

8. List three major health problems among Cuban-Americans.

9. If you were the health education specialist at the clinic, what would you teach the staff about Cuban culture to help them render culturally competent care?

10. Discuss traditional childrearing practices among Cuban-Americans.

## Acknowledgment

The author wishes to thank graduate students Eric Estape, Susan Brenton, and Sallieanne Brewer for some interview data used in this chapter.

## *References*

Bang, K. M., Gergen, P. J., & Carroll, M. (1990). Prevalence of chronic bronchitis among US Hispanics from the Hispanic Health and, Nutrition Examination Survey, 1982–84. *American Journal of Public Health, 80*(12), 1495–1497.

Becerra, J. E., Hogue, C. J. R., Atrash, H. K., & Perez, N. (1991). Infant mortality among Hispanics: A portrait of heterogeneity. *Journal of the American Medical Association, 265* (2), 217–221.

Bernal, G. (1994). Cuban families. In M. Uriarte-Gaston & J. Canas-Martinez (Eds.), *Cubans in the United States* (pp. 135–156). Boston: Center for the Study of the Cuban Community.

Black, S. A. & Markides, K. S. (1994). Aging and generational patterns of alcohol consumption among Mexican Americans, Cuban Americans and Mainland Puerto Ricans. *International Aging and Human Development, 39*(2), 97–103.

Blank, R. & Slipp, S. (1994). *Voices of diversity.* New York: American Management Association, pp. 63–64.

Boswell, T. D. (Ed.). (1991). *South Florida: Winds of change.* Miami, Florida: American Geographers Association.

Boswell, T. D. & Curtis, J. R. (1983). *The Cuban-American experience: Culture, images, and perspectives.* Totowa, New Jersey: Rowman & Allanheld.

Brandon, G. (1990). Sacrificial practices in santeria, an African-Cuban religion in the United States. In J. E. Holloway (Ed.), *Africanisms in American culture* (pp. 119–147). Bloomington: Indiana University Press.

Brewer, S. (1995). *Conception, pregnancy and childbirth rituals, taboos and beliefs within the Filipino and Cuban cultures.* Unpublished manuscript. Miami: Florida International University.

Caudle, P. (1993). Providing culturally sensitive health care to Hispanic clients. *Nurse Practitioner, 18*(12), pp. 40–51.

Council on Scientific Affairs, American Medical Association (1991). Hispanic health in the United States. *Journal of the American Medical Association, 265*(2), 248–252.

Delgado, M. (1981). Hispanic cultural values. Implications for groups. *Small Group Behavior, 12*(1), 69–79.

Diaz, G.M. (1980). *Evaluation and identification of policy issues in the Cuban community.* Miami, Florida: Cuban National Planning Council.

Estape, E. (1995). *The Cuban culture: Folk remedies and magicoreligious beliefs.* Unpublished manuscript. Miami: Florida International University.

Feinsilver, J.M. (1993). *Healing the masses: Cuban health politics at home and abroad.* Berkeley: University of California Press.

Fernandez, R.G. (1977). El cuento Cubano del exilio: Un enforque. Unpublished doctoral dissertation, Florida State University, Tallahassee, Florida.

Fox, G.F. (1979). *Working-class emigres from Cuba.* Palo Alto, California: R & E Research Associates.

Gallagher, P.L. (1980). *The Cuban exile: A sociopolitical analysis.* New York: Arno Press.

Ginzberg, E. (1991). Access to health care for Hispanics. *Journal of the American Medical Association, 265*(2), 238–241.

Gomez, M. R. (1990). Biculturalism and subjective mental health among Cuban Americans. *Social Service Review, 64*(3), pp. 375–389.

Gonzalez, A.M. (1995, June 11). Santeria still shrouded in secrecy. *The Miami Herald,* pp. 1B–5B.

Gonzalez-Whippler, M. (1982). *Santeria: The religion.* New York: Harmony Books.

Grenier, G. J. & Stepick, A. (Eds.) (1992). *Miami*

*now! Immigration, ethnicity, and social change.* Gainesville: University Press of Florida.

Grossman, D., Massey, P., Blais, K., et al. (in press). Cultural diversity in Florida nursing programs: A survey of deans and directors. *Journal of Nursing Education.*

Ismail, A. I. & Szpunar, S.M. (1990). The prevalence of total tooth loss, dental caries, and periodontal disease among Mexican Americans, Cuban Americans, and Puerto Ricans: Findings from HHANES 1982–84. *American Journal of Public Health, 80,* 66–70.

Jorge, A., Suchlicki, J., & Leyva, A. (Eds.) (1991). *Cuban exiles in Florida: Their presence and contributions.* Miami, Florida: University of Miami.

Juarbe, T. C. (1995). Access to health care for Hispanic women: A primary health care perspective. *Nursing Outlook, 43,* 23–28.

Lantigua, J. (1995, June 11). Get your potions here: Botanicas' appeal grows. *The Miami Herald,* pp. 1B, 5B.

Lopez, L. M. (1993). Body fatness, socioeconomic status, and food stamp use in Hispanic women. *Health Values, 17*(4), 3–10.

Lopez, L. M. & Masse, B. R. (1993). Income, body fatness, and fat patterns in Hispanic women from the Hispanic Health and Nutrition Examination Survey. *Health Care for Women International, 14,* 117–128.

Martinez, J. C. (1984). The Cuban immigrant of 1980: An exploration of psychosocial issues in the migration exprience. In M. Uriarte-Gaston & J. Canas-Martinez (Eds.), *Cubans in the United States* (pp. 181–184). Boston: Center for the Study of the Cuban Community.

Martinez, R. & Wetli, C. (1982). Santeria: A magico-religious system of Afro-Cuban origin. *The American Journal of Social Psychiatry, 2*(3), 496–503.

Mendez, A. (1994). *Cubans in America.* Minneapolis: Lerner Publications.

Mendoza, F. S., Ventura, S. J., Burciaga Valdez, R., et al. (1991). Selected measures of health status for Mexican-American, Mainland Puerto Rican, and Cuban-American children. *Journal of the American Medical Association, 265*(2), 227–232.

Mintzer, J. E., Rubert, M. P., Loewenstein, D., et al. (1992). Daughters caregiving for Hispanic and non-Hispanic Alzheimer patients: Does ethnicity make a difference? *Community Mental Health Journal, 28*(4), 293–303.

Murphy, J.M. (1988). Santeria. An African religion in America. Boston: Beacon Press.

National Center for Health Statistics (1989). Anthropometric data and prevalence of overweight for Hispanics: 1982–84. (DHHS Publication No. 89–1689). Hyattsville, MD: Department of Health and Human Services.

National Commission for Employment Policy (1982). *Hispanics and jobs: Barriers to progress.* (Report No. 14.) Washington, DC: Author.

Olson, J. S., & Olson, J. E. (1995). *Cuban Americans: From trauma to triumph.* New York: Twayne Publishers.

Pachter, L.M. (1994). Culture and clinical care: Folk illness beliefs and behaviors and their implications for health care delivery. *Journal of the American Medical Association, 271* (9), 690–694.

Pappas, G., Gergen, P. J., & Carroll, M. (1990). Hypertension prevalence and the status of awareness, treatment, and control in the Hispanic Health and Nutrition Examination Survey (HHANES), 1982–84. *American Journal of Public Health, 80*(12), 1431–1436.

Perez, L. (1984). *The Cuban population of the United States. The results of the 1980 U.S. census of population.* Keynote address at meeting of the Institute of Cuban Studies, Miami, Florida.

Perez, L. (1994). Cuban families in the United States. In R. L. Taylor (Ed.), *Minority families in the United States: A multicultural perspective* (pp. 95–112). Englewood Cliffs, New Jersey: Prentice Hall.

Pletsch, P. K. (1991). Prevalence of cigarette smoking in Hispanic women of childbearing age. *Nursing Research, 40*(2), 103–106.

Portes, A. & Bach, R.L. (1985). *Latin journey: Cuban and Mexican immigrants in the United States.* Berkeley: University of California Press.

Portes, A. & Clark, J. (1980). *Cuban immigration to the United States, 1972–79: A preliminary report of findings.* North Carolina: Duke University.

Portes, A. & Stepick, A. (1993). *City on the edge. The transformation of Miami.* Berkeley: University of California Press.

Portes, A. & Zhou, M. (1994). Should immigrants assimilate? *The Public Interest, 116,* 18–33.

Queralt, M. (1984). Understanding Cuban immigrants: A cultural perspective. *Social Work, 29*(2), pp. 115–121.

Richmond, M.L. (1980). *Immigrant adaptation and family structure among Cubans in Miami, Florida.* New York: Arno Press.

Rojas, D. (1994). Leadership in a multicultural society: A case in role development. *Nursing and Health Care, 15*(5), 258–261.

Sandoval, M. C. (1979). Santeria as a mental health system: An historical overview. *Social Science and Medicine, 13B,* 137–151.

Sandoval, V. A. (1994). Smoking and Hispanics: Issues of identity, culture, economics, prevalence, and prevention. *Health Values, 18*(1), 44–53.

Scott, C.S. (1981). Health and healing practices among five ethnic groups in Miami, Florida. In G. Henderson & M. Primeaux (Eds.), *Transcultural health care* (pp. 102–114). Menlo Park, California: Addison-Wesley.

Smart, J. & Smart, D. (1992). Cultural issues in the rehabilitation of Hispanics. *Journal of Rehabilitation, 58*(2), pp. 29–36.

Smith, P. B. & Weinman, M. L. (1995). Cultural implications for public health policy for pregnant Hispanic adolescents. *Health Values, 19*(1), 3–9.

Solis, J. M., Marks, G., Garcia, M., & Shelton, D. (1990). Acculturation, access to care, and use of preventive services by Hispanics: Findings from HHANES 1982–84. *American Journal of Public Health, 80* (Suppl.), 11–19.

Stroup-Benham, C. A. & Trevino, F. M. (1991). Reproductive characteristics of Mexican-American, Mainland Puerto Rican, and Cuban-American women. *Journal of the American Medical Association, 265*(2), 222–226.

Suarez, Z. E. (1993). Cuban Americans. From golden exiles to social undesirables. In H. P. McAdoo (Ed.), *Family ethnicity: Strength in diversity* (pp. 164–176). Newbury Park, CA: Sage Publications.

Szapocznik, J. & Hernandez, R. (1988). The Cuban American family. In C. H. Mindel, R. W. Habenstein, & R. Wright (Eds.), *Ethnic families in America* (3rd ed, pp. 160–172). New York: Elsevier.

Szapocznik, J., Scopetta, M.A., Aranalde, M.A., & Kurtines, W. (1978). Cuban value structure: Treatment implications. *Journal of Consulting and Clinical Psychology, 46*(5), 961–970.

Szapocznik, J., Kurtines, W., & Fernandez, T. (1980). Bicultural involvement and adjustment in Hispanic American youths. *International Journal of Intercultural Relations, 4*, 353–366.

Thomas, J. T. & DeSantis, L. (1995). Feeding and weaning practices of Cuban and Haitian immigrant mothers. *Journal of Transcultural Nursing, 6*(2), 34–42.

Trevino, F. M., Moyer, E., Valdez, R. B., & Stroup-Benham, C. A. (1991). Health insurance coverage and utilization of health services by Mexican Americans, Mainland Puerto Ricans, and Cuban Americans. *Journal of the American Medical Association, 265*(2), 233–237.

U.S. Department of Commerce, Bureau of the Census (1989a). *March 1989 Current population survey.* Washington, DC: U.S. Government Printing Office.

U.S. Department of Commerce, Bureau of the Census (1990). *Census of the population: General population characteristics, Florida* (28th ed.) Gainesville: University Press of Florida.

U.S. Department of Commerce, Bureau of the Census (1994). *Statistical abstract of the United States* (114th ed.). Washington, DC: U.S. Government Printing Office.

Williamson, E. (1992). *The Penguin history of Latin America.* London: Penguin Books.

# Egyptian-Americans

*Afaf Meleis and Mahmoud Meleis*

---

• Key terms to become familiar with in this chapter are:

| | |
|---|---|
| *Adab* | Nubians |
| *Amal* | *Qur'an* |
| *Arwah* | Ramadan |
| Bedouins | *Saiidis* |
| Copts | *Sikkeenah* |
| Great Eid | Small Eid |
| *Hegab* | *Waham* |
| *Itkhad* | *Zar* |
| *Jenn* | |

## OVERVIEW, INHABITED LOCALITIES, AND TOPOGRAPHY

### Overview

About 1 million Egyptians in the United States are permanent residents, citizens, or in the process of becoming permanent residents. Because of the recency of their arrival, limited scholarly literature is available about this immigrant group and its health-care needs (Keck, 1989). This chapter is based on that literature in conjunction with the authors' own experiences. One of the authors has been professionally involved with health care for this population for 30 years as part of a project designed to provide health-care services to Middle Eastern communities in San Francisco. Both authors have been insiders to Middle Eastern and Egyptian communities in Los Angeles and San Francisco. They have participated in many community celebrations, experienced immigrants' grief over the loss of one of their family members, provided social and emotional support during times of crisis, and counseled many immigrants. Finally, both authors were born in Egypt and came to the United States in the early 1960s to complete their graduate education. Therefore, data in this chapter are from our lived experiences in the two worlds that Egyptian-Americans claim as their own—Egypt and the United States. Some of the similarities between Egyptians, Arabs, and Middle Easterners allowed the authors to use writings related to these other two groups to support their findings.

Because only the most common patterns of responses and experiences of Egyptian-Americans with regard to health and illness are presented in this chapter, diversity among Egyptians is not well depicted, nor does this description represent a universal profile. Egyptians have immigrated under many different circumstances and represent different educational, cultural, and economic backgrounds, which ultimately influence their responses to health and illness. By attempting to define their similarities, the authors' goal is to stimulate interest in a more systematic scholarship about this unique community, their lifestyles, health, and health-care practices.

Egypt enjoys a mild climate throughout the year. The Mediterranean region of Egypt experiences most of the country's rainfall during the winter season. The northern summers are balmy with moderate temperatures and 80 percent humidity. The southern part of Egypt (Upper Egypt) enjoys mild and fairly warm winters and hot summers with temperatures as high as 115°F and little to no humidity. Except for a few hills outside Cairo, Egypt has a flat terrain on both sides of the southern Nile valley and the Sinai Peninsula. The Nile river, a main artery for Egypt and an orientation point for its terrain, runs through the center of the country from south to north to the Mediterranean Sea. The Nile, considered Egypt's lifeline, provides water and supports agriculture.

Most Egyptians live on 5 percent of Egypt's land with a high concentration in large cities and on the banks of the Nile (Beshara, 1981), although in the last 20 years, several new cities have been established in areas not previously inhabited. Approximately 50 percent of Egyptians live in urban Egypt, with 50 percent of the urban population living in Cairo and its vicinity and 50 percent living in Alexandria and its vicinity. Immigrants to the United States come primarily from these two cities.

## Heritage and Residence

The Egyptian people have a strong sense of identity with their own country and demonstrate pride in coming from a civilization over 8000 years old (Metz, 1990). Within the expanse of Egyptian history, the most prominent historical event was the unification of the southern and northern parts of Egypt, during the sixth millennium B.C., led by King Menes of Lower Egypt. Rule of the whole country by one king, who presented himself as a God, was the beginning of highly organized societies.

The ancient Egyptians were the first to believe in life after death, mummify bodies, and build elaborate tombs to preserve and protect these bodies for the afterlife. Egyptians also developed the plow, a system of writing, and medical skills such as surgical operations.

The Arab conquest of Egypt around 641 A.D., which spread the Islamic and Arabic culture among the Egyptians, has lasted to this day. The minority (Christian) **Copts,** who preserved the African-Asiatic language of ancient Egypt, now use the Arabic language and are assimilated into the Arabic culture.

The Ottoman Turks invaded Egypt in 1517, adding it to their vast empire. While living under the Turkish rule, Egypt enjoyed religious and cultural stability because the Turks shared the Islamic and Arabic cultures. In the last two centuries, Egypt has experienced invasions by the French under Napoleon, followed by the British in 1882, who remained in the country until 1954. In 1952, an Egyptian army group led by Lieutenant Colonel Gamal Abdel Nasser took control of the government and removed King Farouk from power. Since then, Egypt has been an independent state (Metz, 1990).

An influential part of modern Egyptian history is the Arab-Israeli conflict. The conflict between Egypt (as part of the Arab League) and Israel ended in 1979 when the two countries signed the Camp David Accords. Anwar Sadat was the president of Egypt at the time. Egypt continues to be involved in diplomatic efforts to arrive at peace between Israel and its neighboring Arab countries. This long history and the diversity of populations have influenced the value systems, beliefs, and explanatory frameworks that Egyptians use in their daily lives and have contributed to the diverse thinking processes that they use to resolve issues and conflict in their lives.

The highest concentration of Egyptian immigrants is found in and around New York, Los Angeles, Washington, D.C., Chicago, and San Francisco. Egyptians prefer to work in large urban areas and usually choose suburban areas for living. However, there is no single geographic area where they live in large and concentrated numbers.

## Reasons for Migration and Associated Economic Factors

Many Egyptians immigrated to the United States in an attempt to escape economic stagnation during President Gamal Abdel Nasser's regime and his failed economic policies that nationalized all privately owned companies and enterprises. The United States offered an economic incentive that rewarded hard-working individuals. After the 1952 military revolution, Egyptians immigrated in two main waves. The first wave consisted of graduate students who came to the United States to obtain advanced degrees. After the defeat of the Egyptian army by the Israelis in 1967, many of these students, believing the totalitarian military regime of Egypt did not offer hope for economic recovery, changed their status to immigrant. For most, this ensured a promising future for their children, even though they would have been assured decent positions in Egypt because of their American education.

The second wave of immigration resulted from the heightened mass dissatisfaction, hopelessness, and anger toward the government of the educated and professional community after the 1967 war. A lenient government policy made it easy and safe for anyone who wanted to leave the country, resulting in the largest exodus of Egyptians out of Egypt in modern history. Included in this wave were many Coptic and other Egyptian Christians (Norden, 1993).

## Educational Status and Occupations

The majority of the first-wave Egyptian immigrants were highly educated individuals with graduate and postgraduate degrees earned in the United States. This group was able to obtain teaching and research positions in universities or work in industries (Sonn, 1989). Some joined companies or started their own businesses in the high-technology industries.

Egyptians in the second wave were more diverse in their educational backgrounds, although most of them were college graduates. Second-wave immigrants worked as engineers, physicians, dentists, accountants, and technicians; however, some with college degrees initially accepted employment as gas station attendants, cab drivers, security guards, and other blue-collar jobs to ensure employment. After improving their language skills and obtaining degrees from American universities, many obtained professional jobs. A small minority were never able to achieve an occupational status equivalent to their original training. Many from this group returned to their home country or plan for such a return.

## COMMUNICATIONS

### Dominant Language and Dialects

The dominant language of Egyptians is Arabic, a Semitic language. It is a common language understood by all Arab nationals who hear it in the popular Egyptian movies, songs, and television programs. The written Arabic language is the same in all Arab countries, but spoken Arabic is dialectal and does not necessarily follow proper Arabic grammar.

A number of Arabic dialects are spoken in Egypt. The **Saiidis** (Egyptians south of Cairo) have a different dialect from the northerners. The **Nubians** (who live around and south of Aswan) have another very different dialect. The **Bedouins** (living in the deserts) have their own unique dialect. Despite these different dialects and their distinct vocabularies, neither Egyptians nor Egyptian-Americans have any noticeable communication barriers among themselves.

For Egyptian immigrants in the United States, English is the language of communication in business and contact with American society. Within their own gatherings, they speak a mixture of Arabic and English, switch with great ease from one language to another, and sometimes speak a mixture of Arabic, English, and French. Egyptian social gatherings usually involve large numbers of people, with multiple conversations occurring simultaneously. In discussing subjects such as politics or religious issues, the level of excitement heightens and the tone of the speech is sharpened, so an outside observer may mistakenly characterize the exchanges as chaotic or angry.

## Cultural Communication Patterns

Several values govern interaction patterns among Egyptians. The first is respect *(Ihteram)*. Respect is expected when speaking with those who are older and those who are in higher social positions. Respect is demonstrated in the Arabic language by differentiation in the words used to address those who are equal in age or position and those who are older in age or higher in position (see Format for Names).

A second important value, politeness (**Adab**) is related to what is appropriate, expected, and socially sanctioned. Truth and reality may be sacrificed for what is appropriate and polite. Politeness results in a preference for more indirect modes of communication (Cohen, 1987). Sharing negative news directly or asking for things directly is not polite. Therefore, a poor prognosis of an illness is not immediately shared; calamities should be slowly and deliberately introduced and shared in stages.

Significant value is related to the status of insiders and outsiders, the private and public spheres. Private spheres are reserved for immediate family, some members of the extended family, and friends who are elevated to the status of family. The public sphere includes acquaintances, public officials, and the rest of the world. Those who occupy a public sphere may get completely different communications and versions of the same events or incidents.

Because Egyptian-Americans tend to be externally driven, they are concerned about what others think of their behaviors (Keck, 1989), which are considered a direct reflection on their entire family. Therefore, parents tend to be overzealous and anxious about the good or bad behaviors of children and adult sons and daughters. These behaviors reflect a measure of how well or how badly parents have raised their children.

Egyptian-Americans tend to be in touch with their inner feelings and are highly expressive of them; however, this expression is governed by external orientation, spontaneity, and the differences between private and public spheres. Egyptian-Americans tend to share the most minute details about their lives and problems with their trusted circle of insiders. However, because they are externally oriented, they tend to look outside for explanations of their feelings, rather than to focus on their own actions.

Egyptians tend to be comfortable and generous in sharing ideas and giving advice to others who might be family members or friends. This behavior stems from close family ties and trust that ensures the family will always be there to provide help. Advice is offered (even when not requested), out of love, care, and a sense of loyalty for friends or relatives. They do not shy away from becoming involved in the problems, trials, and tribulations of those in their private sphere. The extent and depth of involvement is less for those who are in the public sphere.

Although these behavior patterns are a part of the lifestyle of first-generation immigrants, they may not necessarily be maintained by second-generation immigrants. Egyptian-Americans of lower socioeconomic status continue to maintain the older, deep-rooted patterns of behavior, whereas the more affluent middle and upper classes, who are occupied with professional endeavors, have more limited time for family closeness and involvement with friends.

Egyptian-Americans' nonverbal communication patterns are vivid. Because their personal space tends to be small, they stand and sit very close to each other. In spite of their preference for closeness, personal space during interactions is used differently by women and men. Women tend to keep male friends as far away as male strangers (Sanders, Hakky, & Brizzolara, 1985). Distance is kept as a sign of uncertainty in the relationship. Egyptian-Americans speak with their mouth, face, and hands, and their entire body communicates the meaning of their language. Their facial expressions are mirrors of their internal processes and reflections of their inner evaluations of their situations. They tend to touch each other frequently and easily, and touch is both reflexive and deliberative. For example, they tend to touch others while speaking to solicit attention, concentration, and emphasis. To demonstrate trust, increase trust, or emphasize a point, they tend to touch each other on the hands, arms, legs, and shoulders.

Men, whether strangers or acquaintances, touch each other. Similarly, it is acceptable for women to touch. However, it is unacceptable for women and men to touch each other. Touch between the sexes is accepted in private and only between husbands and wives, parents and children, and adult brothers and sisters.

Family members and friends of the same gender always hug and kiss on both cheeks. Friends of different sexes normally shake hands. Devout Muslim males and females do not touch each other; even a handshake is not practiced. In these situations, a head nod substitutes for physical greetings. Among devout Muslims, only *mahrams*, those individuals who are not permitted to marry (for example, sisters and brothers), are permitted to greet each other with hugs. Among Christians and westernized Egyptians and Egyptian-Americans, greetings usually include formal courteous hugs and kisses on the cheeks.

In Egypt, it is very common to see Egyptian males or females walking in public places holding hands or embracing each other. Egyptian-Americans are more self-conscious about touching members of the same sex. In the United States, Egyptians are comfortable touching other non-Egyptians on the arm or shoulder as an expression of care, assuring them that one is a friend. Some Westerners find these gestures strange and express their discomfort with them.

Egyptians have their own nonverbal facial expressions. A momentary wide-eyed gaze to a child means "stop it now." A wink to an adult means "watch what you are saying" or "change the subject because you are treading on dangerous ground." Dissatisfaction is demonstrated by intentionally looking through the person or by avoiding eye contact.

Egyptians think of those who do not maintain eye contact or have shifty eye contact as people who should not be trusted. Because Egyptians tend to stand in close proximity to each other, eye contact is automatic for them. However, women and men who are strangers may avoid eye contact out of modesty and respect for religious rules; the situation is different if the communication is between men and women related by marriage or by blood. Children are taught not to *tebarrak*, "stare," which denotes disrespect for those who are older or who are higher in status.

Egyptians tend to be congenial and personable, injecting humor to lighten stressful encounters or business meetings. They may exaggerate and overly assert judgments of events and situations (Cohen, 1987).

An Egyptian greeting involves every person in a room standing and shaking hands within gender norms. Males' or females' not standing can be considered an insult. A greeting may be just a nod or a few words. Similar greetings are practiced in the United States among immigrants.

## Temporal Relationships

Older Egyptians cherish the past, remembering the days when life was simple and easy. Younger Egyptians live in the present, with its decreased availability of options, and in the future, with its potential, realizing that acquisition of goods comes with a high price tag. Thus, this generation is preoccupied with maximizing their incomes, often working two or three jobs to afford available luxuries. For Egyptian immigrants who are professionals, working hard has been their ticket to upward mobility and living the good life.

In Egypt, social time is a high priority, and engagements are not concluded because of other scheduled appointments; therefore, guests are expected to arrive late. If a friend drops by as another is getting ready to leave for an appointment, the appointment is missed and the friend is not told about the prior engagement. It is customary to arrive at a social gathering, such as a lunch or dinner, as much as 1 or 2 hours late and to be late for business appointments because of heavy traffic and unanticipated and uncontrolled delays.

A social custom is to offer coffee, tea, or a soft drink when businesses are visited. Therefore, a 10-minute office visit usually takes more time. Egyptian-Americans' perception of time is in the context of the nationality of the group. Therefore, they follow "American time" and are punctual for business engagements and meetings with non–Egyptian-Americans but prefer to use Egyptian time for Egyptian-American gatherings. Sanders, Hakky, and Brizzolara (1985) reported that American and Egyptian students construed time similarly and that Egyptians describe time in more favorable terms than Americans, who think of time in terms of predictability.

## Format for Names

In all Arab countries, both male and female children are given a first name, and the father's first name is used as the middle name; the last name is the family name. In the Middle East, a person is called formally by the first name, such as Mr. William.

Respect for individuals is demonstrated in the use of certain titles. *Inta* (you) is saved for those in equal or lower positions, and *hadretak* (you) is reserved for those in higher-ranking positions or for older persons. There are more flowery and more exaggerated variations of both of these appellations, such as *seyadtak*, which is reserved for the highest-level officials. *Inta,* used in place of *hadretak,* is an insult to elderly persons and, more important, a reflection of bad manners and the poor upbringing of the young. Older people should never be called by their first names without an adjective or title attached to the name. The accepted custom in the United States of addressing clients by their first name may be insulting to people from other countries. An adjective, such as aunt, uncle, ostaz (Mr., Madame, Mrs.), or an adjective that denotes a profession, such as bashmohandes (engineer, doctor, physician, or a doctoral degree), may be used with the name. Friends of the family are addressed by both younger and adult children as uncle and aunt. Parental relatives are either called aunt or uncle or a special designation such as *ammeti*, "sister of father"; *ammy*, "brother of father"; *khalty*, "sister of mother"; or *khali*, "brother of mother."

## FAMILY ROLES AND ORGANIZATION

### Head of Household and Gender Roles

The man is formally considered the head of the household. The demands of life on immigrants and nuclear families drive couples to share responsibilities and decision making. Many Egyptian-American men, however, tend to control family budgets, which gives them more power in the family and causes many interpersonal conflicts and much distress for Egyptian-American women.

Egyptian-American family roles change considerably after immigration. The fast pace and complexity of life in America, the multiple demands of childrearing, and the absence of an extended family to preserve traditional roles contribute to a more egalitarian family organization. Husbands and wives experience greater fluidity in their roles, substitute for each other when needed, and participate fully in all family matters. Egyptian-American women tend to work both in temporary occupations and in career positions (Meleis, 1991; Meleis & Rogers, 1987). Many who do not work outside the home consider their situation temporary, are between jobs, or are retooling their skills to be congruent with American job opportunities. Egyptian-American women who are not working outside the house tend to be more stressed than those who are employed. Unemployment brings with it economic limitations, social limitations in terms of developing a support network, or both. In the absence of extended families, lack of this support network increases vulnerability, isolation, and stress.

Although couples may share daily household chores, the norm is similar to that of other educated middle-class families in America. The woman is responsibile for the daily management of family affairs (Keck, 1989; Meleis, 1991). The man is the major breadwinner for the family. Husbands, however, participate in shopping, cleaning, and in activities related to entertaining with their wives. Fathers also participate proactively in activities and education with their children.

## Prescriptive, Restrictive, and Taboo Behaviors for Children and Adolescents

Children are central to Egyptian families; they are treasured in the present and viewed as security for their parents' future. During their early years, they are expected to be studious and goal-oriented (Hattar-Pollara & Meleis, 1995), respectful, and loyal to the family. When they become adults, they are expected to take care of their elderly parents.

However, second-generation Egyptians tend to blend with European-Americans, African-Americans, and Hispanics. Their sense of responsibility toward their parents is a topic of major concern among Egyptian-Americans. Egyptian children are not permitted to use foul language or swear in the home or in front of parents, although this is true to a lesser degree in the United States. Answering back to parents is not condoned and is seen as rude and disrespectful. Some families adjust better than others to the Western style of childrearing, which permits and encourages children's right to question their parents' instructions. Families that allow their children more freedom to express their opinions and ask questions often end up with more well-adjusted children and better preserve family unity as their children grow into adulthood. Religious beliefs and teachings forbid premarital sex and adultery for both Egyptian Muslims and Christians.

As girls reach puberty and the questions of dating, courting, and prom night arrive, some parents cannot cope with the freedom allowed within American society (Aswad, 1993). They worry more about the consequences of dating and their daughter's getting pregnant and fleeing the home, than raising a healthy and well-adjusted young woman. In the extreme, a few families send their daughters with their mothers back to Egypt to complete their education through college under more restrictive conditions or to get married. Some families opt to return for good rather than to raise their daughters in the American culture. Egyptian Muslim and Christian families usually have a hard time giving their young daughters enough space to grow.

Hattar-Pollara and Meleis (in press) found that Egyptian-American parents fear their daughters' losing their virginity, and this represents a major stress in their daily lives. The greatest calamity that may happen in a Christian or Muslim Egyptian-

American household is to have a daughter lose her virginity prematurely. This fear stems from a potential lack of marriageability of the daughter, loss of face for the father, and gossip within the Egyptian-American community. Therefore, parents tend to be restrictive about their daughters' movements and to monitor their whereabouts carefully. Similar restrictions are placed on teenage sons, although they are allowed more freedom and more autonomy in decision making. Most parents prefer that their sons not date and discourage sexual activities. However, if sons disobey the rules of the household, the incident is not regarded as gravely as when daughters do. In spite of these restrictions, Sanders (1986) reported that Egyptian-American students perceive their parents to be more patient, relaxed, and serious than American students perceive theirs. He also reported that the restrictive and authoritarian image of Egyptian fathers is unsupported.

Second-generation Egyptian-Americans are rather philosophical about these restrictions. The open communication in the family allows children to see restrictions as temporary or to devise ways to do what they want without their parents' knowledge. While similar situations may occur in their original country, the difference is that an extended family in the homeland may help mediate when confrontations between parents and children become inevitable. Without extended families, Egyptian-Americans are at a loss for help in resolving family issues. The option of going to counselors or health-care professionals for advice is rarely exercised. Preserving family secrets and honor is more important than external support. Just as families have a strong need for virginity to be preserved, teen pregnancy is not openly discussed in the community. Because of the many restrictions placed on daughters' movements and the limited opportunities for teenage daughters to go out without chaperons, such pregnancies rarely occur. Birth control is not usually discussed in families until marriage, and Pap smears are not sought or accepted until after marriage. Egyptian-American children are expected to marry Egyptian-Americans. However, because many second-generation Americans do not reside in areas with an abundance of Egyptian-Americans, cross-cultural marriages are becoming a trend. Many first-generation Egyptian-Americans return to their home country to get married.

## Family Roles and Priorities

The family is the most sacred institution to Egyptian-Americans. Although Egyptians in their own country have extended families, Egyptian-American families tend to be more nuclear. As compared with other Arabs in the United States, most Egyptian-Americans immigrated individually, were joined later by a bride, or immigrated as nuclear families. In some families, brothers, sisters, nephews, and nieces may arrive later. Even when extended families arrive later, they tend to live apart (Keck, 1989; Meleis, 1981).

Job opportunities dictate living choices and patterns of living among Egyptian-Americans. Egyptians in their own country view the relocation of sons or daughters for education or an occupation with trepidation and concern. However, once children move, even though not bound by extended families, they remain connected with them and reluctant to remain anywhere else permanently. In their home country, Egyptians tend to include the extended family in activities and consult them for advice. In the absence of such a family in the United States, they either resort to close Egyptian-American friends or seek counseling from extended families in their home country. Christian families may resort to religious leaders in their church or community for assistance.

The most important goal for Egyptian-American families is to raise children who are well educated, employable, and able to secure occupations that allow career mobility, financial security, and an acceptable social status. To that end, many other goals are subordinated. Because of this goal, parents may uproot and move to areas with better school systems and are willing to withstand financial or other hardships for the sake of their children.

Another goal of Egyptian-American families is to keep children geographically close, if not living at home, until they get married to the right partner. Parents consider it their responsibility to assist their children, especially daughters, to find a suitable marriage partner, and they support children financially through wedding preparations. Raising children who are considered *moaddabeen* by Egyptian standards is important. A child who is *moaddab* is one who respects parents, defers to them for decisions, is mindful of elderly persons, does not drink or indulge in immoral acts, listens to parents' advice, and does not answer back during conflict.

One final goal of Egyptian families is to maintain a good face in public. This goal is achieved when children do not bring shame by engaging in activities forbidden by their parents, such as drinking, smoking, or going somewhere without their parents' permission.

As Egyptians become older, they are considered richer in experiences and wiser and command more respect. They are treated with gentleness and never made to believe that their usefulness is limited just because they are retired. Their children and extended family are obligated to care for them. The elderly do less by choice and expect more services, respect, and reverence from family members and subordinates. Women gain status with age and with childbearing. Young women know that inequities they may suffer as young brides are more than compensated for when they get older. Elderly women, however, are expected to care for the elderly men in the family.

Because most of the Egyptian-American community immigrated as young adults, as they advance in age they are the first generation to experience growing old in the United States. Many parents have a morbid fear that they may be forced to move into a nursing home. Many are considering a return to their home country to avoid the humiliation of aging in America with the potential loss of home, family care, and respect. Egyptian-Americans do not believe that they can expect or hold their children responsible for becoming their caregivers during old age. Growing old in America is surrounded by many images of abandonment, humiliation, loss of respect, and above all, loneliness. Those who adapt to a life without extended family and create an extended family will likely establish a new means to deal with their old age. Health-care professionals may consider alternative ways to support this community and enhance their self-care activities to help them avoid feelings of loneliness and a sense of abandonment in old age.

Many Egyptian-Americans are part of a network of Egyptian-American friends. New friends become their new extended families, and they share their celebrations and their calamities with them. Where mosques or a Middle Eastern Orthodox church exist, these organizations are used to promote social gatherings. In the absence of such organizations, Egyptian cultural clubs promote meetings, discussions, and sharing news from the homeland. During social gatherings, Egyptians are recognized by their elegant clothes, the hustle and bustle of children playing, adults chattering, and fine Egyptian food.

Egyptian-Americans prefer family gatherings over adult gatherings for celebrations such as **Ramadan** (the month of fasting), the *Eid* feast celebrations, Christmas, and New Year's. Most often they include extended family and their new networks of friends. Social networks are connected by their heritage, rather than by their occupations (Abraham, 1989; Meleis, Lipson, & Paul, 1992). Without these large gatherings, loneliness and a sense of deprivation are exaggerated at times of crises or during normal developmental events such as birthing a baby (El Sayed, 1986) or the death of a family member.

In Egypt, extended family members play a strong role in the life of a family. It is an important goal of family members to live in the same city. Extended family members provide backup and support for working women by providing child care and for nonworking women with multiple children as they need tangible support.

Families raise children, not mothers or fathers. Advice on childrearing is freely given by all family members (Keck, 1989).

In the United States, Egyptian immigrants do not usually have extended family members living with them, but they continue to consider the extended family living abroad as their support network (May, 1992). For those who have extended family members and who are professionals with careers, the relationship tends to be more limited by time, responsibilities, and other demands.

Social status is gained through professional accomplishments, financial success, and involvement in Egyptian community affairs. Respect is given to community leaders who give of themselves and share life experiences. No caste system exists based on color, familial lineage, or ancestry either among Egyptians or Egyptian-Americans. In some communities, Egyptian-Americans are divided by religion, Muslims and Copts, and by professional status, clubs for professionals and others for blue-collar and other white-collar workers (Keck, 1989).

## Alternative Lifestyles

The divorce rate among Egyptian immigrants is low, a pattern similar to that in Egypt. In cases of divorce where one parent raises the children, the Egyptian community supports the single parent, including his or her own parent(s). Divorce is not seen as a stigma, but an unfortunate situation in which the children pay the greatest price. In second marriages, partners work hard to make a new life together and are committed to raising each other's children as if they were their own.

Communal and same-sex families is a concept that does not exist in Egyptian societies. Although there is a community of gays, homosexuality is not disclosed nor collectivized (Dunne, 1990). They do have meeting places that are ignored or intentionally overlooked. To be gay or lesbian is considered immoral and is not accepted by any Arab or Middle Eastern religions. To discover a gay son or lesbian daughter is akin to a catastrophic event for Egyptians and Egyptian-Americans.

## WORKFORCE ISSUES

### Culture in the Workplace

Egyptian-American nurses, who usually hold a minimum of a bachelor's degree, cope well with the demands inherent in providing nursing care in the United States. In the beginning of their careers in the United States, however, they encounter three challenges. First, Egyptian-American nurses frequently expect detailed and careful communication of all steps and aspects of nursing care. This expectation is inherent in both cultural patterns and their educational preparation. Although interactions and communications come naturally to Egyptian-Americans, this naturalness is usually reserved for family and close acquaintances. In addition, their professional preparation does not emphasize communication skills for interacting with clients. Because Egyptian clients do not expect detailed information from physicians and nurses, the routine of informing clients about the rationale for interventions may challenge Egyptian-American nurses.

The second challenge relates to the systematic and careful recording and documentation of nursing care. Egyptians are inclined to an oral tradition; therefore, the need to document in writing what can be shared verbally seems foreign to Egyptian-American nurses.

The third challenge relates to the work environment itself. For Egyptians, the work environment is also their social environment where friendships are built and life experiences and personal issues are shared with a selected few. The emphasis on privacy and separating work and social life expected in American work settings seems artificial to Egyptian-Americans. Therefore, they tend to view American work relationships as superficial and often experience a sense of loss in terms of close, meaningful work relationships and a supportive collegial network. This feeling is similar to how women in other professions view satisfying and stressful aspects of their work situation. For example, in studies on women in clerical jobs, the most satisfying aspects of jobs were related to interpersonal relationships (for example, Meleis, et al., 1989).

Egyptian-American social networks are formed outside their work environments and are largely made up of immigrants (Keck, 1989). Thus, much like other Arab and Middle Eastern immigrants, those who do not assimilate into the American social network live a double life—a well-acculturated life at work and an Egyptian life with perceptible traces of Americanization in the home and community (Bragdon, 1989; Abu-Laban, 1989).

Many Egyptian communities in the United States form Egyptian cultural clubs to which a small percentage of these immigrant nurses belong. Such clubs help to decrease their sense of marginality (Abraham, 1989). Activities usually include parties, dinners, picnics, and dances. Some of these clubs offer Arab language classes for the children. The more religious socialize around their local mosques and churches, which is a good and safe forum for their teenage sons and daughters to meet prospective marital partners.

Egyptian immigrants to the United States work hard at becoming integrated into the Western work environment. They thrive on professional satisfaction, defining success in terms of advancement. They tend to be team players and effective contributors to the society at large. They are usually punctual and follow work rules and procedures. Being well assimilated, they create a close network of colleagues.

## Issues Related to Autonomy

Most Egyptians prefer to work in a job setting where they are employees of an organization. They do not experience difficulty in reporting to a superior and following instructions. These cultural patterns do not preclude their being professionally motivated to work hard and advance their careers within respective organizations. As managers, leaders, or supervisors, they bring a personal touch and demonstrate human interest in their dealings with subordinates and coworkers. They demand loyalty and respect. On the whole, their religious affiliations do not pose problems for them when dealing with coworkers outside their own religions. However, the long history of Egyptian and Arab–Israeli animosity causes some of them to approach their dealings with Jewish coworkers cautiously. Egyptian immigrants tend to be respectful of female coworkers, and often their protective responses may be interpreted as patronizing by some females. They treat women as sisters or daughters.

Few Egyptians are entrepreneurial by nature. Those who opt to start their own businesses struggle to make them work. Egyptian-Americans in general value job and economic security over the risk-taking inherent in operating a business. Therefore, they join established organizations with long-term goals.

Egyptians learn British English in schools and universities. On immigrating to the United States, they are confronted with unfamiliar slang and idioms. When viewed from an immigrant's point of view and basic knowledge of British English, some of these expressions are hard to interpret and could be construed as insults. An example of this type of misunderstanding happened to one of the authors (MHM). As he narrates it:

> When I arrived in the United States (over 30 years ago) as a graduate student in engineering, I had an occasion to be studying at a University of California Los Angeles library on a weekend day with my wife, a graduate student in nursing. When we decided to go to the local school cafeteria for a cup of tea, we noticed

one of her psychology professors in the library whom we knew very well inside and outside of the school. I approached him, greeted him, and asked if he would like to join us for a cup of tea. He responded by saying, "No, I don't care to have a cup of tea now." This, of course, is a very simple and totally acceptable American response. For me, a recent Egyptian immigrant (less than a year), this was a personal insult. The words, "I do not care . . ." meant to me that he did not care about *me,* not the process of having tea. We discussed this conversation a year later as he and I became close friends and laughed about it. He obviously meant no insult, and I just did not know enough about the idioms and commonly used expressions to "get it."

With increasing exposure to the media and life in the United States, it does not take long for a new immigrant to understand and accurately interpret idioms and commonly used expressions.

## BIOCULTURAL ECOLOGY

### Skin Color and Other Biologic Variations

Most Egyptians have olive skin tones, some are fair-skinned, and others dark-skinned. Northern Egyptians exhibit a fairer complexion than most other Egyptians. Southern Egyptians (Nubians) are generally black, with very fine facial features. Upper Egyptians have a darker complexion. The average height of Egyptian males is about 5'10", whereas females have an average height of 5'4".

### Diseases and Health Conditions

Several risk factors are peculiar to life along the banks of the Nile. Egyptians suffer from a host of parasitic diseases; the most common is schistosomiasis, known as *bilharzia* in Egypt. Schistosomiasis has been endemic in Egypt throughout history and has been found in mummified bodies from the pharaonic era. A high percentage of the Egyptian rural population are infected with *Schistosoma mansoni* or *Schistosoma haematobium.* The life cycle of schistosomiasis includes snails and human beings as hosts. Microscopic cercariae leave the snail in the warmth of the midday sun and penetrate the skin of humans who enter the shallow canals to irrigate crops, wash dishes or clothes, or swim. The cercariae migrate to areas near the liver, in the case of infection with *Schistosoma mansoni,* or near the bladder, in the case of infection with *Schistosoma haematobium.* The parasitic worms mature, mate, reproduce, and are expelled with urine or stools. If urine or stools are deposited in or near fresh water canals or rivers where snails live, the eggs seek out a snail to begin the cycle again (Sun, 1988).

In human hosts, as the female worm expels the eggs, some of them flow with the blood and become lodged in the liver or around the urinary tract. The body, treating the eggs as foreign irritants, surrounds them with granular tissue, leading to cirrhosis, liver failure, portal hypertension, esophageal varices, bladder cancer, and renal failure (Markell, Voge, & John, 1992). Filariasis may be the second most challenging parasitic disease after schistosomiasis (National Academy of Science, 1979).

Rates of blindness in Egypt are among the highest in the world. Trachoma and other acute eye infections affect 5 percent of the rural and 2 percent of the urban population (National Academy of Science, 1979). Trachoma, a chronic infection of the lining of the eyelids caused by infection with *Chlamydia trachomatis* (Lane, 1987), is most common among children and can have severe disabling consequences in adulthood. The active inflammatory stage is characterized by gel-like lymphoid follicles that subside over time, leaving residual scarring of the inner eyelids. In the most severe cases, trichiasis, an end stage complication of chronic trachoma, occurs when scarring shrinks the lid lining and turns the eyelashes inward, scratching the cornea. This painful condition often leads to corneal ulceration, opacity, and eventual blindness. Injuries and corneal ulcers secondary to other infections are also common causes of blindness in Egypt (Lane, 1987).

Other infectious diseases include typhoid and paratyphoid fevers, which are more frequent in urban than rural areas. Streptococcal disease and rheumatic fevers are frequent among children, and tuberculosis continues to be a major problem in Egypt. Egyptian-Americans who have positive tuberculin tests should be questioned about a history of BCG vaccination.

Diarrheal diseases result from environmental conditions and family lifestyles. Heat contributes to the development of bacterial diseases, and dehydration results from diarrhea and vomiting caused by bacterial infections. Programs and campaigns using rehydration packets with water, salt, and sugar have drastically decreased mortality rates caused by diarrheal diseases. These endemic diseases are more common in rural areas than in urban areas. Egyptian immigrants come mainly from urban areas and therefore do not usually suffer from these diseases. However, some may have family members with complications due to one of these diseases who may come to the United States for treatment. Kidney diseases, lack of proper hydration, and eating habits may contribute to kidney failure and the subsequent need for kidney transplantation. Clinicians in the Middle East suspect that fasting during Ramadan increases the potential of dehydration, contributing to kidney problems.

The people of Egypt currently suffer from diseases that are common to developing countries, such as undernutrition and malnutrition, and diseases resulting from overindulging in foods with high-fat and high-sugar contents. Modern diseases such as obesity, hypertension, and lower back pain affect a high percentage of Egyptians. Similarly, cardiovascular diseases resulting from stress, obesity, lack of exercise, and hypertension are on the rise. Egyptians who immigrate to the United States are more likely to become victims of these diseases of modernization than of rural diseases. Type II diabetes is of concern to Egyptians and is further complicated by obesity. In addition, Egyptians are at a genetic risk for $\beta$-thalassemia, which can be detected from a molecular genetic standpoint through carrier screening and prenatal diagnosis (Hussein, et al., 1993).

## Variations in Drug Metabolism

The literature reports few studies related to variations in drug metabolism and specific drug interactions among Egyptian-Americans. Some evidence indicates that Egyptians are poor metabolizers of beta-blockers (Levy, 1993). More research is needed in this area to provide better health care to Egyptian-Americans.

## HIGH-RISK BEHAVIORS

Certain behaviors may increase the risk of illness for Egyptians in America. One of these is the lack of regular exercise. Information about exercise has just begun to appear in the media in Egypt, and health clubs and gyms have begun to spring up in Cairo and Alexandria. This is a new phenomenon that began well after many Egyptians immigrated to America. Although exercise and fitness are regularly included in the curricula of schools and colleges, exercise is not part of the daily lives of adult Egyptians and, even less so, among Egyptian-Americans.

Overeating food delicacies high in fat, sodium, and sugar; sedentary lifestyles; and an entertainment style based on eating contribute to obesity and immobility. Although no data exist on health risk factors for Egyptian-Americans, the authors suspect that if such data were obtained, it would demonstrate an increased risk for coronary artery diseases, diabetes, and esophageal hernias. The few premature deaths in Egyptian-American communities are due to massive heart failure. Egyptians came to the United States as young adults; as the community of Egyptian-Americans ages, questions related to sedentary lifestyles, overindulgence in food, and genetic makeup should be of interest.

Egyptian-Americans are at risk for stomach and intestinal problems that include heartburn, flatulence, constipation, and hemorrhoids and fecal impaction. These conditions result from limited roughage, lack of fluids, and their rapid consumption of food. Another factor contributing to constipation may be their expectations and the meaning they attach to regularity that prompts them to push and strain to force a bowel movement prematurely.

Like many developing countries, Egypt responded with zeal to campaigns launched by the cigarette industry. Cigarette smoking is on the rise in Egypt, mostly among men, but it is also increasing among women. However, it appears that this is not a major risk factor among the majority of Egyptian-Americans. The few who smoke, smoke heavily and are unwilling to quit.

One of the most dangerous risk factors among Egyptians in Egypt is their driving behavior. Most Egyptians drive recklessly and aggressively, they do not wear seat belts, and they drive without respect for speed limits. However, the extreme traffic congestion in Egypt provides a safety cushion for them. It takes Egyptian immigrants a number of years in America to learn to respect traffic rules, wear seat belts, and drive cautiously.

## Health-care Practices

Two conditions increase the utilization of preventive health care by Egyptian-Americans: having health insurance and having a health-care provider with whom they can develop a trusting and responsive relationship (Laffrey, et al., 1989). Egyptian-Americans like prompt and personal attention; they are usually among the most compliant clients if these conditions are met.

One reason for Egyptian-Americans' seeking health care is a perception that they are experiencing high blood pressure. They believe it is important to have frequent readings but prefer to treat hypertension with medications rather than with changes in diet or lifestyle. Hypertension, the silent killer of many Americans, may not be so silent for Egyptians. Whether they can detect fluctuations in their blood pressure remains to be carefully studied. However, this behavior of reading one's own body cues should be encouraged and promptly addressed by health-care professionals.

Pap smears and mammograms tend to be new preventive health practices for Egyptian-Americans. Education about the importance of these tests promotes compliance with regular check-ups. As mentioned earlier, Pap smears for unmarried women are discouraged and considered totally unacceptable because of the expectations for preserving virginity until marriage. Gynecologic examinations are only given to married women, usually during the check-up for a first pregnancy.

## NUTRITION

### Meaning of Food

Food is an important component of Egyptian social life. Egyptians entertain lavishly and enjoy good food. Food represents nurturing, and the more food one provides the more love is portrayed. Egyptians develop trust in each other by having a meal together. The saying *Akalt eish wa malh maa baad* literally means "eating bread and salt together" and symbolically signifies trust, care, and truthfulness.

Some beliefs surrounding meals may increase health risks. For example, Egyptians prefer not to drink water or fluids with meals because they believe that fluid displaces the volume that could be used for food, decreasing their appetite for solid nutrients. Some believe that fluids dilute the stomach "juices," make digestion difficult, and cause indigestion.

In addition to being part of Egyptian social life, food is associated with health. The more food a person eats, the greater the potential expectation for health. Thus, children tend to be overfed.

Food is also associated with the ability of the head of the family to provide for family members. Therefore, parents take pride in the amount and the quality of food they bring to their families. Because food is associated with caring and nurturing, mothers and wives spend much time and effort shopping and cooking family meals.

Finally, food is associated with generosity and giving. To offer food and to accept food are indications of friendship.

## Common Foods and Food Rituals

Egyptian food is tasty, well done, and well seasoned. Egyptian-Americans take pride in the food they serve and the way they present it. Although in Egypt vegetable dishes are considered main dishes to be complemented by meat and rice dishes, this conception has changed for most Egyptian-Americans. Preferred meats are lamb, chicken, beef, and veal. Favorite vegetables are peas, green beans, cauliflower, and molokhia, a green vegetable that is cooked like soup. The meat dishes are considered by the majority as main dishes, complemented by vegetables and rice. Rice, a main staple, adorns dinner or lunch tables on a daily basis even when potatoes are served. Tomato-based red sauces are popular, and some pasta and vegetable dishes are dressed with rich white sauces such as *bechamel*. They use lentils, fava beans, and bulgur in their cooking. Whole-wheat bread is the preferred bread.

Egyptians acquired a taste for tea from their years under British rule and drink strong tea with hot milk several times a day. Those who prefer tea without milk drink it black or with mint leaves. They tend to use several teaspoons of sugar to sweeten their tea. Although it is not easy for them to decrease their sugar intake, they do so if they understand its relationship to caloric intake, insulin requirements for those who are diabetic, or for other health considerations. Egyptians drink coffee, a habit acquired from Turkish rule. The coffee is thick, strong, and served in small demitasse cups, with or without sugar. Egyptians also consume a large quantity of soft drinks.

Hostesses insist on giving guests excessive amounts of food and act insulted if guests refuse the food. Those who understand the ritual may insist on refusal or may take the food and not eat it. It is more polite to leave some food on the plate than to refuse it. If the plate is completely emptied it might be an indication that the guest did not have enough to eat. Egyptian-Americans use modified versions of this ritual, depending on the guests and their length of time in the United States.

In Egypt, three main meals a day are served with a late afternoon or early evening snack of sweets with tea (a remaining English tradition). The main meal is lunch, usually consumed at the end of the working day between 2 and 3 P.M. It is a complete meal after which there is usually a period of rest when many take an afternoon nap. Working men and women in the current economic climate of Egypt either return to work in the early evening between 5 and 6 P.M. or have a second job or business for the remaining part of the evening. Supper, usually a lighter meal, is eaten after 9 P.M.

On religious holidays, certain foods are prepared and shared with family and friends. An example is baking a variety of cookies at the end of the holy month of Ramadan, a time when Muslims fast daily from sunrise to sunset, and during the **Small Eid** feast (also called the *Small Barrium*). During the **Great Eid** feast (also called the *Big Barrium*) a sheep is sacrificed; its meat is given to needy families and some is kept for consumption by the family during that feast. Most of these rituals are modified in the United States. For example, Egyptian immigrants follow American eating habits of a small meal for lunch and then dinner at home after work between 6 and 7 P.M. Some immigrant families still make cookies at end of Ramadan, but very few have a sheep slaughtered. Whether in Egypt or in America, the most devout Muslims do not consume pork or drink alcohol. Egyptian Copts may consume both in moderation.

For Egyptian-American Muslims, many rituals are revived during the month of Ramadan. The month of Ramadan is the ninth of 12 Islamic months that follow the lunar calendar. Therefore, Ramadan does not coincide with a particular month in the Christian calendar; instead it rotates and can fall on any of the Christian calendar months. Ramadan rituals are based on the teaching of the **Qur'an** (Koran) that calls for a month of fasting to experience the plight of the poor and the underprivileged. Fasting precludes taking anything by mouth or intravenously and abstaining from sexual activities. Muslims are expected to donate food for those in need, and they may eat modestly from sunset to sunrise. Egyptian-American Christians fast for a varied number of days for several major religious celebrations. For them, fasting constitutes not eating any animal products.

Ramadan is a month of prayers and family festivities with many food rituals. At sunset, families gather to eat lavish meals consisting of several kinds of meat and poultry, rice, dried fruits, and desserts such as *konafa* (shredded filo dough stuffed with nuts and raisins and soaked in honey) and *kataif* (pancakelike dough) dressed with nuts, raisins, and sugar and smothered in honey. The meals are usually high in protein, fat, sugar, salt, and calories. Just before sunrise, they consume a lighter meal in preparation for a day of fasting. Some Egyptian-American Muslims follow these rituals in the United States. Even those Egyptian-Americans who do not follow and abide by the teachings of Islam during the year consider this month a holy month, and they become more devout Muslims during Ramadan. Some Egyptian-Americans join others in social clubs and plan weekly potluck "sundown Ramadan breakfasts." During these gatherings, Egyptian-Americans, their friends, and children exchange stories related to Ramadan, read from the *Qur'an,* and indulge in eating delicacies that are specific to Ramadan.

## Dietary Practices and Rituals

Egyptian-Americans do not mix hot and cold nor sweet and sour foods. For example, the accepted habit in America of eating ice cream as desert with coffee was a foreign concept for Egyptians during the early stages of their immigration. However, it is a food habit to which they easily accommodate. Some Egyptian-Americans grew up believing that mixing fish and milk may cause digestive problems or create behavioral problems. Therefore, dairy products and fish are generally avoided in combination. Some may have practiced drinking milk with yeast to increase their vitamin B complex, a popular custom in Egypt.

Most Egyptian Muslims do not eat pork, as proscribed by the *Qur'an.* They eat only well-cooked meat and do not touch rare meat. Recent Egyptian immigrants find it strange to eat cooked corn, which is only barbecued in their country. Most are partial to their own cooking, preferring not to eat in restaurants. They prefer kosher meat, trusting the dietary restrictions and food preparation practices of the Jewish population. In the absence of kosher meat, they use regular supermarkets.

## Nutritional Deficiencies and Food Limitations

Egyptians, particularly those who live in rural and poor communities, experience vitamin and iron deficiency anemias. They eat more fresh vegetables, fresh fruits, and enriched or whole-wheat grain breads. Egyptians in the United States may resort to eating more processed foods and high-protein diets in the form of red meats because of increased availability. They also tend to eat more junk foods, preferring sweets. Therefore, Egyptian-Americans may have a greater tendency to have diets higher in fat and consume fewer fresh fruits and vegetables. No literature exists about the changes in dietary habits and the effects on vitamin and mineral deficiencies among Egyptian-Americans.

## PREGNANCY AND CHILDBEARING PRACTICES

### Fertility Practices and Views toward Pregnancy

An Egyptian family is not complete until they have a child. Systematic and concerted efforts have been initiated to develop and implement birth control practices in urban and rural areas of Egypt. Although these have met some success, birth control is far more apparent in urban Egypt. While Egyptian-Americans may practice family planning and birth control, these are never advocated before conceiving the first child. Family planning is practiced through a variety of methods, including birth control pills, condoms, and early withdrawals. Abortion is used in Egypt, as in other countries, as a method of birth control. Desirable family size in urban Egypt is three or four children, whereas desirable family size in the United States among Egyptian-Americans is two or three children. Women take an active role in limiting pregnancies; they are willing to use any method of birth control to achieve and maintain a small family size (Fouad, 1986; Keck, 1989).

Families in general and women in particular are usually under stress until they conceive their first baby (Meleis & Hatar-Pollara, in press), fearing marriage instability due to lack of childbearing. Even if their husband is the cause of delayed or permanent infertility, women are threatened by the potential of divorce and are expected to conceive within their first year of marriage (Meleis & Aly, 1992). Egyptian-American families are under less stress and pressure to conceive because of the absence of extended family (Fouad, 1986), although extended families continue to pressure their daughters and sons through letters and telephone calls.

Pregnancies cement marriages, ensure a more lasting relationship, and are a way of getting men and women to mature in their relationship. Pregnancy brings women a sense of security and their husbands' and in-laws' respect. The status and power of women are considerably strengthened by birthing, particularly a son. Pregnancy gives women permission to decrease their responsibilities.

### Prescriptive, Restrictive, and Taboo Practices in the Childbearing Family

Women are expected and advised to curtail physical activities during pregnancy for fear of miscarriage. Women are also advised to eat more because they are feeding two. Some Egyptian-American women have strong craving urges (**waham**) for certain foods that may extend to such scarce foods as out-of-season strawberries. It is believed that if these foods are not consumed, babies may be marked with the shape of foods that were craved. Therefore, every effort is made to provide the pregnant woman with the needed foods.

Providing support during labor and delivery is reserved for the woman's relatives, particularly her mother. Egyptian-Americans invariably request that a female family member accompany the birthing mother. If an Egyptian-American woman goes into labor with only her husband in attendance, it is considered an emergency. Acculturated Egyptian-American men want to be included in the birthing experience, which may offend Egyptian newcomers. In Egypt, men are excluded from the birthing process because, it is believed, men lack the ability to witness this highly emotional and painful process and the experience to support their wives.

The cold and hot theory for health and illness prevents women from bathing during the postpartum period. Bathing or washing hair could expose them to colds and chills. Egyptian-Americans respond well to a sound rationale for bathing in a hot tub or taking a shower that dispels beliefs about the potential for infection. Chicken and chicken broth are expected to help women during their postpartum transition. The postpartum period lasts 40 days, during which new mothers are expected to rest, eat well, be confined to the house with their babies, and not engage in any sexual activities. They are usually cared for by family members and not expected to have any demands put on them. This practice is eroding, however, due to increasing demands on women and the migration of families (Lane & Meleis, 1991). Information related to birth control is always welcomed after the first pregnancy, although it is not sought during the postpartum period (El Sayed, 1986).

# DEATH RITUALS

## Death Rituals and Expectations

Among Muslims in Egypt, Islam calls for burial of the deceased as soon as possible. The burial ritual includes cleaning the body and wrapping it in a white cotton wrap. Verses from the *Qur'an* are read and a special prayer recited at the mosque before the body is buried underground in a simple tomb. Islam prohibits fancy tombstones; only a simple stone with the name of the deceased written on it is placed above ground. The simple stone suggests that individuals are equal in death when meeting their creator. On the night of the burial, friends and family gather in a large tent outside the deceased's home to give their condolences and respect to the grieving family. No food is served, but Turkish coffee is usually offered. Forty days after the burial, another mourning ritual takes place in the home of the deceased's family. Family members listen while passages from the *Qur'an* are read by a religious man and console the family. Thereafter, a similar ritual takes place on the anniversary of the death. Egyptian Christian death rituals in Egypt and the United States are similar to American Christian death rituals.

For Egyptian immigrants, some cultural rituals are followed. For instance, the Islamic burial rituals are carried out in designated cemeteries. The evening before the burial, the *Qur'an* is recited and occasionally the mourning ritual forty days after burial is observed. The annual death observance ritual is rarely carried out. Some Muslim families insist on having the deceased buried in Egypt, which is a very costly process involving approval from both countries and transporting the deceased in a special casket. Abdel-Khalek and Ahmed (1986) found that Egyptian-Americans have slightly higher anxiety about death than Americans. Health-care providers may be involved in and bewildered by the decision-making processes that families go through on the death of family members.

## Responses to Death and Grief

Egyptians in Egypt and the United States react vigorously and dramatically to the loss of a family member, expressing their grief outwardly. Wailing and public crying occur on first learning of death. This public reaction is an expected demonstration of their grief; otherwise the community may regard them as lacking affection for the deceased. Death is seen as inevitable, although any loss brings shock and despair. Older people speak calmly about their own impending death. Egyptian-Americans with a strong religious foundation do not fear the nearness of death but rather view it as a journey to the other world, which is believed to be better. Egyptian Muslims and Christians believe in an afterlife and expect rewards for good deeds accomplished in their first life. They anticipate reuniting with those who preceded them.

## SPIRITUALITY

### Religious Practices and Use of Prayer

Religious practices for Egyptian-Americans are performed during marriage, death, and religious holidays. Egyptian-Americans participate in two wedding ceremonies: one is a religious and civil ceremony performed by the Mosque's *imam* and the other a social ceremony in which friends and family gather for a gala evening. Both could be performed on the same day or days, months, or years apart. A separation after the religious ceremony is considered a divorce, but it is customary for brides and grooms to live together only after the social celebration has taken place. Egyptian-American Christians have one religious marriage ceremony.

Prayers, even for the nondevout Muslim or Christian, are significant during times of illness. Egyptian-Americans may bring the *Qur'an* or the bible to their hospital beds, and they usually put it under the pillow or on the bedside table. Prayers may be recited by the individual, in groups for Muslims, or in religious settings such as Mosques or churches. Families and friends pray for each other, invoking good health, cure of illness, and peace. Prayers during holidays are enjoyed particularly in groups and in religious settings.

### Meaning of Life and Individual Sources of Strength

Religious Egyptians achieve inner peace through practicing their respective religious rituals, including individual or collective prayers, reading from the *Qur'an* or bible, and other religious texts written by religious scholars. Muslims who can afford the expense and are in good health make the pilgrimage to Mecca sometime during their lifetime, which provides a source of inner fulfillment. Similar patterns of fulfillment through participation in religious activities are common in the United States.

### Spiritual Beliefs and Health-care Practices

Most Egyptian-Americans talk about their religious teachings during episodes of illness. They derive comfort, strength, and meaning from verses in the *Qur'an* and of prophets. Family members use these verses to remind them that they are at the mercy and under the control of God and that God may have a particular reason for their suffering. To lose hope may mean that they are losing faith in God and His abilities.

## HEALTH-CARE PRACTICES

### Health-seeking Beliefs and Practices

The health-care practices of Egyptian-Americans can be best understood by looking at the historical roots and the meanings of health and health care for Egyptians. The pharaohs are credited with introducing medicine to the world, as evidenced by the writings on papyri from 4000 B.C. The practice of mummification, perfected to ensure that the pharaohs' bodies were preserved to wait for the return of the departed spirit, may have helped the pharaohs to understand the intricate anatomy of the body. Papyri writings have been found describing body organs, gynecologic conditions, surgery, and signs and symptoms of illnesses. There are indications that the early Egyptians also had dental knowledge and had developed treatments for dental problems. Pharaonic writings introduced the idea of body parts and segmentation.

Egyptian health care is also influenced by Greek medicine, *unani medicine.* The most famous medical library in the world was built in Alexandria during the reign of Alexander the Great; it housed almost all the medical knowledge of the ancient world. The books contained in this library, which was later burned, chronicled numerous diseases and treatments. The Greeks combined medicine and philosophy and expanded the understanding of anatomy. Their texts influenced the entire region. As early as the 10th century A.D., medical schools were established by the Arabs based on unani medicine. Texts known as the laws of medicine were written by early Arab scholars that embodied the teachings of the previous eras of preventive and curative health care.

Egyptian beliefs about health care are also influenced by humoral systems described in Greek documents. The principles behind the humoral system are based on dividing many aspects of life into four: the year into four seasons; matter into fire, air, earth, and water; the body into black phlegm, black bile, yellow bile, and blood; and the environment into hot, cold, moist, and dry. Diseases follow these humors with treatments based on opposite humors. The pharaohs introduced the principle of balance and imbalance as cause of illness. Egyptians believe that illnesses are caused by cold and moist environments, by changes from cold to hot or vice versa. The opposite humor is used for treating the illness.

Other influences on the Egyptian health belief system came from the colonization of Egypt by the Turks, French, and British (Lane, 1987). In addition to illnesses being caused by humoral imbalances, Egyptians believe them to be caused by being presented with bad news suddenly (***Itkhad,*** "without preparing") or by a fight. While a person's mental and physical health are intricately interwoven, treatment sought from the health-care system is focused on physical or biomedical treatment. Mental health problems are usually handled outside the health-care system by family or religious persons. Egyptians tend to manifest symptoms of mental health problems somatically. Therefore, they seek medical care to deal with the physical manifestations of mental illnesses.

While Egyptian-Americans are usually well educated, their views are colored by beliefs about the influence of imbalances, the evil eye, and Islamic beliefs about the role that God plays in their illness (Morsy, 1993). However, they are firm believers in Western medicine's miraculous ability to treat and cure illnesses. None of their beliefs prevents them from seeking or complying with the prescriptions of Western medicine. If they practice the belief of balancing or of warding off the evil eye, it is done in conjunction with Western medicine.

## Responsibility for Health Care

The *Qur'an* and the sayings of Mohammed, the prophet of Islam, have made a major contribution to health care. In particular, preventive health care is embodied in many of Mohammed's prophetic sayings. Cleanliness and hygiene are integral to practicing Muslims. A number of elaborate prayer rituals are also related to health care and prevention of illness. For example, before praying, Muslims must engage in a purification ritual, which consists of washing every exposed body part. Prayer, required five times daily, consists of elaborate bending and kneeling movements in systematic ways, increasing a person's range of movements, limbering stretches, and meditative poses. Religion and prayers are believed to be protective from illnesses (Walsh, 1980).

Egyptians come from a country where health care is available free or at low cost for all citizens. A government health insurance policy allows every citizen to receive free care, treatments, and medications. However, Egyptians believe that to receive better-quality health care, they must shop, bargain, and negotiate. In the process, they learn that quality care means fees. If they can afford it, they prefer quality care. Most Egyptian-Americans join an HMO or have private medical insurance. While they may refuse to have life insurance (Islam does not condone insurance), they realize the importance of quality health care. Newcomers, however, may wait to develop financial security before they join a health insurance plan. Typically, Egyptian-Americans experiencing a health problem consult family members and friends before visiting a trusted health-care professional. Once in the health-care system, they prefer immediate, personalized attention (Reizian, 1985). They value tests and prescriptions for their illnesses and follow medical regimens and prescriptions carefully, particularly if they consist of medications, injections, or both (Lipson, Reizian, & Meleis, 1987). However, they tend to be skeptical of treatments such as weight reduction, exercise, and diet restrictions.

The family of a client expects and prefers to be involved in all health-care decisions. Their focus on human relations and interpersonal contact make it difficult for Egyptian-Americans who encounter changing staff and assignments during treatments. They believe that they have a better chance of receiving quality care if trusting relationships are formed. Thus, constancy and consistency of contacts decrease potential conflicts in their relationship with the health-care system.

Egyptian-Americans may practice self-medication. They tend to share medications freely and use Western medications and home remedies such as herbs, hot compresses, and hot fluids and foods. Many Egyptians keep a very active medicine cabinet filled with antibiotics, tranquilizers, sleeping pills, and pain medications. They also believe that vitamins given intramuscularly and intravenously are more effective than vitamins taken in pills. In Egypt, vitamin B complex injections and iron supplements are common self-medicating activities. Some common herbal and home remedies are boiled mint leaves for a stomachache; boiled cumin for gas; boiled caraway for coughs; and hot pads for aches, pains, and boils.

Regulation of prescription drugs in the United States restricts the use of prescriptions, prompting some Egyptian-Americans to get their supply of medications from their home country or friends. Use of illegal drugs is minimal in this community. Although some Egyptian-Americans may overindulge in alcohol, the teachings of Islam prohibit its use. Many who drink alcohol tend to do so socially and in limited quantities.

## Folk Practices

According to Islam, illnesses are caused by lack of hygiene, exposure to diseases, or environmental conditions, although it is up to God who gets sick and who does not, and people are expected to care for themselves and work at preventing illnesses when possible. In addition, beliefs related to the healing powers of shrines and holy men or saints and the counterpowers of the devil (*Jenn*) and evil spirits (*arwah*) influence health care. Thus, ceremonies are designed to eliminate the devastating powers of the *Jenn*; among them is the famous **Zar** ceremony and the **Hegab**. The *Zar* ceremony includes gathering friends and relatives around a sick person, with loud music playing and drums beating to increase the frenzy of dance and movement. The energy of the group and their solidarity help to eliminate the bad spirits from the body, taking with them the illness or the handicapping condition. *Zar* is rarely practiced among Egyptian-Americans. The *Hejab,* an amulet with sayings from the *Qur'an*, is worn by a person who is trying to get rid of an illness. There is also the **Amal**, which is designed to bring bad luck or illness to an unloved person.

Egyptians believe that the evil eye is responsible for personal calamities. The evil eye is cast by those who have blue eyes, by those who tend to speak of an admired person or object in a boastful manner, or by the mere description of beauty, wealth, or health without saying some verses from the *Qur'an* or bible. These verses protect the person from losing whatever good they possess. Some Egyptian-Americans use blue beads or religious verses inscribed on charms to protect them or their children from the evil eye. Children are particularly at risk for the evil eye and need more protection than adults (Harfauche, 1981).

## Barriers to Health Care

A barrier to health care among Egyptian-Americans is related to economics, work demands, and full schedules. Fitting appointments into their schedules proves to be somewhat difficult, particularly in families where a spouse is working long hours and the family owns only one car. When the family has two working members, access to the health-care system at designated times is even more challenging.

Another barrier is the difference in explaining health problems. The degree of specificity required in the U.S. health-care system, the narrative storytelling nature of Egyptians, and the contextual way in which Egyptians view a situation contribute to a frustrating experience for both the immigrant and the health-care professional.

## Cultural Responses to Health and Illness

Egyptians avoid pain at all costs by seeking prompt interventions. They tend to be verbally and nonverbally expressive about pain; moaning, groaning, sighing, and holding tight the painful body part are common expressions of pain. As Reizian and Meleis (1987) demonstrated, Arab-Americans tend to respond to an episode of pain depending on the intensity, severity, and their audience. Although they tend to be more constrained in front of health-care professionals or other "strangers," they are quite expressive in front of family members, grunting, pushing, screaming, using guttural sounds, or gasping for air. These conflicting behaviors are confusing to health-care professionals when family members insist that the client needs pain relief. The absence of these responses in front of health-care professionals makes verification of the intensity of pain difficult.

Egyptian descriptions of pain also may not be as specific as the Western health-care system prefers. Egyptians present a more generalized description of pain, regardless of whether it is localized. They usually describe general weakness, dizziness, or overall tension and stress associated with pain (Reizian & Meleis, 1987). They also use metaphors reflecting humoral medicine such as earth, rocks, fire, heat, and cold to describe their pain.

Age and birth order correlates significantly with individual responses and descriptions of pain. Younger children and first-borns are often more expressive about pain. Higher intensities of pain are also associated with increased behavioral responses in children. Egyptian children tend to describe their pain with sensory descriptors such as **sikkeenah**, or "it's like a knife" (Essaway, 1987). Giving birth is associated with severe pain, not to be endured alone. Therefore, birthing mothers tend to be highly expressive of the intensity of their pain. It is helpful for Egyptian-Americans to have a close family member present during the pain episode. Children prefer their mothers (Essaway, 1987), whereas adult women and men prefer female family members who are more nurturing, caring, and capable of comforting a person in pain (Meleis & Sorrell, 1981).

Although mental illness has been considered a stigma that should not be disclosed, there is more tolerance of emotional problems in modern Egypt (Meleis & Warshaw, 1984). Rural Egypt explains mental health problems within supernatural frameworks, including the *Amal*, "a curse," or *Jenn*, "the devil." Urban Egyptians explain emotional problems in terms of grief, losses, wrongdoing by others, or by blaming the victims for not being able to control and snap out of their distress. Mental and emotional issues tend to be expressed somatically, and therefore psychosomatic interventions are more effective than psychologically based interventions. Although

Egyptians may seek therapy and counseling, they prefer to seek the advice of family members or trusted friends rather than go to strangers. They also do not like to call treatments psychotherapy or analysis. Egyptians tend to place the blame externally, looking for external actions or events to explain the situation. Because Egyptians are more community oriented, they tend to seek the approval and sanction of others; therefore, shame rather than guilt tends to explain their actions and their reactions (Budman, Lipson, & Meleis, 1992).

Disabilities are not hidden from public view. While there is public sympathy and acceptance of the disabled, families still tend to be protective and shield them from public display. Families assume responsibility for the care of their disabled members and usually do not expect help or services from society. Egyptian-Americans, however, tend to hide their disabled family members from other Egyptian-Americans for fear of evoking reactions of pity. They are open, however, with health-care professionals in the hope of receiving better health care.

There is a general belief that chronic illnesses can be controlled by the scientific sophistication of Western medicine. Therefore, health-care professionals and clients have a general pattern of cooperation on long-term treatments (Lipson & Meleis, 1983). Less regard is held for complementary therapies and the demand is greater for scientifically supported remedies, regardless of their intrusiveness. Egyptian-Americans tend to be hopeful, persistent, and optimistic about their prognoses (Meleis & Jonsen, 1983). Therefore, they may shop around for health care that promises a better prognosis. Rehabilitation programs that include drastic changes in lifestyles are less appealing unless the programs are scientifically supported.

Egyptian families take care of their sick members. Promotion of self-care is viewed with suspicion by Egyptian-Americans, just as by other Arab-Americans, and sick persons are not expected to participate in programs to enhance their self-care capabilities. Rather, they are expected to preserve their energy for healing. Attempts to engage Egyptian clients in self-care by promoting responsibility for daily care, for example, by keeping a colostomy incision clean, are resisted and perceived as a request to decrease the work of the nurse and the other staff (Meleis & Warshaw, 1984). Sick persons are also relieved from making major health-care decisions (Lipson & Meleis, 1985). Their families make all health-care decisions for them.

## Blood Transfusion and Organ Donation

Egyptian-Americans have no taboos against blood transfusions or organ transplants. All measures needed to heal, cure, or prolong life are welcomed. Their trust and respect for the health-care system and health-care professionals facilitate their decision making, and they support recommendations offered by the health-care provider. They are hesitant, however, to pledge their own organs to others or permit an autopsy. Because of their belief in the afterlife, they favor being buried whole.

## HEALTH-CARE PRACTITIONERS

### Traditional Versus Biomedical Care

Egyptian-Americans may consult family members and friends about their health and illness, but they do not consult traditional or folk practitioners. In fact, they may be reluctant to seek health care from anyone but physicians. Using the services of acupuncturists, podiatrists, chiropractors, and physical therapists is foreign to those not integrated into the American culture. Some folk practices are built on traditional values, such as avoiding drafts and cold, protecting clients from the evil eye through amulets, and advising clients not to share their news about good fortunes to protect themselves.

In general, members of the Egyptian-American community have a positive perception of the U.S. health-care system. They believe that physicians and nurses are experts, caring and responsive to the needs of their community. Egyptian-Americans are in awe of Western medicine, its scientific basis, and its vast resources. One of their most common responses is, "We were lucky to be in the United States when the illness occurred" (Meleis, 1981). For some Egyptian-Americans, however, the meticulous diagnostic approaches practiced by American physicians may be misinterpreted. Accustomed to Egyptian physicians whose clinical judgments and skills have been developed within a system that lacks adequate resources for meticulous diagnoses, some may misperceive the American physicians' meticulousness as a lack of experience or appropriate knowledge. Therefore, they may shop for physicians whose clinical judgments are congruent with their cultural expectations of a prompt and firm diagnosis. Others may view the laborious and involved diagnostic process, which uses many resources and tests, as an indication of the gravity of the diagnosis.

A recent trend in Egypt is to consider gender as an important variable in the selection of health-care professionals. Although rural and less educated urbanites have always valued this, religious influences have prompted a renewed preference for health-care providers of the same gender. Many Egyptian-Americans immigrated before the wave of Islamic fundamentalism and its influence on life patterns and expressions. Therefore, first- and second-wave Egyptian-Americans may not consider gender as an important criteria in the selection of their health-care providers. Third-wave immigrants may prefer gender-congruent health-care providers, although this preference may be mitigated by their respect for Western medicine. In addition to religious fundamentalism, modesty may influence the desire for gender-congruent health care. For some Egyptian-Americans, sharing the intimate details of their health history is enhanced if the health-care provider is the same gender. Egyptian-Americans may also view older female physicians as more experienced and therefore more trustworthy than younger female physicians (Lipson & Meleis, 1985)

## Status of Health-care Providers

Physicians are highly respected by Egyptians and Egyptian-Americans. As in most health-care systems throughout the world, Egyptian physicians expect to be the head of the health-care team and the primary decisionmakers for all aspects of clinical care. Egyptian-Americans prefer physicians affiliated with large, respected organizations because they believe them to be more experienced. For some, the physician's age, years of experience, and position in the organization may indicate better qualifications.

As in the United States, nurses in Egypt are educated at many different degree levels and have similar patterns of practice. The majority graduate from high school programs developed to meet the nursing shortage. Limited resources, an overabundance of physicians, limited educational preparation of the majority of nurses, low pay scales, and long work hours contribute to poor nursing care in Egypt. Consequently, nursing care in Egyptian hospitals is left to family members, who usually surround the client every waking moment. They are expected to carry out most of the care and act as advocates for the client.

Egyptians' contacts in the homeland with nurses who are knowledgeable and expert in their fields have been minimal. Consequently, their expectations of nurses are usually far below their experiences in the U.S. health-care system. They view U.S. nurses as well educated and well qualified and are grateful for their expertise and for their attention.

Egyptian-American physicians tend to be impressed with U.S. nursing. Their limited views and expectations of nurses based on Egyptian experiences are drastically altered after short contact with U.S. nursing practices. They consider nurses in the United States to be well educated and view their expertise as enhanced by years of experience and availability of resources. The emphasis on higher levels of education for U.S. nurses is congruent with the high value Egyptians place on education. Egyptian physicians also believe that the better pay for U.S. nurses is congruent with better education and better expertise.

## CASE STUDY

The Fayez family came to the United States from Cairo, Egypt, in 1976. After spending 6 months with distant relatives in Daly City, California, Anwar and his wife Fatma moved into an apartment of their own, and Anwar continued the job his Uncle Hussain had helped him get in the construction business. Fatma has never worked outside the home. In 1979, Mr. and Mrs. Fayez had their first child, a son named Sherief. In 1980, they had their second child, a daughter named Randa. Two years ago, Fatma miscarried in her 4th month of pregnancy and lost a male child. At this point in their lives, Fatma is 6 months pregnant, and Anwar owns and operates his own small construction and roofing company in the Richmond area of San Francisco. Sherief is a healthy-looking boy who does well in school, and Randa is in the first grade.

The public health nurse—family nurse practitioner assigned to the Fayez family for their well-child and prenatal care—has made two visits to the family's home. On both occasions the nurse noticed that Mrs. Fayez looked very fatigued and short of breath. Both Sherief and Randa were very quiet during the visits. Anwar boasted often of his son's achievements in school and said little about Randa. Fatma was showing some slight edema in both feet, and the nurse noticed during these visits (both in the evening) that Fatma was frequently getting up to serve the family tea and food. Mr. Fayez described how Sherief's teachers complain about his "aggressive behaviors in school." Mrs. Fayez was concerned about her daughter's "finicky" eating habits. During both visits the nurse noticed an older, conservatively dressed woman who sat quietly during the early part of the visit and communicated to family members in Arabic. She always left the room soon after the nurse arrived and the nurse sensed that the family acknowledged her with a great deal of respect. The house (apartment) was nicely furnished, and no educational toys or books visible were visible.

## STUDY QUESTIONS

1. Identify the strengths in the Fayez family that may support and enhance their health.
2. What problems do you think are inherent in the situation?
3. What assessments do you think need to be made?
4. What might some of your goals as a nurse be?
5. Identify priorities for health care and give rationales for these priorities.
6. Identify three cultural factors that influence the health of the Fayez family.
7. Describe two strategies you might use to help the Fayez family deal with their son's "aggressive behaviors."

*continued on page 242*

8. Describe two strategies you might use to help the parents deal with their daughter's "finicky" eating habits.

9. Discuss your intervention plans for Mrs. Fayez's pregnancy.

10. Discuss a culturally competent approach to assessing and intervening with the health-care concerns of the Fayez family.

11. Describe and discuss three areas of at-risk behaviors that you might want to explore preventively with the Fayez family.

12. Compare and contrast first-wave and second-wave Egyptian immigrants in America according to their reasons for immigration.

13. Identify potential communication concerns in the American workforce with newer Egyptian-American immigrants.

14. Identify infectious conditions that may be common with newer Egyptian-American immigrants.

15. Identify culturally congruent bereavement patterns for Egyptian-Americans.

16. Identify counseling strategies for Egyptian-Americans in regards to self-medicating practices.

## References

Abdel-Khalek, A., & Ahmed, M. (1986). Death anxiety in Egyptian samples. *Personality and Individual Differences, 7*(4), 479–483.

Abraham, N. (1989). Arab American marginality: Mythos and praxis. *Arab Studies Quarterly, 11*(2–3), 17–43.

Abu-Laban, S. M. (1989). The coexistence of cohorts: Identity and adaptation among Arab-Americans. *Muslim Arab Studies Quarterly, 11*(2–3), 45–63.

Aswad, B. C. (1993). Arab Americans: Those who followed Columbus. *MESA, 27,* 5–22.

Beshara, A. (1981). Planning new development regions in Egypt: Settlement planning related to economic development. *Third World Planning Review, 3*(2), 234–249.

Bragdon, A. L. (1989). Early Arabic-speaking immigrant communities in Texas. *Arab Studies Quarterly, 11*(2–3), 83–102.

Budman, C., Lipson, J., & Meleis, A. (1992). The cultural consultant in mental health care: The case of an Arab adolescent. *American Journal of Orthopsychiatry, 62*(3), 359–370.

Cohen, R. (1987). Problems of intercultural communications in Egyptian American diplomatic relations. *International Journal of Intercultural Relations, 11,* 29–47.

Dunne, B. W. (1990). Homosexuality in the Middle East: An agenda for historical research. *Arab Studies Quarterly, 12*(3–4), 55–82.

El Sayed, Y. A. (1986). *The successive-unsettled transitions of migration and their impact on postpartum concerns of Arab immigrant women.* Unpublished doctoral dissertation, University of California, San Francisco.

Essaway, M. A. H. (1987). *The relationship of certain factors an the expression of pain among hospitalized surgical school age children.* Unpublished doctoral dissertation, Alexandria University, Alexandria, Egypt.

Fouad, N. A. (1986). *Family planning behavior of Arab American women.* Unpublished doctoral dissertation, University of California, San Francisco.

Harfauche, J. K. (1981). The evil eye and infant health in Lebanon. In A. Dundes (Ed.), *The evil eye: A folklore casebook.* New York: Garland Publishing, Inc.

Hattar-Pollara, M., & Meleis, A. I. (1995). Parenting adolescents: Jordanian immigrant women in California. *Health Care for Women International 16*(3), 195–211.

Hattar-Pollara, M., & Meleis, A. I. (1996). The daily lived experiences of Jordanian immigrant women in the United States: Stress of immigration. *Western Journal of Nursing Research 17*(5), 521–539.

Hussein, I. R., Temtamy, S. A., El-Beshlawy, A., Fearon, C., Shalaby, Z., Vassilopoulos, G., & Kazazian, H. H. J. (1993). Molecular characterization of beta-thalassemia in Egyptians. *Human Mutations, 2*(1), 48–52.

Keck, L. T. (1989). Egyptian Americans in the Washington DC area. *Arab Studies Quarterly, 11*(2–3), 103–126.

Laffrey, S., Meleis, A., Lipson, J., Solomon, M., & Omidian, P. (1989). Assessing Arab-American health care needs. *Social Science and Medicine 29*(7), 877–883.

Lane, S. D. (1987). *A biocultural study of trachoma in an Egyptian hamlet.* Unpublished doctoral dissertation, University of California, San Francisco.

Lane, S. D., & Meleis, A. I. (1991). Roles, work, health perceptions and health resources of women: A study in an Egyptian delta hamlet. *Western Science and Medicine, 33*(10), 1197–1208.

Levy, R. (1993). Ethnic and racial differences in response to medicines: Preserving individualized therapy in managed programmes. *Pharmaceutical Medicine, 7,* 139–165.

Lipson, J. G., & Meleis, A. I. (1985). Culturally appropriate care: The case of immigrants. *Topics in Clinical Nursing, 7*(3), 48–56.

Lipson, J. G., & Meleis, A. I. (1983). Issues in health care of Middle Eastern patients. *Western Journal of Medicine, 139*(6), 854–861.

Lipson, J. G., Reizian, A. E., & Meleis, A. I. (1987). Arab American patients: A medical record review. *Social Science in Medicine, 24*(2), 101–107.

Markell, E. K., Voge, M., & John, D. T. (1992). *Medical parasitology.* Philadelphia: W. B. Saunders.

May, K. M. (1992). Middle-Eastern immigrant parents' social networks and help-seeking for child health care. *Journal of Advanced Nursing, 17,* 905–912.

McLeod, A. E. (1992, Spring). Hegemonic relations and gender resistance: The new veiling as accommodating protest in Cairo. *Signs,* 533–557.

Meleis, A. I. (1981). The Arab American in the health care system. *American Journal of Nursing, 81,* 1180–1183.

Meleis, A. I. (1991). Between two cultures: Identity, roles and health. *Health Care for Women International, 12,* 365–378.

Meleis, A. I., & Aly, F. (1992). A global perspective. In J. McCloskey & H. Grace (Eds.), *Current Issues in Nursing,* (4th ed.). St. Louis, MO: C. V. Mosby.

Meleis, A. I., & Jonsen, A. (1985). Ethical crises and cultural differences. *The Western Journal of Medicine 138*(6), 889–893.

Meleis, A. I., Norbeck, J. S., Laffrey, S., Solomon, M., & Miller, L. (1989). Stress, satisfaction, and coping: A study of women clerical workers. *Health Care for Women International, 10,* 319–334.

Meleis, A. I., Lipson, J. G., & Paul, S. (1992). Ethnicity and health among five Middle Eastern immigrant groups. *Nursing Research, 41*(2), 98–103.

Meleis, A. I., & Rogers, S. (1987). Women in transition: Being vs. becoming or being and becoming. *Health Care for Women International, 8,* 199–217.

Meleis, A. I., & Sorrell, L. (1981). Arab American women and their birth experiences. *American Journal of Maternal Child Nursing, 6,* 171–176.

Meleis, A. I., & Warshaw, C. (1984). Arab Americans and psychiatric care. *Perspectives in Psychiatric Care, 22*(2), 72–76, 85–56.

Metz, C. H., (Ed.). (1990). *Egypt: A country study.* Washington, DC: Federal Research Division, Library of Congress.

Morsy, S. A. (1993). *Gender, sickness, and healing in rural Egypt: Ethnography in historical context.* Boulder, CO: Westview Press.

National Academy of Sciences. (1979). *Health in Egypt: Recommendations for U.S. assistance.* Report of a study by a committee of the Institute of Medicine, Division of International Health. Washington, DC: National Academy of Sciences.

Norden, E. (1993, June). America's oldest (and newest) Christians. *The American Spectator,* pp. 24–28.

Reizian, A. (1985). *Illness behavior and help-seeking behavior among Arab Americans.* Unpublished doctoral dissertation, University of California, San Francisco.

Reizian, A. E., & Meleis, A. I. (1987). Arab Americans' perceptions of and responses to pain. *Critical Care Nurse, 6*(6), 30–37.

Sanders, J. L., Hakky, U. M., & Brizzolara, M. M. (1985). Personal space amongst Arabs and Americans. *International Journal of Psychology, 20*(1), 13–17.

Sanders, J. L. (1986). Egyptian and American university students' attitudes toward parents and family. *Journal of Social Psychology, 126*(4), 459–463.

Sonn, T. (1989). Arab Americans in education: Cultural ambassadors? *Arab Studies Quarterly, 11*(2–3), 127–139.

Sun, T. (1988). *Color atlas and textbook of diagnostic parasitology.* New York: Igakushoin.

Walsh, A. (1980). The prophylactic effect of religion on blood pressure levels among a sample of immigrants. *Social Science in Medicine, 14b,* 59–63.

# Filipino-Americans

*Beatriz F. Miranda, Magelende R. McBride,*
*and Zen Spangler*

---

• Key words to become familiar with in this chapter are:

| | |
|---|---|
| *Amor propio* | *Ibang tao* |
| *Bathala* | *Manong* |
| *Galang* | *Pabasa* |
| *Hilot* | Pilipino |
| *Hindi ibang tao* | Tagalog |
| *Hiya* | Tag-Lish |

## OVERVIEW, INHABITED LOCALITIES, AND TOPOGRAPHY

### Overview

With a U.S. population of 1,450,000 *(U.S. Statistical Abstracts: 1995)* and a Canadian population of 157,250 *(Statistics Canada: Ethnic Origins, 1993),* Filipinos are the fastest growing Asian group in North America. The Filipino diversity in North America is evident in the more than 100 languages spoken by the estimated 75 ethnolinguistic groups representing the Philippines. Regional variations are reflected in belief systems, values, and behaviors represented by such identity labels as "**Tagalog**," "Ilocano," "Bisaya," "Moro," and others. Interracial marriages and travel for economic purposes influence population characteristics in the Philippines and North America. Cultural norms among Filipino-Americans vary in degree and according to primary and secondary characteristics of their culture (see Chapter 1).

In this chapter, people who relocate from the Philippines to North America are referred to interchangeably as Filipinos or Filipino-Americans. The latter designation, however, is frequently used by immigrant Filipinos to identify American-born persons of Filipino ancestry. The term **Pilipino** has been adapted by the Philippine government to refer to the languages of the country. The term may also be used to refer specifically to the Tagalog language, the primary language of the country. On some parts of the West Coast, the term Pilipino is used by community organizations whose goals are linked with empowerment, capacity building, and the labor movement. The information and cultural norms described in this chapter may not pertain to all Filipinos. Therefore, health-care providers should use them only as a guide to add depth to standard practices used for clinical and cultural assessment of Filipino-American clients.

The Philippine archipelago is located slightly north of the equator and consists of 7107 islands with a land mass of 300,000 square kilometers, an area slightly larger than Nevada. Only about 14 percent of the islands are inhabited (Agoncillo & Guerrero, 1987; Pido, 1986). The western region is bound by the South China Sea, the east by the Pacific Ocean, the south by the Sulu and Celebes seas, and the north by the Bashi Channel (*Philippine Statistical Yearbook,* 1995). The three major island groups—Luzon, Visayas, and Mindanao—are traversed by bodies of water and volcanic mountain ranges, many of which remain active today. Natural resources are plentiful. The tropical climate is suitable for year-round agriculture and fishing.

## Heritage and Residence

The Filipino people are predominantly of Malayan ancestry, influenced by the neighboring Chinese, Japanese, Asian Indian, Indonesian, Malaysian, and Arab cultures. In the late 1300s, Islam was introduced to the southern part of the archipelago, mostly in Mindanao and Sulu. Between 1521 and 1898, Spanish colonization transformed the religious, cultural, economic, sociopolitical, and intellectual development of the people. The Filipino Moslems of Mindanao refused to embrace Catholicism, choosing instead to preserve their culture and traditions.

In addition to the Hispanization of Filipinos, the Americanization of the Philippines began immediately after the Spanish-American war. The introduction of American-style education, alliance with the U.S. Armed Forces in World War II, Hollywood movies, and television have influenced the culture, values, and practices, some of which can be observed in many Filipino-American communities today.

Immigrants, rather than U.S.-born Filipinos, constitute the majority of Filipinos in the United States. Immigration trends are expected to continue, having a major impact on Filipino-American communities well into the 21st century. The first Filipinos in the United States, originally part of the labor force in Spanish galleons, settled in Louisiana as early as 1753 and introduced the dry shrimp industry to the United States (Espina, 1988). The first major wave of Filipino immigration to America occurred around the early 1900s, soon after the Philippine-American war (1899 to 1902). At that time, the Philippines was a U.S. territory and Filipino migration was not restricted. Exclusionist policies in the Immigration Act of 1924 significantly restricted Filipino immigration (Wong & Hirschman, 1983). The second wave came between 1935 and the mid-1960s. The third wave of immigration started in 1965 (Tompar-Tiu & Sustento-Sereniches, 1994; McBride, Mariola, & Yeo, 1995) when the Immigration and Nationality Act Amendment of 1965 eliminated the quota system for the Philippines. The majority who came after 1965 were middle class with professional education and experience and the relatives of earlier immigrants. First-wave immigrants settled in California, Hawaii, and Alaska. Second-wave and third-wave immigrants settled in urban areas of California, New York, New Jersey, Illinois, and Texas.

Health-care providers must recognize the social and cultural distinctions between the earlier and more recent Filipino immigrants. These different groups bring unique social and cultural backgrounds and experiences that influence their beliefs, values, and attitudes toward health and health-care services.

## Reason for Migration and Associated Economic Factors

The first wave of immigrants consisted mostly of single male laborers from the rural areas of the Philippines who were brought over by the U.S. government to work on plantations in Hawaii, farms in California, and canneries in Alaska. These men, unlike the more recent Filipino immigrants, endured much discrimination. They were considered "inassimilable," prevented from owning or leasing land, denied union membership, and banned from becoming U.S. citizens (Almirol, 1985; Bulosan, 1973; Catapusan, 1936, 1939, 1940; Kitano & Daniels, 1988; Lasker, 1931; McWilliams, 1964; Melendy, 1972). Filipino laborers in Hawaii called themselves the *sakadas* and were contract workers. Farm and domestic workers and others who worked menial jobs on the West Coast called themselves *pinoys* (Tompar-Tiu & Sustento-Seneriches, 1994). This group, referred to as **manongs** (older brothers) or "old-timers" by recent immigrants, is aging and frail. They bear the scars of their distressed past and humiliating experiences. Many remain traditional, poor, and without families (McBride, Mariola, & Yeo, 1995). In Hawaii and on parts of the West Coast, many *manongs* live in small rented rooms with a communal kitchen and bathroom, supplementing their meager incomes with whatever low-paying jobs they can find (Caringer, 1977).

The Filipinos who came during the second and third waves have fared better. The majority are highly educated professionals from the urban middle class, consisting of farm workers, students, World War II veterans and their families, U.S. Navy recruits at the height of the cold war, and young professionals. This middle-class exodus has resulted in a "brain drain" in the Philippines.

In the third wave, women outnumbered men by a large margin. Mostly professionals in health-care, education, and engineering, they were able to arrange employment and housing before immigrating. Thus, their need for support from family and kin who immigrated earlier became less important (Requisa, 1974). As they became economically stable and began to raise families, many brought their aging parents to the United States under the family reunification provisions of the present immigration law (McBride & Parreno, 1996; Yeo & McBride, 1995). With the declaration of martial law in 1972, Filipinos left the Philippines with tourist, business, student, and refugee visas to legally enter the United States, with hopes of converting their temporary visas into long-term immigrant status.

The last group of third-wave immigrants to arrive in the United States were 3000 to 4000 Filipino World War II veterans, who were granted citizenship without veterans benefits. Many settled on the West Coast, reluctantly supporting themselves with Supplemental Social Security Income (commonly referred to as SSI) and Medicaid. They continue to advocate for veterans benefits, refuse to consider themselves as welfare recipients, and search for ways to meet their primary goal of improving the future of their families in the Philippines (Chinn, 1993; McBride, 1993).

## Education Status and Occupations

For the majority of Filipino-Americans, educational status and employment are closely linked with their immigration history. Dropout rates are high in the younger generation, which is a serious concern for leaders in the Filipino community (Pilipino Mini-Health Forums Committee, 1993).

High educational attainment of native-born and immigrant Filipinos does not guarantee their entry into well-paying or high-status jobs (Almirol, 1985; Kuo, 1981; Pido, 1986). Many encounter difficulties finding jobs that match their education and experience. Competition in the labor market limits their success even when competing for low-level jobs for which many are overqualified (Pido, 1986). Teachers become salespeople or secretaries, accountants become clerks, and engineers become draftsmen or insurance agents. In a New Jersey study, although 52 percent of Filipino immigrants had undergraduate or graduate education, they worked in low-paying service jobs, such as office workers, salespersons, maintenance workers, bank tellers, or cashiers (Garde, Spangler, & Miranda, 1994). Only those educated in health-care fields found jobs that were consistent with their education. However, even those in health-care fields encounter a general lack of recognition of their college education, which has affected their career mobility. In the 1960s and 1970s, immigrant Filipino nurses were required to complete a course in American history and a language proficiency examination before they could take the professional licensing examination.

## COMMUNICATION

### Dominant Language and Dialects

Pilipino, or Tagalog, is the national language of the Philippines, and English is the second official language (Lamzon, 1978; Yraola-Westfall, 1986). Although the society is multilingual, eight languages or "dialects" are spoken by distinct ethnic groups. They are Tagalog (29.6 percent), Cebuano (24.2 percent), Ilocano (10.3 percent), Ilonggo (9.2 percent), Bicolano (3.5 percent), Waray (4 percent), Kapampangan (2.8 percent), and Pangasinenses (less than 1 percent) (Lamzon, 1978; Enriquez, 1994; Tompar-Tiu & Sustento-Seneriches, 1994).

Filipinos commonly conduct business in English, **Tagalog**, or "**Tag-Lish**," a combination of both languages mixed in the same sentence (Karnow, 1989; Pascacio, 1971; Yraola-Westfall, 1986). For example, a health instruction such as "Gamitin ang kapi na walang caffeine" may be used in client education. English is the language for school instruction beyond third grade, formal correspondence, meetings, political and business campaigns, and diplomacy (Karnow, 1989). Although many Filipinos speak English, the cadence and inflection of the English words are often influenced by their ethnic language or dialect.

Health-care providers may interact with Filipino immigrants from various regions of the Philippines who differ in their ability to enunciate the English language or have strong preferences for one of the Pilipino languages. In addition, Filipinos may converse only in English because of regional differences and the inability to speak Tagalog. However, Tag-Lish is a common practice among immigrants and American-born Filipinos and in local television programs. In multigenerational Filipino-American families, different languages may be used to communicate with family members and friends. Thus, part of the health assessment should include the language used between parents and their children, between adult children and their aging parents, and during other types of interactions.

Traditional Filipino communication is highly contextual. Many Filipinos are observant, displaying an intuitive feeling about the other person and the contextual environment during their interactions. Within the family, each member develops an intuitive knowledge of the other so that words are unnecessary to convey a message. A Filipino describing her upbringing said, "At home, we did not have to be told. One look from our father and we knew what he meant."

Filipinos accustomed to high-context communication are often puzzled and sometimes offended by the precision and exactness of American communication. They may respond in silence to Americans' need to know what they are thinking "in words." To many traditional Filipinos, actions speak louder than words. They value respect and might find questions like "Do you understand?" or "Do you follow?" disrespectful. Health-care workers should ask indirectly whether the Filipino client understands and have the person or family member do a return demonstration of a procedure or repeat an instruction rather than question his or her comprehension.

### Cultural Communication Patterns

Social scientists (Barnett, 1966; Eggan, 1971; Guthrie, 1971; Lynch, 1964) have observed that Filipino interpersonal and social life operates by indirection aimed at maintaining a smooth interpersonal relationship. According to Guthrie (1971) and Eggan (1971), Filipinos may sacrifice clear communication to avoid stressful interpersonal conflicts and confrontations.

Lynch (1964) introduced the phrase "smooth interpersonal relationship" to translate *pakikisama,* a Filipino value for getting along. Enriquez (1986, 1994), a Filipino social psychologist explains that *pakikipagkapwa,* or "being one with others," originates from the core value *kapwa* and is the superordinate Filipino value of relationships. Eight levels of social interactions for the concept *pakikipagkapwa* have been proposed. They fall within two domains: **Ibang tao** (external or outsider), a domain with five levels of interaction, and **Hindi Ibang Tao** (internal or one-of-us), a domain with three levels. Relationships may evolve within a hierarchical structure moving from *pakikitungo* (civility, level 1), *pakikisalimuha* (interacting, level 2), *pakikihalok* (participating, level 3), *pakikibagay* (conforming, level 4), *pakikisama* (adjusting, level 5), *pakikipagpalagayang loob* (understanding and accepting, level 6), *pakikisangkot* (getting involved, level 7), and *pakikiisa* (being one with, level 8) (Enriquez, 1986, 1994; McBride & Parreno, 1996; PePua, 1990; Enriquez & Santiago, 1976; Tompar-Tiu & Sustento-Seneriches, 1994). Achieving a working relationship with a Filipino-American may be possible at the point of *pakikilahok.* For example, a Filipino postsurgical client who agrees to ambulate for the first time is participating in the treatment plan. The health-care provider may think of the interaction as a threshold where other ambulating strategies might gradually be introduced. Qualitative clinical studies on Filipino-Americans using this interaction model are needed to further clarify and understand the process within the context of provider and client interactions.

In explaining Lynch's (1964) construct of smooth interpersonal relationship, Enriquez (1994) suggested that Lynch may have been successful in penetrating the highest level of social interaction for the *Ibang-Tao,* the outsider's domain. Although *pakikisama* is valid, it only explains a portion of Filipino social interaction values, which are established according to socially defined rules of behaviors. He proposed that *kapwa* (in which the closest English equivalent is "others") encompasses the categories of *sariling tao* (insider) and *ibang tao* (outsider) and depicts a person's ties with fellow human beings. Because of *kapwa's* importance, the Philippine language has two pronouns for the English "we": *tayo,* an inclusive we, and *kami,* an exclusive we.

While concern for others and maintaining good relationships may still be paramount to Filipinos residing in the United States, the insider and outsider delineations may be less important, especially among recent immigrants. Highly educated Filipino-Americans take pride in their outlook, perceiving themselves as global people. Unlike other immigrants who settle in ethnic enclaves, more recent Filipino immigrants acculturate, finding it easy to ally with people from various cultures (Awanohara, 1991).

Eye contact may vary among Filipino-Americans depending on the degree of acculturation, length of time in America, age, and education. Some individuals may avoid prolonged eye contact with authority figures and older persons as a form of respect. Older men may refrain from maintaining eye contact with young women because it may be interpreted as flirtation or a sexual advance (Orque, 1983). Filipinos are comfortable with silence and may allow the other person to initiate verbal interaction as a sign of respect. Nodding during a verbal interaction, such as client teaching, must be evaluated carefully. The nonverbal behavior may not always mean comprehension or agreement. The message may be "Yes, I hear you," "Yes, we are interacting," "Yes, I can see the instructions," or some other message that may be difficult for the person to disclose.

## Temporal Relationships

Filipinos, who represent an amalgam of many cultures, are relaxed in their temporal outlook. They have a healthy respect for the past, the ability to enjoy the present, and hope for the future. They are cognizant of their cultural history and draw much from their past. They enjoy their families, fiestas, and life and spend generously to make family events memorable and enjoyable. However, they are also ambitious and dream of the good life, which they believe can be realized through hard work, education, and some luck.

Filipinos refer to "Filipino time," which is a context-dependent approach to appointments or schedules. For social events and family gatherings, it is acceptable to be 1 to 2 hours late. However, a non-Filipino guest who arrives at the appointed time is warmly welcomed. The focus is on the gathering rather than on the schedule. While many Filipinos preserve this approach to time in social events, they adapt well to the American value of punctuality in their work lives.

## Format for Names

Filipinos use the same format for names as the Americans, where the given name comes first followed by the family name. The wife and children take the husband's family name (for example, Santos). The child uses the mother's last name as a middle name (for example, Kalaw) in addition to a true middle name (for example, Lucila). Thus, the name is recorded as *Maria Lucila Kalaw Santos*. This naming practice has a significant social value. Kinship and family affinity can be legally and spiritually claimed equally from both sets of families, giving the child the identity and extended family that assures a "good" future (Medina, 1991).

Many Filipino surnames are of Spanish origin, such as de la Cruz, Lopez, Villa, and so forth. Although the name Maria is often given to girls, some traditional Catholic families have used it for the first name of a male child followed by a male Christian name. Thus, a male name might be written in legal documents as *Ma. Santiago Kalaw Santos*. Early immigrants to the United States who experienced discrimination with Spanish surnames tried to protect their families by identifying with other racial groups on official documents such as census forms, thus influencing the sociopolitical development of the Filipino-American community. As interracial marriages occur among Filipino-Americans and the practice of adapting the male spouse's surname continues, one can expect more Filipino-Americans with surnames reflecting the ethnic origins of the father. Few Filipino-American women keep their own surname after marriage, although this may increase among the second-generation and third-generation Filipinos.

## FAMILY ROLES AND ORGANIZATION

### Head of Household and Gender Roles

Before the Spanish settlement of the Philippines, Filipino women were held in high regard, having rights equal to those of men (Agoncillo & Guerrero, 1987). In today's Filipino family, although the father is the acknowledged head of the household and naming is patronymic, authority in the family is considered egalitarian (Medina, 1991). The mother plays an equal role in decisions regarding health, welfare, and family finances.

Egalitarianism is also evidenced in gender-neutral Tagalog words such as *asawa*, "spouse"; *kapatid*, "brother or sister," *anak*, "son or daughter"; *manugang*, "child-in-law," and *biyenan*, "parent-in-law"; and in the absence of he or she pronouns. Gender is specified by indicating *anak na lalaki*, "male child or son" or *anak na babae*, "female child or daughter." The idealized Hispanicized Filipino woman is Maria Clara, a lady who epitomizes demureness, femininity, and modesty (Nakpil, 1978), created as a fictional character and perpetuated by the famous literary works of Jose Rizal. However, this image of womanhood has undergone major metamorphosis. While contemporary Filipino women in the Philippines maintain their femininity, they vigorously pursue formal education and careers. Since the 1950s, women represent close to 50 percent of university enrollments, with careers in medicine and law being customary. Traditional parents of second-generation Filipino-Americans tend to incorporate this belief system in their parenting roles.

## Prescriptive, Restrictive, and Taboo Behaviors for Children and Adolescents

The family and one's family role define and order authority, rights, obligations, and modes of interaction. *Galang,* or "respect," is a dominant value that is taught from childhood and practiced by many immigrant Filipino families. Maintaining respect is a sign of good upbringing and is manifested in words and in deeds. Within the family, seniority accords certain rights and obligations. For example, older siblings assume the role of second parents; in return, they can expect the respect of younger siblings. Friends of Filipino children are expected to greet adult members of the family when they visit.

The ultimate sign of respect is filial piety, "honor and respect for one's parents." Children are expected to show their respect by caring for their aging parents. To neglect this prime cultural value is to lose face and incur *hiya*, "shame."

Young daughters are advised that a short courtship period may suggest that she is "easy to get" and that a young man with sincere intent must strive to get on the good side of the family. Some immigrant Filipino mothers may have courtship histories of having been wooed through their parents and having bride gifts arranged before the wedding. Modernization, industrialization, and urbanization have changed the social mores in the Philippines, yet many Filipino-Americans families are still perceived by younger family members as having an overly protective attitude towards children in matters of "hanging out" with friends, dating, and courtship.

## Family Goals and Priorities

The Filipino family is predominantly monogamous. However, polygamous families exist among Moslem Filipinos. The basic kinship unit is the nuclear family, consisting of a father, a mother, and children. The family is consanguineous, keeping blood ties that extend to distant cousins, and bilateral by descent. This provides a close association of the children with relatives from both maternal and paternal family lines.

For the more acculturated family member, tensions and conflicts may arise when the preferred approach to caregiving is nontraditional. Superio (1993) reported that middle-aged immigrant Filipino parents raising families on the West Coast indicate that they do not expect to live with their children in their old age. In contrast, a younger group of immigrant and native-born Filipinos believe that children should take care of their elderly parents.

Education is of paramount importance to the Filipino family and is seen as an important mechanism for professional and social advancement. Many families, especially in the Philippines, sacrifice to help their eldest sons or daughters obtain an education leading to a well-paying job. Older children who have received their education are obligated to help younger siblings obtain theirs. Parents who have been successful in sending their children to college proudly display framed diplomas in their living rooms. Some families even exhibit printed signage of children's degrees so neighbors and others can see the accomplishments of their children.

Education and democracy, the American legacy to Philippine society, served to attenuate the authoritarian and hierarchical approach to setting societal norms acquired from the Spanish influence of 300 years. In whatever form the Western influence expresses itself in the Filipino culture, there is a pervading attitude that acquiring Western ways (that is, the ways of white American culture) is a legitimate achievement. Having a "stateside (American) education," marrying a *Kano* or *puti* (American or white), and having facility with American slang may create a veneer of a Westernized image for many Filipino immigrants that may be puzzling to someone who is unfamiliar with the culture.

Respect for self and others, especially for those who are older and those in positions of authority, is highly valued. Respect is shown in deferential behavior for one's elders, who may be only a few years older. This basic value is expressed in kinship hierarchical terms of respect for older brothers and sisters: *kuya,* "eldest brother"; *dikong, sangko,* and *singko,* "next three older brothers"; and *ate(i),* "eldest sister," *ditse, sanse,* and *sinse,* "next three older sisters"; *na,* "aunts or older women"; *ta,* "uncles or older men." A young person who disagrees with an older person does not answer back. Extreme familiarity with older persons or persons in positions of authority meets with disapproval.

In the field of gerontology, Filipino elders who came after 1965 are referred to as "followers of adult children" (McBride & Parreno, 1996; McBride, Mariola, & Yeo, 1995). They resettled in America to be with their families, expecting to have a significant role in the household; however, this seldom happens. Many find their lives different from what they anticipated; experiencing culture shock and being unable to drive cause many to feel isolated and lonely. Almost all social activities are with families and close friends. Community and cultural events that elders enjoyed in the Philippines may not be available in the area where they live. Many multigenerational Filipino households have both parents working, and the grandparents become babysitters or surrogate parents for their grandchildren. Many accept this role gladly, whereas others feel the need to be more independent from their family. This dependency may cause a Filipino elder to miss medical appointments because of transportation problems or to not take prescribed medications because the elder may not want to discuss the transportation problems or expenses with the adult child.

In the extended family network, blood relatives often extend to third cousins with a clear structure and network of relationships. In addition to blood relations, it is possible to establish relationships through religious ceremonies such as baptism

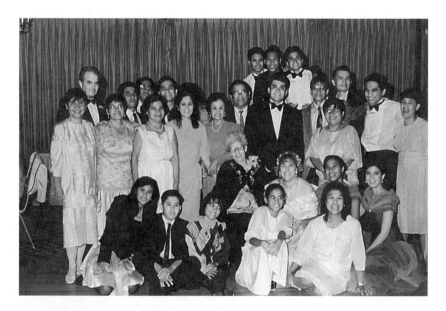

**Figure 10–1.** Three generations of Filipino-Americans celebrate a wedding.

and marriage. Filipino-Americans who left families or relatives in their home country forge close relationships through these ceremonies. Friends are often asked to be the godparents of their children. During times of illness, the extended family provides support and assistance. Sometimes a family visit to the hospital takes on the semblance of a family reunion. Fortunately, most institutions tolerate these visits, and a few even appreciate the therapeutic value of supportive relationships. Hospital rules regarding visitors should be examined on an individual basis, considering the family's cultural values.

Although a disparity between the rich and the poor persists among Filipinos, democratic values nurture hopes that everyone, regardless of their initial station in life, can advance to a higher social strata. An advanced degree is viewed as the means of obtaining higher social status.

## Alternative Lifestyles

Although the literature reports no studies specific to alternative lifestyles for Filipino-Americans, homosexual relationships probably occur at a frequency similar to that in the rest of society. With the high rates of human immunodeficiency virus (HIV) infection among Filipinos, culturally specific education geared to the unique needs of Filipinos is needed. Some intervention for the gay and lesbian community is available through the Filipino Task Force on AIDS in San Francisco. In addition, the office of the Philippine Ministry of Health has developed community acquired immunodeficiency syndrome (AIDS) education programs.

Although sex education is seldom provided by parents in the Philippines, chastity is valued and young women are expected to remain virgins until marriage. The tenets of the Catholic Church have a direct bearing on sexual mores for Filipino-Americans, yet in a report to the San Francisco Health Commission, the incidence of teenage pregnancy is high among Filipino youth. The majority of Filipino parents do not provide sex education at home (Medina, 1991), which may partially explain pregnancy rates among Filipino-American teens.

## WORKFORCE ISSUES

### Culture in the Workforce

Filipinos who are observant, adaptable, ambitious, and intelligent quickly learn how to meld their values with the values and expectations of the mainstream culture and workforce. In a study of Filipino nurses in New York (Spangler, 1991a), one nurse described the immigrant acculturation experience as follows:

> I must mention that our appearance influences our adjustment. We can change some of our outlook, our values, but we cannot change our looks, our accents. No matter how egalitarian Americans claim to be, we know that they are not color blind. Americans feel that they are advanced. They sometimes look down on people who come from the third world where technology and economic resources are not great. We on the other hand are here to better ourselves, not unlike the ancestors of the Americans who look down on us now. We are the new kid on the block who must prove himself *[sic]*. We work hard. We put up with a lot more because we want to be accepted. We learn to adjust. It is not that we feel inferior, but we are aware that we are different. We were brought up differently and some of our values are different. In the process of adjusting, we evaluate what values to keep and what American ways we should adapt. It [acculturation] is a slow process. Despite the pain, you stay open. As you gain confidence, you are able to draw from yourself

and your traditions again. You learn that there are some things from your ways that are good and can be blended with the new. (p. 208)

Although the 1965 Immigration Act brought many Filipino nurses to the United States, most of them practice in tertiary health-care systems or acute care hospitals in urban areas. Negligible numbers are in advanced practice and primary care settings where the need is greatest. The Philippine Nurses Association of America (PNAA) is redirecting Filipino nurses to primary care, assisting them to obtain graduate degrees, and preparing them to work in primary care settings.

Some barriers to gaining employment are language and experience. Some allegations are made that employing foreigners takes jobs away from Americans. The barriers to equitable employment become especially acute during periods of economic retrenchment. As immigrants, Filipinos often believe that they have fewer rights or at least have no grounds to complain about their situation in the United States. After all, they reason, they have voluntarily chosen to immigrate, and as nonwhites, they are likely to be subjected to discrimination (Pido, 1986; Spangler, 1991a).

## Issues Related to Autonomy

Although Filipinos speak, write, and understand English, their pronunciation may inhibit their ability to convey ideas clearly. In a study of Filipino and European-American nurses in a New York hospital, language difference was one of the major sources of conflicts between groups (Spangler, 1991a, 1992, 1993). The European-American nurses complained that the Filipino nurses were cliquish and isolated themselves by speaking Tagalog. The Filipino nurses asserted that they spoke Tagalog only when no other cultural groups were present. They further stated that they did not want to exclude or offend others when they spoke Tagalog; however, they expressed a need to speak in their native language to articulate their ideas, feelings, and humor among themselves.

The hierarchical authoritarian structure of the Philippine cultural system is reflected in Filipinos' interactions with people in authority positions. In the Philip-

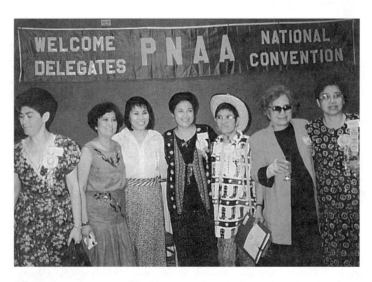

**Figure 10–2.** Filipino nurses have been recruited from the 1950s through the 1990s. These nurses are attending a national convention of the Philippine Nurses Association of America in San Antonio, Texas.

pines, positions in society may be acquired by wealth, education, marriage, a distinguished position, or by biologic age. Although this value has weakened among younger Filipinos, respect for the elderly and those in positions of power is firmly entrenched among most Filipinos.

Within traditional upbringing, Filipinos are taught not to answer back or show open disagreement. Studies (Beyers, 1979; Miraflor, 1976; Spangler, 1991a, b) report that Filipino nurses are reluctant to question physicians or administrators. Americans who uphold egalitarianism and candid expression of feelings and ideas are perplexed by the Filipino deference to authority. The less acculturated Filipino may not understand the directness of Americans and, thus, may find it insulting. In Spangler's (1991a, b) study, European-American nurses saw the quiet, observant, tactful, patient, and slow-to-respond behaviors of Filipino nurses as unassertive. The Filipino nurses saw outspoken, impatient, bold, and fast-moving behaviors of European-American nurses as crass and insensitive. A Filipino may say "yes" to avoid hurting other people's feelings. Pascacio (1971) suggested that a Filipino's response of yes must be examined in context to interpret its true meaning.

Filipinos are proud people, and it is important to maintain *amor propio,* "pride" and dignity by saving face and avoiding *hiya,* or "shame." Their delicacy, sensitivity, and attention to other people's feelings are often exhibited as indecisiveness, which many Americans interpret as lack of assertiveness.

## BIOCULTURAL ECOLOGY

### Skin Color and Other Biologic Variations

Given the ethnic, cultural, and racial intermingling among Filipinos dating back at least 40,000 years, the genetic composition of Filipinos varies. Thus, the health-care provider must keep in mind a range of anthropomorphic, physical, and biophysiological characteristics of Filipinos.

Some common physical features are jet black to brunette or light brown hair, dark to light brown pupils with eyes set in almond-shaped eyelids, deep brown to very light tan skin tones due to high melanin content, and mildly flared nostrils and slightly low to flat nosebridge. The eye structure may challenge health-care providers when observing pupillary reactions for increased intracranial pressure, measuring ocular tension, evaluating peripheral vision, and other assessments involving the eye. The flat nosebridge may be overlooked by opticians when fitting and dispensing eyeglasses. The high melanin content in the integumentary system and mucosa may pose problems for health-care providers when assessing jaundice, cyanosis, and pallor and when diagnosing retinal abnormalities and gum-related or oral tissue problems.

Health-care professionals performing skin assessments should consider the complexion and skin tone of the Filipino client. Anemia, which is usually manifested by pallor and jaundice, may be better assessed in the conjunctiva. Newborns may have Mongolian spots, bluish-green discolorations, on their buttocks, which are normal and eventually disappear.

Physical size ranges from under 5 feet to the size of the average American. One of the Filipino ancestral ethnic tribes, the Aeta, is negroid and petite in stature. They are believed to have migrated from Africa through land bridges during the Ice Age *(Philippine Statistical Yearbook,* 1995). However, like other tribal groups in the Philippines, they are now a numerical minority. The typical native-born or immigrant Filipino in the United States may be of Malay stock (brown complexion) with blended multiracial genetic background. It is important to note that intermarriage or consanguineous relationships between Filipinos and persons from African-American, Asian Pacific Islander, European-American, Spanish, and Native-American backgrounds occur among many Filipino communities across North America. In clinical assessments, a family genogram identifying ethnic or racial blending is useful in tracking predisposition to genetic disorders.

Body weight varies according to nativity; length of stay in North America; and factors tied to nutrition, physical activity, and heredity. No definitive Filipino studies relate nutrition and standard height and weight measures for this population in America. Therefore, it is essential to assess for weight changes.

The youthful facial features of Filipinos are a frequent first impression that non-Filipino observers have of this group. Physical signs of aging may not readily provide the health-care provider with an estimate of biologic age.

Approximately 40 percent of Filipinos have blood type B and a low incidence of the Rh-negative factor (Anderson, 1983). As more interracial families emerge in the Filipino-American community, their serologic profile can be expected to change.

## Diseases and Health Conditions

Endemic diseases in the Philippines are related to the natural terrain and climate. The tropical climate increases risks for malaria, pneumonia, tuberculosis, and gastrointestinal diseases associated with bacteria and parasites. Injuries and physical disabilities occur during natural disasters such as tropical storms, volcanic eruptions, and coastal flooding. The leading causes of mortality and morbidity are pneumonia, tuberculosis, heart disease, diarrheal diseases, cancer, cerebrovascular accidents, traumatic accidents, bronchitis, and nutritional deficiencies (Anderson, 1983).

On the basis of the limited scientific literature on health risk factors among Filipinos in the United States, immigrants are at high risk for developing coronary heart disease, hypertension, and diabetes at midlife and old age (Anderson, 1983; Gerber, 1980; Nora & McBride, 1996; Stavig, Igra, & Leonard, 1988; McBride, Mariola, & Yeo, 1995), renal stones and hyperuricemia, and gout (Guillermo, 1993). A shift from a traditional Filipino diet to an American diet increases the occurrence of hyperuricemia, with some older Filipinos developing gout (McBride, Mariola, & Yeo, 1995). Breast, cervical, prostate, thyroid, lung, and liver cancers are major threats to this population. A high prevalence of late-stage breast and cervical cancers at diagnosis has been reported for Filipino women in the northern California region (Northern California Cancer Center, 1990, 1991). Liver cancer tends to be diagnosed in the late stages of the disease and appears to be associated with the presence of the hepatitis B virus. Silent carriers of the virus are common among Asians, and its presence is detected only when other problems are being evaluated. Health-care providers should routinely screen for hepatitis B virus, especially among recent immigrants. A high incidence of glucose-6-phosphate dehydrogenase, $\alpha$-thalassemia, and lactose intolerance and malabsorption exists among the Filipino population (Anderson, 1983).

A study assessing cardiovascular risk factors of Asians in California shows that Filipino men and women have the highest prevalence of hypertension when compared to the Chinese, Japanese, and other Asians (Klatsky & Armstrong, 1991). In a New Jersey study (Garde, Spangler, & Miranda, 1994), 23 percent of the 262 respondents reported hypertension. A health survey of 89 newly arrived Filipino World War II veterans, aged 62 to 86, identified hypertension and arthritis as their major health concerns (McBride, 1993).

## Variations in Drug Metabolism and Interaction

In aggregate data of pharmacological research on Asians, Levy (1993) reported that Asians require lower doses of neuroleptic drugs such as haloperidol than do whites. In addition, Asians are more sensitive to the adverse effects of alcohol than are whites (Levy, 1993). Araneta (1993) suggested that Filipino-Americans have a lower tolerance for alcohol. More research is needed to determine pharmacodynamics among Filipinos, including gender differences. Thus, health-care providers need to assess each person individually when administering and monitoring medication therapies for Filipino-Americans.

## HIGH-RISK BEHAVIORS

Filipinos show a greater tolerance and acceptance of high-risk health behaviors related to alcohol, drugs, cigarettes, and sex among Filipino men than among women. Although alcohol was identified as a popular drink at social gatherings, in the PNAA's study of Filipino health behaviors in New Jersey, 67 percent of respondents reported that they did not drink alcohol. Only 1 percent reported having three or more drinks per day (Garde, et al., 1994). A study of drinking patterns among Filipinos, Chinese, and Japanese in California reveals that men from all three ethnicities have roughly the same percentage of heavy drinkers (28 percent), whereas less than 4 percent of Filipino women are heavy drinkers (Chi & Kitano, 1989). Because denial is closely associated with alcoholism, the frequency and the amount of alcohol imbibed is generally underreported. Thus, the actual number of users may be slightly higher than reported but probably still lower in comparison with the Western standard.

Cigarette smoking is more prevalent among Filipino men than women, although the rates varied for each study (Burns & Pierce, 1992; Klatsky & Armstrong, 1991). Factors that may influence smoking rates include limited education and personal income of less than $15,000 (Garde, et al., 1995); tendency to think or speak in a Filipino language (Asian American Health Forum, 1991); and, for females, being born in the United States. In San Francisco, the majority of the Filipino youth reported living with an adult who smoked, and their first substance of choice was cigarettes followed by alcohol and inhalants (Pilipino Mini-Health Forums Committee, 1993).

The incidence of AIDS among Asians has increased in the past few years. Filipinos have the highest incidence of AIDS among Asian Pacific Islanders living in San Francisco, New York, and Los Angeles. At risk are American-born Filipino youth. Low knowledge scores on HIV transmission underscores the urgency of HIV and AIDS education. Unprotected sex with multiple partners requires immediate intervention for AIDS prevention (Gock, 1994).

### Health-seeking Behaviors

Studies related to health-seeking behaviors among early Filipino-American immigrants report that they do not seek health care until the illness is quite advanced (Anderson, 1983; Caringer, 1977). Aside from culture, their social and economic circumstances may have more to do with underutilization of health services. Early Filipino immigrants were prevented from joining the cultural mainstream. They were poor when they came to the United States, and many remained poor and felt shunned and rejected as they grew older. Being part of the ethnically underserved elderly population in American, many are unaware of or feel reluctant to access social and health services, particularly when culturally sensitive, bilingual providers are unavailable (Nora & McBride, 1996; McBride, Mariola, & Yeo, 1995). Lack of transportation, fear of the area where services are located, and inappropriate program design may be other reasons for low utilization rates for many underserved Filipinos (Pilipino Mini-Health Committee, 1993).

A study of newer Filipino immigrants contrasts significantly with information on early Filipino immigrants. For example, in the New Jersey study, 78 percent of Filipinos had private or prepaid health insurance, 10 percent were on Medicare or Medicaid, and 7 percent had no insurance. Participants reported seeing a health-care provider at least every year. Only 2 percent had not seen a physician for more than 5 years (Garde, Spangler, & Miranda, 1994). However, a group of older widowed Filipino women living in New York compared their functional capacity with that of peers to determine their level of wellness and possible need for health-care services (Valencia-Go, 1989). The differences are likely due to variations in education, income, adjustment to the host culture, and acculturation experiences. Encouraging a Filipino-American client to identify and describe the formal and informal resources that are accessed for health promotion can provide the health-care provider with a more realistic profile of the person's current health practices.

## NUTRITION

### Meaning of food

Fernandez (1986) provides an in-depth exploration of food and the meaning of food among Filipinos. Food is more than nourishment for the body; it is a fundamental form of socialization. Food punctuates life and celebrations in both the Philippines and the United States. Whether eating a small sandwich or a feast, the more traditional Filipino may feel compelled to invite others to share it. A lunch pack may be prepared for the possibility of sharing lunch with a coworker.

### Common Foods and Food Rituals

Food, viewed as *biyaya ng lupa,* "bounty of the earth," is to be savored fresh with little adulteration. The indigenous cuisine before Spanish and American influences used boiling, steaming, roasting, broiling, or sour stewing to preserve the fresh and natural taste of food. *Sawsawan,* "sauces," which are generally salty, include *patis, bagoong,* soy sauce, and sour vinegar with tomatoes, garlic, pepper, and sliced green mango served as side dishes. Filipino chefs view cooking as a partnership between the cook and the diner. They often remark, "Why drown the fresh taste in heavy sauces?" The chef's role is to preserve and bring out the freshest natural-occurring taste of the food. The diner's role is to complete the chef's creation by using sauces to taste.

The sense of obligation to share food is strong in the Filipino's home and takes on a certain ritual. Anyone who arrives at mealtime or other times when food is being served is offered some. Even more symbolic is the food served to guests. Guests, who are considered *ibang tao,* are served Western food like bread; *relleno,* "roasted chicken"; and *paella,* "Spanish rice with saffron, sausages, and seafood." *Hindi ibang tao* are served native cuisines like *sinigang* with *sawsawan,* "boiled meat or fish"; *paksiw,* "sour stew"; or *inihaw,* "broiled dishes." A guest's being allowed to help in the kitchen is an expression of acceptance, *sariling tao,* or "one of us." The expression *hindi ka na bisita,* "you are no longer a guest," means inclusion into the insiders' circle.

In highly agricultural regions of the Philippines, a heavy breakfast of rice, meat, or fish and vegetable dishes or dinner leftovers is preferred because of heavy farm work. The breakfast beverage may be coffee, chocolate, or *kapi,* a special brew from roasted rice. In urban areas, Western-style meals are more common, and breakfast may include eggs, sausages, *ensaimada* (Spanish sweet pastry), and rice. For many Filipinos, breakfast, lunch, and dinner are not complete without steamed or fried rice served with fish, meat, especially pork, and vegetables.

Except for babies and young children, milk is almost absent in the adult Filipino diet, partly due to lactose intolerance. However, milk in desserts such as the *leche plan,* "egg custard," and ice cream seems to be tolerated. Snacks of bananas, yams, *sweet bibingka* (rice cake), *puto bumbong* (rice flour cake), and others are served as *merienda*, "midday snacks between meals and before bedtime." Salt and vinegar are popular ingredients used to preserve meat and fish because cold storage is not readily available to many households in the Philippines. The high incidence of hypertension among immigrant Filipinos may be associated with high intake of salt and animal (pork) fat (Nora & McBride, 1996).

Because of the tropical climate of the Philippines, many types of plant and animal life flourish on the land and in the waters. The waters constitute the most immediate source of food for the everyday Filipino diet, which revolves around fish and seafood. Filipinos tend to have particular standards to determine freshness of fish, that is, a fresh fish is a live fish. Fish on ice is considered inferior and purchased only if live fish is unavailable. Animals, especially cows and water buffalo, are used for farming more than for food. After fish, chicken and pork are common sources of animal protein. Special delicacies are made with goat meat in certain regions. As in many Asian countries, dog meat is considered a delicacy by some Filipinos. In farms and villages, children and adults may drink fresh milk from water buffalo and goat, but canned evaporated milk and canned sweetened concentrated milk are easily available to families throughout the country. Some poor families may add water to canned milk.

Plant life is the second most important food source in the Philippines, including a variety of seaweeds, edible roots, delicate leaves, tendrils, tropical fruits, seeds, and some flowers. The contemporary Filipino palate prefers simple and fresh dishes that have been adapted to the Chinese, Spanish, and American cuisines. Regional variations in food preparation and use of spices are practices that may be found in Filipino-American households today. Nutrition counseling should take into account these variations when a Filipino needs to alter dietary patterns because of hypertension, diabetes, or other health problems.

## Dietary Practices for Health Promotion

Filipinos believe that health is maintained by moderation. Although Filipinos enjoy food and love to eat, they adhere to the wisdom that too much of a good thing can be harmful. In some parts of the Philippines, it is considered polite to leave food on one's plate. For many Filipino-Americans, moderation in food intake is a special challenge. Better-quality products, easy access, and multiple choices at reasonable costs create difficult situations for new immigrants. Often, significant change in weight and dietary patterns are observed in the early years among new immigrants.

The abundance of plant life provides many medicinal plants and herbs for people in the Philippines. Filipino households may keep potted medicinal plants that are used for common colds, stomach upsets, urinary tract infections, and other minor ailments. Many of these plants are soothing, or innocuous at best, and serve as comfort herbs. Garlic and fresh ginger root are most popular. Unfortunately, very few of these plants have been analyzed for their medicinal qualities. However, use of certain herbs and spices continues to be popular among immigrants and their families.

## Nutritional Deficiencies and Food Limitations

The nutritional status of Filipinos, especially in the Philippines, is greatly affected by economic factors and social class. Nutritional deficiencies are common among the poor and less educated. Access to land that the poor depended on to grow food has diminished greatly, in part due to global export industries that are often controlled by a few affluent families and large international corporations.

In the United States, many Filipino immigrants may be at risk for nutritional deficiencies during their adjustment period, especially when they come with limited resources and without a support network of family and friends. Some of the groups who may be at risk for nutritional deficiencies include the **manongs** who live in substandard housing, World War II veterans who lack benefits, patients with AIDS who lack a support network, and infants and toddlers of families with both parents working who are being raised by aging, less educated, immigrant grandparents. Knowledge about nutrients in American food products, Filipino dishes served at mealtime and *merienda,* and sources of baseline knowledge on nutrition are important data to include in nutritional assessment to determine nutritional risk.

Indigenous Filipino foods are readily available in Asian-American stores. Many cities on the East and West Coasts and the Midwest have Filipino stores and restaurants that provide native and Westernized Filipino foods. Although these places offer many of the exotic plants and tropical fruits not ordinarily found in American grocery stores, they are not able to supply the variety of fresh live fish that is harvested from the Philippine waters. However, frozen, salted, and dried or smoked fish are available.

## PREGNANCY AND CHILDBEARING PRACTICES

### Fertility Practices and Views toward Pregnancy

The Catholic faith of Filipinos influences their beliefs and practices related to fertility. In marriage, the only accepted mode of contraception is the rhythm method. Abortion is considered a sin and generally not supported. While these beliefs have a stronghold on many Filipinos, education, global communication, and modernization are changing these convictions, particularly in metropolitan cities such as Manila. Recent Filipino immigrants who come from large urban areas are more educated and less committed to the Catholic church's position on birth control and premarital sex. Being a child-centered culture, abortion evokes strong reactions even to a liberal Filipino-American. Some may support the right to get an abortion but may have difficulty and feel guilty in considering this option for themselves.

Pregnancy is considered normal and is a time when a woman can demand attention, pampering, and solicitude from her husband and family members. Healthcare providers who do not understand this special period for the pregnant Filipino woman have commented on the laziness of their pregnant Filipino clients (Stern, 1985). Pregnancy and childbirth is a time for the Filipino family to draw closer together. Everyone assists in anticipation of the new baby, especially the pregnant woman's mother, who has great influence during this period. For mother and daughter, this is a special event in which the bond between them becomes closer. In the Filipino-American community, women openly give advice to pregnant women, share their own birthing experiences, and ask personal questions that may be considered rather intrusive by someone who is unfamiliar with the culture.

### Prescriptive, Restrictive, and Taboo Practices in the Childbearing Family

Filipino practices surrounding pregnancy are influenced by Westernized practices. In the Philippines, most pregnant women are willing to see health-care providers who received training in Western obstetrics, nursing, and midwifery. Pregnant women are followed and monitored during their prenatal period by community health nurses. The expectant mother may also consult the local **hilot**, "massage therapist," for physical, spiritual, and psychological advice and guidance. Although these health-care providers are trained in Western methods, they are sensitive and cognizant of the folk health beliefs and practices related to pregnancy, childbirth, and the postpartum period. For example, pregnant mothers are cautioned against taking medications, which are believed to harm the fetus. Stern (1985) reported that pregnant Filipino women in California refused to take vitamins because they were afraid that vitamins could deform the fetus.

Some believe that when pregnant women crave certain foods, especially during the first trimester, the craving should be satisfied to avoid harm to the baby. Filipino-Americans may continue to believe that the baby takes on the appearance of the craved food. Thus, if the mother craves dark-skinned fruit or dark-colored food, the infant's skin will be dark. Pregnant women are protected from sudden fright or stress because of the belief that this may harm the developing fetus. Becoming aware of the pregnant Filipino woman's network of family and community health advisors whose opinions she respects is important for building trust and rapport in the client-provider relationship.

Most women in the Philippines give birth in hospitals or periculture centers, small birthing centers prevalent in smaller cities, although home birthing is still practiced. Therefore, recent immigrants can be expected to be familiar with child-birth in a hospital. Some women prefer to have their mothers rather than their husbands in the delivery room. The mother of the pregnant woman serves as coach and teacher. The daughter defers to her mother's experience and knowledge. Indeed, the mother may have more influence on her pregnant daughter than the health-care professional. This may be puzzling to the professional, who views pregnancy as an emancipating event. Conflicts are likely to occur if the coach and teacher believes in practices that are contrary to Western childbearing practices. After childbirth, pampering of the new mother continues. Relatives help with the new baby and in running the household. Lactating mothers are encouraged to take plenty of soup, especially chicken soup, because it is believed to induce milk production. Showers are not encouraged for this may cause *pasma ng ugat* (arthritis). However, a sponge bath with aromatic oils and herbs is given by the woman's mother, or a *hilot* gives an aromatic herbal steam bath followed by full body massage including the abdominal muscles, stimulating a physiological reaction that has both physical and psychological benefits. Filipino women who experience this special attention after childbirth talk with nostalgia about this traditional ceremonial practice that is a rarity in many Filipino-American communities.

# DEATH RITUALS

## Death Rituals and Expectations

After a death, a wake is planned. The wake may last from 3 days to 1 week (to wait for the arrival of a relative) and is usually held in the home, although funeral parlors are used in Filipino-American communities. Families and friends gather to give support and recall the special traits of the deceased. Food is provided to all guests throughout the wake and after the burial.

The burial rites are consistent with the religious traditions of the family, which may be Judeo-Christian, Muslim, Buddhist, or other religions. When resources are available among Catholic families, 9 days of **pabasa,** "novenas," are held in the home or in the church. These special prayers ask God's blessing for the deceased. Food and refreshments are served after each prayer day. Sometimes the last day of the novena takes on the atmosphere of a *fiesta* or a celebration. Filipino families in the United States follow variations of this ritual according to their social and economic circumstances.

On the first-year anniversary of the death, family and friends are reunited in prayer to celebrate this memorable event. Most Filipino women wear black clothing for months or up to a year after the death. The one-year anniversary ends ritualistic mourning. Memories and love for the deceased continue to be manifested during All Soul's Day, a Catholic feast day, when families visit and decorate the graves of their loved ones. Filipino-American families may continue these traditions, particularly when strong kinship is present and the clan lives in close proximity. Many who die in the United States are buried in the Philippines; thus, the tradition is continued by the family in that country.

Beliefs related to cremation vary according to individual preference. Ordinarily, bodies are buried, but cremation is acceptable to avoid the spread of disease. In America, some Filipinos who wish to return their deceased family members to the Philippines may choose cremation for practical and economic reasons.

## Response to Death and Grief

Death, as in most cultures, is greeted with much sorrow. The expression of grief varies from region to region and by socioeconomic class. The affluent, educated classes have learned to moderate their expressions of grief, but many Filipinos still accept emotional outbursts of grief exhibited through uncontrolled crying. Sometimes fainting is a common bereavement practice.

## SPIRITUALITY

### Religious Practices and Use of Prayer

Considered the only Christian country in the Far East, the Philippines is about 80 percent Christian, of which 90 percent is Roman Catholic. Membership in the *Iglesia ni Christo* and the *Aglipay* churches is gradually increasing, and a small minority of Filipinos are returning to their ancestral religion **Bathala**, God worship with a *babaylan*, "spiritual guide or priest," usually a woman (Enriquez, 1994; Tompar-Tiu & Sustento-Seneriches, 1994). About 4 percent of the population practices Islam, including traveling to the Middle East to observe religious traditions (Nora & McBride, 1996; Pido, 1986; Tompar-Tiu & Sustento-Seneriches, 1994).

With the introduction of Christianity in the Philippines, the people adapted and reshaped the new religion to fit their ancient rituals. Some of these are the *moro-moro* (folk religious drama), *santakrusan* (May religious celebration), *moriones* (elaborate and colorful masks depicting the crucifixion of Christ), and others. Many contemporary Filipinos have a personal and intimate relationship with their religion, which is a source of strength in their daily lives.

Although Filipinos seek medical care, they believe that part of the efficacy of a cure is in God's hands or by some mystical power. Novenas and prayers are often made on behalf of the sick person. Families may bring religious items such as rosaries, medals, scapulars, and *anting anting* (talismans) for the sick person to wear. Health-care workers must be sensitive to the needs of those who express their faith in God or a spiritual power in this manner.

### Meaning of Life and Individual Sources of Strength

Some Filipinos are considered fatalistic in that they tend to accept fate easily, especially when they feel they can do little about a situation. However, acceptance of fate or destiny emanates from their close relationship and healthy respect for nature. Living in islands that are subjected to the whims of nature, Filipinos have known earthquakes, torrential monsoons, cataclysmic tides, and volcanic eruptions. These natural adversities are but the other face of the natural blessings that include temperate climate and rich flora and fauna, for which they are grateful. Therefore, they accept the blessings and banes of nature with equanimity.

The acceptance of events they cannot change is tied to their religious faith. A common expression uttered by Filipinos is *bahala na*, originating from *bathala na*, "it is up to God." Enriquez (1994) explained that *bahala na* is often used when the person has used all resources to deal with a problem, and it is up to a higher power to take care of the rest. Nevertheless, there is an element of individualism among Filipinos, manifested by being confident that the situation is within their sphere of influence. An excellent example is Filipinos' belief in the ability of education to change their lives.

To the ancient Filipinos, nature was a living force, holding the divine and magical properties of nature, other humans, and ancestor gods. To the traditional Filipino, strength comes from an intimate relationship with God, family, friends, neighbors, and nature. The concept of self is formed from the relationship with a divine being and the social collective. Thus, the self is an important extension of the gods, fellow beings, and nature.

## Spiritual Beliefs and Health-care Practices

Deeply religious Filipinos believe that events, including illness, happen for reasons that they often entrust to God or a higher power. While they believe in objective causes of diseases and in personal responsibility for one's wellness and illness (for example, exposing oneself to illness), the predominant belief may be that something happens because it is the "will of God." Others believe in the power of good spirits to sustain health or to eliminate illness and evil spirits that induce illness.

## HEALTH-CARE PRACTICES

## Health-seeking Beliefs and Practices

Beliefs about health and illness include indigenous and modernistic views. Filipinos who have benefited from the Western public health system are receptive to modern medicine along with folk health beliefs and practices. Thus, a dual system of personal health care exists for many Filipinos, including those who are established in American communities. The differentiation between formal and informal behaviors extends to biomedical knowledge and interaction with health-care workers. On the formal level, Filipinos may accept and adhere to medical recommendations. On the informal level, they may use alternative sources of care. Very often, they adhere to Western medicine and indigenous medicine simultaneously, creating more choices to deal with their own or their family's health issues.

The central traditional Philippine health concepts are balance and moderation. Health is the result of balance, and illness is the consequence of imbalance. Imbalances that threaten health are thought to be brought about by personal irresponsibilities or irregularities. Prudent care of the body through adequate sleep, rest, nutrition, and exercise is essential for staying healthy. A high value is also placed on personal cleanliness. Keeping oneself clean and free of unpleasant body odors is viewed as good for one's health and face-saving. To be slovenly and disorderly is to be shamelessly irresponsible (Anderson, 1983). Aromatic baths are taken both for pleasure and to restore balance.

Traditional Filipinos believe that people reap what they sow—that everything balances out. If one foments negativity, injustice, or untruths, the venom created is greater within oneself than in the person to which the malice is directed. Illness can therefore be self-induced or may thus occur as a divine retribution. Responsibility, moderation, and clear conscience are keys to good health.

## Responsibility for Health Care

The germ theory is part of the Filipino's beliefs about disease causation, but this view is moderated by the concept of host susceptibility and timing (Himes, 1971). Timing is not always under a person's control, but host susceptibility is something one can control through the practice of regularity and balance. Thus, the indigenous interpretation of the germ theory incorporates an inherent value for personal responsibility, using one's resources to their limits, then allowing a higher power to resolve a health problem or health crisis.

Parents may seek all possible assistance that they can personally generate from family, friends, the church, community, and the formal health-care system (often in that order) for a child who has cancer, eventually accepting the inevitability of death. From a Western perspective, the outcome may be slightly different than if formal services were accessed as early as possible. As Himes (1971) noted, belief in accidental causation is paramount. Filipinos do not see themselves as victims, but rather as part of the larger cosmos, subject to both the controllable and uncontrollable forces of nature.

In the Philippines, it is possible to buy nearly all types of medicines without a prescription. Many Filipinos informally consult a physician, nurse, pharmacist, or neighbor who had similar symptoms. Once the person finds the brand name of the "effective" medicine, the person can easily purchase the drug. Bringing a supply of medicines from the Philippines, asking family or friends to purchase medication in the Philippines, hoarding prescription drugs, and sharing medicine may be practiced by Filipinos in the United States (Pilipino Mini-Health Committee, 1993). Those who do not believe in wastefulness or those who believe that office visits are expensive may choose to engage in these behaviors.

When educating Filipino-American clients about medication, health-care professionals should stress that medications need to be taken as prescribed, medications are ordered specifically for each ailment, unused drugs should be discarded, and the use of medications by persons other than the intended may have serious consequences. Assessing these behaviors and delivering the message in a respectful, courteous, and unhurried manner may enhance the client-provider relationship, especially for traditional Filipino clients.

## Barriers to Health Care

Early studies of Filipinos in the United States indicate that Filipinos generally do not seek care for an illness until it is quite advanced. The reasons for not seeking early medical care are many. Some take minor ailments stoically and consider them natural imbalances that will run their normal course and disappear. Others claim to watch the progress of their illness so that the appropriate health-care provider can be consulted (Anderson, 1983). Still others may not seek help because of economic reasons, distrust of the health-care system, religious reasons, lack of knowledge, or an inability to articulate their needs (Pilipino Mini-Health Forums, 1993; McBride, Mariola, & Yeo, 1995; Tompar-Tiu & Sustento-Seneriches, 1994).

Some Filipinos may not have a primary health-care provider and thus rely on emergency services. Many Filipinos are reluctant to participate in health promotion programs such as cancer screening and health education. The early Filipino immigrants, unlike recent immigrants, did not have adequate health benefits through their place of employment. Thus, they may have been used to postponing illness care until the illness was quite advanced. Some recent immigrants appear to behave differently, as described in a study of Filipino households in New Jersey in which almost 76 percent of the sample had seen a physician within the last year and approximately 92 percent had health insurance (Garde, et al., 1995).

Conversely, in a survey of newly arrived aging Filipino World War II veterans, many who seek health-care services relate experiences of being denied services or being referred to various nonprofit community clinics because they do not have veterans benefits (McBride, 1993). Health-care providers who practice in different parts of the United States should expect wide variations in health behaviors among Filipino-American clients. Most important, a nonjudgmental approach to history-taking regarding previous actions taken to deal with a health concern should be documented in the most accurate and fair manner. Turning on the "multicultural ear" and listening with care to the context of these actions can provide insight for practitioners, particularly when the practitioner is under time pressure to process clients.

## Folk Practices

Personalistic or magicoreligious beliefs about illness fit the general conceptualization of balance among traditional Filipinos. For example, in sorcery, disease is believed to be caused by a poison or a noxious substance introduced into the body, disturbing the normal equilibrium. This is treated by extracting the offending object or by counter sorcery. Nydegger (1983), an anthropologist who studied the Tarongs of the Ilocos region, described the phenomena called "soul loss." The soul leaves the body under conditions of fear, shock, or intense longing, causing a loss of balance. To return the soul, rituals involving prayers, feast, or exorcism alone or in combination are performed to placate the souls or spirits.

Balance and moderation extend to humoral, activity, temperature, and dietary balances. The ideal environment is warm, moderate, and balanced. The underlying principle is that changes should be introduced gradually. Sudden changes from hot to cold, from activity to inactivity, from fasting to overeating, and so forth, introduce undue bodily stresses, which can cause illness. Some Filipinos in the United States avoid hand washing with cold water after ironing or heavy labor. After strenuous physical activity, a rest should precede a shower; otherwise the person could develop *pasma ng ugat*, "arthritis." Cold drinks or foods such as orange juice or fresh tomatoes are not served for breakfast to prevent *masisikmura*, "stomach upset." Exposure to sudden cold drafts may induce colds, fever, rheumatism, pneumonia, or other respiratory ailments.

## Cultural Responses to Health and Illness

Filipinos view pain as part of living an honorable life. Some view this as an opportunity to reach a fuller spiritual life or to atone for past transgressions. Thus, they may appear stoic and be tolerant of a high degree of pain. Health-care providers may need to offer, and in fact encourage, pain-relief interventions for the Filipino client who does not complain of pain despite physiological indicators. Others may have a strong sensitivity to the "busyness" of health-care providers, quietly diminishing their own need for attention so that others can receive care, or they may simply have little knowledge of how pain management can be maximized. Filipino clients who display visible evidence of their religiosity such as religious medals or prayer cards can be encouraged to incorporate their prayers or rituals into the pain management program. Pain assessment can include the role of prayer by the patient and members of the support network. Questions such as "Do you have someone praying for you?" or "Is there a special prayer to help you deal with pain?" may provide vital information for individualizing a Filipino client's care.

Most Filipinos believe that mental illness carries a certain amount of stigma, and some believe that mental illness is hereditary. If an emotional problem is manifested, family members may choose to take care of their own sick relative rather than to seek mental health care. The few studies on Filipino mental health support the underutilization of mental health services. A study of psychiatric admission records of Queens Medical Center in Hawaii (Wedge & Abe, 1949) found that Filipinos, based on their number in the population, were underrepresented. However, hospitalized Filipinos manifested more bizarre behaviors and dramatic delusions of grandeur and persecution. Weiner and Marvit (1977) reported a moderate incidence of schizophrenia among Filipinos compared with other ethnic groups. They noted that the psychopathologies appeared at a somewhat later age than in other groups. Perhaps Filipinos in this study used informal systems of care until the symptoms became severe and difficult to handle.

In a study of Filipinos in San Francisco, Shon (1972) reported a higher proportion of Philippine-born women with psychopathologies. For most, the symptoms were precipitated by a loss in self-esteem, loss of status, and shame. The problems were related to the stresses of immigration, such as family separation, inability to find suitable employment, uncertainty, lack of money, and other relocation stressors.

Valencia-Go's (1989) study of aging and role integration among elderly immigrant Filipino widows in an upstate New York suburb reported the perception of wellness as a component of the participants' definition of mental health. Many indicated that staying active, being involved with family activities, being true to one's faith, and comparing one's functional capacity with that of their peers were strategies for maintaining wellness.

A Hampton Roads, Virginia, study indicates that major adjustment problems such as loneliness and inability to get around results in depression, (Welch, 1987). In contrast, financial difficulty was the primary cause of depression given by participants in a study of adult Filipinos with depression living in the San Francisco Bay area (Tompar-Tiu & Sustento-Seneriches, 1994).

In 1978, a mental health survey of Filipinos in the New York metropolitan area suggested that respondents were fairly healthy emotionally based on a 12 percent response rate (Amaranto & Reyes, 1978). However, it was theorized that the low response rate may be associated with the Filipinos' attitude toward mental health and mental illness. Nevertheless, the sample cited lack of language ability, work, and money as significant problems. The study confirmed that high educational attainment and underemployment among Filipinos created serious psychological reactions. Only 15 percent indicated that they would avail themselves of mental health services. The study suggested that this group may have difficulty accepting emotional problems. In the San Francisco depression study, when asked who would be the best person to treat their condition, the first two choices were a loved one or a caring family member, followed by a health professional (Tompar-Tiu & Sustento-Seneriches, 1994). Talking to a trusted family member or friend, psychotherapy, staying involved, support and prayer groups, employment, and medication were the preferred treatment approaches.

Using sociocultural behaviors learned early in life, Filipinos have a remarkable ability to maintain a proper front to protect their self-esteem and self-image. However, this front may be fragile, and chronic repression of resentment and anger may build up and erupt violently. Mental health providers should recognize that despite the possibility of a Filipino client's refusing professional mental health services, involving a trusted family member or friends, conducting the initial contact with a Filipino mental health worker, especially a Filipino physician, or both practices may increase the odds of getting the person into a culturally compatible treatment program (McBride, 1994, 1996; Nora & McBride, 1996; Tompar-Tiu & Sustento-Seneriches, 1994).

Deference to authority may successfully bring the Filipino client into treatment with the client's expectation that the authority figure will fix the problem. A family therapy framework that considers the Filipino's cultural views on mental illness and the meaning of the illness to the person and the family can have a more beneficial outcome (Kim, 1985; McBride, 1996; Tompar-Tiu & Sustento-Seneriches, 1994; Tsui & Schultz, 1985).

The literature reports no studies on Filipino perceptions of physical and mental disability. Major concerns over hereditary diseases are associated with the selection of marriage partners. The birth of a developmentally disabled child may be viewed as God's gift, an opportunity to become a better person or family, a curse from some unknown "angry spirit," negligence while pregnant, or a family matter that should be kept private (Tompar-Tiu & Sustento-Seneriches, 1994). American-born Filipinos may be more inclined to accept rehabilitation services through a home-care program than through institutional placement, such as special schools and long-term care facilities.

The Filipino family plays an important role during illness. The sick person assumes a dependent role, and the family's responsibility is to protect and care for the needs of the sick person, who makes decisions in consultation with the family. In some instances, the family makes unilateral decisions. The role of the family becomes more prominent in events where a significant and unpleasant piece of information needs to be disclosed, for example, a bad prognosis. Unlike the Western approach of full disclosure, the Filipino family prefers to be informed of the bad news, and they in turn gradually share the information with the sick member; however, in cases when a long-term care placement is inevitable and family members concur, the health-care provider, particularly the attending physician, may be asked to take responsibility for the decision and to inform the client. Thus, the family feels able to continue a comfortable relationship with the disabled family member.

Living wills and advance directives put the belief systems of many Filipinos in a major collision course with the American health-care and legal system. Anticipating death or facilitating the termination of life, no matter how futile the situation looks, may be the least acceptable way of presenting the need to make decisions. As unpleasant and culturally incompatible as it may feel, most Filipino families take action when the issue is discussed within the context of caring values, kinship, and spirituality rather than as an institutional or legal necessity.

## Blood Transfusion and Organ Donation

The value of blood transfusion is recognized and accepted by Filipinos. However, organ donation may be less acceptable, except perhaps in cases where a close family member is involved. Many Filipinos, who follow Catholic traditions, may believe that keeping the body intact as much as possible until death is a reasonable preparation for the afterlife. Eighty-eight percent of respondents in the New Jersey health study did not carry an organ donor card or know of the program. When asked if they would be willing to sign an organ donor card, only 29 percent responded affirmatively. Explanations offered were related to the rarity of organ donation and transplantation and limited technological support for the procedures in the Philippine health-care system (Garde et al., 1995). From this survey, no cultural or religious reasons were identified that might dissuade Filipinos from donating organs or receiving transplants.

## HEALTH-CARE PRACTITIONERS

## Traditional Versus Biomedical Care

Western medicine is familiar and acceptable to Filipinos. Moreover, many recent Filipino immigrants are educated in the health-care field. By their sheer number alone, many Filipinos in the United States know or are related to a health-care worker. Nevertheless, some Filipinos accept the efficacy of folk medicine and may consult both Western-trained and indigenous healers. Folk healers are less common in the United States, with the exceptions of the West Coast and Hawaii. When available, they contribute by facilitating cultural rapport between the health-care provider and the client and by increasing utilization of needed health-care services. For example, the *hilot*, whose authority is respected by the Filipino who seeks his or her service, is often willing to be included in the counseling session, support advice to consult a physician, follow treatment regimens, or use prescribed medications. The *hilot* may provide a special prayer to be incorporated into the medically prescribed treatment plan to increase the client's sense that all available resources are being mobilized. In some areas on the West Coast, the *hilot* has a distinct role and function in the Filipino community. A few Filipino health professionals have learned the *hilot's* art, skills, and spiritual approach, which they blend into their professional practice (McBride, 1994).

A practitioner of the same gender and the same culture may encourage more Filipinos to take advantage of health prevention services. The availability of Filipino primary care providers and, whenever possible, a bilingual person are critical to improving health care for Filipino elderly persons, who are predominantly immigrants in the United States.

## Status of Health-care Providers

The Filipino perception of health-care practitioners is similar to that of the rest of American society. One difference is that many consider the physician as the primary leader of the health-care team and other providers are expected to defer to the physician as they do for their family. In addition, the expectation may be that the physician can fix the problem. As Filipino families become more acculturated and aware of how health-care services are accessed in the United States, changes in attitude and behavior may be expected.

When ill, Filipinos may first consult a family member or a friend who is a physician or other professional before arranging a medical appointment. Some prefer physicians from their own region, when possible, whereas others indicate preference for physicians who are knowledgeable, competent, and have good bedside manners regardless of culture or ethnic background (Spangler, 1985). In San Francisco, a group of middle-aged immigrant Filipino women shared some criteria for choosing a health-care provider. They were concern for privacy, feelings of modesty, approval from family members (especially the spouse), and most important, the overall caring environment in the system (McBride, 1995).

---

### CASE STUDY

In 1990, Jose Bisigan, aged 87, and his wife Carmen, aged 85, sold their small restaurant and immigrated to Los Angeles from a small town in the Visayan region. They came to join their firstborn, daughter-nurse, Felicia, aged 54, her husband, and their three children aged 10 to 18. Mr. Bisigan speaks limited English and is in a poststroke rehabilitation unit. Since the stroke, he has had mild aphasia, mild confusion, and bladder and bowel continence problems. His hypertension and long-standing diabetes is controlled with medication and diet. His wife, daughter, and grandchildren have been supportive of him during this first hospitalization experience. Mr. Bisigan's family has cooperated with the health team, often agreeing with minimal resistance to the prescribed treatment management. The rehabilitation team recommended subacute rehabilitation treatment as part of the discharge plan.

As a businessman and the elder in the family household, Mr. Bisigan is looked to for counsel by the immediate and extended family. Mr. Bisigan's status, however, has caused friction between Felicia and her husband, Nestor, an American-born Filipino who works as a machinist. Nestor has accused Felicia of giving excessive attention to her mother and father. Felicia's worries about her parents' health have made Nestor very resentful. He increased his already daily "outings with the boys." Felicia maintains a full-time position in acute care and a part-time night shift position in a nursing home.

Mr. Bisigan's discharge is pending and a decision must be made before Medicare coverage runs out. Felicia has to consider the possible choices available to her father and the family circumstances and expectations. Mrs. Bisigan, who is being treated for hypertension, has always deferred decisions to her husband and is looking to Felicia to make the decisions. Because of her work schedule, the absence of a responsible person at home, her mother's health problems, and intergenerational friction, Felicia considers nursing home placement. She is, however, reluctant to broach the subject with her father, who expects to be cared for at home. Mrs. Bisigan disagrees with putting her husband in a nursing home and is adamant that she will care for her husband at home.

Felicia delayed talking to her father until the rehabilitation team requested a meeting. At the meeting, Felicia indicated that she could not bring herself to present her plan to put her father in a nursing home because of her mother's objection and her own fear that her father will feel rejected. Feeling very much alone in resolving the issue about nursing home placement, she requested the team to act as intermediary for her and her family.

## STUDY QUESTIONS

1. Identify cultural family values that are contributing to the conflicts experienced by each family members.

2. Identify a culturally competent approach that the team can use when discussing nursing home placement with the Bisigans.

3. How might the rehabilitation program be presented to Mrs. Bisigan and still allow her to maintain her spousal role?

4. Discuss at least three communication issues in the family that are culture-bound and suggest possible intervention.

5. Identify psychocultural assessments that should be done by the rehabilitation team to have a greater understanding of the dynamics specific to this family.

6. Identify and explain at least two health promotion issues for each family member that are complicated by cultural beliefs and practices.

7. How might the family and the rehabilitation team benefit from consultations with a geriatric nurse practitioner or a transcultural clinical nurse specialist?

8. What food preferences in the traditional Filipino diet might be detrimental to Mr. and Mrs. Bisigan's health?

9. Identify health promotion counseling that might be discussed with the Bisigan's grandchildren.

10. List at least five culturally sensitive communication guidelines for talking with Mr. and Mrs. Bisigan.

11. Identify and explain major sources of stress for each member of this household.

12. What cultural belief system complicates the family members' responses and may contribute to the discharge plan for a subacute rehabilitation program?

## *References*

Agoncillo, T., & Guerrero, M. (1987). *History of the Filipino people* (7th ed.). Manila, Philippines: Garcia Publishing.

Almirol, E. B. (1985). Exclusion and acceptance of Filipinos in America. *Asian Profile, 13*(5), 395–408.

Amaranto, E. A., & Reyes, F. (1978). *Mental health study of Filipino immigrants in the New York metropolitan area.* (Rep. No. 13.) Asian American Mental Health Research Center.

Anderson, J. N. (1983). Health and illness in Pilipino immigrants. *Western Journal of Medicine, 139*(6), 811–819.

Araneta, E. G. (1993). Psychiatric care of Pilipino Americans. In A. C. Gaw (Ed.), *Culture, ethnicity, and mental illness* (pp. 377–411). Washington, DC: American Psychiatric Press.

Awanohara, S. (1991, February 7). High growth, low profile. *Far Eastern Economic Review,* 39–40.

Barnett, M. L. (1966). Hiya, shame, and guilt: Preliminary consideration of the concepts as analytical tools for Philippine social science. *Philippine Sociological Review, 15*(4), 276–281.

Beyers, M. (1979). *Exploration of factors affecting the achievement of licensure for foreign-educated nurses.* Unpublished doctoral dissertation, Northwestern University, Chicago.

Bulosan, C. (1973). *America is in the heart.* Seattle: Washington University Press.

Burns, O., & Pierce, J. (1992). *Tobacco use in California, 1990–1991.* Sacramento, CA: California Department of Health Services.

Caringer, B. (1977). Caring for the institutionalized Filipino. *Journal of Gerontological Nursing, 3*(5), 33–37.

Catapusan, B. T. (1936). Filipino repatriates in the Philippines. *Sociology and Social Research, 21,* 72–77.

Catapusan, B. T. (1939). Filipino immigrants and public relief of the United States. *Sociology and Social Research, 23,* 546–554.

Catapusan, B. T. (1940). Leisure time of Filipino immigrants. *Sociology and Social Research, 24,* 541–549.

Chi, I. & Kitano, H. H. L. (1989). Asian Americans and alcohol: The Chinese, Japanese, Koreans, and Filipinos in Los Angeles. *Alcohol use among U.S. ethnic minorities* (Research Monograph No. 18). Bethesda, MD: National Institute on Alcohol Abuse and Alcoholism.

Chinn, S. (1993, December 20). Filipino veterans poor in the land they fought for. *The San Francisco Examiner,* p. A20.

Eggan, F. (1971). Philippine social structure. In G. M. Guthrie (Ed.). *Six perspectives on the Philippines* (pp. 1–47). Manila: Bookmark.

Enriquez, V. G., & Santiago, C. (1976). *Tungo sa makipilipinong pananaliksik* [About Philippine soul searching]. Manila, Philippines: *Sikolohiyang Pilipino: Mga ulat at balita, 1*(4).

Enriquez, V. G. (1986). Kapwa: A core concept in Filipino social psychology. In V. G. Enriquez (Ed.), *Philippine worldview* (pp. 6–19). Singapore: Institute of Southeast Asian Study.

Enriquez, V. (1994). *From colonial to liberation psychology: The Philippine experience.* Manila, Philippines: De La Salle University Press.

Espina, M. E. (1988). *Filipinos in New Orleans.* New Orleans: Laborde & Sons.

Fernandez, D. G. (1986). Food and the Filipino. In V. G. Enriquez (Ed.), *Philippine worldview* (pp. 20–43). Singapore: Institute of Southeast Asian Study.

Garde, P., Spangler, Z., & Miranda, B. (1994). *Filipino-Americans in New Jersey: A health study* (Final Report of the Philippine Nurses' Association of America to the State of New Jersey Department of Health, Office of Minority Health).

Gerber, L. (1980). The influence of environmental factors on mortality from coronary heart disease among Filipinos in Hawaii. *Human Biology, 52,* 269–278.

Gock, T. S. (1994). Acquired immunodeficiency syndrome. In N. Zane, D. Takuechi, & K. Yong (Eds.), *Confronting critical issues of Asian Pacific Islander Americans* (pp. 247–265). Thousand Oaks, CA: Sage Publications.

Guillermo, T. (1993). Health care needs and

service delivery for Asian and Pacific Islander Americans: Health policy. *LEAP: The state of Asian Pacific America–Policy issues to the year 2020* (Asian Pacific Public Policy Institute and Asian American Studies Center). Los Angeles, CA: University of California Los Angeles Press.

Guthrie, G. M. (1971). The Philippine temperament. In G. M. Guthrie (Ed.), *Six perspectives on the Philippines,* (pp. 49–83). Manila: Bookmark.

Himes, R. S. (1971). *Tagalog concepts of causality: Disease* (IPC Paper No. 10). Manila, Philippines: Ateneo de Manila University Press.

Hinds, M. W., Kolonel, L. N., & Lee, J. (1980). Association between cancer incidence and alcohol cigarette consumption among five ethnic groups in Hawaii. *British Journal of Cancer, 41,* 929–940.

Karnow, S. (1989). *In our image: America's empire in the Philippines.* New York: Random House.

Kim, S. (1985). Family therapy for Asian-Americans: A strategic structural framework. Psychotherapy, 22(2s).

Kitano, H. & Daniels, R. (1988). *Asian-Americans.* Englewood Cliffs, NJ: Prentice Hall.

Klastky, A. L., & Armstrong, M. A. (1991). Cardiovascular risk factors among Asian Americans living in Northern California. *American Journal of Public Health, 8*(11), 1423–1428.

Kuo, W. H. (1981). Colonized status of Asian-Americans. *Asian Groups, 3,* 227–251.

Lamzon, T. (1978). *Handbook of Philippine language groups.* Quezon City, Philippines: Manila University Press.

Lasker, B. (1969). *Filipino immigration to continental United States and Hawaii.* New York: Arno Press.

Levy, R. A. (1993). Ethnic and racial differences in response to medicines: Preserving individualized therapy in managed pharmaceutical programmes. *Pharmaceutical Medicine, 7,* 139–165.

Lynch, F. 0. (1964). *Social acceptance: Four readings on Philippine values* (IPC Papers No. 2). Manila, Philippines: Ateneo de Manila University Press.

McBride, M. (1993). *Health status of recently naturalized Filipino WWII Veterans.* Paper presented at the annual conference of the American Society on Aging, Chicago, IL.

McBride, M. (1994). *Intergenerational issues and mental health in Filipino American families.* Paper presented at the summer conference of Filipino Americans in Medicine, University of California, Irvine.

McBride, M. (1996). *Mental health issues and Filipino American women.* Paper presented at Asian American Health Forum, San Francisco: University of California San Francisco.

McBride, M., Mariola, D., & Yeo, G. (1995). *Aging and health: Asian Pacific Islander American elders.* Stanford, CA: Stanford Geriatric Education Center.

McBride, M., & Parreno, H. (1996). Filipino American families and caregiving. In G. Yeo & D. Gallagher-Thompson (Eds.), *Ethnicity and the Dementias.* Washington, DC: Taylor & Francis.

McWilliams, C. (1964). *Brothers under the skin.* Boston: Little Brown & Co.

Medina, B. (1991). *The Filipino family.* Quezon city, Philippines: University of the Philippines Press.

Melendy, B. (1972). California's discrimination against Filipinos, 1927–1935. In R. Daniels & S. C. Olin (Eds.), *Racism in California.* New York: MacMillan.

Miraflor, C. G. (1976). The Philippine nurse: Implications for orientation and in-service education for foreign nurses in the United States. Unpublished doctoral dissertation, Loyola University, Chicago.

Nakpil, C. G. (1978). The Filipino woman in legend and history: Perspective Philippines. *Philippines Herald: New Years Supplement,* p. 9.

Nora, R., & McBride, M. (1996). Health needs of Filipino Americans. *Asian Pacific Islander American Journal of Health.*

Northern California Cancer Center (1990). Prostate cancer incidence in the Bay Area. *Bay Area Cancer Registry Report, 2* (1).

Northern California Cancer Center (1991). Cervical cancer incidence among women in the San Francisco and Monterey Bay Area. *Bay Area Cancer Registry Report, 3*(3).

Nydegger, C. N. (1983). Multiple causality: Consequences for medical practice. *Western Journal of Medicine, 138*(3), 430–435.

Orque, M. (1983). Nursing care of Filipino-American patients. In M. Orque, B. Bloch, & L. Monrroy (Eds.), *Ethnic Nursing Care: A Multicultural Approach.* St. Louis, C. V. Mosby.

Pascacio, E. M. (1971). Communications breakdowns. *Silliman Journal, 18*(3), 312–319.

PePua, R. (1990). Pagtatanung-tanong: A method for cross-cultural research. In V. Enriquez (Ed.), *Indigenous Psychology: A Book of Readings.* Quezon City, Philippines: New Horizons Press, Akademya ng Sikolohiyang Pilipino.

*Philippine Statistical Yearbook* (1995). Malcati, Philippines: National Statistics Information Center: National Statistical Coordination Board.

Pido, A. J. A. (1986). *The Pilipinos in America: Macro/micro dimensions of immigration and integration.* New York: Center for Migration Studies.

Pilipino Mini-Health Forums Committee (1993). *Executive report: Pilipino health assessment report to the San Francisco health commission.* San Francisco, CA:Author.

Requisa, M. C. (1974, June 10–14). *The role of social networks in Filipino immigration to the east coast of the United States.* Paper presented at the conference on International Migration from the Philippines, East-West Center, Honolulu, Hawaii.

Shon, S. P. (1972). *The Filipino community and mental health: A study of Filipino Americans in mental health district 5 of San Francisco.* San Francisco, CA: Langley Porter Neuropsychiatric Institute, Community Mental Health Training Program.

Spangler, Z. (1985). *Coping with cancer: Comparison of Philippine and American cancer patients.* Unpublished qualitative interviews.

Spangler, Z. (1991a). Culture care of Philippine and Anglo-American nurses in a hospital context. In M. L. Leininger (Ed.), *Culture care diversity & universality: A theory of nursing* (pp. 119–146). New York: National League for Nursing Press.

Spangler, Z. (1991b). *Nursing care values and caregiving practices of Anglo-American and Philippine-American nurses.* Unpublished doctoral dissertation. Wayne State University, Detroit, Michigan.

Spangler, Z. (1992). Transcultural nursing care values & caregiving practices of Philippine-American nurses. *Journal of Transcultural Nursing, 4*(2), 28–37.

Spangler, Z. (1993). Generic and professional care of Anglo-American and Philippine-American nurses. In D. A. Gaut (Ed.), *A global agenda for caring* (pp. 47–62). New York: National League for Nursing Press.

*Statistics Canada: Ethnic Origins* (1993). Minister of Industry, Science, and Technology. Ottawa, Canada.

Stavig, G. R., Igra, A., & Leonard, A. (1988). Hypertension and related health issues among Asians and Pacific Islanders in California. *Public Health Reports, 103,* 28–73.

Stern, P. N. (1985). A comparison of culturally approved behaviors and beliefs between Pilipina immigrant women, U.S.-born dominant culture women, and Western female nurses of the San Francisco Bay Area:

Religiosity of health care. *Issues in Health Care,* 123–133.

Superio, E. (1993). *Beliefs held by Pilipinos regarding filial responsibility.* Unpublished master's thesis, California State University, San Jose, CA.

Tompar-Tiu, A., & Sustento-Seneriches, J. (1994), *Depression and other mental health issues: The Filipino American experience.* San Francisco: Jossey-Bass.

Tsui, P., & Schultz, G. (1985). Failure of rapport: Why psychotherapeutic engagement fails in treatment of Asian clients. *American Orthopsychiatric Journal, 35*(4).

U.S. Bureau of the Census (1995). *Statistical Abstracts of the United States.* Washington, DC: U.S. Government Printing Office.

Valencia-Go, G. (1989). *Integrative aging in widowed immigrant Filipinos.* Unpublished dissertation, Adelphi University, Garden City, NY.

Wedge, B., & Abe, S. (1949). Racial incidence of mental disease in Hawaii. *Hawaii Medical Journal, 8,* 337–338.

Weiner, B. P., & Marvit, R. C. (1977). Schizophrenia in Hawaii: Analysis of cohort mortality risk in a multi-ethnic population. *British Journal of Psychiatry, 131,* 497–503.

Welch, A. (1987). *Concepts of health, illness, caring, aging and problems of adjustment among elderly Filipinos residing in Hampton Roads, Virginia.* Unpublished doctoral dissertation, University of Utah, Salt Lake City, UT.

Wong, M., & Hirschman, C. (1983). The new Asian immigrants. In A. C. Gaw (Ed.), *Culture, ethnicity, and identity* (pp. 381–403). New York: Academic Press.

Yraola-Westfall, E. (1986). Tagalization of Spanish and English: A case study of code switching and mixing. *Dissertation Abstracts, 47*(4), 1309-A.

# French Canadians

*Ginette Coutu-Wakulczyk, Ann C. Beckingham,
and Denise Moreau*

---

• Key terms to become familiar with in this chapter are:

| | |
|---|---|
| Acadia | *Joual* |
| Acadian | *Métis* |
| *Fayots* | Québec |
| Francophone | Quebecer (*québécois*) |

## OVERVIEW, INHABITED LOCALITIES, AND TOPOGRAPHY

### Overview

Canada, with over 3,800,000 square miles and a population of 27 million, is larger than the entire United States but has only one-ninth the population. The land mass covers six time zones and has fertile agricultural land, a vast tundra, dense forests, and mountain ranges. The country is rich in minerals, coal, oil, and gas. Only 20 percent of the land is habitable (*Canadian Almanac and Directory,* 1995).

Canada, a self-governing member of the Commonwealth Nations, is a federation of 10 provinces and two territories. The Constitution Act of 1981 transferred the Parliament from Britain to Canada. Even though the Queen of England is also the queen of Canada, the Canadian constitution is entirely in the hands of the Canadians. Each province is nominally headed by a lieutenant governor who is appointed by the federal government. The 10 provinces in descending order of population are Ontario, **Quebec**, British Columbia, Alberta, Manitoba, Saskatchewan, Nova Scotia, New Brunswick, Newfoundland, and Prince Edward Island. The Northwest Territory is larger than the Yukon Territory. Canada's largest cities are Toronto (3.9 million persons), Montreal (3.2 million persons), Vancouver (1.6 million persons), and the capital, Ottawa (921,000 persons) (*Canadian Almanac and Directory,* 1995).

### Heritage and Residence

Before the 1960s, people with French as their mother tongue were identified as French Canadians, referring to France as their country of origin. Today, people living in Canada using French as their first language are referred to as **Francophones,** independent of their country of origin. This designation, based on language, permits a broader regrouping of the multiethnic and cultural mosaic of the Canadian population. However, the French-speaking population of Canada is far from homogeneous. French-speaking areas of Canada are inhabited by diverse cultural and ethnic groups, including the *métis* communities with a mixture of French, Native-American, and other cultural groups. The St. Boniface, Manitoba, community, where Louis Riel (1844 to 1885) fought for land rights and is considered a hero, is a good example of French Canadians' determination to keep French as the mother tongue. More recently, Francophones from former colonies under French rule, such as Haiti, Lebanon, and Vietnam, have added to the French population of Canada.

During the last 20 years, many Quebec families have adopted young children from Latin America and the Middle East. This practice has contributed to the development of an ethnic mosaic within the younger adult population. Although the vast majority of French Canadians live in the province of Quebec, the French language is used daily for communication within families and communities from coast to coast and as far north as the Yukon. Another major portion of the French-speaking population in Canada comprises **Acadians** residing in the Maritime provinces. They include descendants of the early colonists, mainly persons of west central French origin who settled in the Maritimes (Roy, 1995).

New settlers arriving by ship brought with them the French dialect, characteristics of the French people, customs, songs, stories, and games, which have been enriched over the centuries by contact with native tribes, Basque, Scots, and Irish. Therefore, assessments must be carefully completed to avoid generalizations based on language and physical or racial traits.

Between 1981 and 1991, 37,375 (3 percent) of Canadian immigrants reported French as their mother tongue, in comparison with 28,975 (2.3 percent) of immigrants before 1961. This increase in recent years validates the growth in regional ethnocultural diversity for the total French-speaking immigrant population (Badets & Chui, 1994). Most Canadians are aware that Canada has an official policy of multiculturalism; however, far fewer understand its history and its implications (Kulig, 1995). The Multiculturalism Canada Act of 1988 provides guidelines for implementing this policy (Fleras & Elliott, 1992).

To understand French culture in a Canadian historical perspective, some attention must be focused on New (Nouvelle) France, the name given to Canada when it was first settled. In the 17th century, Portugal, Spain, Holland, France, and England vied for the colonization of New France. Although religious influences played a part in colonial policies, the mercantile system stimulated the colonials to penetrate the North American wilderness and develop trading companies (Wesber, Wesley, & Danhier, 1944). French immigration to North America resulted in transplantation of their developed civilization to a relatively unpopulated but fertile continent. Two independent settlements were established simultaneously without much contact between each other, largely because of geographic location. Soon after settling in Quebec City in 1608, one of the first permanent colonies in Canada, these French settlers moved up the St. Lawrence River and established other settlements such as Vile-Marie (Montreal) in 1642. They explored the Great Lakes (out of which the St. Lawrence flows), opened fur trading centers, and converted the natives to Christianity. In 1718, the French settled in New Orleans at the opposite end of the continent. In 1750, by moving up the Mississippi River, approximately 80,000 French lived within the vast area between the mouths of the St. Lawrence and the Mississippi Rivers. A large part of Canada and cities such as St. Louis and New Orleans in the United States still reflect the French influence (Wesber, Wesley, & Danhier, 1944).

Around 1603, other groups of settlers established themselves in **Acadia**, north of what Giovanni da Verrazano in 1534 referred to as Arcadia (note the "r"). This region is known today as Delaware, Maryland, and Virginia (Daigle, 1995). After a devastating experience on the Ile Sainte-Croix where half of the 80 colonists died during the first winter (1604 to 1605), the settlers moved to the Bay of Fundy and founded Port-Royal, which was to become the first coastal settlement and capital of

Acadia (Cormier, 1994). By the middle of the 1700s, the Acadians numbered 13,000 persons who descended from small clusters of families. Caught in the crossroads of imperial rivalries, Acadian lands became strategically vital to the ambitions of England, France, and inhabitants of the American colonies. During the 17th century, the Acadian colonies changed hands 14 times before finally being absorbed into the British Empire (Griffiths, 1973).

Struggles between France and England began in Europe and North America in 1689 and led to a series of treaties that left France with only two small fishing islands off the coast of Newfoundland, St. Pierre and Miquelon. With the Treaty of Utrecht in 1713, England secured Newfoundland, Acadia, (renamed Nova Scotia), and the extensive region drained by the rivers flowing into the Hudson Bay. The French and Indian War in 1754 settled the issue between France and England in North America when Wolfe defeated Montcalm under the walls of Quebec during the final battle. With the Treaty of Paris in 1763, France relinquished all its North American possessions east of the Mississippi River to England. Spain, which had been involved in the war, ceded Florida to England in exchange for the French territories west of the Mississippi River (Wesber, Wesley, & Danhier, 1944). Thus, as a geographic area, Nouvelle-France became only a memory. Yet, the French culture, language, and religious institutions remain as an everlasting tribute to the past. The heritage and early French architecture is well preserved through concentrated efforts and pride in restoration. Publication of information about monuments, houses, churches, and ramparts around Quebec City keep the public informed about the area's rich French heritage.

Throughout the period of uncertainty, the Acadians insisted on neutrality by maintaining a friendly relationship with the English and the Micmac natives, reserving their emotional loyalty for their families, their villages, and their lands. As a result of unresolved controversy over several highly contentious oaths of allegiance to the English, between 1755 and 1762, a massive deportation occurred. Referred to as *le grand dérangement,* 8000 French-speaking Catholic Acadians were removed from their homes in Nova Scotia and New Brunswick and were dispersed in many locations, namely Massachusetts, New York, Pennsylvania, Maryland, Virginia, the Carolinas, Georgia, and Louisiana. Some fled to Quebec, others took refuge in the woods, and many died.

Although distinctly different from the French Canadians, 1.7 million Americans of French descent live in scattered populations throughout the United States along the Mississippi River and the Champlain Valley in New York, Vermont, Connecticut, and Massachusetts (*Canadian Almanac and Directory,* 1995).

In 1774, some exiled Acadians returned to the Maritimes and attempted to re-create their lives. Unable to secure their former lands because of British occupancy, they directed their energies to forming new areas and gradually explored new activities such as fishing and forestry (Daigle, 1995). Today, 90 percent of the Acadians reside in northern and eastern New Brunswick, southern Nova Scotia, the Acadian region of Cape Breton, and the Evangeline region of Prince Edward Island (Beaudin & Leclerc, 1995).

The civil law code (Code Napoléonien) is still in effect in the province of Quebec, whereas other parts of Canada have adopted the common law code. Nevertheless, religious institutions and language provide commonalities among traditions and culture within Canada. The emerging identity and roots of regionalism were formed between 1763 and 1867 when the British North America Act established the Confederation of Canada. These roots of regionalism are still distinctive in modern Canada. Since the beginning of the French colony to 1763, 25,000 individuals came to Quebec from France. Of these, only about 8500 settled permanently (Boleda, 1984; Harris & Matthews, 1987). Today, French Canada has grown to over 6 million inhabitants, unevenly distributed across Canada with the majority (5 million) living in Quebec (*Statistics Canada,* 1992).

The most profound changes in Canada came with an influx of English Loyalists starting between 1774 and 1775. Thirty thousand settled in Nova Scotia around the St. John River and the Bay of Fundy. After the dispersal of the Acadians, British authorities divided Acadia geographically and politically into three Maritime provinces: Nova Scotia in 1763, Prince Edward Island in 1769, and New Brunswick in 1784 (Couturier Lebanc, Godin, & Renaud, 1995). Migration of another 10,000 Loyalists brought settlements to the Lower St. Lawrence and Great Lakes region. In 1791, the province of Canada had two divisions: Upper Canada (later Ontario) and Lower Canada (later Quebec). From 1820 to the mid-1850s, a British immigration wave brought 800,000 people from all segments of society primarily into Upper Canada. A planned settlement of Scottish Highlanders on the Red River (Manitoba) in 1811 suffered tragedies yet survived (Careless, 1970). Thus, Canada's multicultural society was already apparent by 1850. The settlement's heterogeneous Manitoban population of 5000 included a majority of French métis supplemented by Scottish Indian métis, English and Scottish settlers, some Americans, and some Upper Canadians (French and British early settlers). By 1895, French Canadians, responding to gold rush fever, settled as far as the Yukon. By the end of the 19th century, these regions showed disparate environmental and societal development (McInnis, 1969).

Although the majority (80 percent) of Canadian Francophones live in the province of Quebec, not everyone answers to French ancestry. According to Henripin and Martin (1991), only 40 to 45 percent are *Québécois de souche*, descendants of earlier settlers from France. French Canadians living in Quebec with French as the official language are the majority; however, outside the province of Quebec, they become a minority. Nevertheless, health services provided in the French language are protected by law in the provinces of Quebec, Ontario, and New Brunswick.

Throughout Canada, important regional differences related to ethnicity exist among the French-speaking population. Outside Quebec, the French-speaking population within each province or territory has its own association, which is organized nationally under the *Fédération des communautés Francophones et Acadiennes du Canada (FCFA du Canada)*.

An important consideration when the health-care provider assesses a family's cultural background is the number of mixed marriages leading to the adoption of English as the language spoken in the home and by the majority. The combination of acculturation and the steadily declining fertility rate of Canadians of French ancestry since the 1930s, currently at 1.82 nationally and 1.6 for Quebec, could cause the French-speaking Canadian population to "disappear by the year 2786" if immigration does not continue (Health and Welfare Canada, 1989, p. 2). French-speaking Canada has become an increasingly diverse society composed of various ethnocultural groups. In the 1991 census, 31 percent of the population reported ethnic origins other than British or French (Ministry of Industry, Science and Technology, 1993).

## Reasons for Migration and Associated Economic Factors

Economic reasons, including the desire to cultivate the land and exploit fisheries, were the most frequent motivations for early French Canadian settlers in the 17th century (Griffiths, 1973). The majority of these settlers originated from the French regions of Normandy, Perche, Poitou, and some from Aunis, Brittany, Ile de France, and Saintonge. During the 17th century in France, many nobles lost their fortune owing to France's feudal system, and colonization of the New France offered possibilities for regaining their prestige and land for their vassals. The richness and the quality of pelts available in the New World promoted fur trading with the Native-Americans and attracted merchants and their employees. In addition, missionaries and religious orders were among the earlier settlers.

## Educational Status and Occupations

Although the overall official literacy rate in Canada approaches 99 percent (*Canadian Almanac and Directory,* 1995), the functional literacy rate is lower, and the educational levels of French Canadians represent a broad spectrum, depending on age group and geographic location. The Office of Francophone Affairs of Ontario (1994) faces many challenges related to education: 50 percent of Francophone students do not complete high school, with illiteracy reaching 50% in some regions, especially among the elderly. The postsecondary education rate for Francophones is approximately half of the provincial rate for Ontarians. More recently, educational opportunities at all levels have become available in the French language in Ontario. Although a student dropout rate of 50 percent could reflect a phenomenon of the era rather than a provincial problem, the rate reaches 40 percent in some areas of Quebec. Nevertheless, the lack of professionals prepared for the delivery of services in French, as prescribed by the 1989 Ontario government, jeopardizes the development of a full network of services in some regions.

A population trend analysis in 1983 showed that despite the improved legal status of the French in Ontario, sociological conditions, particularly urbanization and economic pressures, are contributing to a decline in French-speaking Ontarians. This decrease is more noticeable in southern Ontario, with less decline in the north and the eastern counties bordering Quebec (Gill, 1983). As a result of urbanization, the distribution of Francophones in Ontario has become fragmented, although regional cohesion of French-speaking Ontario has remained strongly supported by active networks at the local and provincial levels (Gilbert, 1991).

Despite the constitutional guarantee of the right of Francophones to receive instruction in their native language, in British Columbia, the most western province in Canada, bilingual education for French Canadians was neglected in the past (Robillard, 1986a). Political decisions that restricted the use of French between 1885 and the mid-1960s led to a decline in Francophones in Saskatchewan (Genuist, 1986). In addition, a progressive loss of the linguistic rights of French-speaking Albertans suffered from 1892 to 1985 (Robillard, 1986b). Genuist (1986) parallels this situation to that of the Bretons, showing that the fate of ethnocultural minorities depends on their will to survive and their treatment at the hands of the majority. Although representing only 5 percent of Manitoba's population, Francophones have flourished within the context of modern civilization and continue to defy complete assimilation (Annandale, 1988). Indeed, many Francophone writers grew up in Manitoba. Paradoxically, Franco-Manitobans, as defined by their mother tongue, are decreasing since their rights have been reinstated. Nevertheless, Manitobans' behavior has been influenced by and continues to be consistent with Ontario law and practice (Wiseman, 1992).

Since 1969, the Official Languages Act of New Brunswick guaranteed the availability of government services and education in French and English at all educational levels. Although the act has increased the political and social utility of French, it has not reversed Acadians' use of the English language or the decline in the proportion of Francophones in the province (Gill, 1980). In an effort to prevent linguistic assimilation, a new policy for language teaching is used in the Francophone schools of heavily anglicized regions. English as a second language is only taught beginning in grade 5 rather than in earlier grades (Peronnet, 1995). The 1976 Canadian census revealed that in all provinces except New Brunswick, where the French are the minority (one-third of the population), a disproportionate number of young French Canadians are assimilated into the majority English society (Castonguay, 1980). In contrast, on Prince Edward Island the struggle to obtain education in French remains an ongoing issue, relying on *La Voix Acadienne,* a weekly newspaper, to keep the French-speaking population's subculture alive (Arsenault, 1981).

The issue most threatening to the cultural survival of French-speaking minorities is directly related to education (Huel, 1986). The dilemma associated with minority status in Saskatchewan is most keenly perceived by French Canadian clergy, who feel that assimilation entails a loss of the Catholic faith. Thus, clergy actively promote activities that unite and organize the French-speaking population to defend and enhance their linguistic and educational privileges. The clergy were instrumental in establishing the journal *Le patriote de l'Ouest,* which provides a means for communicating with dispersed French populations. Through its pages, the concepts of union and organization as means of ensuring survival are supported.

At the beginning of colonization, major occupations such as agriculture, fur trading, and fisheries were important for survival. In the later part of the 19th century, French-speaking Canadians joined the developing movement of the industrial labor force. Factories, mining, forestry, and fisheries took advantage of the numerous hands available among the fertile Canadian families of French ancestry. Despite language barriers, this was a time when the borders of Quebec did not stop young families from moving across Canada for work. Throughout Canada, even in the Yukon, the origins of early French-speaking Canadian settlements can be traced to these years. Today, French-speaking Canadians are represented in all trades and professions. However, the elderly population may have a different life history depending on their region of origin such as Gaspésie, Abitibi, Beauce, Acadia, and the cities of Montreal and Quebec. According to Vaillancourt and Saint-Laurent (1981), the reduced differences in average income for Quebec's ethnic groups is due to improved production by Canadian workers of French origin, controlled economic activities, and advanced education.

## COMMUNICATIONS

### Dominant Language and Dialects

Bilingual Canada has two official languages, French and English. Regional differences exist in accent, vocabulary, and degree of anglicization. However, French Canadians do not have difficulty understanding one another because the original French spoken in Canada includes some old 17th-century French words and expressions that are no longer used in France. Oral communication, in particular, has undergone assimilation with Native-American words combined through the common use of English. English words are incorporated into a syntax and grammar that is essentially French, resulting in a dialect, *joual,* which is spoken primarily by lower socioeconomic and undereducated groups (Tétu de Labsade, 1990).

Préfontaine (1981) studied French-speaking persons in Manitoba who were isolated from the main French-speaking population centers and concluded that Manitoban French are truly international, despite colloquialisms. Nevertheless, according to Lachapelle (1986), assimilation is insidiously at work throughout Canada. Between 1971 and 1981 in northwestern New Brunswick where 58 percent of the population is of French descent, 10 percent of Canadians whose maternal language had been French, abandoned it as their primary language. In southeastern and northeastern Ontario where 25 to 35 percent of the population is of French ancestry, abandonment of the French language reached 25 percent. In Newfoundland, Prince Edward Island, Nova Scotia, southern New Brunswick, northwestern Ontario, and Manitoba, anglicization occurred in 40 to 60 percent of the French populace. Further north and west, anglicization exceeded 60 percent. Maintaining French depends mostly on the strength of the local French community. As for other culturally diverse clients, health-care providers must respect the client's preference in choice of language by seeking interpreters when possible; gearing health teaching to the educational level of the client; and supplementing written directions with verbal instructions, demonstrations, and pictures.

## Cultural Communications Patterns

Conversations among **Quebecers** may be conducted with high voice crescendos, which do not necessarily mean anger or violence. Volume can increase with the importance and the emotional charge invested in the content of the message. Non-verbal communication patterns for French Canadians resemble that of their Latin and Mediterranean ancestors, which encourage sharing their thoughts and feelings. In contrast, the Acadians are more reserved (quieter) and shy, even self-effacing, and are less likely to share their thoughts and feelings than people of Quebec. Gesturing by using their hands frequently for emphasis when speaking is common. Facial expressions for men and women of all ages are a part of communication, often replacing words.

Health-care providers working with French-speaking Canadians, especially aged clients, mothers, and children, need be attentive to nonverbal and paraverbal communication. These observations provide much of the information on affect, emotion, and mutual understanding between the health-care provider and the client.

Spatial distancing for French-speaking Canadians differs among family members, close friends, and the public. When in the intimacy zone, people may touch frequently and converse in close physical space; however, they tend to avoid physical contact in the public arena. When greeting another person, men usually shake hands, which is recommended for health-care providers. Close female friends and family members may greet each other with an embrace. However, in public and more formal situations such as the health-care environment, this is not a recommended practice. When receiving intimate care, many women tend to be modest, especially the elderly. The health-care provider needs to respect their modesty and provide privacy when delivering physical care.

Before radio and television reached the Port au Port Peninsula of Newfoundland, there was a public tradition of storytelling. Narrators were invited to a home where several families had gathered and an entire evening of storytelling took place (Thomas, 1980). These public performances were time consuming, followed stylistic conventions and formulas, and made dramatic use of gesturing. Since the 1960s, private storytelling has substantially replaced the public tradition. Stories are told within the confines of a single family or small group, and usually last less than an hour, about the length of a television episode. Narrators no longer use stylistic devices, literary formulas, or dramatic gesturing (Thomas, 1980; Butler, 1985).

## Temporal Relationships

French-speaking Canadians of Quebec have a past, present, and future orientation in their worldview. Balancing the three dimensions depends on traditionalism, generation, religiosity, and urbanization (Pronovost, 1989). More traditional people and many from rural backgrounds attach primary importance to living in the present and accepting day-to-day occurrences in a context of fatalism. Many elderly with a strong religious background maintain a future worldview regarding life after death and a past orientation celebrating death anniversaries of family members and other events. However, many of the younger generation reject past traditions and attempt to balance enjoying the present and working and planning for their future (Paquet, 1989; Pronovost, 1989).

## Format for Names

Traditionally, until the late 1970s, women and children took the father's surname. Today, under Quebec law, a women keeps her maiden name throughout her lifetime, although in other parts of Canada this practice is decided between the spouses. This situation has created tension and self-identity difficulties for some elderly. As for children, a **québécois** family of two spouses and children may well include four different surname combinations: one child may have the father's surname or the mother's surname alone or a hyphenated or nonhyphenated surname composed of those of the father and mother. For a second child, the surnames are the same, but in reverse order (Eichler, 1988). The decision for using surnames rests entirely with the parents and must appear on the birth certificate. Today, very few parents adhere to the official use of multiple surnames for children. Women married for several years before the new law often added their maiden name hyphenated with that of their husbands.

Many French-speaking Canadians have dropped the custom of naming the oldest son after the father or the grandfather. The custom of adding Joseph to male infants' and Mary to female infants' names that prevailed until recently in Quebec is declining. Until 10 to 15 years ago, the custom was to use only one name without initials, except on legal documents, which used all three or four names as they appeared on the birth certificate. Another recent change is using names other than those of saints. All of these factors should alert the health-care practitioner to the potential for confusion in the name format for client cultural identification.

## FAMILY ROLES AND ORGANIZATION

### Head of Household and Gender Roles

The profound social changes encountered after the "Quiet Revolution" of the late 1960s and early 1970s brought important modifications in education and industrialization and increased the roles of women in economic activity. Women not only became producers of domestic goods in the household, but they could also become productive outside the home environment. Traditionally, in French-speaking Canadian families, the male was responsible for material well-being and the female for household activities, child care, and health care (Thibaudeau & Reidy, 1985). By the end of the Quiet Revolution, marriages changed fundamentally, moving towards equality of husbands and wives but not necessarily of children and parents (Henripin & Martin, 1991). Using the husband's income as an index for comparing the quality of communication and relative independence on marital adjustment among 180 French speaking-couples, Aube and Linden (1991) found that the degree of marital discord was similar across different socioeconomic levels. However, quality of communication accounted for 16 percent of the variance in marital satisfaction among men and only 13 percent of the variance among women. From a socioanthropological perspective, a national survey with 5614 females and 10,965 males addressed income differences between genders. Inequality attributable to career interruptions in the female was estimated along with the importance of such factors as education, occupation, socioeconomic status, and hours worked per year. The income difference by gender among native and linguistic minorities in Canada showed that the inequality between the sexes was smaller among French-speaking Canadians than other groups (Goyder, 1981).

### Prescriptive, Restrictive, and Taboo Behaviors for Children and Adolescents

The greatest source of pride for French Canadian families is to see their children well established with a good education. On this issue, the majority of the present political elite, educated through religious colleges, share the values and beliefs of their religious professors, not the prescribed behavior for their offspring.

## Family Roles and Priorities

Traditional French Canadian intergenerational relationships are rapidly disappearing (Fig. 11–1). Urbanization, particularly without adequate social security measures, results in social dislocation of the young and old. Strategies for maintaining cohesion between the generations are required to avoid intergenerational conflict related to competition for scarce resources when survival challenges are real.

Today, French Canadian families follow the same pattern of declining birth rates as other Canadians. In Canada, many of the social policies are under provincial jurisdiction. Quebec has done the most in formulating a family policy and stimulating a widespread popular debate on the issue (Eichler, 1988). Family policy, when geared toward protecting and fostering a particular type of family, contributes to the detriment of other types of families and becomes a prescribed structure for acceptance. For example, because children born out of wedlock were being penalized on the basis of their parents' relationship, the legal category of illegitimate children has been abolished in Quebec and in most other Canadian provinces (Eichler, 1988).

French-speaking Canadian family membership is known for its closeness, and some families are a "closed" family system. Urbanization and smaller families along with the Quiet Revolution in Quebec have encouraged people to open their borders and expand their circle to include others by broadening their family perspective. Nevertheless, within the microcosm of the French Canadian population, the physical

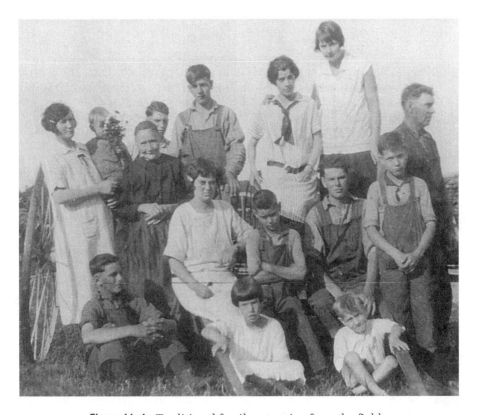

**Figure 11–1.** Traditional family returning from the fields.

and social quality of the microenvironment is more critical to health and survival than wealth and a mechanical connection (Evans & Stodart, 1994). House, Lanais, and Umberson (1988) reported widespread and strong correlations between mortality and social support networks—friends and family keep French Canadians alive! The sheer number of contact persons one has is protective, regardless of the nature of the interaction (Evans, 1994).

Lambert et al. (1986), using the 1984 national election study of 3377 Quebec inhabitants, explored cognitive differences from a social class perspective. English-speaking and French-speaking residents of Quebec were surveyed regarding their perceptions on (1) social class, (2) the importance of using characteristics to describe people from diverse social classes, and (3) differentiation of the most important characteristics of social class. Approximately 45 percent stated that the idea of social class had no meaning to them or that they were unsure of its meaning, with English-speaking Canadians being more likely to give this response. Generally, people who said they understood the concept believed that social classes differed materially, whereas those who did not understand the concept preferred to evaluate persons on individual characteristics. French-speaking respondents defined social class in a materialist sense of income and wealth, whereas English-speaking Canadians emphasized individuals in terms of character and ambition and used ascriptive criteria such as country of origin, birth, or ancestry.

## Alternative Lifestyles

At present, there is a growing trend for couples to live together without marrying. Many young couples will answer that they cannot financially afford to get married. Yet, many of these same couples insist on having their children baptized and raise them according to Catholic Church principles.

Hobart (1992) studied sexual behaviors and attitudes toward sex, sexually transmitted diseases, and acquired immunodeficiency syndrome (AIDS) among 1775 Anglophone and 493 Francophone Canadian postsecondary students, surveying their expectations about condom usage with different sexual partners. Results imply that women's patterns of sexual behaviors were more predictive than men's, but the relationships between variables were neither consistent nor strong. The most powerful predictors of safe sex practices were the size of the home community and romantic love beliefs among Francophone women.

## WORKFORCE ISSUES

### Culture in the Workplace

Among Canadians, workforce issues often correspond to educational background. However, the overall educational level of French-speaking Canadians is lower than that of their English-speaking counterparts. In addition, the proportion of part-time and casual workers among French-speaking Canadians is higher, especially in Quebec hospitals. Labor unions support part-time and casual work as being shared work. However, many male workers are beginning to resent this approach, calling it "shared poverty." The strong laws to protect French in Quebec may have created another problem for its population. While promoting a pseudosense of security by maintaining the dominance of the French language, a large portion of Quebec's French-speaking population lack sufficient knowledge of the English language to access the workforce outside their province and have difficulty in higher education programs where readings are mostly in the English language.

Hofstede (as cited in Punnett, 1991) examined the preferred leadership styles among 113 Anglophone and 77 Francophone managers in Ottawa from a language and cultural values perspective. The two groups were similar on their preferred style of leadership but differed significantly in terms of individualism. Differences between this group and an earlier Canadian sample suggest that organizational influences may have more impact on expressed cultural values than language differences. To a large extent, outside the province of Quebec, French-speaking Canadian's patterns of acculturation are intermeshed with educational and work opportunities. From an educational perspective, in the 1970s a vast movement for French immersion classes across Canada started changing the views of the younger generation. Also, the long battle for the administrative French School Board system has reduced the acculturation process in many areas of Canada without stopping it. The availability of higher education in the French language outside of Quebec completes the realm of factors necessary to reverse acculturation and assure health services for French-speaking Canadians wherever they live.

## Issues Related to Autonomy

Bilingualism, multiculturalism, and a focus on open-mindedness are the dominant themes in the Canadian workplace. With the exception of the Quebec province's position regarding French as the official language, very few places of employment want to identify an official language. However, geographic and regional aggregates shape the language of services offered.

Nurses' roles and activities remain consistent across Canada; however, changes in the mode of care and the language used in delivering services are apparent. Opportunities for Francophone nurses to function successfully outside Quebec are limited if they have not mastered the English language. Frustration occurs among Francophone nurses when the time and effort put into mastering and delivering services in both official languages are not recognized. In addition, the number of Francophone nurses academically prepared to serve in decision-making positions is limited outside of the province of Quebec. This hinders the type and mode of services offered when decisions are translated into public health policies.

## BIOCULTURAL ECOLOGY
### Skin Color and Biologic Variations

Canadians of French descent are white; however, Francophones as a linguistic group represent a mosaic of ethnocultural characteristics, including racial differences. Thus, persons must be assessed individually according to their racial heritage.

## Disease and Health Conditions

Given the limited population density, multiculturalism, and regionalism factors affecting Canadian society, specific risk factors for Canadians of French ancestry are the same as those of other minority groups, except for those in Quebec. The primary causes of death among the Quebec population are cardiac diseases, lung cancer in men, breast cancer in females, (*Rapport de la Commisssion d'Enquête sur les Services de santé sociaux,* 1988), premature birth rates (Coté, 1992), and trauma for those under age 30 years. In this assessment, however, Quebec is not different from Ontario and the rest of Canada.

In addition, suicide rates in Quebec are greater than in the United States, Japan, and Sweden (*Rapport de la Commisssion d'Enquete sur les Services de santé sociaux*, 1988). In 1978, approximately four times more Canadian men than women committed suicide (Health Canada, 1994). The suicide rate for men increased fivefold between 1950 and 1990, moving suicide from the ninth to the first place in Canada for all causes of death. A Quebec study by Cormier and Klerman (1985) showed a correlation between unemployment and suicide rates among men between the years 1950 and 1981, and women between the years 1966 and 1981. Platt (1984) concluded that there is a potential link between unemployment and suicide. However, in practice, this situation is not observed in other regions where prevalence of unemployment is chronically high. The high rate of suicide and suicide ideation, particularly among adolescent and young adult males, is one aspect of mental health that health-care practitioners have yet to address adequately.

Today's French Canadian population suffers from the same endemic conditions and sensitivities to environmental diseases as the Canadian population as a whole. The harsh topography and low winter temperature are responsible for 19 percent of the population's osteoarthritic disorders; 13 percent of the allergies are related to urban air pollution, smog, and poor air circulation in public buildings (Pampalon et al., 1990).

A number of hereditary and genetic diseases that are more common among Quebecers of French origin can be traced to early colonists. Familial chylomicronemia resulting from the lipoprotein lipase (LPL) deficiency, hyperlipoproteinemia type I, is an autosomal recessive disorder with a prevalence of 1 in 1 million persons (Brunzell, 1989). Through genealogical research, this hereditary disorder has been traced to migrants from the Perche region of France (DeBraekeler & Dao, 1994a, 1994b). The distribution of LPL deficiency among French Canadians of Quebec is the highest frequency worldwide (Ma et al., 1991). Within the French Canadian population of Quebec, its prevalence is especially high in the eastern part of the province (Gagné et al., 1989). Two separate mutations in the LPL gene introduced by French immigrants in the 17th century have been identified. Although the birthplaces of the obligate carriers were scattered throughout the province, three geographic clusters were identified: the Trois-Rivières-Mauricie region, the Saguenay-Lac-St.-Jean-Charlevoix region, and Beauce region (Dionne et al., 1993). The carrier rate of LPL deficiency is estimated to be 1 in 139 persons in the province as a whole but 1 in 85 persons in eastern Quebec, with a peak of 1 in 47 persons in Saguenay-Lac-St.-Jean (Dionne et al., 1993). With the discovery of a mutation in the human LPL gene, scientists have identified the most common cause of familial chylomicronemia in the French Canadian population (Ma et al., 1991). Furthermore, a single mutation of the fumarylacetoacetate hydrolase gene can lead to hereditary tyrosinemia type I (Grompe et al., 1994).

Findings related to familial hypercholesterolemia leading to coronary thrombosis support the French origin of the French Canadian deletion. One century after settlement in North America, the founders originating from Perche had a large number of descendants. Among the 50 or more fertile couples, 14 came from Perche (Charbonneau et al., 1987). However, it is suggested that the high frequency of this mutation among French Canadian clients with hypercholesterolemia is due to a founder effect rather than to a high frequency within the population (Fumeron et al., 1992).

A province-wide, long-term longitudinal study on all newborns identified a rare genetic disease among French Canadians. Profiles of phenylketonuria (PKU) in Quebec populations show evidence of stratification and novel mutations (Rozen et al., 1994). To date, five mutations account for almost 90 percent of PKU diagnoses among French Canadians from eastern Quebec (John et al., 1992). Time and space clusters of the PKU mutation can be traced to France (Lyonnet et al., 1992).

In addition, an increased incidence of cystic fibrosis occurs among French-speaking Canadians (Howell et al., 1991; Rozen et al., 1992). Muscular dystrophy, with a worldwide frequency of 1 in 25,000 persons, occurs in 1 in 154 French Canadians of the Saguenay region (DeBraekeleer, 1991). Health-care providers working with this specialized population of Quebecers must screen for these genetic diseases and provide genetic counseling for clients expressing an interest.

## Variations in Drug Metabolism

Research literature supporting differences in drug metabolism related to race and ethnicity is beginning to identify genetic mutations among descendants of French Canadian settlers from specific areas of France (DeBraekeler & Dao, 1994a, 1994b). Although these findings may produce data related to drug metabolism, thus far, little has been published.

# HIGH-RISK BEHAVIORS

Risk factors affecting French-speaking Canadians tend to be related to type of work, geographic region, communication, education, and age groups. In view of these risk factors, special attention must be given to Francophone elders living outside Quebec.

Abuse of alcohol, tobacco, and psychotropic drugs are major health problems among Francophone Quebecers. Although the number of people who use tobacco is decreasing, 35 percent of men and 31 percent of women continue to smoke (*Rapport de la Commisssion d'Enquete sur les Services de santé sociaux,* 1988). Alcohol dependency is highest among the 20- to 24-year-old age group (Coté, 1992). Lapp's (1984) study on 132 female and 84 male college students in Montreal found that the use of psychotropic drugs is primarily among females. However, drug use is not associated with personality factors or depression when measured by Rotter's Internal-External Locus of Control Scale Depression Inventory. Tobacco and alcohol use was highest among French-speaking males and is associated with masculine sex roles, higher self-esteem, and an external locus of control. Nonmedical drug use, primarily marijuana and hashish, most frequently involved males and was related to an internal locus of control.

## Health-seeking Behaviors

Beliefs about methods for improving one's health are seen as influential factors in health-seeking behaviors. Edwards and Rootman's (1993) analysis of data from Canada's health promotion survey 1990 on Canadians aged 15 and older identified the following practices for improving health: smoking cessation (81 percent), increased relaxation (69 percent), increased exercise (65 percent), income security (45 percent), quantity of time spent with family (45 percent), weight loss (42 percent), better dental care (27 percent), job changes (22 percent), reduced drinking (16 percent), moving (14 percent), and reduced drug use (9 percent).

Responses of French-speaking Canadians throughout Canada correlated more with the province in which they lived than with the selected cultural group. This correlation could be due to the method of data collection, which is less accurate with a small response rate. The higher proportion of respondents from Quebec and New Brunswick may have skewed the statistical outcome. Overall, age was a factor associated with beliefs about one's ability to achieve an improved health status. Results imply that elderly persons focus more on personal well-being than on health practices.

Feather and Green's (1993) study on health behaviors and intentions found that good health practices are more prevalent among Canadian males under the age of 25 years and over the age of 65 years than among men in their middle adult years. In contrast to males, the prevalence of good health practices among Canadian females increases until the age of 65 years and then decreases. In addition, these practices are positively correlated with levels of education in both sexes, adequate income for women, and managerial or professional occupations of men.

# NUTRITION

## Meaning of Food

The strong influence of nutritional status on health prompted the inclusion of questions on nutritional behaviors and diet changes in the 1990 health promotion survey to identify data among high-risk groups (Craig, 1993). In this survey, body mass index was used to calculate the ratio of weight relative to height and determine the potential for health risk. Age, gender, and education rather than culture were identified as positive influences on the practice of reading labels for nutritional value of food. Regardless of the reason, this practice demonstrates the importance individuals attribute to food in relation to health.

## Common Foods and Food Rituals

Common vegetables enjoyed by French Canadians include potatoes, turnips, carrots, asparagus, cabbage, lettuce, and tomatoes. Apart from citrus fruits, all other edible fruits and berries grown in gardens or the wild are prepared and preserved by French Canadians for winter. Meat choices are mainly beef, pork, and poultry. Until the late 1960s, fish was often perceived as a Friday food. However, for the younger generation, this belief is no longer practiced. Increased immigration and fast food availability have influenced food choices and customs to the point of transforming French Canadians' customs and food practices.

In Acadia, due to the proximity of the coastal areas, fresh fish and seafood are part of the diet. Common foods include *fricot* (stew made with a special spice called summer savory). Traditional foods such as *poutine râpées* (balls of dough made from grated potatoes) and *râpure* (grated potato) are not part of the regular diet but are still enjoyed during special events. The equivalent to the French Canadian pea soup is named *fayots* soup in Acadia.

## Dietary Practices for Health Promotion

Most men and women report reading nutritional labels on food packages. This behavior is a good predictor of diet changes during the preceding year. As a whole, more Quebecers than other Canadians report eating breakfast. Only 10 percent of the French-speaking Canadians report skipping breakfast, which is significantly lower than among respondents from the rest of Canada (Craig, 1993).

## Nutritional Deficiencies and Food Limitations

In an industrialized country like Canada, six times as many women as men are underweight, yet half as many women as men rated themselves as underweight (Craig, 1993). However, one-third of all Canadians are trying to lose weight. The 1990 health promotion study demonstrates that being overweight is inversely proportionate to education and income for both men and women. For men, there was no association between being underweight and education and income, whereas for women, with the exception of the very poor, there was a positive correlation between being underweight and increased income (Craig, 1993).

# PREGNANCY AND CHILDBEARING PRACTICES

## Fertility Practices and Views toward Pregnancy

Until the middle of the 20th century, French Canadians maintained high fertility rate, which is uncommon for a population living in an industrial country. This phenomenon, called the "revenge of the cradles," has never been explained. According to Fournier (1989), classic interpretations based on the economy, religion, or education do not hold up to scientific examination. The historical co-occurrence of the power of the church and high birth rates do not prove a causal link. Instead, the "overfertility" of French Canadians appears to be a response to socialization that is distinguished by the prevalence of extended family ties (Fournier, 1989).

For many years, French Canadian fertility practices have been closely tied to the Catholic religion. Before the 1960s, the only acceptable birth control method was abstinence, resulting in a high fecundity rate. In 1851, Quebec families had a mean of 6.84 children per family, which was maintained until the 1960s, when the number of children per family started to decline from 3.1 in 1965 to 1.5 in 1990 (Henripin & Martin, 1991) with a recent record of 1.2 (Statistics Canada, 1992).

Effective contraception and family planning methods such as the pill, intrauterine device, and tubal ligation have become available to all women. By 1985, the pill was used by 44 percent of women and remains the primary reversible method for birth control (Health and Welfare Canada, 1989). On the basis of relative frequency, tubal ligation and vasectomy follow the pill as nonreversible methods of fertility control.

Diaphragms, foams, and creams are not commonly used for birth control, partially because perceptions imply that women are not supposed to or do not like to touch their genitals. Men are still reluctant to use prophylactics because they associate their use with prostitution. The beliefs that prophylactics reduce the level of sexual feeling during intercourse or that contraception is not a male responsibility are inversely proportionate to the age of men. Among French-speaking Canadians, abortion is still considered morally wrong but is legally practiced. The number of annual abortions by language or cultural subdivision is unavailable. However, figures published by province under the obstetric or gynecologic classification other than birth, show that the frequency of abortion is greater than the frequency of rape and incest. Finally, new reproductive technologies are available and used by a small number of French-speaking Canadians, more because of scarcity than cultural denial or restriction.

Although pregnancy is considered a normal life event, fear of labor and delivery prevails. This learned fear is transmitted to women from childhood and often reinforced by the health-care system. Midwives have officially been accepted by the government, but the use of midwives and maternity houses (maison des naissances) are far from being the custom.

## Prescriptive, Restrictive, and Taboo Practices in the Childbearing Family

From a clinical perspective, prenatal medical visits are recommended once a month until the end of the seventh month, twice during the eighth month, and weekly during the last month. Since the mid-1970s, prenatal classes are attended by most couples. These classes are generally free of charge and focus on information regarding health and hygiene during pregnancy and on preparation and exercises for labor and delivery.

Alcohol and tobacco use are discouraged for the duration of pregnancy and the breast-feeding period. Intercourse restrictions are not commonly applied during pregnancy unless required for medical reasons. For the last 30 years, fathers have been encouraged to be present in the case (delivery) room. They are invited to assume an active role by assisting the mother and the physician, receiving the baby, and cutting the cord. The vast majority of Canadian women of French descent still deliver their baby in a dorsal position, despite the fact that lying on the back has been shown to be antiphysiological (ASPQ, 1980). However, with the advent of birthing rooms, more women are delivering their babies in half-sitting or side-lying positions.

In regard to home delivery by a midwife, more women are talking about the desire to deliver at home, but the number who actually use the services of a midwife throughout labor and delivery at home is quite low. The use of analgesics, local anesthetics such as epidural for delivery, or both remain high. Very few French Canadians practice natural childbirth.

During hospitalization, cohabitation of the mother and child is a relatively new practice. Many hospitals have made cohabitation a generalized practice, unless the child or mother necessitate special treatment. Breast-feeding has regained importance after years of bottle feeding. The mother's general hesitation relates to not having sufficient milk, experiencing sore nipples, losing breast firmness, and muscle wasting after the breast-feeding period. In practice, once the mother has made a decision regarding breast-feeding, the father's support and encouragement are key for a successful outcome.

Differences exist between English-speaking and French-speaking women with respect to breast-feeding. During the Health Survey of 1990, 44 percent of Canadian mothers reported breast-feeding their last child. Of these, 48 percent were Anglophones and 26 percent were Francophones. Craig (1993) found a significant difference in practices among regions of the country. Approximately one-quarter of women from the Maritimes, one-third from Quebec, and one-half from Ontario and the western provinces breast-feed their babies.

Women who breast-feed their babies to please the fathers or their families or those who find it more comfortable to hide and isolate themselves to breast-feed the babies are bound to fail. Mothers should not be made to feel guilty if they do not breast-feed. Bottle feeding in these circumstances may be the best choice.

Maternity and paternity leaves are available and range from 6 to 20 weeks. In practice, however, fathers often take only a few days to a few weeks of leave to help the mother care for the new baby and other children.

In general, French Canadians are particularly distinctive in terms of taboo behaviors. Some taboo practices related to pregnancy have persisted throughout the years. Although the movement used in washing a floor resembles that of an exercise aimed at strengthening the perineal muscles, this activity in the past was associated with the onset of labor and early or preterm deliveries. Another belief, which is shared by some nurses, is that the full moon plays a role in the onset of labor once the full-term period has been reached. This belief applies to pregnant women that are 2 weeks predate or postdate. A much less generalized taboo is that pregnant women who experience hyperglycemia give birth to boys and that lack of salt announces the birth of girls.

## DEATH RITUALS

### Death Rituals and Expectations

French Canadians do not differ from Canadians of European origin on issues related to death and death rituals. Expectations are closely related to Christian religious practices, in particular, those of the Roman Catholic Church, of which most French Canadians are members. Whether one is an active member in the Church or not, religious funerals are the norm and general practice. Values and beliefs related to life after death, the soul, and God vary dramatically across the age span among French Canadians and, even more so, among Francophones. Thus, it is essential to assess each family individually when it comes to death rituals and expectations.

For many years, cremation was seen by the Catholic Church as a ritual left for specific circumstances. Currently, the Catholic Church advocates cremation as an acceptable practice.

## Responses to Death and Grief

During the second half of the 20th century, long grief and mourning rituals imposed by social norms have adapted to modern lifestyles. One aspect that has shaped the traditional responses to death and mourning periods is influenced by the place women hold in the workforce. Currently, the expression of grief among French Canadians is similar to the stages described by Kübler-Ross (1974). Support for those who have lost a family member include openly acknowledging the family's right to express grief, being physically present, making referrals to appropriate religious leaders, and encouraging interpersonal relationships.

## SPIRITUALITY

### Religious Practices and Use of Prayer

Because most French Canadians are Roman Catholic, they are usually baptized at birth and may or may not remain active church members. However, a growing number of children are registered through civilian channels rather than through the traditional Catholic registry and baptismal. Despite the sharp decline in actively practicing Catholics, the majority of people from all socioeconomic levels turn to their church for important life events such as marriage and funerals. In some cases, even in a civil ceremony involving previously divorced spouses, the couple may ask a priest to say a mass and bless the union because the religious marriage and exchange of solemn vows is not permitted by the Catholic Church.

Religious holidays honored as civic holidays are New Year's day, Good Friday, Easter and Easter Monday, and Christmas. In the province of Quebec, St. John the Baptist Day (June 24) is a civic holiday, and in most Acadian institutions, the national Acadian holiday feast of the Assumption is celebrated on August 15. All Saints Day, November 1, and Epiphany, January 6, were dropped in the 1970s.

Older adult generations are more inclined to use prayers for finding strength and adapting to difficult physical, psychological, and social health problems. In times of illness and tragedy, French-speaking Canadians use prayer to help recovery. Many of the younger generation are not strongly influenced by religious values and beliefs and faith practices. Yet, many French Acadians still request the sacrament of the sick and a visit from the priest.

## Meaning of Life and Individual Sources of Strength

Traditional French Canadians who view themselves as the core (gyron) of the family and who believe that the well-being of their children is more precious than their own life have faded proportionally with the prevalence of divorce. For hard-working men and women of previous generations, leisure activity was a trivial expression. The little time that could be spared on holidays was dedicated to visiting distant relatives.

## Spiritual Beliefs and Health-care Practices

Although modern health promotion theories suggest that spiritual needs are a critical factor in comprehensive client care (McSherry & Nelson, 1987; Rukholm et al., 1991a), this aspect of family needs has received little attention among French-speaking Canadians. Many health-care providers still equate spirituality with religion; this is often reflected in the patient history at the time of admission. According to Rukholm et al. (1991a), the most important issues are knowing that the patient is valued, recognizing the family, and respecting the client's values and spirituality. Their study of French and English cultural differences in family needs and anxiety in an intensive care unit (ICU) in three hospitals of northeastern Ontario found that spiritual needs and anxiety explained 33 percent of the variations in family needs.

## HEALTH-CARE PRACTICES

## Beliefs That Influence Health-care Practices

In the earlier part of the 20th century, sick people did not readily enter hospitals because mortality rates were high and care was often inhumane. Resources and preventive health care before the Confederation rested in the hands of religious sisterhoods, United Empire Loyalists, church groups, and local authorities (Allemag, 1995). As pioneers in health services, the Gray Nuns visited the sick and opened hospitals such as St. Boniface in Manitoba in 1847 and Bytown in Ontario in 1845. In 1860, they extended their services to an Indian settlement 400 miles north of Saskatoon and to Fort Providence on Great Slave Lake (1867).

Beckingham, Coutu-Wakulczyk, and Lubin's (1993) study on rural elderly Francophones and Anglophones living in Ontario and Quebec showed that 20 percent of Ontarians rated their health as excellent, compared with 14 percent for Quebecers. However, 71 percent of Ontarians rated their health as excellent or good, compared with 62.9 percent of Quebecers. In Bourque et al.'s (1991) study on New Brunswick Francophone elderly adults, 58.5 percent of respondents rated their health as good or excellent. Using the same scales, Bellehumeur (1994) found similar results on a randomized sample of French Canadian elderly adults living in northeastern Ontario.

St.-Amant and Vuong (1994) surveyed 57 elderly former psychiatric clients from 14 organizations in New Brunswick on the relation between cultural affiliation, gender, and satisfaction with health-care services. The findings revealed that women's mental health was more fragile than men's. A positive correlation and higher satisfaction with services was found among those with longer institutionalization. The authors concluded that Francophones in New Brunswick rely more on an informal family support network, whereas Anglophones rely more on professional services.

Results of a 1990 Canadian health survey show that residents of British Colombia and Ontario reported the most favorable assessments of their health, with almost 3 out of 10 reporting excellent health. Lower levels of health were reported in eastern Canada where one in five Nova Scotians reported excellent health. Canadians from New Brunswick, followed by those from Quebec, were more likely to report fair or poor health, with only 17 percent and 16 percent, respectively, reporting excellent health (Stephens & Fowler Graham, 1993b). Good health was related to education and income, occupation, or both. However, lifestyle showed an inconsistent relationship with income. Among younger adult and older men, social class had little effect on income, whereas among women, the effect of income dominated over social class. Syme and Berkman (1976) suggested that rather than attempting to identify risk factors for specific diseases, it may be more meaningful to identify those factors that affect general susceptibility to risk factors.

# Responsibility for Health Care

Canada's national government-administered health system ensures free, universal health coverage at any point of entry into the system. A survey conducted by Renaud, Jutras, and Bouchard (1987) showed user satisfaction reaching 80 percent. However, many people in the upper socioeconomic classes call on their family physicians instead of the *Centre locaux de services communautaires (CLSC)* (in Quebec) or community center (also free). Among the lower socioeconomic classes of Quebec and the Maritimes, many do not seek health care until their health is in a crisis situation.

The famous Canadian white paper "A New Perspective" (Lalonde, 1974) proposed that the determinants of health status are lifestyle, environment, human biology, and health-care organizations. According to Evans and Stoddard (1994), the assumption is that lifestyle and, to a lesser extent, living environments are chosen by the person. Corin (1994) offers a matrix of stressors for identifying high-risk behaviors within a perspective that avoids victim blaming. Lifestyle behaviors are readily perceived as being under the control of the individual. The broad set of relationships encompassed under the label of "stress" and predictive factors against stress have demonstrated the importance of social relationships for preventing disease and mortality (Dantzer & Kelly, 1989; Sapolsky, 1990).

The government of the province of New Brunswick, in establishing the New Brunswick Extra-Mural Hospital in 1980, opened a novel delivery program to provide home-care services (acute and chronic) to a largely rural province with a small population density and limited financial resources (Robichaud, 1985). Because the willingness of clients and family members to participate actively in a plan of care is critical to the success of community-based services, the Extra-Mural Hospital program strongly encouraged self-care with strong family involvement. Unlike other community initiatives in Canada such as *CLSC,* the Ontario Home Care Program, the Extra-Mural Hospital does not restrict services within specific boundaries and offers a comprehensive, province-wide delivery system via a single-agency approach (Cormier-Daigle et al., 1995). However, as of June 1996, the Extra-Mural Hospital came under the jurisdiction of the hospital corporations rather than the central administration. The delivery system remained the same.

The link between health promotion and community health nursing with conceptual and practical issues was raised by Hagan, O'Neill, and Dallaire (1995). In Quebec, the infrastructure for public health is different from that in other provinces. The CLSCs emerged from the Castonguay-Nepveu reform of health and welfare services in the early 1970s. The *Fédération des CLSC du Québec's* (1992) mission is to provide health and social services for primary and secondary prevention and rehabilitation (Hagan et al., 1995). In a survey on health education roles and activities of some 631 nurses, Hagan (1991) found that 89 percent of nurses have a humanistic vision of health education. This vision was defined as "teaching and establishing a helping relationship aimed at facilitating individuals' choices of strategies for improving or maintaining their global health" (p. 278).

French-speaking Canadians have joined the current trend toward over-the-counter drug use. However, from the health survey of 1990, their use of analgesics and tranquilizers shows strong provincial differences (Adlaf, 1993). As compared with the national average for the use of narcotic analgesics (11 percent), Quebec residents' use is only 5 percent. Residents of Quebec (67 percent) are less likely to use aspirin than the average Canadian (76 percent). However, the use of tranquilizers among Quebecers is slightly higher than the Canadian average (8 percent versus 5 percent). Drug use followed a pattern similar to that found in the healthy lifestyle practice. Despite the move towards healthy lifestyles, French Canadian elderly adults have not changed dramatically in comparison with younger age groups. In addition, in the 1990 health survey, the leisure time physical activity (LTPA) index reported a positive relation between adoption of health lifestyles and socioeconomic status, although not a smooth linear one. In particular, the daily LTPA index decreased with increasing education.

## Folk Practices

Saillant (1992) analyzed the importance, characteristics, and mechanics of women's knowledge of folk medicine in Quebec Francophone families at the beginning of the 20th century. This anthropological study focused on domestic activities. The ethnographic data were drawn from 4000 medical receipts dealing with the knowledge of women in folk-healing practices in Quebec and abroad to enhance the understanding of the roles played by women in rural society folk-healing tradition. The numerous connections between the culinary and therapeutic realms of activities bring one to rethink the link between nutrition and health practiced in the early years of the colony.

## Barriers to Health Care

Current views towards multiculturalism include removing barriers so that all citizens have equal access and opportunities and so that cultural diversity needs are considered in decision making and resource allocation (Fleras & Elliott, 1992). For many French Canadian elderly adults raised outside the province of Quebec, French was the language used in daily living within their cultural environment, except for educational services. In their childhood, they attended English-speaking schools because the public school system was all that was available outside Quebec. This situation and other issues present challenges in organizing transcultural heath-care delivery: the spoken language is French, yet reading skills (or what is left of them) are often English. Thus, in view of these facts, the health-care team may need to supplement written messages and instructions with verbal instructions to ensure understanding (Coutu-Wakulczyk & Beckingham, 1993).

## Cultural Responses to Health and Illness

Choinière and Melzack (1987), using the McGill Pain Questionnaire and a visual analogue intensity scale, assessed acute and chronic pain differences between 68 French-speaking and English-speaking people with hemophilia. The results showed a similarity in the sensory, affective, and evaluative properties between the two types of pain. However, acute pain was described as more intense than chronic pain. French-speaking subjects rated their pain as more intense and more affectively laden than the English-speaking group. From a different perspective, Rukholm, Bailey, and Coutu-Wakulczyk (1991b), studying French and English cultural differences in family needs and anxiety in an ICU, found that English-speaking subjects rated their distress at seeing a relative in pain more highly than French-speaking subjects. Though puzzling, this finding deserves attention and additional research to better understand and plan health-care interventions and to assist family members involved with ICU services.

Adam (1989), as part of a broader package of health promotion, developed, implemented, and evaluated a 15-hour community program for French-speaking women living in minority situations, many of whom were socially and economically disadvantaged. The program was designed to increase the participants' ability to take charge of their lives and better manage their physical and mental health. After presenting the program to some 29 groups, evaluations showed that women generally reported satisfaction as the program progressed. Most subjects were satisfied with their broader understanding of stress and relaxation techniques for controlling daily stress.

Covered under federal and provincial laws in Canada, the physically and mentally disabled are protected from discrimination and abuse with the vast deinstitutionalization movement of the 1970s. Physically disabled people, regardless of their ethnicity, benefit from equal opportunity regulations. Throughout Canada, official general acceptance and an increased awareness have lead to the physical adaptation of the environment to facilitate access for the disabled. However, the homeless mentally disabled raise different concerns in regard to the cost of maintaining this segment of the population in the community for lack of adequate organized services.

Transcultural validation on self-reported assessment instruments provides another perspective when mental health issues are addressed. For example, Fortin, Coutu-Wakulczyk, and Engelsmann's randomized study (1989) to validate Derogatis' Symptom Check List-90-Revised (SCL-90-R) instrument on French-speaking women found that the women in their sample generally obtained higher raw scores than those reported by Derogatis (1977) on American women in the general population for the nine symptom scales and the three global scores. This higher rate of self-reported symptoms corresponds to the Canadian health survey (Statistics Canada, 1981), which also yielded higher scores for Quebec women on the Bradburn test measuring a lack of psychological well-being.

The sick role among French Canadians was studied from a clinical anthropological perspective by Saillant (1990). This author explored the relation between discourse, knowledge, and the experience of cancer within the life story of a patient suffering from cancer. The underlying theoretical model drew on a cultural hermeneutic approach. The client's discourse was analyzed for cognitive and symbolic models used to understand the experience of cancer. The results of this study highlighted the gap between the client's actual medical knowledge and the health profession's perception of the client's experiences and discourse about cancer.

## Blood Transfusion and Organ Donation

As a cultural group, French Canadians have no official proscriptions against receiving blood or blood products. Those who are members of a religious group that prohibits the acceptance of blood transfusion are rare in Canada. Organ donation and transplant are relatively new treatments in Canada. The decision to donate or receive an organ is an individual decision without any cultural influence for French Canadians.

## HEALTH-CARE PRACTITIONERS

### Traditional Versus Biomedical Care

French Canadians have discarded the idea that one goes to the hospital to die. With a fully public-administered health-care system since the 1960s, the population has benefited with increased accessibility to health care. However, financing this "welfare state" (*état providence*) has imposed a tremendous burden on taxpayers. Although the overall impact on health-care services is minimal, alternative therapies are gaining popularity, which may reflect disillusionment with the biomedical model in Quebec.

Males have been members of the nursing profession since the early 1970s, at which time the second "I" was added in the AIIC (*Association des infirmières et infirmiers du Canada*), the French name for the Canadian Nurses Association, and the OIIQ (*Ordre des infirmières et infirmiers du Québec*). Although male nurses receive the same training as female nurses, they still account for less than 10 percent of professional nurses in Canada. While bedside nursing is gaining in popularity for men, the vast majority hold administrative or teaching positions.

A transcultural study of self-concept using Fitts' (1965) Tennessee Self-Concept Scale (TSCS) was conducted on the 399 undergraduate nursing students of two bilingual programs. Results showed significant differences in the dimensions of total self-esteem ($p<.05$), self-identity ($p<.001$), moral-ethic self ($p<.001$), and family self ($p<.05$) between Francophone and Anglophone students when controlling for the language spoken at home, language of high school study, and province of origin (Coutu-Wakulczyk et al., 1992).

## Status of Health-care Providers

In Canada as a whole, health-care practitioners cover a broad realm of specialties and disciplines, each working within an interdisciplinary and intersectorial approach to well-being. However, the system is not ideal and tension does occur within and among disciplines. Health-care providers hold a favorable status in the eyes of French Canadians, especially among elderly persons. At the beginning of the century, parents and grandparents were pragmatic and practical people, sharing views about God's power over everyday life. For example, a mother would pray to have at least a priest and a nun among her children, and a physician or a nurse was next in her wish to God.

Today, folk and traditional practitioners are almost nonexistent. Professionals throughout Canada are vigilant in trying to avoid exploitation by traditional and folk healers, who are viewed as practicing against the law. A major deterrent to traditional and folk practitioners is that the current universal health insurance system makes the folk practitioners less appealing.

---

**CASE STUDY**

Mr. Latrémouille, a retired 72-year-old electrician, lives in a second-floor dwelling with his wife, aged 72. Mrs. Latrémouille has recently experienced an exacerbation in her Parkinson's disease, which she has had for many years. She is experiencing problems with walking and needs assistance getting in and out of the bathtub. She insists on doing light housework and preparing meals. Mr. and Mrs. Latrémouille manage by themselves.

The community health nurse was called by the eldest daughter, who lives in a nearby village. The daughter wishes to see her parents move into a nursing home because she works during the day and cares for her own grandchildren in the evening while her son goes to school. Her daughter-in-law works the evening shift. The Latrémouilles' other children do not share this view because Mr. and Mrs. Latrémouille strongly resent leaving their home and becoming dependent. Although Mr. Latrémouille is bilingual, Mrs. Latrémouille grew up in a French-speaking community, never mastered the English language, and does not understand or speak much English, which is the language used in the nursing home in the town where they live.

## STUDY QUESTIONS

1. What are the major obstacles to health and well-being for this elderly couple?

2. What are the major obstacles to independence? How do these differ from those that interfere with health and well-being?

3. How do the meanings that people attach to health and well-being, the control they assume or wish to assume over their health, and the objective features of health reflect cultural differences in later life?

4. Discuss the role of the public health nurse and the implications for independent living of this couple at risk for institutionalization.

5. What are the types of assistance and relationships between generations that are important in maintaining this family unit?

6. How important are kinship ties in minority settings with regard to the adjustment and morale of older adults?

7. Are cultural factors more important for older adults than for other age groups?

## *References*

Adam, D. (1989). Women and stress: A community prevention and health promotion program. *Canada Mental Health, 37*(4), 5–8.

Adlaf, E. (1993). Alcohol and other drug use. *Health and welfare Canada: Canada's health promotion survey 1990—Technical report* (Cat. No. H39–263/2–1990E). Ottawa: Minister of Supply and Services Canada.

Allemag, M. M. (1995). Development of community health nursing in Canada. In M. J. Stewart (Ed.), *Community nursing: Promoting Canadians' health* (pp. 2–36). Toronto: W. B. Saunders Canada.

Annandale, E. T. (1988). A dynamic minority: Francophone culture in a Western Canadian province. *Contemporary French Civilization, 12*(2), 194–206.

Arsenault, J. E. (1981). La voix acadienne: Un hebdomadaire au service des acadiens de l'Île du Prince-Edouard. *Vie Française (Canada), 33*(7–9), 49–53.

ASPQ (1980). Accoucher ou se faire accoucher. Colloques sur l'humanisation des soins en périnatalité. Québec: Bureau de l'Éditeur officiel du Québec.

Aube, N., & Linden, W. (1991). Marital disturbance, quality of communication and socioeconomic status. *Canadian Journal of Behavioral Science, 23*(2), 125–132.

Badets, J., & Chui, T. W. (1994). *Canada's changing immigrant population* (Cat. No. 96–311E). Ottawa: Statistics Canada and Prentice-Hall Canada.

Beaudin, M., & Leclerc, A. (1995). The contemporary Acadian economy. In J. Daigle (Ed.), *Acadia of the Maritimes: Thematic studies from the beginning to the present* (pp. 1–44). Moncton, NB: Université de Moncton: Chaire d'études acadiennes.

Beckingham, A. C., Coutu-Wakulczyk, G., & Lubin, B. (1993). French-language validation of the DACL and MAACL-R. *Journal of Clinical Psychology, 49*(5), 685–695.

Bellehumeur, N. (1994). Influence de l'auto-évaluation de la santé et de l'humeur dépressive sur l'observance du régime thérapeutique auprès de personnes âgées à domicile. Unpublished master's thesis, Faculté des Lettres et Sciences Humaines, Université de Sherbrooke.

Boleda, M. (1984). Les migrations au Canada sous le régime français (1608–1760). *Cahier Québec Démographe, 13*, 23–40.

Bourque, P., Blanchard, L., Sadeghi, M. R., & Arseneault, A. M. (1991). État de santé, consommation de médicaments et symptômes de la dépression chez les personnes âgées. *Canadian Journal on Aging, 10*(4), 309–319.

Brunzell, J. T. (1989). Familial lipoprotein lipase deficiency and other causes of the chylomicronemia syndrome. In C. R. Scriver, A. L. Beaudet, W. S. Sly, & D. Valle (Eds.),

*The Metabolic basis of inherited disease* (pp. 1165–1180). New York: McGraw-Hill.

Butler, G. R. (1985). Supernatural folk belief expression in a French-Newfoundland community: A study of expressive form, communicative process, and social function in L'Anse-à-Canards. Unpublished doctoral dissertation, Memorial University, St. John, Newfoundland.

Canadian Almanac & Directory Publishing (1995). *Canadian Almanac & Directory 1995.* Toronto: Author.

Careless, J. S. M. (1970). *Canada: A story of challenge.* Toronto: Macmillan of Canada.

Castonguay, C. (1980). La position des minorités francophones en 1976. *Action Nationale (Canada), 69*(10), 825–829.

Charbonneau, H., Desjardins, B., Guillemette, A., Landry, Y., Légaré, J., & Nault, F. (1987). *Naissance d'une population: Les Français établis au Canada au XVII siècle.* Paris: Institut National d'Études Démographiques.

Choinière, M., & Melzack, R. (1987). Acute and chronic pain in hemophilia. *Pain, 31*(3), 317–331.

Clifton, R. A. (1982). Ethnic differences in the academic achievement process in Canada. *Social Science Research, 11*(1), 67–87.

Corin, E. (1994). The social and cultural matrix of health and disease. In R. G. Evans, M. L. Barer, & T. R. Marmor (Eds.), *Why are some people healthy and others not? The determinants of health of populations,* (pp. 93–132). New York: Aldine De Gruyter.

Cormier, H. J., & Klerman, G. L. (1985). Unemployment and male-female labor force participation as determinants of changing suicide rates of males and females in Quebec. Social Psychiatry, 20, 109–114.

Cormier, Y. (1994). L'Acadie d'aujourd'hui: guide des provinces maritimes francophones. Moncton, NB: Editions d'Acadie.

Cormier-Daigle, M., Baker, C., Arseneault, A.M., & MacDonald, M. (1995). The Extra-Mural hospital: A home health care initiative in New Brunswick. In M.J. Stewart (Ed.), *Community nursing: Promoting Canadians' health* (pp. 163–179). Toronto: W.B. Saunders Canada.

Coté, M. (1992). *Health and welfare policy.* Québec: Le Ministère.

Coutu-Wakulczyk, G. & Beckingham, A. C. (1993). Ethnicity and aging. In A. C. Beckingham & B. W. DuGas (Eds.), *Promoting healthy aging: A nursing community perspective* (pp. 370–394). Toronto: Mosby.

Coutu-Wakulczyk, G., Larochelle, C., & Black, R. (1992). Perception de soi des étudiants de premier cycle: Étude transculturelle. Ottawa: Université d'Ottawa. Rapport de recherche.

Couturier LeBlanc, G., Godin, A., & Renaud, A. (1995). French education in the Maritimes, 1604–1992. In J. Daigle (Ed.), *Acadia of the Maritimes: Thematic studies from the beginning to the present* (pp. 523–562). Moncton, NB: Université de Moncton: Chaire d'études acadiennes.

Craig, C. L. (1993). Nutrition. In T. Stephens & D. Fowler Graham (Eds.), *Canada's health promotion survey 1990—Technical report*

(Cat. No. H39–263/2–1990E) (pp. 125–137). Ottawa: Health and Welfare Canada, Minister of Supply and Services Canada.

Daigle, J. (1995). Acadia from 1604 to 1763: An historical synthesis. In J. Daigle (Ed.), *Acadia of the Maritimes: Thematic studies from the beginning to the present* (pp. 1–44). Moncton, NB: Université de Moncton: Chaire d'études acadiennes.

Dantzer, R., & Kelly, K. W. (1989). Stress and immunity: An integrated view of relationships between the brain and the immune system. *Life Sciences, 44,* 1995–2008.

DeBraekeleer, M. (1991). Deleterious genes. In G. Bouchard & M. DeBrackeleer (Eds.), *History of a geonome: Population and genetics in Eastern Québec* (pp. 343–363). Québec: Presses de l'Universite de Québec.

DeBraekeleer, M. & Dao, T. N. (1994a). In search of founders. Pt. 1. Hereditary disorders in the French Canadian population of Québec. *Human Biology, 66*(2), 205–224.

DeBraekeleer, M. & Dao, T. N. (1994b). Contribution of Perche (migrants from Perche, France). Pt. 2. Hereditary disorders in the French Canadian population of Québec. *Human Biology, 66*(2), 225–250.

Dionne, C., Gagné, C., Julien, P., Murthy, M., Roederer, G., Davignon, J., Lambert, M., Chitayat, D., Ma, R., Henderson, H., Lupien, P. J., Hayden, M. R., & DeBraekeleer, M. (1993). Genealogy and regional distribution of lipoprotein lipase deficiency in French Canadians of Québec. *Human Biology, 65*(1), 29–40.

Edwards, P., & Rootman, I. (1993). Supports for health. In T. Stephens & D. Fowler Graham (Eds.), *Canada's health promotion survey 1990—Technical report* (Cat. No. H39–263/2–1990E) (pp. 43–63). Ottawa: Health and Welfare Canada, Minister of Supply and Services Canada.

Eichler, M. (1988). *Families in Canada today* (2nd ed.). Toronto: Gage Educational Publishing.

Evans, R. G. (1994). Introduction. In R. G. Evans, M. L. Barer, & T. R. Marmor (Eds.), *Why are some people healthy and others not? The determinants of health of populations* (pp. 3–26). New York: Aldine De Gruyter.

Evans, R. G. & Stoddart, G. L. (1994). Producing health, consuming health care. In R. G. Evans, M. L. Barer, & T.R. Marmor (Eds.), *Why are some people healthy and others not? The determinants of health of populations* (pp. 27–66). New York: Aldine De Gruyter.

Feather, J., & Green, K. L. (1993). Health behaviours and intentions. In T. Stephens & D. Fowler Graham (Eds.), *Canada's health promotion survey 1990—Technical report* (Cat. No. H39–263/2–1990E) (pp. 225–235). Ottawa: Health and Welfare Canada, Minister of Supply and Services Canada.

Fédération des CLSC du Québec. (1992). *Les services infirmiers en CLSC: Document de réflexion.* Montréal: Author.

Fleras, A. & Elliott, J. L. (1992). *Multiculturalism in Canada: The challenge of diversity.* Toronto: Mosby.

Fitts, W. H. (1965). *The Tennessee Self-Concept Scale Manual.* Nashville, TN: Counselor Recording and Tests.

Fortin, M. F., Coutu-Wakulczyk, G., & Engelsmann, F. (1989). Contribution to the validation of the SCL–90–R in French-speaking women. *Health Care for Women International, 10*(1), 27–42.

Fournier, D. (1989). Pourquoi la revange des berceaux? L'hypothèse de sociabilité. *Recherches Sociographiques, 30*(2), 171–198.

Fumeron, F., Grandchamp, B., Fricker, J., Krempt, M. Wolf, L. M., Khayat, M. C., Boiffard, O., & Apfelbaum, M. (1992). Presence of the Canadian deletion in a French patient with familial hypercholesterolemia. *New England Journal Medicine, 326*(1), 69.

Gagné, C., Brun, L. D., Moorjani, S., and Lupien, P.J. (1989). Primary lipoprotein-lipase-activity deficiency: Clinical investigation of a French Canadian population. *Canadian Medical Association Journal, 140*(4), 405–411.

Genuist, P. (1986). Être ou ne pas être fransaskois. *Études Canadiennes (France), 12*(21, Pt. 1), 67–73.

Gilbert, A. (1991). L'Ontario français comme région: Un regard non assimilationniste sur une minorité, son espace et ses réseaux. *Cahiers de Géographie du Québec (Canada), 35*(96), 501–512.

Gill, R. M. (1980). Bilingualism in New Brunswick and the future of l'Acadie. *American Review of Canadian Studies, 10*(2), 56–74.

Gill, R. M. (1983). Federal and provincial language policy in Ontario and the future of Franco-Ontarians. *American Review of Canadian Studies, 13*(1), 13–43.

Goyder, J. C. (1981). Income differences between sexes: Findings from a national Canadian survey. *Canadian Review of Sociology and Anthropology, 18*(3), 321–342.

Griffiths, N. (1973). *The Acadians: Creation of a people.* Toronto: McGraw-Hill Ryerson.

Grompe, M., St-Louis, M., Demers, S. I., Al-Dhalimy, M., Leclerc, B., & Tanguay, R. M. (1994). A single mutation of the fumarylacetoacetate hydrolase gene in French Canadians with hereditary tyrosinemia type I. *New England Journal of Medicine, 331*(6), 353–358.

Hagan, L. (1991). Analyse de l'exercice de la fonction éducative des infirmiers et des infirmières des Centre locaux de services communautaires du Québec. Unpublished doctoral dissertation, Faculty of Education Sciences, Université de Montréal.

Hagan, L., O'Neill, M., Dallaire, C. (1995). Linking health promotion and community health nursing: Conceptual and practical issues. In M. J. Stewart (Ed.), *Community nursing: Promoting Canadians' health* (pp 413–429). Toronto: W.B. Saunders Canada.

Harris, R. C., & Matthews, G. (Eds.). (1987). *Historical Atlas of Canada (Part I): From the beginning to 1800.* Toronto: University of Toronto Press.

Health and welfare Canada (1989). Charting Canada's future: A report of the demographic review. Ottawa: Minister of Supplies and Services Canada.

Health Canada (1994). *Suicide in Canada: Update of the report of the task force on Suicide in Canada.* (Cat. No. H39–107/1995E). Ottawa: Ministry of Supply and Services Canada.

Henripin, J. & Martin, Y. (1991). La population du Québec d'hier *à demain.* Montréal, Québec: Presses de l'université de Montréal.

Hobart, C. (1992). How they handle it: Young Canadians, sex and AIDS. *Youth and Society, 23*(4), 411–433.

House, J. S., Landis, K.R., & Umberson, D. (1988). Social relationships and health. *Science, 241,* 540–545.

Howell, W.M ., Sage, D. A., Evans, P.R ., Smith, J. L., Francis, G. S., & Haegert, D. G. (1991). No association between susceptibility to multiple sclerosis and HLA-DPB1 alleles in French-Canadian population. *Tissue Antigens, 37*(4), 156–160.

Huel, R. (1986). When minority feels threatened: The impetus for French Catholic organization in Saskachewan. *Canadian Ethnic Studies, 18*(3), 1–16.

John S. W., Rozen, R., Laframboise, R., Laberge, C., Scriver, C. R. (1992). Five mutations at the PAH locus account for almost 90% of PKU mutations in French-Canadians from eastern Quebec. *Human Mutation, 1*(1): 72–74.

Kübler-Ross, E. (1975). *Death: The final stage of growth.* Englewood Cliffs, N.J.: Prentice-Hall, Inc.

Kulig, J. C. (1995). Culturally diverse communities: The impact on the role of community health nurses. In M. J. Stewart (Ed.), *Community nursing: Promoting Canadian's health.* Toronto: W. B. Saunders Canada.

Lachapelle, R. (1986). La démolinguistique et le destin des minorités françaises vivant à l'extérieur du Québec. *Transactions of the Royal Society of Canada, 1,* 123–141.

Lalonde, M. (1974). *A new perspectve on the health of Canadians.* Ottawa: Department of National Health and Welfare.

Lambert, R. D., Brown, S. D., Curtis, J. E., & Kay, B. J. (1986). Canadians' beliefs about differences between social classes. *Canadian Journal of Sociology/Cahiers canadiens de sociologie, 11*(4), 379–399.

Lapp, J. E. (1984). Psychotropic drug and alcohol use by Montréal college students: Sex, ethnic and personality correlates. *Journal of Alcohol Drug Education, 30*(1), 18–26.

Lyonet, S., De Braekelee, M., Labramboise, R., Rey, F., John, S. W., Berthelon, M., Berthelot, J., Journel, H., & Le Marec, B. (1992). Time and space clusters of the French-Canadian MIV phenylketonuria mutation in France. *American Journal of Human Genetics, 51*(1), 191–196.

Ma, Y., Henderson, H., Ven Marthy, M. R., Roederer, G., Monsalve, M. V., Clarke, L. A., Normand, T., Julien, P., Gagné, C., Lambert, M., Davignon, J., Lupien, P. Jé, Brunzell, J., & Hayden, M. R. (1991). A mutation in the human lipoprotein lipase gene as the most common cause of familial chylomicronemia in French Canadians. *New England Journal of Medicine, 324*(25), 176–182.

McInnis, E. (1969). *Canada: A political and social history.* Toronto: Holt, Rinehart & Winston of Canada.

McSherry, E. & Nelson, W. A. (1987). The DRG era: A major opportunity for increased pastoral impact or crisis for survival? *Journal of Pastoral Care, 16*(3), 201–211.

Ministry of Industry, Science & Technology (1993). *Ethnic origin: The nation.* Ottawa: Statistics Canada.

Pampalon, R., Gauthier, D., Raymond, G., & Beaudry, E. (1990). *Health map: A geographical distribution of the Québec Health Survey.* Québec: Ministere de la Santé et des Services Sociaux.

Paquet, G. (1989). *Health and social inequality: Cultural gap.* Québec, QC: Institut Québecois de Recherche sur la Culture.

Peronnet, L. (1995). The situation of the French language in Acadia: A linguistic perspective. In J. Daigle (Ed.), *Acadia of the Maritimes: Thematic studies from the beginning to the present* (pp. 451–484). Moncton, NB: Université de Moncton: Chaire d'études acadiennes.

Platt, S. (1984). Unemployment and suicidal behavior: A review of the literature. *Social Science and Medicine, 12*(2), 93–115.

Préfontaine, R. (1981). Aux frontières de la francophonie: Le Manitoba français. *Vie Française (Canada), 35*(4–6), 36–48.

Pronovost, G. (1989). Transformation in work time and leisure time. In G. Pronovost & D. Mercere (Eds.), *Time and socities* (pp. 37–61). Québec: Institut Québecois de Recherche sur la Culture.

Punnett, B. J. (1991). Language, cultural values and preferred leadership style: A comparison of Anglophones and Francophones in Ottawa. *Canadian Journal of Behavioural Science, 23*(2), 241–244.

*Rapport de la Commission d'Enquete sur les Services de santé et les Services sociaux.* (1988). Québec: Institut Québecois de Recherche sur la Culture.

Renaud, M., Jutras, S., & Bouchard, P. (1987). Solutions brought forth by quebecers concerning social and health problems. Paper presented at the Inquiry Commission on health and social services. Québec: Les Publications du Québec.

Robichaud, J. B. (1985). *La santé des francophones* (Tome 1). Moncton, NB: Éditions d'Acadie.

Robillard, J. D. (1986a). La Colombie Britanique et ses francophones. *Action Nationale (Canada), 75*(6), 496–509.

Robillard, J. D. (1986b). Les Franco-albertans. *Action Nationale (Canada), 75*(5), 422–433.

Roy, M. (1995). Demography and demolinguistics in Acadia, 1871–1991. In J. Daigle (Ed.), *Acadia of the Maritimes: Thematic studies from the beginning to the present* (pp. 125–200). Moncton, NB:

Université de Moncton: Chaire d'études acadiennes.

Rozen, R., De Braekeleer, M., Daigneault, J., Ferrire-Rajabi, L., Gerdes, M., Lamoureux, L., Aubin, G., Simard, F., Fujiwara, T. M., & Morgan, K. (1992). Cystic fibrosis mutations in French-Canadians: Three CFTR mutations are relatively frequent in a Québec population with elevated incidence of cystic fibrosis. *American Journal of Medical Genetics, 42*(3), 360–364.

Rozen, R., Mascisch, A., Lambert, M., Laframboise, R., & Scriver, C. R. (1994). Mutation profiles of phenylketonuria in Québec populations: Evidence of stratification and novel mutations. *American Journal of Human Genetics, 55*(2), 321–326.

Rukholm, E., Bailey, P., Coutu-Wakulczyk, G., & Bailey, W. (1991a). Needs and anxiety levels in relatives of intensive care unit patients. *Journal of Advanced Nursing, 16,* 920–928.

Rukholm, E., Bailey, P., & Coutu-Wakulczyk, G. (1991b). Needs and anxiety in ICU: Cultural differences in northeastern Ontario. *Canadian Journal of Nursing Research, 23*(3), 67–81.

Saillant, F. (1990). Discourse, knowledge and experience of cancer: A life story. *Culture Medicine and Psychiatry, 14*(1), 81–104.

Saillant, F. (1992). Savoir et pratiques des femmes dans l'univers ethnomedical québécois. *Canadian Folklore (Canada), 14*(1), 47–72.

St.-Amand, N., & Vuong, D. (1994). Quand la langue fait une différence: Ce que des "bénéficiaires" pensent du système de santé mentale. *Sociologie et Sociétés, 26*(1), 179–196.

Sapolsky, R. M. (1990). Stress in the wild. Ottawa: Policy, Analysis and Research Directorate Multiculturalism. *Scientific American, 262*(1), 116–123.

Statistics Canada (1986). *Census.* Ottawa: Ministry of Supply and Services Canada.

Statistics Canada. (1992). *Home language and mother tongue: 1991 Census of Canada* (Cat. No. 93–317). Ottawa: Industry, Science and Technology Canada.

Stephens, T., & Fowler Graham, D. (1993a). *Canada's health promotion survey 1990—Technical report* (Cat. No. H39–263/2–1990E). Ottawa: Health and Welfare Canada, Minister of Supply and Services Canada.

Stephens, T., & Fowler Graham, D. (1993b). Overview. In T. Stephens & D. Fowler Graham (Eds.). *Canada's health promotion survey 1990—Technical report* (Cat. No. H39–263/2–1990E) (pp. 3–7). Ottawa: Health and Welfare Canada, Minister of Supply and Services Canada.

Syme, S. L., & Berkman, L. F. (1976). Social class, susceptibility and sickness. *American Journal of Epidemiology, 104*(1), 1–8.

Tétu de Labsade, F. (1990). *Québec: A country, a culture.* Montréal: Boréal.

Thibaudeau, M., & Reidy, M. (1985). A nursing care model for the disadvantaged family. In

M. Stewart (Ed.), *Community health nursing in Canada.* (pp. 269–286). Toronto: Gage Publishing.

Thomas, G. (1980). Public and private storytelling situations in Franco-Newfoundland tradition. *Arv (Sweden), 36,* 175–181.

Vaillancourt, F., & Saint-Laurent, P. (1981). Les déterminants de l'évolution de l'écart de revenu entre canadian-anglais et canadian-français: Québec 1961–1971. *Journal of Canadian Studies (Canada) 1980–81 15*(4), 69–74.

Wesber, H., Wesley, E. B., & Danhier, E. (1944). *World civilization.* Toronto: The Copp Clark Co.

Wiseman, N. (1992). The questionable relevance of the constitution in advancing minority cultural rights in Manitoba. *Canadian Journal of Political Science (Canada), 25*(4), 697–721.

# Greek-Americans

*Toni Tripp-Reimer and Bernard Sorofman*

---

• Key terms to become familiar with in this chapter are:

| | |
|---|---|
| *Endropi* | *Pappou* |
| *Giagia* | *Philotimo* |
| *Koumbari* | *Phylactos* |
| *Magissa* | *Practika* |
| *Matiasma* | *Vendousas* |
| *Nerva* | |

## OVERVIEW, INHABITED LOCALITIES, AND TOPOGRAPHY

### Overview

Greece, a small country in southern Europe with a climate similar to that of Southern California, covers slightly more than 50,000 square miles. The land is very mountainous with small patches of fertile land separated by hills, mountains, and sea. The main crops are wheat, grapes, olives, cotton, and tobacco. Geopolitical boundaries have shifted dramatically over time. Greeks struggled under 400 years of Turkish rule which ended in 1829. At that time, the Peloponnese, central Greece, and some of the Aegean Islands were freed. Later, Thessaly, Macedonia, Crete, the Ionian Islands, Epirus, Thrace, and the Dodecansese were incorporated into Greece's boundaries.

The characteristics of members of a Greek community vary considerably according to the time of immigration (with earlier immigrants being predominately younger rural males), the characteristics of site of immigration (rural, island, or urban), and the number of generations since initial immigration. Despite considerable temporal and geographic variation, several core themes are common to persons who retain affiliation with a Greek community; these include emphasis on family, honor, religion, education, and Greek heritage.

The core values of *philotimo*, "honor and respect" and *endropi*, "shame," are key when considering the experience of Greeks. While values of honor and shame are found in all societies, they attain immense importance among Mediterranean groups. Although *philotimo* is a characteristic of one's family, community, and nation, it most centrally implies concern for other human beings (Campbell, 1964). *Philotimo* is a Greek's sense of honor and worth that is derived from one's self-image, one's reflected image (respect), and one's sense of pride. *Philotimo* is enhanced through courage, strength, fulfilling family obligations, competition with other persons, hospitality, and right behavior. Shame results from any conduct that is considered deviant. Campbell (1964) postulated that the system of honor and shame in the Mediterranean countries derives from three central features: complementary opposition of the sexes, the solidarity of the family, and the relationships of hostility and competition between unrelated or unconnected families.

## Heritage and Residence

Today, Greek-America is a composite of three immigrant groups: an older group who came before or just after World War I, a second group who arrived after the relaxation of immigration laws in the mid-1960s and who constitute the main group in the Greek-American community, and the American-born children and grandchildren of these immigrants.

The earlier Greek immigrants congregated for the most part in the western states of Utah, Colorado, and Nevada, where they worked in mines and on railroad crews; in the New England states of New Hampshire, Massachusetts, and Connecticut, where they worked in shoe and textile factories; and in the large northern cities of Chicago, Detroit, Toledo, Milwaukee, Philadelphia, Buffalo, Cleveland, and New York, where they worked in factories or found jobs as shoe shiners or peddlers. The greater proportion of Greek-Americans continue to live in the Northeast and the Midwest.

The majority live in large urban areas such as New York and Chicago. While new immigrants still tend to gravitate toward the established Greek communities in the city proper, many Greek-Americans have relocated to the suburbs (Moskos, 1989). According to the 1990 census, 1,110,000 person report Greek ancestry, with 37 percent residing in the Northeast, 23 percent in the Midwest, 21 percent in the South, and 19 percent in the West (U.S. Bureau of the Census, 1995).

## Reasons for Migration and Associated Economic Factors

Significant Greek migration chiefly occurred during the late 19th and early 20th centuries. During this period, migration depleted the population of Greece by about one-fifth. Economic factors were largely responsible for this mass exodus. In the latter part of the 19th century, Greece suffered a major economic crisis resulting from a nearly complete failure of its major crop, currants; relatively heavy governmental taxation to sustain an army against hostilities with Turkey; and family pressure on fathers and brothers to supply a substantial dowry for unmarried women in the family. Before the 1880s, relatively few Greek immigrants had come to the United States, with only slightly over 2000 arriving in the period from 1881 to 1890. Although this number increased fivefold to almost 16,000 from 1891 to 1900, it was not until the start of the 20th century that massive numbers of Greek immigrants came to America (Moskos, 1989). Between 1900 and 1920, almost 350,000 Greeks came to America, 95 percent of them males (Scourby, 1984). They came with dreams of economic opportunity in America, hoping to make enough money to provide good dowries for their sisters and daughters and to be able to return to Greece with enough money to live comfortably in their villages. At the time, Greece was beleaguered by turbulent internal politics and was a difficult place for the average Greek peasant to earn a descent living.

Early American immigration laws greatly affected the number of Greek immigrants that came into the country. In 1921, 28,000 Greek immigrants came to America. Legislation passed in 1921 and 1924 transformed America's open-door policy toward European immigrants into a closed-door policy. The next year, the first year of the restrictive immigration laws, the quota of Greeks allowed into the country was reduced to 100. This was raised to 307 in 1929, and remained at that level for three decades (Moskos, 1989). Greek immigrants who had cared little about becoming American citizens saw citizenship as the only chance to bring other family members to America or to be able to return to America after visiting Greece. In addition, because of fewer people emigrating from Greece, membership in the Greek-American community consisted of increasing numbers of American-born Greeks.

During most of the 1930s, the numbers of Greeks returning to Greece exceeded the number coming to America (Moskos, 1989). Despite the economic downturn in this country, Greek-Americans managed to invest a great deal of energy in their communities. Greek language schools were started for their children, the Greek Orthodox Archdiocese centralized, and charitable organizations were established for the poor. When the Great Depression came, however, everyone in America was affected, including the Greek immigrants. Many businesses failed, jobs were lost, and fortunes disappeared.

The Italian invasion of Greece in 1940 precipitated Greece's entry into World War II and a great outpouring of support from the Greek-American community for the mother country. After America entered the war in 1941, the intermingling of Greek and American interests produced a combination of American patriotism with Greek ethnic pride, which underscored the great love that Greeks in America felt for both their home and adopted countries. The immigration laws, however, kept the actual number of new Greek immigrants to a minimum, with only 8973 coming to America between 1941 and 1950 (Moskos, 1989; U.S. Immigration and Naturalization Service, 1993).

Although the quota system was maintained, special legislation in 1953 allowed those persons who had been displaced by the war and those who wished to reunite with their families to enter America. In addition, countries were allowed to "borrow" on quotas for future years. As a result, approximately 70,000 Greeks entered the United States between World War II and 1965. During this time, the immigration laws dating from the 1920s were liberalized. This large influx rejuvenated the Greek-American community's ties to Greece and changed the composition of the Greek community from Greeks with American citizenship to Americans of Greek descent. By this time, the third generation of Greek-Americans was being born. When the Immigration Act of 1965 lifted the earlier restrictive quotas, over 15,000 Greeks came annually to America from 1966 to 1971. This eventually stabilized to approximately 9000 per year, with approximately 92,000 Greek immigrants arriving in America between 1971 and 1980.

Since 1980, the number of Greeks immigrating to the United States has dropped considerably, with between 2000 to 3000 coming annually between 1983 and 1991 and less than 2000 coming annually in 1992 and 1993 (U.S. Immigration and Naturalization Service, 1993). While these figures reflect a numerical decline, they also reflect a change, beginning in 1980, in the way the Census Bureau determines ethnicity, which moved from a listing of country of birth and parents' birth to the use of a self-described national origin or descent. Of the 177,000 claiming Greek birth, only 12.8 percent entered America during the period between 1980 and 1990 (U.S. Bureau of the Census, 1994).

The decline in Greek immigration to the United States is attributed to several factors that are largely economic in nature. Improvement of economic conditions in Greece has lessened the impetus to emigrate. Canada and Australia have more lenient visa requirements than the United States. Finally, European economic communities, such as the Federal Republic of Germany and Sweden, have encouraged the immigration of Greek workers (Moskos, 1989).

## Educational Status and Occupations

Early Greek immigrants were male and poor and had limited education. However, they had a very strong work ethic, determination, and ethnic pride. The "achievement syndrome" first discussed by Rosen (1959) and later elaborated by Kunkelman

(1990) is evident in the schooling patterns of Greek immigrants and is fostered by the competitive dimension of Greek character. The Greek child is expected to succeed in school. This attitude is fostered by an achievement orientation, high educational and occupational aspirations, a cohesive family unit that exhorts children to succeed, nationalistic identification with the cultural glories of ancient Greece, and private schools that teach Greek culture (Majoribanks, 1994; Rosen 1959). Typically this pattern of achievement continues into adulthood and is reflected in career success. A majority of third-generation Greeks have attended college with considerable diversity in areas of study. During the 1965 immigration, several thousand Greek immigrants represented a different category of immigrants, which included educated professionals and students in professional fields such as engineering, medicine and surgery, and other academic areas (Moskos, 1989; Scourby, 1984).

A common theme (repeated so often it has become an archetype) is that of Greek parents who came from an impoverished land with no money or education. Lacking English language skills, most of these immigrants had no recourse except to accept low-paying jobs as peddlers pushing carts and shoe shiners. Greek men disliked working for others and considered it a violation of pride *(philotimo).* They were industrious and frugal and eventually saved enough money to start their own businesses, such as restaurants and cigar and candy stores (Lovell-Troy, 1990). They take pride in controlling their own businesses and have done very well economically. Initially, they sought these opportunities to save more money to return to their homeland sooner, but the more successful Greek immigrants became, the more likely they were to put down roots in America. Those Greek immigrants who earned only marginal wages were more likely to return to Greece. This description represents the typical pattern in the East and North. In the West, men worked on railroads and in mines and exhibited greater rates of outmarriage because of their smaller numbers in more remote communities. Often once they had settled, worked hard, and acquired some capital, these Greeks too became entrepreneurs, opening shops and small businesses and eventually acquiring American citizenship.

In the United States, Greek immigrants attained middle-class status more rapidly than most of their fellow immigrants. As America grew more affluent in the 1920s, so did the Greek immigrants. During the 1950s, even more Greek-Americans ascended into the middle class. American-born Greeks held mostly white-collar jobs, and the majority of Greek immigrants were small businesspersons. Professions such as engineering, medicine, pharmacy, scientific research, and teaching predominate as those favored by Greek-Americans (Kunkelman, 1990).

## COMMUNICATIONS

### Dominant Language and Dialects

In Greece, language is a fluid and complex issue with strong political overtones. The language spoken by most Greeks and used by contemporary novelists is *demotic Greek.* Demotic Greek is not the same as the official language of Greece, which is *puristic* or *Katharevousa,* and is used in government reports, scholarly journals, and university lectures. Entirely different words with different roots are used in the two language systems. Further, each of these systems has undergone considerable revision, so that the demotic language of the 1800s is considerably different than that of present day; various forms of *katharevousa* have also evolved. Most early immigrants knew only the demotic form from the 1880s because puristic Greek was generally learned in school. More recent immigrants, who tend to have received more education, often know both forms. There is considerable regional variation of local dialects spoken in villages (Bien, Rassias, & Bien, 1972). Greek newspapers printed in the United States and radio programs tend to use the demotic form; the language used in Greek Orthodox churches varies and is determined by local preference.

## Cultural Communication Patterns

Because Greeks value warmth, expressiveness, and spontaneity, northern Europeans are often viewed as "cold" and lacking compassion. Within the Greek family, there is little value placed on privacy. Protection of family members and maintenance of family solidarity tends to be foremost among Greeks. As a consequence, Greeks are often friendly but somewhat superficial and distant with those considered "outsiders" (Collings, 1991).

While many have a deep commitment to honesty among family and in personal relationships, the "white lie" is a customary manipulation used to avoid embarrassment or to minimize intense feelings (Welts, 1982). Similarly, Greek speech patterns employ greater use of an indirect conversational style. In health-care situations, patients often appear to be compliant in the presence of the health-care worker, but this may be only superficial compliance, which is employed to ensure "smoothness" in the relationship (Tripp-Reimer, 1981). Actual deeds are considered to be much more important than what one says.

Greeks tend to be expressive in both speech and gestures. They embrace family, friends, and others to indicate solidarity. Eye contact is generally direct, and speaking and sitting distance is closer than that of other European-Americans. Greeks use their hands more in gesturing while talking, and they have more specific gestures than Anglos (Patterson, 1989). While innermost feelings such as anxiety or depression are often shielded from outsiders, anger is an emotion that has high expression, sometimes to the discomfort of those from less expressive groups.

## Temporal Relationships

Greeks demonstrate a variety of temporal orientations. First, they are oriented to the past as they are highly conscious of the glories of ancient Athens. They are present oriented with regard to *philotimo,* family life, and situations involving family members. Finally, they tend to be future oriented with regard to educational and occupational achievements.

Greek-Americans differentiate between "Greek time," which is used in family and social situations, and "American time," which is used in business situations. Greek time emphasizes participating in activities until they reach a natural breaking point, whereas American time emphasizes punctuality.

## Format for Names

It is customary for honorific titles to be given to members of the community who are elders or otherwise deemed for respect. Terms such as *Thia,* aunt; *Kyria,* Mrs.; or *giagia,* grandma, may be used (Kroger, Wood, & Beam, 1984). For Greek-Americans, having a Greek name is an important sign of their heritage. First names are names of saints or holy days and are derived from those already used in English or those translated directly from Greek to English, for example, Eleni to Helen. The first name reflects the saint whose birthday is honored. Ideally, first daughters are named for the mother's mother, and first sons for the father's father. Following tradition, middle names are the first name of the father; thus, all children of Stavros might carry his first name as their middle name.

## FAMILY ROLES AND ORGANIZATION

### Head of Household and Gender Roles

The father is considered the head of the household in the Greek family. However, the complexity of household dynamics is noted in the well-known folk phrase "the

man is the head, but the wife is the neck that decides which way the head will turn."
This saying gives credence to the primacy of fathers in the public sphere, but the
strong influence of women in the private sphere. In recent years, there has been
increased recognition of a trend toward more equality in decision making.

Gender roles of Greek-Americans reflect those of rural Greece where there is a
socially delineated division of labor. Most important, however, in consideration of
gender roles is the complementary values of honor *(philotimo)* and shame *(endropi)*.
These core values tend to set the pattern for the family and for the enactment of
gender roles. Although the educational levels of women often matched those of their
brothers in the past, women often did not work outside the home, particularly after
they married. A woman, however, may have worked in her husband's store or restaurant. Women of later generations who obtained professional degrees tended to
work after their children were in school. The roles of husband and wife are characterized by mutual respect (a partnership). However, their relationship is less significant than that of the family as a unit. Fathers are responsible for providing for the
family, whereas women are responsible for the management of the home and children. Traditionally, the cleanliness and order of the home reflected the moral character of the woman. However, the values that were central to female identification
in Greece can be a liability after immigration as women identify and are prepared for
roles outside the home (Lock, 1990).

## Prescriptive, Restrictive, and Taboo Practices for Children and Adolescents

The close family is adult centered rather than child centered. However, children are
included in most family social activities and tend not to be left with babysitters. The
child is the recipient of intense affection, helpful interventions, and strong admiration. The child may be disciplined through teasing, which is thought to "toughen"
children and make them highly conscious of public opinion. The family environment
has been identified as strongly pressuring for dependence and achievement. The
family goals of achievement are directed toward and internalized by the children
(Ehiobuche, 1988; Marjoribanks, 1994; Papps et al., 1995).

The Greek-American family stays intact longer than other American families
because adolescents, particularly females, tend to reside with their parents until they
get married. Formerly, males did not marry until their sisters' *prika*, "dowry," was
established and they had married. Among first-generation immigrants, single males
often returned to Greece for a bride. These marriages were usually arranged by a
*proxenia*, "matchmaker," and the families, pending the approval of the adolescent
involved. Today, spouse selection is left to the adolescent, with parental approval.

Females have considerably less freedom in dating than their brothers, and it is
common for them to be prohibited from dating until they are in the upper grades in
high school. Adolescents in more traditional families may experience stress as incongruence in family and peer values and preferences precipitate family conflict. In
fact, suppression of personal freedom by parents is a major risk factor for suicidal
attempts in Greek adolescent girls (Beratis, 1990). Additional areas identified as high
stress for Greek adolescents include extreme dependence on the family, intense pressure for school achievement, and a lack of sexual education in the home (Ierodiakonou, 1988).

## Family Roles and Priorities

Greek families are closer than those of many other groups. Within the family, members are expected to express unlimited respect, concern, and loyalty. *Symbetheri*,

"in-laws," are considered first-degree relatives. Family solidarity is the context in which the values of honor and shame are measured. Prestige is connected to the idea that honor is not individualistic, but collective. Because a person loses honor if kin act improperly, the honor of each family member is a matter of concern for all family members.

Elders hold positions of respect within the Greek community. Their stories, whether pioneers, veterans, or hard-working businessmen, are well known throughout the community. Their notable deeds are heralded and documented in community histories, which are usually maintained by the Greek Orthodox churches in each local community. Treatment of the *giagia*, "grandmother," and the *pappou*, "grandfather," reflect the themes of closeness and respect emphasized in the family. Grandparents tend to participate fully in family activities. Families strongly feel the responsibility to care for their parents, particularly mothers, in old age and children are expected to "take in" widowed parents. Failure to do so results in a sense of dishonor for the son and guilt for the daughter. If the elder is ill, living with the family is the first preference for elders followed by residential care facilities; living alone is the least preferred residential pattern. While there is some concern for the parent being cared for by *xeni*, "strangers," it is worse to be alone (Tripp-Reimer & Schrock, 1982). Of all members of the community, Greek-American widows experience the greatest degree of social marginality, which is exacerbated if they do not have close contact with their children (Kozaitis, 1987).

One of the most important roles is that of fictive kin, termed *koumbari*, "coparents." *Koumbari* serve as sponsors in either (or both) of two religious ceremonies: baptism and marriage. Ideally, the marriage sponsor also serves as the sponsor of the child's baptism. The relationship of parents with koumbari is closer than of sponsors to baptized child. The relationship of sponsor is so important that families who are joined by this bond of fictive kinship are prohibited from intermarrying.

The basis of social status and prestige is family *philotimo* and cohesiveness. However, social status is also received from attributes such as wealth, educational achievement, and achievements of its members. Honor is the social worth of the family as judged by the community. The status and integrity of other families is validated when a family is stricken with a misfortune such as poverty or dishonor.

## Alternative Lifestyles

Greek communities tend to be relatively conservative in orientation. As a consequence, alternative lifestyles such as divorce and same-sex relationships are considered sources of concern for family members and the community.

## WORKFORCE ISSUES

### Culture in the Workplace

In the United States, the high achievement orientation and work ethic have resulted in Greeks serving as a "model" ethnic group. In England and Canada, more recent immigrants with little education have not been as upwardly mobile. Workforce issues in which the interplay between gender and poverty is at work have been well described (Lock, 1990). Although there were many incidents of discrimination and segregation early in this century, including acts of physical violence and murder directed at Greek immigrants, there is virtually no discrimination in the workplace today. The Greek-American's rapid, selective acculturation has been addressed in earlier sections on migration, occupation, and education.

## Issues Related to Autonomy

Probably no single characteristic applies so completely to members of the Greek community as the emphasis on self-reliance within a family context. This trait is stressed by Greeks in Greece as well as those in the United States, Canada, England, Australia, and Sweden. It is seen as reluctance to be told what to do and is given as a major reason for the Greeks' pattern of establishing their own businesses as soon as possible.

After the first generation, virtually all Greek-Americans speak English fully. However, there is considerable effort to retain fluency in Greek by attending Greek language schools, maintaining (but diminishing) use of Greek in Church services, and communicating with and traveling to the homeland.

## BIOCULTURAL ECOLOGY

### Skin Color and Other Biologic Variations

Greeks are most commonly of medium stature, shorter than northern Europeans but taller than other populations of southern Europe. Although there are blue-eyed blond Greeks, usually from the northern provinces, the majority are dark haired and dark skinned. However, even these distinctions do not tap into regional differences. Greeks from the south central area tend to have dark eyes and curly hair; those from Epirus have lighter eyes, less hair, and a characteristic skull formation; those from Thrace have primarily dark eyes and little hair growth. West Macedonians have the lightest eyes and skin, and Aegeans are the tallest regional group.

### Diseases and Health Conditions

Early Greek immigrants, who predominantly emerged from the poorer, rural mainland areas of Greece, often suffered from malaria, tuberculosis, or both; however, these conditions are rare among either settled or immigrant members of the community. Hepatitis A and B, tetanus, and typhoid are relatively common, particularly in the rural areas. Malaria, pulmonary tuberculosis, and dysentery have been controlled since the end of World War II. Typhoid has been reduced from its previously epidemic proportions. Current causes of death are those of developed countries and include cancer and cardiovascular and cerebrovascular diseases (WHO, 1994). Health-care providers need to assess recent immigrants for health conditions such as typhoid and Hepatitis A and B.

Two important genetic conditions, thalassemia and glucose-6-phosphate dehydrogenase (G-6-PD), are seen in relatively high proportions among Greek populations. They likely result from the selective advantage against malaria that these diseases confer on hemizygotic carriers. In the red blood cell, G-6-PD is a key enzyme in the hexose monophosphate shunt, which prevents oxidation of hemoglobin to methemoglobin. This pathway is essential in maintaining the integrity of the red blood cell and in preventing hemolysis. G-6-PD is important in the metabolism of glutation, an antioxidant agent. G-6-PD deficiency leads to hemolysis, which is generally well tolerated except under specific circumstances, including exercise, infections, and the presence of oxidant drugs. The genetic locus for the deficiency is on the X chromosome, making it more common among males than females. The possibility of G-6-PD deficiency should be considered in Greek clients with unconjugated jaundice (Missiou-Tsagaraki, 1991; Sodeinde, 1992; Todd, Samaratunga, & Pembroke 1994; Tripp-Reimer, 1980).

Thalassemia is a set of genetic disorders manifested by a quantitative defect in the synthesis of hemoglobin A or B chain. In the homozygous state, serious anemia results, leading to early death in untreated thalassemia A cases. The genetic frequency of $\beta$-thalassemia is 20 percent in some Greek populations. Features of $\beta$-thalassemia include diarrhea, recurrent fever, and progressive enlargement of the spleen. $\beta$-Thalassemia is treated with transfusion and chelation therapies (Pearson, Rink, & Guiliotis, 1994; Schrier, 1994; Schwartz & Luddy, 1992; Tegos, Voutsakakis, & Karmas 1992; Tripp-Reimer, 1984).

## Variations in Drug Metabolism

Glucose-6-phosphate dehydrogenase deficiency can result in a life-threatening hemolytic crisis after oxidating drugs are taken. These drugs include primaquine, quinidine, thiazolsulfone, dapsone, furzolidone, nitrofural, naphthalene, toluidine blue, phenylhydrazine, and chloramphenicol. Even common medications such as aspirin can induce a hemolytic crisis. This crisis is sufficiently severe that the World Health Organization recommends that all hospital populations in areas with high proportions of Greeks be screened for G-6-PD deficiency before drug therapy (Missiou-Tsagaraki, 1991; Sodeinde, 1992; Todd, Samaratunga, & Pembroke, 1994).

## HIGH-RISK BEHAVIORS

Greeks in Greece, the United States, Canada, and Australia demonstrate less nontherapeutic drug use, alcoholism, and high-risk sexual behaviors than those in other European or North American countries (Beratis, 1991; Hyphantis et al., 1991; Kokkevi & Stafanis, 1991; Patterson, 1989; Powles et al., 1991; Rosenthal, Moore, & Buzwell, 1994). These patterns are not due to an emphasis on health promotion but rather to a hyperawareness of the social consequences of these behaviors for the family. For example, alcohol is most often considered a food item and is consumed with meals. However, losing control by being "under the influence" engenders considerable gossip and social disgrace, focused not only on the individual, but also on the family (Tripp-Reimer & Sorofman, 1994).

Concern for the reputation and standing of the family is a prime deterrent to many high-risk behaviors. On the other hand, high-risk behaviors such as obesity among both sexes and smoking among males are higher among Greeks (Wilson et al., 1993). Knowing these behavioral characteristics can assist health-care providers in planning interventions that are culturally sensitive.

## Health-care Practices

Although they are usually very healthy, Greeks have tended to disregard standard health promotion behaviors. Regular annual physicals are often viewed as unnecessary. Safety measures for adults, such as seat belts and helmets, are often viewed as infringements on personal freedom and are often ignored.

## NUTRITION

### Meaning of Food

Greeks describe their culture as an "eating culture." By this, they mean that food is a centerpiece of everyday life as well as of social and ritual events. Greek hospitality nearly always includes a ritual of food and drink.

Fasting is an integral part of the Greek Orthodox religion. General fast days are

Wednesdays and Fridays. During strict fasts, it is forbidden to eat meat, fish, and animal products such as cheese and milk, wine, and oil. However, persons with health conditions and small children are exempt from fasting. Most Greek-Americans observe a modified fasting schedule. The four major fasting periods are:

The Great Fast, Lent, for 7 weeks before Easter

The Fast of the Apostles, from Monday 8 days after Pentecost to June 28, the eve of the Feast of the Saints Peter and Paul

The Assumption fast, from August 1 to August 14

The Christmas fast, from November 15 to December 14

## Common Foods and Food Rituals

Greeks have based their diet on cereals, pulses, vegetables, fruits, olive oil, cheese, milk, and some fish and meat. Both Greeks and Greek immigrants are relatively high consumers of sweets and snacks. In Greece, there has been a pattern of decreased consumption of pulses, such as lentils and peas, and an increased consumption of meats. The consequences of this trend are not yet known (Trichopoulou, Katsouyanni, & Gnardellis, 1993).

For adults, dairy products are consumed in the form of yogurt or cheeses such as feta, kopanisti, kefaloteri, and kaseri. Fats are consumed in the form of olive oil, butter, and olives. Meats include chicken and lamb or, in the United States, beef

Table 12–1 • **Common Greek Foods**

| Name | Description | Ingredients |
|------|-------------|-------------|
| *Avgholemono* | Soup | Chicken stock, eggs, lemon, rice |
| *Hummus* | Thick sauce for dipping bread | Chick peas (mashed), *tahini* sauce (sesame and olive oil) |
| *Maroulousalata* | Salad | Lettuce, onions, cucumbers, radishes, parsley, tomatoes, feta cheese, olives, anchovies, olive oil |
| *Tsatziki* | Salad | Cucumbers, yogurt, vinegar, mint, onions, sugar |
| *Spanakopita* | Cheese tarts | Spinach and feta cheese in phyllo dough pastry |
| *Dolmathes* | Stuffed grape leaves | Meat, rice, grape leaves |
| *Keftedes* | Meatballs | Ground beef, onions bread, parsley, oregano, eggs, garlic |
| *Souvlaki* | Meat | Marinated beef on skewer |
| *Moussaka* | Casserole | Eggplant, ground lamb, onions, tomato, garlic, parsley, white sauce |
| *Pastichio* | Casserole | Ground beef, macaroni, cinnamon, white sauce, cheese, parsley, tomato sauce, butter |
| *Psiti kota* | Lemon chicken | Chicken, lemon, egg, flour, oil |
| *Loukomades* | Pastry | Flour, water, honey, oil, sugar, cinnamon |
| *Kourambiethes* | Wedding cookie | Flour, almonds, cloves, powdered sugar, egg, brandy |
| *Baklava* | Sweet dessert | Phyllo dough, pecans, honey, sugar, cinnamon, cloves, butter |
| Greek coffee | Coffee | Greek coffee, sugar |

adaptations. Eggs, lentils, fish such as shrimp and other shellfish, white fish, and anchovies are additional sources of protein.

Vegetables such as eggplant, grape leaves, spinach, garlic, onions, peas, artichokes, cucumbers, asparagus, cabbage, and cauliflower are common Greek food choices. Bread choices include pita, crescent rolls, yeast, and egg breads. Carbohydrates include rice, tabouli, macaroni, and farina.

Common seasonings used by Greeks are anise, basil, cumin, cinnamon, citron, clove, coriander, dill, fennel, ginger, garlic, lemon, marjoram, mint, mustard, nutmeg, oregano, parsley, rose, sage, sesame, thyme, vinegar, bay leaf, and honey. Fruit preferences include grapes and currants, figs, prunes, oranges, lemons, peaches, and apricots. Beverages such as coffee, tea, chocolate milk, and wine are common choices. Common food items are listed in Table 12–1.

The earlier pattern of eating four meals a day—breakfast, lunch, afternoon meal, and dinner—was described by Homer in 900 B.C. However, the customary pattern today is three meals. Breakfast is a small meal with milk, sugar, or cocoa served early in the morning. Lunch is taken after noon, and dinner is served considerably later, between 7:30 and 9 P.M., when situations permit (Neiderud, 1989; Neiderud & Philip, 1990).

Specific foods are linked with different holidays or ceremonies throughout the year. For example, there are several different special breads that are served at traditional ceremonies: New Year's bread, *vasilopita;* Easter bread, *tsoureki;* Christmas bread, *chistosomo;* and traditional breads for weddings and funerals, *koliva.*

## Dietary Practices for Health Promotion

Although there is no specific classification of foods for health or illness, a general consensus is that persons will naturally choose foods that are healthy. Therefore, an effort is made to provide ill persons with the food that they request. This pattern is most pronounced for pregnant women. In fact, numerous folk prescriptions exist regarding the provision of food for pregnant women, even if they are not close family or friends.

## Nutritional Deficiencies and Food Limitations

Although nutritional deficiencies per se are rare among Greeks, two important enzymatic conditions merit attention. For persons with G-6-PD deficiency, broad beans (fava beans) can induce hemolysis and an acute anemic crisis when ingested (Riepl et al., 1993). Second, the prevalence of lactose maldigestion in Greek adults is about 75 percent; however, milk intolerance is rarely seen in children (Ladas & Katsiyiannaki-Latoufi, 1991; Spanidou & Petrakis, 1972). Health-care providers should use this knowledge when counseling clients with these conditions.

Virtually all food items used in the traditional Greek diet are available in the United States, Australia, and Canada. Even specialty items such as phyllo dough for pastries and appetizers, grape leaves in brine, and olives can be found in specialty areas of major supermarkets. There has, however, been a trend away from lamb to beef for many dishes. The popularity of Greek food is evidenced in the success of Greek restaurants wherever there is a Greek community.

## PREGNANCY AND CHILDBEARING PRACTICES

### Fertility Practices and Views toward Pregnancy

In both European and American Greek populations, limitation of family size is stressed. The trend in Greece for smaller families has been noted since at least the turn of the century. In large part, this decreased fertility has resulted from the desire of parents to provide adequately for their children and to have them educated so they can achieve professional status (Friedl, 1962).

In the United States, family size has been deliberately limited to adequately care for and educate children. However, the method of limiting pregnancies has changed from control of gestation to control of conception. In Greece, abortions were not legal but were commonly performed by physicians. In the United States, a wide variety of birth control measures, such as intrauterine devices, birth control pills, and condoms, are preferred (Tripp-Reimer, 1982). The Greek Orthodox Church has issued encyclicals condemning birth control; however, each local priest may interpret these differently. Generally, the attitude of the church is lenient and practical with regard to birth control. However, abortion is regarded as murder. Adoption is rare among Greeks, both in Greece and in the United States.

While the family may experience shame and dishonor if an unmarried woman becomes pregnant, it is also of concern when married couples are infertile. For infertile couples, the reputation of the husband is put at risk, and the woman is unable to achieve her highest role. Infertile couples are reported to experience mental stress evidenced as depression for woman and anxiety for men (Tarlatzis et al., 1993). In a group with such a strong emphasis on fertility, there is a very positive and protective attitude toward the pregnant woman.

## Prescriptive, Restrictive, and Taboo Practices in the Childbearing Family

Pregnancy is a time of great respect for women and a time when they are given special considerations. For example, strangers may offer a pregnant woman their seat. Other proscriptions include not attending funerals or viewing a corpse, refraining from sinful activity as a precaution against infant deformity, and praying to St. Simeon (Tripp-Reimer, 1981). However, the majority of pregnancy admonitions are related to diet. Pregnant women are encouraged to eat large quantities; foods high in iron and protein are particularly important. A number of tales surround the provision of food to pregnant women. It is commonly believed that giving meat to a pregnant woman makes the dish turn out well. In addition, if a pregnant woman remarks that a food smells good, or if she is hungry for that food, it should be offered to her; otherwise the child may be "marked."

During childbirth in rural Greece, a woman is generally attended by a midwife and female kin. The pattern of the noninvolvement of the fathers still holds in immigrant generations (Dragonas, 1992) but is being replaced with greater participation.

After delivery, the mother, termed *lahoosa*, is considered by most traditional Greeks ritually impure and particularly susceptible to illness for 40 days. During this time, she is admonished to stay at home and not attend church. At the end of the 40 days, the mother and child attend church and receive a ritual blessing. For breast-feeding mothers, early showering is sometimes thought to result in the infants' developing diarrhea and becoming allergic to milk.

Newborns are generally breast-fed, and solids are not introduced early. When a child is visited by relatives in the hospital, silver objects or coins may be brought and placed in the crib for good luck (Tripp-Reimer, 1981).

## DEATH RITUALS

### Death Rituals and Expectations

Last rites are administered in the Sacrament of Holy Communion given by a priest or occasionally a Deacon (Moskos, 1989). On the death of a community member, close relatives are notified in person, while other community members are notified by telephone. The wake, *klama*, is held in the family home or, more commonly today, in a funeral home. All relatives and friends are expected to attend for at least a brief time. Even persons with whom there was considerable strife are expected to attend. The wake ends when the priest arrives and offers prayers. The funeral, *kikhia*, is held the following day at the Orthodox Church with internment in a cemetery. After internment, family and friends gather for a meal of fish, symbolizing Christianity; wine; cheese; and olives in the family home or a restaurant.

On the basis of the Orthodox belief in the physical resurrection of the body, Greeks often reject cremation (Kyriacou, 1983). However, there is considerable diversity in the degree of adherence to this precept.

## Responses to Death and Grief

After a death, pictures and mirrors may be turned over. During the wake, women may sing dirges or chant. In some regions, there is the practice of "screaming the dead," in which the lament, *miroloyi*, is cried. This ritual involves screaming, lamenting, and sobbing by female kin (Moskos, 1989; Seremetakis, 1990; Stewart, 1992). After death, family and close relatives, who may stay at home, mourn for 40 days.

Black is the color of mourning dress and is often worn by family members throughout the 40-day mourning period; for widows it may be worn longer. Formerly, a widow was expected to wear black and no jewelry or makeup for the rest of her life. While black armbands are still worn in Greece, that custom is virtually nonexistent in immigrant communities. Widows generally look to their family for support; widowers often remarry. These practices should be encouraged and respected by health-care providers.

A memorial service follows 40 days after burial and at 3 months, 6 months, and yearly thereafter. At the end of this service, *koliva*, boiled wheat with powdered sugar, is served to participants and mourning is conducted with joyful reverance.

Dreams have special importance to family members after a death. It is not unusual for family members to experience visitations by the deceased in their dreams. Often, these dreams provide reasons for the deceased to leave the earth.

## SPIRITUALITY

### Religious Practices and Use of Prayer

Greek-Americans are affiliated with the Greek Orthodox Church, although many are not overly pious. The central religious experience is the Sunday morning liturgy, which is a high church service with icons, heavy incense, and singing or chanting by the choir. Services that previously lasted over 3 hours are now generally shortened to 1½ hours.

The Greek Orthodox religion emphasizes faith rather than specific tenets. Unlike most Protestant denominations, Greek faith does not emphasize bible reading and study. While some parishioners attend church services weekly, others attend only a few times a year. Easter is considered the most important of holy days, and nearly all Greek-Americans attempt to honor the day. In addition, Greek-Americans attend special services for baptisms or deaths.

Daily prayers may be offered to the saints. Faith is often considered an important factor in regaining health, particularly by women. Family members may make "bargains" with saints, such as promises to fast, be faithful, or make church donations if the saint acts on behalf of the ill family member. They may call individual's namesake or a saint believed to have special affinity with healing. Two saints frequently invoked are Cosmas and Damian, early Christian physicians. In invoking the saint, the supplicant may say special prayers, light candles, place small gold medals at the base of the icon, or carry out some combination of these rituals. There is also a strong belief in miracles, even among third-generation Greek-Americans (Collings, 1989).

## Meaning of Life and Individual Sources of Strength

The world is viewed as a cosmic battleground in which the individual must be continuously vigilant and resourceful. Based on the principle of limited good, one family's gain is another's loss. Only within the bonds of the family can an individual find protection from a dangerous world. The primary set of relationships, even in an extended household, is between members of the nuclear family. From this central group, relationships radiate outward, lessening in strength to include all affinity, consanguineous, and *koumbaros* relationships to the second degree (e.g., second cousins).

Life has meaning as family roles are enacted successfully. Parents strive to provide for their children, and in turn, they expect the children to achieve success in academic and occupational endeavors. Through wrong behaviors or misfortunes individuals can bring public sanction and shame *(endropi)* on the family.

The Greek concept of self is constituted from the interrelationship of the three values: self-respect, a sense of freedom, and the concept of the ideal person. The self emerges through relationships with other persons, but primarily from the family (Blue, 1993). Freedom is a central element in the self-concept. Self-reliance, that is, nonreliance on persons outside the family, is a virtue. For Greeks, sources of strength are the family, the close network of extended family and friends, and the history of the glories of ancient Greece. Particularly in immigrant communities, the Greek Orthodox Church serves as a base for spirituality, language, social and political organization, and an ongoing identity with Greece and continental Greeks.

## Spiritual Beliefs and Health-care Practices

A distinctive feature of the Greek Orthodox religion is the place it assigns to icons, such as paintings of saints, the Virgin Mary, and Christ. These icons are not religious art but have sacred significance as sources of connection to the spiritual world. Icons grace the walls and ceilings of the church cathedrals and are also found in personal altars in homes. In the homes, holy vigil candles are kept burning. To ensure safety and health, many begin each day by kissing the blessed icons and making the sign of the Greek cross. When a person is ill, the icon of the family saint or the Virgin Mary may be placed above the bed. Greek-Americans also may sprinkle their homes with holy water from Epiphany Day church services to protect the members of their household from evil.

## HEALTH-CARE PRACTICES

## Health-seeking Beliefs and Behaviors

The degree of acceptance and use of biomedicine is highly related to one's level of education and generation of immigration. For example, although fourth-generation Greek-Americans in Ohio are highly traditional in many aspects of their lives, such as religion, language retention, and food preferences, they have not retained many of the folk beliefs and practices concerning health care (Tripp-Reimer, 1983). The traditional practices discussed subsequently tend to apply to earlier immigrant generations.

Among Greek immigrants, there tends to be an anxiety about health, a lack of trust of health professionals, and a reliance on family and community for advice and remedies. Problems are seen as originating outside the individual's control and are attributed to God, the devil, spirits, and envy or malice of others. The gods may punish the nonreligious with illnesses such as *anthenia or arrosita*, but more often the forces of evil are believed to cause illness. Another example of an external cause of illness is that of the *matiasma* (evil eye), which is often unintentionally caused through the envy of others (Tripp-Reimer, 1983).

To be healthy means to feel strong, joyful, and content; to be able to take care of oneself; and to be free from pain (Rosenbaum, 1991; Tripp-Reimer & Sorofman 1989). Threats to health result from a lack of balance in life; departure from family; neglect of education or work; and failure to demonstrate right behaviors, such as respect toward parents, sharing with family, upholding religious precepts, and staying out too late (Kanitsaki, 1993; Tripp-Reimer & Sorofman, 1989).

## Responsibility for Health Care

Central to issues of responsibility are the orientations toward honor, independence, and distrust of persons outside the family. In traditional thought, the cause of illness and misfortune falls outside the person. The family generally assumes responsibility and care for a sick member and works to control interactions with health professionals.

In the United States, insurance enrollment among Greek-Americans is high, which correlates with high rates of employment among this group. Even when coverage is available, however, there is often a delay in seeking professional care. Greek-Americans are extremely reluctant to use welfare services or other forms of governmental assistance to meet their health-care needs. Reliance on public assistance would indicate that the sick person and family are not self-reliant. Greek-Americans are also reluctant to rely on Greek community organizations, such as the women's Philoptochos Society (Friends of the Poor), for support.

## Folk Practices

Three traditional folk healing practices are particularly notable: *matiasma*, "bad eye or evil eye"; *practika*, "herbal remedies"; and *vendousas*, "cupping." *Matiasma* results from the envy or admiration of others. While the eye is able to harm a wide variety of things including inanimate objects, children are particularly susceptible to attack. Common symptoms of *mati* include headache, chills, irritability, restlessness, and lethargy; in extreme cases, *mati* has resulted in death.

Greeks employ a variety of preventive mechanisms to thwart the effects of envy, including protective charms in the form of *phylactos*, amulets consisting of blessed wood or incense, or blue "eye" beads, which "reflect" the eye. When the diagnosis of *matiasma* is suspected, the most common method of detection consists of placing olive oil in a glass of water. If the oil disperses, then the eye has been cast. Subsequent treatment consists of physical acts, such as making the sign of the Greek cross over the glass of water or reciting ritual prayers passed on in families by members of opposite sex. In particularly severe cases, the Orthodox priest may recite special prayers of exorcism and use incense to fumigate the afflicted person (Tripp-Reimer, 1981, 1983).

*Practika* are herbal and humoral treatments used for initial self-treatment. Chamomile, the most popular herb, is generally used in teas for gastric distress or abdominal pain, including infant colic and menstrual cramps. It is also used as an expectorant to treat colds. Liquors, such as anisette, oozo, and *mestika*, are used primarily for colds, sore throats, and coughs and are consumed alone or in combination with

### Table 12–2 • *Practika* Used in Greek Folk Medicine

| Practice | Indication |
|---|---|
| *Frascomilo* (sage) tea | Colds |
| *Moroha* | Stomachache |
| Linden tea | Stomachache |
| Mustard plasters | Colds |
| Rice (boiled) | Diarrhea |
| Cinnamon tea | Menstrual cramps |
| Tobacco | Inhibition of infection |

*Source: Adapted from Tripp-Reimer, T. (1981). Ethnomedical beliefs among Greek imigrants: Implications for nursing interventions. Transcultural Nursing Care 6, 129–140; and Tripp-Reimer, T., & Sorofman, B. (1989). Illness related self-care responses in four ethnic groups: Final Report #R01Nu 1101. (Submitted to National Institute of Nursing Research. Bethesda, MD: National Institutes of Health.)*

tea, lemon, honey, or sugar alone or in some combination. Occasionally, liquors are used for treatment of "nerves," *nevra*. Raw garlic is used as a prevention for colds and cooked garlic for blood pressure and heart disease. Other *practika* include those described in Table 12–2.

*Vendousas* is a healing practice known throughout the circum-Mediterranean area. Most frequently, it is used as a treatment for colds, but other indications include high blood pressure and backache. The technique consists of lighting a swab of cotton held on a fork, then placing the swab in an inverted glass creating a vacuum in the glass, which is then placed on the back of the ill persons. The skin on the back is drawn into the glass. This procedure is repeated 8 or 12 times. An alternative method, for particularly serious cases, is the *kofte*, "cut *vendousa*." Here, the same procedure is followed, except that a cut in the shape of a cross is made on the skin. When the glass is placed over this cut, blood is drawn into the glass. The therapeutic rationale for using vendousas surrounds its counterirritant effect; the technique increases and revitalizes the circulation, draws out poisons and "cold," and prevents coagulation of blood. *Vendousas* are rarely used by fourth-generation community members (Tripp-Reimer, 1981, 1983).

## Barriers to Health Care

The primary barriers to health care for Greek-Americans include a reliance on self-care in the family context and a general distrust of bureaucracies. Self-medicating behaviors are normative, with herbal remedies and over-the-counter medications used widely for specific symptoms. Self-care, however, is usually undertaken with the advice of family members.

In Greece, pharmacies are a common source of self-medication. In Greece, pharmacies have considerably greater authorization to prescribe and dispense medications. Self-treatment is still used as a first line response to illness (Tripp-Reimer & Sorofman, 1989). As a result, immigrants may not be used to seeking physicians care in a primary setting. When self-care fails, families often bring the ill person to a specialist rather than a primary care physician. The use of all physicians is lower for Greeks than for other groups of European descent; however, their low use of physicians for primary care is remarkable (Tripp-Reimer & Sorofman, 1989).

Whenever possible, bureaucratic organizations are avoided because they serve as threats to independence and the privacy of the family. Mistrust of professionals is discussed further in the section on health-care practitioners.

## Cultural Responses to Health and Illness

Mental illness is accompanied by social stigma with negative consequences for the afflicted person as well as the family and relatives. The shame *(endropi)* originates in the notion that mental illness is hereditary; afflicted persons are viewed as having lifelong conditions that "pollute" the bloodline (Blue, 1993). The stigma is so wide ranging that persons labeled as mentally ill and their families may experience the loss of friends and social isolation (Tripp-Reimer & Lively, 1993). As a result, families place a wide variety of behaviors within the range of "normal" to delay receiving the stigmatized label. Persons with mental illness often present with somatic complaints such as dizziness and parathesias on initial visits to health-care practitioners (Marmanidis, Holme, & Hafner, 1994). Recent immigrants tend to have higher rates of mental disorders, which likely results from the stress of culture change (Adamopoulou et al., 1990; Mavreas, Bebbington, & Der, 1990).

There is, however, a folk model for *nevra* (nerves) that is a socially acceptable and a culturally condoned medium for the expression of otherwise unacceptable emotions. *Nerva* is experienced most commonly by those in positions of least power, such as women and persons living in poverty. It encompasses a wide variety of symptoms and provides a metaphor for social disorder, such as conflict between close kin or intergenerational conflict (Clark, 1989; Dunk, 1989; Lock, 1990). Ideally, *Nerva* is treated through medications for the relief of symptoms instead of through talk therapy.

Greek culture socially stratifies persons by the nature of their disorders. Persons with physical illnesses such as asthma, diabetes, and arthritis are most accepted, followed by persons with disfiguring illnesses such as cerebral palsy. Persons and their families experiencing mental retardation, psychiatric illness, and acquired immunodeficiency syndrome are less accepted. However, persons in the most stigmatized group are those with social deviance, such as addictions or delinquency (Westbrook, Legge, & Pennay, 1993).

*Ponos*, "pain," is the cardinal symptom of ill health. It is not viewed as something to be endured, but as an evil that needs eradication. Pain mobilizes considerable family concern. The person in pain is not expected to suffer quietly or stoically in the presence of family. The family is relied on to find resources to relieve the pain or, failing that, to share in the experience of suffering. However, in the presence of outsiders, the lack of restraint in pain expression suggests lack of self-control and therefore is an opportunity for *endropi*. Although the experience of physical pain is acknowledged publicly, emotional pain is hidden within the privacy of the family.

The key aspect of the sick role is for sick persons to fully rely on the family to sustain them. Solitude is considered unpleasant and is avoided even when persons are well. When ill, it is considered particularly important that the individual not be left alone. Sick persons are often surrounded by a small crowd of family and neighbors. Family and visitors provide advice regarding appropriate treatments and recall similar situations experienced by themselves or others.

When hospitalization occurs, family members expect to stay with sick persons, even during examinations and therapeutic procedures. They are expected to ensure that sick persons are not harmed and are receiving the best care possible. Protection of sick persons even includes shielding them from a serious diagnosis such as cancer until the family feels they are ready to learn about the diagnosis (Kanitsakis, 1993; Ierodiakonou, 1988; Tripp-Reimer, 1992).

## Blood Transfusion and Organ Donation

On the basis of the Orthodox belief in the physical resurrection of the body, Greeks often reject the concept of autopsy and do not readily accept organ donation. However, blood transfusions are wholly acceptable and are common for persons with thalassemia.

## HEALTH-CARE PRACTITIONERS

### Traditional Versus Biomedical Care

In Greece, a number of lay practitioners, including herbalists who peddle herbs and tonics around neighborhoods, midwives, and bonesetters. A woman who cures, particularly the evil eye, is known as *magissa*, which is usually translated as "witch" but means "magician"; they may also be called doctor.

In the United States, however, this diversity of lay healers is not available. Most lay healing is conducted by "wise women" from one's own family. Occasionally, for particularly difficult cases of *matiasma,* Greek-Americans call on a woman with particular gifts in diagnosis and healing. The priest may also be called on for advice, blessings, exorcisms, and direct healing, depending on the generation of the Greek-American and characteristics of the priest.

### Status of Health-care Practitioners

Many Greeks display a general distrust of all professionals other than family members, and physicians, in particular, are distrusted and avoided as long as possible. Considerable "shopping around" for physicians and other professionals to obtain additional opinions is relatively common. This is particularly true if the sick person does not receive the diagnosis or the degree of sympathy judged appropriate by the family. Inconsistencies in opinions or recommendations result in further concern. In addition, use of multiple physicians simultaneously may result in untoward drug interactions from multiple drug use.

Hospitals are a particular source of mistrust both for Greeks and immigrants. When hospitalizations occur, the family may be perceived by staff as demanding or "interfering" as they enact their protective advocacy roles. Mothers may demand to sleep with their children and fear they may not receive appropriate care. There is also a fear that the sick person's blood may be sold or that they may be used as subjects for experimentation (Anderson, 1985; Kanitsakis, 1993; Kozaitis, 1987; Tripp-Reimer & Sorofman, 1989).

---

### CASE STUDY

Mr. X is a 76-year-old immigrant from Athens, Greece. In 1940, at the request of his father, Mr. X migrated to Chicago, Illinois. Greece had just entered World War II, and the father wanted Mr. X to "earn some money for the family." In fact, Mr. X believes that his father sent him away so that he would not have to enter the war as a soldier. Avoiding conscription in the Greek military is somewhat of an embarrassment. So Mr. X moved to Chicago to the home of his mother's sister and then, after a short time, to the Quad Cities between Iowa and Illinois to be near two of his father's brothers.

For a number of years, Mr. X worked as a waiter and later as a manager of his uncle's business. On three occasions, second jobs were taken to send extra money home. When possible, Mr. X traveled to Greece to see family. After he became a United States citizen, he married a woman from Athens and she joined him in Davenport, Iowa. There they raised a family of four and, shortly after the second child was born, Mr. X went into the wholesale pharmaceutical distribution business and became very successful.

Shortly after the death of his wife, Mr. X retired. At the age of 75 years, he sold his business to a nephew because all of his children went to college and received graduate professional degrees unrelated to his business. Although financially able to live alone, he lives with his eldest son's family in Moline, Illinois. His son is an engineer and owns his own firm. Both Mr. X and his son are financially able to manage Mr. X's health-care needs. The rest of Mr. X's children also live in the area. He has a rich social life centered around the Greek Orthodox Church.

Mr. X visited the Family Health Medical Clinic in October complaining of headaches and lightheadedness. His son said that he had been irritable. Some days ago, he had a dark urine stream. A health history further uncovered that he was sure that it was not what he called *"matiasma."* Unusual in his history is that he reported never going to a physician until this time. He only recently began to feel ill, diagnosing his condition as arthritis and taking "several pills a day" for the last few weeks. Nothing else in the history was remarkable.

A urine culture was negative. However, a preliminary diagnosis of urinary tract infection was made, and Mr. X was sent home with sulfisoxazole (500 mg four times a day).

Mr. X appeared in the emergency room complaining of severe abdominal and back pain and weakness several days after the clinic visit. He appeared in distress. Additional health data obtained in the emergency room indicated that Mr. X consumes approximately two glasses of wine and an after-dinner drink each evening, has a 50-pack-per-year history of smoking, and has been relatively compliant on the antibiotic medication prescribed during his clinic visit.

Clinical laboratory results indicate severe anemia. A subsequent laboratory analysis for G-6-PD deficiency indicates that Mr. X has this deficiency. He is treated for anemia, and the sulfa drugs and aspirin are removed from his therapy. He remains in the hospital for only 2 days. The illness and hospitalization is hard on Mr. X, and one social worker recommends that he be discharged to an intermediate nursing facility for recovery. On the evening before his discharge, he had an argument with his son and his daughter-in-law over whether Mr. X should continue to reside in their home. Mr. X is discharged to home with an instruction to no longer treat his self-diagnosed and unconfirmed arthritis.

## STUDY QUESTIONS

1. List some social values presented in the case that are common to members of the Greek community.

2. The migration of Mr. X to the United States served as both an obligation and a source of shame. How might this be explained?

3. In what ways was Mr. X's immigration pattern similar to other persons of Greek heritage?

4. U.S. immigration laws in the early half of the 20th century instituted quotas for Greek immigrants. Examining the basic values of Greek immigrants, how might you explain the shift to U.S. citizenship by Greek residents?

5. From a clinical perspective, the influence of the two drugs aspirin and sulfisoxazole uncovered a hereditary medical problem, G-6-PD. Discuss that problem.

6. What reasons might account for the fact that the disease did not occur until late in life?

7. How does Mr. X's pattern of family life demonstrate core cultural values of Greek-Americans?

8. What is the folk illness in this case, and why did Mr. X think it might be important?

9. How does Mr. X's health-seeking pattern fit with Greek values?

10. One issue in this case is where Mr. X will reside. Discuss this issue in the context of family and residential preferences of older Greek-Americans based on their heritage.

## References

Adamopoulou, A., Garyfallos, G., Bouras, N., & Kouloumas, G. (1990). Mental health and primary care in ethnic groups: Greek Cypriots in London. *International Journal of Social Psychiatry, 36,* 244–251.

Anderson, J. M. (1985). Perspective on the health of immigrant women. *Advances in Nursing Science, 8,* 61–76.

Beratis, S. (1990). Factors associated with adolescent suicidal attempts in Greece. *Psychopathology, 23,* 161–168.

Beratis, S. (1991). Suicide among adolescents in Greece. *British Journal of Psychiatry, 159,* 515–519.

Bien, P., Rassias, J., & Bien, C. (1972). *Demotic Greek.* Hanover, NH: University Press of New England.

Blue, A. (1993). Greek psychiatry's transition from the hospital to the community. *Medieval Anthropology Quarterly 7*(3), 301–318.

Clark, M. H. (1989). Nevra in a Greek village: Idiom, metaphor, symptom, or disorder? *Health Care for Women International, 10,* 195–218.

Collings, D. M. (1991). *Ethnic identification: The Greek Americans of Houston, Texas.* New York: AMS Press.

Dragonas, T. G. (1992). Greek fathers' participation in labour and care of the infant. *Scandinavian Journal of Caring Sciences, 6*(3), 151–159.

Dunk, P. (1989). Greek women and broken nerves in Montreal. *Medical Anthropology, 11,* 29–45.

Ehiobuche, I. (1988). Obsessive-compulsive neurosis in relation to parental child-rearing patterns amongst the Greek, Italian, and Anglo-Australian subjects. *Acta Psychiatrica Scandanavia 344*(Suppl.), 115–120.

Friedl, E. (1962). *Vasilika: A village in modern Greece.* New York: Holt, Rinehart, & Winston.

Hyphantis, T., Koutras, V., Koakos, A., & Marselos, M. (1991). Alcohol and drug use: Family situation and school performance of adolescent children of alcoholics. *International Journal of Social Psychiatry, 37*(1), 35–42.

Ierodiakonou, C. S. (1988). Adolescent's mental health and the Greek family: Preventive aspects. *Journal of Adolescence, 11,* 11–19.

Kanitsaki, O. (1993). Transcultural human care: Its challenge to and critique of professional nursing care. In D. A. Gaut (Ed.), *A global agenda for caring* (pp. 19–45). New York: National League of Nursing Press.

Kokkevi, A., & Stefanis, C. (1991). The epidemiology of licit and illicit substance use among high school students in Greece. *American Journal of Public Health, 81,* 48–52.

Kozaitis, K. A. (1987). Being old and Greek in America. In D. E. Gelfand & C. M. Barresi (Eds.), *Ethnic dimensions of aging* (pp. 179–195). New York: Springer.

Kroger, R. O., Wood, L. A., & Beam, T. (1984). Are the rules of address universal? Greek usage. *Journal of Cross-Cultural Psychology, 15,* 259–272.

Kunkelman, G. A. (1990). *The religion of ethnicity: Belief and belonging in a Greek-American community.* New York: Garland.

Ladas, S. D., & Katsiyiannaki-Latoufi, E. (1991). Lactose maldigestion and milk intolerance in healthy Greek school children. *American Journal of Clinical Nutrition, 53*(3), 676–680.

Lock, M. (1990). On being ethnic: The politics of identity breaking and making in Canada, or nevra on Sunday. *Culture, Medicine, and Psychiatry, 14,* 237–254.

Lovell-Troy, L. A. (1990). *The social basis of ethnic enterprise: Greeks in the pizza business.* New York: Garland.

Marjoribanks, K. (1994). Cross-cultural comparisons of family environments of Anglo, Greek, and Italian Australians. *Psychological Reports, 74,* 49–50.

Marmanidis, H., Holme, G., & Hafner, R. J. (1994). Depression and somatic symptoms: A cross-cultural study. *Australian and New Zealand Journal of Psychiatry, 28,* 274–278.

Mavreas, V., Bebbington, P., & Der, G. (1990). Acculturation and psychiatric disorder: A study of Greek cypriot immigrants. *Psychological Medicine, 20,* 941–951.

Missiou-Tsagaraki, S. (1991). Screening for glucose-6-phosphate deficiency as a preventive measure: Prevalence among 1,286,000 Greek newborn infants. *Journal of Pediatrics, 119*(2), 293–299.

Moskos, C. C. (1989). *Greek Americans: Struggle and success.* London: Transaction.

Neiderud, J. (1989). Greek immigrant children in southern Sweden in comparison with Greek and Swedish children. *Scandinavian Journal of Social Medicine, 17,* 25–31.

Neiderud, J., & Philip, I. (1990). Greek immigrant children in southern Sweden in comparison with Greek and Swedish children. Pt. 2. Meal patterns and food habits. *Acta Pediatrica Scandinavia, 79,* 920–929.

Papps, F., Walker, M., Trimboli, A., & Trimboli, C. (1995). Parental discipline in Anglo, Greek, Lebanese, and Vietnamese cultures. *Journal of Cross-cultural Psychology, 26*(1), 49–64.

Patterson, G. J. (1989). *The assimilated Greeks of Denver.* New York: AMS Press.

Pearson, H. A., Rink, L., & Guiliotis, D. K. (1994). Thalassemia major in Connecticut. *Connecticut Medicine, 58,* 259–269.

Powles, J. W., Macaskill, G., Hooper J. L., & Ktenas, D. (1991). Differences in drinking patterns associated with migration from a Greek island to Melbourne, Australia. *Journal of Studies on Alcohol, 52,* 224–231.

Riepl, R. L., Schreiner, J., Muller, B., Hildemann, S., & Loeschke, K. (1993). Broad beans as a cause of acute hemolytic anemia. *Deutsche Medizinische Wochenschrift, 118,* 932–935.

Rosen, B. (1959). Race, ethnicity and the achievement syndrome. *American Sociological Review, 2,* 1167–1173.

Rosenbaum, J. N. (1991). The health meanings and practices of older Greek-Canadian widows. *Journal of Advanced Nursing, 16*(11), 1320–1327.

Rosenthal, D., Moore, S., & Buzwell, S. (1994). Homeless youths: Sexual and drug-related behaviors, sexual beliefs and HIV/AIDS risk. *AIDS Care, 6*(1), 83–94.

Schrier, S. L. (1994). Thalassemia: Pathophysiology of red cell changes. *Annual Review of Medicine, 45,* 211–218.

Schwartz, A. D., & Luddy, R. E. (1992). Thalassemia screening in Baltimore. *Maryland Medical Journal, 41,* 145–147.

Scourby, A. (1984). *The Greek Americans.* Boston: Twayne.

Seremetakis, C. N. (1990). The ethics of antiphony: The social construction of pain gender, and power in the Southern Peloponnese. *ETHOS, 18,* 481–511.

Sodeinde, O. (1992). Glucose-6-Phosphate dehydrogenase deficiency. *Baillieres Clinical Haematology, 5*(2), 367–382.

Stewart, C. (1992). Strategies of suffering and their interpretations. *Culture, Medicine, and Psychiatry, 16,* 107–119.

Tarlatzis, I., Tarlatzis, B. C., Diakogiannis, I., Bontis, J., Lagos, S., Gavriilidou, D., & Mantalenakis, S. (1993). Psychosocial impacts of infertility on Greek couples. *Human Reproduction, 8,* 396–401.

Tegos, C. N., Voutsadakis, A. J., & Karmas, P. A. (1992). Diagnostic strategy for thalassemias and other hemoglobinopathies: A program applied to the Hellenic Army recruits. *Military Medicine, 157,* 183–185.

Todd, P., Samaratunga, I. R., & Pembroke, A. (1994). Screening of glucose-6-phosphate dehydrogenase deficiency prior to dapsone therapy. *Clinical and Experimental Dermatology, 19*(3), 217–218.

Trichopoulou, A., Katsouyannni, K., & Gnardellis, C. (1993). The traditional Greek diet. *European Journal of Clinical Nutrition, 47*(Suppl. 1), S76–S81.

Tripp-Reimer, T. (1980). Genetic demography of a urban Greek immigrant community. *Human Biology, 52,* 255–267.

Tripp-Reimer, T. (1981). Ethnomedical beliefs among Greek immigrants: Implications for nursing interventions. *Transcultural Nursing Care, 6,* 129–140.

Tripp-Reimer, T. (1982). Cultural influences on the potential for natural selection. *Central Issues in Anthropology, 4*(2), 49–57.

Tripp-Reimer, T. (1983). Retention of a folk healing practice (matiasma) among four generations of urban Greek immigrants. *Nursing Research, 32,* 97–101.

Tripp-Reimer, T. (1984). Reconceptualizing the construct of health: Integrating emic and etic perspectives. *Research in Nursing and Health, 7,* 101–109.

Tripp-Reimer, T. (1992). Cultural assessment. In J. Bellach & B. Edlund (Eds.), *Nursing assessment and diagnosis* (pp. 208–231). Boston: Jones and Bartlett.

Tripp-Reimer, T., & Lively, S. (1993). Cultural considerations in mental health-psychiatric nursing. In R. P. Rawlings, S. R. Williams, & C. K. Beck (Eds.), *Mental health: Psychiatric nursing—A holistic life-cycle approach* (pp. 166–179). St. Louis: Mosby.

Tripp-Reimer, T., & Martin, M. (1983). Knowledge and use of folk remedies among ethnic aged. In G. Felton & I. Alpers (Eds.), *Nursing research: A monograph for non-nurse researchers* (pp. 100–113). Iowa City: University of Iowa Press.

Tripp-Reimer, T., & Schrock, M. (1982). Residential patterns and preferences of ethnic aged: Implications for transcultural nursing. In C. N. Uhl & J. Uhl (Eds.), *1982 Proceedings of the 7th annual Transcultural Nursing Society* (pp. 144–157). Salt Lake City: Transcultural Nursing Society.

Tripp-Reimer, T., & Sorofman, B. (1989). *Illness related self-care responses in four ethnic groups: Final report* #R01Nu 1101. (Submitted to National Institute of Nursing Research. Bethesda, MD: National Institutes of Health.)

Tripp-Reimer, T., & Sorofman, B. (1994). *Drinks, foods, medicines and markers: Alcohol issues in four ethnic groups.* Paper presented at the American Anthropology Association meetings, Atlanta, GA.

U. S. Bureau of the Census (1995). *Statistical abstract of the United States: 1994* (114th ed.). Washington, DC: U. S. Government Printing Office.

U. S. Immigration and Naturalization Service. (1994). *Statistical yearbook of the Immigration and Naturalization Service: 1993.* Washington, DC: U. S. Government Printing Office.

Westbrook. T. M., Legge V., & Pennay, M. (1993). Attitudes toward disabilities in a multicultural society. *Social Science and Medicine, 36,* 615–623.

Wilson, A., Bekiaris, J., Gleeson, S., Papasavva, C., Wise, M., & Hawe, P. (1993). The good heart, good life survey: Self-reported cardiovascular disease risk factors, health knowledge, and attitudes among Greek-Australians in Sydney. *Australian Journal of Public Health, 17,* 215–221.

World Health Organization (1994). *World health statistical annual 1993.* Geneva: Author.

# Iranians

*Juliene G. Lipson and Homeyra Hafizi*

---

• Key terms to become familiar with in this chapter are:

| | |
|---|---|
| *Andarun* | *Khakshir* |
| *Atary* | *Lavash* |
| *Baten* | *Mezaj* |
| *Cheshm-i-bad* | *Nabat* |
| *Doog* | *Naharati* |
| *Eid* | *Neshasteh* |
| *Garm* | *Norooz* |
| *Garmie* | *Sard* |
| *Ghalbam gerefteh* | *Sardie* |
| *Gol-i-gov zabon* | *Ta'arof* |
| *Halal* | *Tabi'at* |
| *Haram* | *Tagdir* |
| *Hejab* | *Zaher* |
| *Jinns* | *Zerangi* |
| *Kashk* | |

## OVERVIEW, INHABITED LOCALITIES, AND TOPOGRAPHY

### Overview

Iranian immigrants in the United States number about one million (Beauchamp, 1988), with some 450,000 living in California (Tyler, 1989). Thirty-nine thousand live in Canada, two-thirds of whom live in Ontario (*Statistics Canada: Ethnic Origin,* 1993). Remarkably little literature is available on the health of this population in the United States, except for clinical descriptions (Ardehali & Backer, 1980; Jalali, 1982) and research on general health and adjustment (Lipson, 1992), concepts of health (Hafizi, 1990), and such mental health topics as depression (Good, 1980), grief (Kashani, 1988), and marital satisfaction (Rezaian, 1989; Vatan, 1991). The dearth of

---

Acknowledgment: We thank Fakhri Rezaian, PhD, and Azita Nabavi, RN, MS candidate, for critically reading this chapter and for providing additional information.

literature necessitated relying on information from Iranians in their home country, which may or may not be accurate for those in the United States.

Despite the focus in this chapter on commonalities among Iranian immigrants, they vary enormously along many dimensions. They range from highly traditional to highly acculturated; their reasons for leaving vary; and they vary in social class, education, religion, and ethnic background. In addition, the U.S. Iranian immigrant population is in transition; therefore, generational differences are great. For example, Hanassab (1991) found that young Iranian women in Los Angeles who left Iran at a younger age and therefore have been away from Iran longer are much more acculturated as evidenced by more liberal attitudes toward sex and intimate relationships and more conflicts about their Iranian and American identities.

Iran, with an area of 636,000 square miles, is about the size of Alaska. Most of Iran is a mountainous plateau around 4000 feet above sea level and surrounded on three sides by mountain ranges, with the highest peak at 18,000 feet. Its neighboring countries are Turkey, Iraq, Armenia, Azerbaijan, Turkmenistan, Afghanistan, and Pakistan. Large salt deserts cover much of the area, but there are also many oases and forest areas. Most of its nearly 65.6 million people live in the north and northwest (*World Almanac,* 1995). The capital, Tehran, has nearly 12 million residents. A large proportion of the population lives in rural areas and small towns. The climate varies from hot and dry in the summer to cold in the winter, particularly in the higher altitudes, with snow in the northern part of the country.

Because many Iranians call themselves Persians for historical and political reasons, the terms *Persians* and *Iranians* are used interchangeably in this chapter. The country's name was changed in 1935 from Persia to Iran (derived from the word *aryana*) to present an image of progress and to attempt to unify into one nation the enormous diversity of urban dwellers and rural tribes, ethnic groups, and social classes.

## Heritage and Residence

Persian culture is very rich and very old. Iranians are proud of their heritage, which includes the Zoroastrian religion and some of the world's greatest poets and leaders in the history of medieval philosophy, astronomy, and medicine; for example, the physician Ibn Sina (Avicenna) (Lewis & Stevens, 1986). The original Persians were an Indo-European group related to the Aryans of India, first invading the area now known as the Middle East around 1500 B.C. The Persian empire, founded by Cyrus the Great in 559 B.C. covered an area from the Hindu Kush (now in Afghanistan) to Egypt, Palestine, Syria, and parts of Asia Minor.

Throughout its history, Persia was subjected for long periods to foreign rulers with customs, languages, and religions vastly different from its own (Lorentz & Wertime, 1980). Alexander the Great conquered Persia in 333 B.C., but Persians regained their independence in the next century under the Parthians. Arabs brought Islam to Persia in the seventh century, and the majority of the Zoroastrian inhabitants were converted to Islam in the next two centuries. Many of the calendars used in the Middle East date from this time, beginning with the flight of the Prophet Mohammed and his Islamic community from Mecca to Medina in 622 A.D. However, predating Islam is **Norooz** (New Year), the beginning of the calendar year that falls on the first day of spring, a non-Islamic Persian holiday.

Persian political and cultural autonomy reasserted itself in the ninth century, and the arts and sciences flourished for the next several centuries. Turks and Mongols in turn ruled Persia from the 11th century to 1502, when a native dynasty regained full independence. The British and Russian empires vied for influence in the 19th century, and Afghanistan was severed from Iran in 1857.

In the past 70 years, Iran has seen the rise and fall of the Qajar dynasty; the Pahlavi dynasty (supported by the British); the short-lived National Front (social democratic organization led by Mossadeq, who rejected the British and returned the oil fields to the Iranians); the return of the Pahlavi dynasty led by Mohammed Reza Shah (supported by the United States); and finally, the current Islamic regime. Every revolution instituted a one-party government that strongly controlled the people of Iran. At the same time, Iran's strategic location and resources have stimulated continuing foreign interest.

Powerful social and economic reforms were fostered by Reza Shah Pahlavi and his son from the mid-1930s to the 1979 revolution. These reforms included national public health and education programs and a more secular society with decreased power for tribal chiefs, clergy, and landed aristocracy. During this period, women were allowed by law to go unveiled, gained access to university education, and were fully enfranchised in 1963. By the late 1970s, women had become senators, cabinet ministers, physicians, and professors (Fischer, 1978). However, despite these economic and social changes, Mohammed Reza Shah showed the same disrespect for democracy as did his father before him; for example, he reinstituted the secret police and had no tolerance for political opposition.

After the conservative Moslem protests that led to the 1978 violence, martial law was declared and a military government was appointed to deal with striking oil workers. Early in 1979, the Shah fled Iran for the United States. The "reform" instituted by the new Islamic government was deeply colored by the religious traditions and ideology of Shi'ia Islam. Since the fundamentalist revolution, Iran has once again come to externally resemble the more conservative Muslim countries. However, the radical social changes of past the four decades could not be erased; some have simply been forced underground. Urban women, for example, are covered and dress conservatively in public, but dress stylishly indoors. The diversity created by these changes are reflected in the diversity of Iranian immigrants to the United States.

In essence, modern Iranian culture is a rural farming culture with a recent overlay of industrialism initiated by the Pahlavi Dynasty. This industrialism did not develop within Iranian culture itself but was imposed from without and based almost entirely on the oil industry. Political instability and the fragility of an economy based on this one industry have led to Iran's current situation of a bankrupt economy, weak production, government subsidy of food and other staples, scarce merchandise (obtainable but prohibitively expensive), high inflation, and a near lack of competition. Iranians have become dependent and insecure in this situation.

Jalali (1982) described three waves of Iranian immigration to the United States. The first wave (from 1950 to 1970) consisted mostly of students from the social elite and with professional backgrounds, many of whom decided to remain in the United States after completing their education. The second wave (from 1970 to 1978) comprised immigrants who were more varied in social class background, but most were predominantly urban and affluent. They came mainly to pursue educational, professional, or economic opportunities or to join family members. Many came to obtain graduate or other university education, and many of these remained. In both first and second waves, familiarity with European-American culture and the ability to gain similar employment to that in Iran facilitated a relatively easy cultural transition. However, they were dispersed throughout the United States and did not establish ethnic enclaves as did many other immigrant groups. The third wave began with the Islamic revolution and included a large number of political exiles and forced migrants, who came mainly for personal or economic security. They are more heterogenous in education, age, social class, religiosity, and exposure to Western culture.

Iranian immigrants have faced considerable ethnic bias from nonimmigrant Americans because of events in Iran. Anger and prejudice toward Iranians reached their heights with the occupation of the U.S. Embassy in Tehran by a group of the Ayatollah Khomeini's followers from November 1979 until January 1981. Postrevolution immigrants and Iranian students at all levels of the educational system became the target of frustration with the hostage crisis. Television news programs covered the hostage crisis for over a year; Americans were barraged daily with such commentary as "Day 414 of the hostage crisis." This daily coverage stirred up continuing hostility toward Iranians in the United States, which manifested itself in threats painted on store windows owned by Iranians immigrants. In the worst cases, Iranians were assaulted or received threatening telephone calls (Lipson, 1992). Some immigrants were afraid to admit that they came from Iran, such as a Turkish-speaking Iranian woman who told people that she was Turkish. The hostage crisis was the most difficult time for Iranians living in the United States. Those not encountering direct personal bias were still distressed by the reports in the media.

While large communities of expatriate Iranians live in Britain, France, and Canada (Tyler, 1989), Los Angeles has the largest concentration of Iranians outside of Iran. The numbers, though hotly disputed, ranged from 74,000 to 300,000 in the mid-1980s (Kelly, Friedlander, & Colby, 1993). The Los Angeles population is ethnically and religiously diverse; while Muslims are still the majority, the minority populations of Armenians, Jews, and Baha'is are far larger than they were in Iran. Iran has alternated between tolerance of ethnic and religious differences and religious persecution, which stimulated emigration among religious minorities.

In most areas of the United States, Iranians do not live in ethnic enclaves that can help newcomers adjust. While many small and cohesive social networks exist, the Iranian population is divided by distrust based on political, religious, and social class differences. The large Los Angeles population has ethnic and religious communities concentrated in different areas, for example, Muslim "Little Tehran" in Santa Monica and Palms, Baha'is in West Los Angeles; Armenians in Glendale; and Jews in Westwood and Beverly Hills (Bozorgmehr, Sabagh, & Der-Martirosian, 1993).

## Reasons for Migration and Associated Economic Factors

The immigration experience is strongly influenced by persons' reasons for leaving their home country and by the opportunities they hoped to pursue in their new homeland, so-called push and pull factors (Peterson, 1958). Most prerevolution Iranian immigrants came to the United States for education and economic opportunities, although some, such as Baha'is and Jews, immigrated to escape religious persecution. The 1975 to 1980 cohort of immigrants included a higher proportion of religious minorities and more women and elderly, who had less education and more problems with English (Sabagh & Bozorgmehr, 1987). Many of those immigrating since the 1979 revolution consider themselves exiles rather than immigrants by choice. Many postrevolution immigrants are ambivalent about having left Iran. While free of the social and political limitations imposed by the Islamic Republic, most still feel guilt and sorrow about leaving their families behind and live in an atmosphere of instability and uncertainty.

The immigration experiences described by Iranians compare with those of most relatively new immigrants to the United States; they frequently experience culture shock and problems associated with poor mastery of English, perceived loss of status, and difficulty finding work comparable to that which they left behind (Lipson, 1992). "Newer" and "older" immigrants experience some of the same stressors, and some different ones as well. The newest Iranian immigrants confront the loss of their culture, habits, and identity. Those who have lived in the United States longer are still concerned about language as well as occupational, financial, and academic functioning, but they also experience more family problems (Lipson, 1992). After 5 or 6 years, many have adjusted to their new home but have become discouraged about their own achievements and consider their exodus as having been "for the sake of the children." Relative stability usually occurs after 10 years, but most, formerly of the upper class, still have not recovered the status they had in Iran (Stein, 1981).

Elderly immigrants more often express their ambivalence about being in the United States and may strongly believe that they are in the United States to care for their children by providing both emotional and financial support. They often feel isolated and do not learn English or participate in American culture; their desire to return home keeps them from making permanent commitments and cementing emotional ties. They are also concerned about their inability to keep their children from becoming too Americanized. They perceive American children as lacking respect for the elderly and having loose family ties.

Many younger people lack social support in the United States. In Iran, friendships and relationships with extended family members are established from birth, and these relationships are sorely missed in the United States. Because most Iranians are highly social and dislike being alone, some spend their time with individuals with whom they have little in common except the language and cultural norms. Thus, national heritage has become a basis for friendship instead of personal history or other shared characteristics.

Financial problems are a source of considerable stress among many newer immigrants. Some wealthy persons lost considerable money in leaving Iran; other new arrivals have run out of savings, and income sources from Iran have dried up. Highly skilled professionals often cannot obtain employment in their fields; as a result, engineers work in gas stations, and journalists and physicians work in restaurants. Despite many having left Iran during or after the revolution because of fear for their safety, the U.S. government recognizes few as refugees; thus, most have no access to social programs designed for refugees. Some are undocumented and live in constant fear of discovery and deportation.

Prerevolution immigrants experience stressors related to close family and cultural ties with Iran, such as fear of never seeing family members again or, during the Iran-Iraq war, fear of receiving the dreaded news that a relative had been killed (Lipson, 1992). Despite their permanent status in the United States, some grieve the loss of their country (Kashani, 1988). Iranians who are relatively financially secure experience more subtle stressors, such as perceptions of hostility and ethnic bias.

## Educational Status and Occupations

Most Iranian immigrants in the United States are from urban rather than rural areas. Iranians are the most highly educated immigrant group in the United States, with 40 percent in 1980 holding a bachelor's or advanced degree (Bozorgmehr et al., 1993). In 1979 to 1980, 51,300 Iranian students resided in the United States, more than any other nationality, with twice as many in California as any other state (Connell, 1981).

Education is highly valued among Iranians and advanced degrees are highly respected; for example, those with doctorates are often consulted for their advice. In Iran, even poor villagers sacrifice their personal comfort to send their children to school (Kelly, 1973). The children of immigrants in the United States are expected to do well in school and to attend college. In Los Angeles, educational status of Iranians varies among ethnic groups: 40 percent of Muslims and 50 percent of Baha'is and Jews have graduate degrees; 33 percent of Armenians have completed at least 4 years of college (Bozorgmehr et al., 1993).

Occupations among Iranian immigrants depend on the opportunities, education, and skills they brought from Iran and time and age of arrival in the United States. Iranians who immigrated before the 1979 revolution often chose to study medicine and engineering, and many professionals comprise the Iranian immigrant population. Of the 20 percent of U.S. practicing physicians who are foreign medical graduates, most are Iranians and Filipinos (Herman & Hojat, 1984). In the 1970s, the "brain drain" of physicians, nurses, and other professionals was of particular concern in Iran. There were 2066 Iranian physicians in the United States, with only 9535 physicians practicing in Iran (Ronaghy et al., 1976). One nursing school lost one-third of its graduates to the United States (Ronaghy et al., 1975).

Those educated in the United States since the revolution represent the range of occupations available through higher education and other means. Many former middle-aged physicians, engineers, professors, army generals, and government officials unable to find comparable work in the United States have gone into business for themselves. Some began with pizza parlors or gas stations, using their business acumen to maintain a middle-class or better lifestyle in the United States. In Los Angeles, 61 percent of Iranian heads of households claimed to be self-employed in 1987 and 1988 (Dallalfar, 1994), with Iranian Jews having a self-employment rate of 82 percent, and only 10 percent reporting employment in blue-collar jobs (Bozorgmehr et al., 1993). Because health-care providers may encounter a jewelry store owner who is a former judge, they must not assume education and social class from occupation alone.

Iranian women are quite active in the ethnic economy in Los Angeles as owners and employees in such diverse small businesses as travel agencies, accounting, and retail businesses; few are waitresses and none were observed working in gas stations or as taxi drivers, an occupation in which Iranian men are quite visible (Dallalfar, 1994). A number of women in Los Angeles have home-based businesses; for example, they might work as seamstresses or clothing outlet operators, pastry makers, beauticians, or makeup specialists. These occupations improve their economic situation and expand or recreate vital social and supportive networks in the Iranian immigrant community (Dallarfar, 1994).

However, occupation remains a major concern for some immigrants, particularly those from the Iran's upper social strata, who cannot get recognition through employment or status in their new country. Jobs that require manual labor are not respected, and some cannot accept that they have to take such menial jobs because of their limited skills in the English language. In a Canadian medical record review of Iranian immigrant psychiatric clients, Bagheri (1982) found that satisfactory employment strongly correlated with emotional well-being and positive mental states. The discrepancy in social status in Canada and Iran for this same group of immigrants was key in the development of psychiatric problems, particularly among middle-aged men.

## COMMUNICATIONS

### Dominant Language and Dialects

Farsi (Persian) is the national language of Iran, and all school children are taught in Persian. An indication of modern Iran's Indo-European heritage is found in words similar to English words; for example, the English word "mother" is a cognate to the Persian word *madar*. However, nearly half of the country's population speaks a different language, for example, Turkish, Kurdish, Armenian, Baluchi, or other Iranian dialects. Well-educated and well-traveled immigrants may speak three or more languages; for example, French as a cultural language or English in business settings.

### Cultural Communication Patterns

Communication among Iranians must be understood within the context of Iranian history, the personality style valued in the culture, and the structure of social relationships. Multiple foreign invasions of Persia and strict control by each ensuing government has influenced Iranians' interaction with outsiders. These foreign governments' disregard for human life led to Iranians' mistrust and suspicion of foreigners. People adapted and assimilated without losing their own identity. The disclosure of personal thoughts to strangers is generally perceived to have detrimental consequences. Not verbalizing one's thoughts is a useful defense, and overt expressions of emotions to strangers may be culturally stigmatized (Jalali, 1982; Beeman, 1988; Kelly, Friedlander, & Colby, 1993).

Iranians greet each other by asking about the family and engaging in social conversation to build rapport before getting down to business. Tone of voice and whether women speak more softly than men depends heavily on rural or urban background and the influence of traditionalism. Among women, patterns of speech may appear restrained or refined to avoid too much self-disclosure or to prevent loss of face, but overall, the situation guides the degree of expressiveness. Iranians tend to tell stories and give considerable detail rather than use blunt and succinct messages.

Bagheri (1992) described valued personality characteristics as indirectness, subdued assertiveness, and attempts to please others through modesty and politeness. Iranians are very concerned with respectability, a good appearance of the home, and a good reputation. They are embarrassed by financial troubles and even conceal such problems from relatives (Ardehali & Backer, 1992). **Zerangi** (cleverness) is valued, but only among nonintimates; it means knowing how to manipulate bureaucratic structures and is used because government organizations were not trusted to function for the good of the people in Iran. The ability to bargain well is an example of *zerangi*. In the public sphere, bargaining is how things get done in Iran; one never accepts the first price quoted or believes that a stated rule cannot be changed. However, it is very important to distinguish between "valued" or common cultural characteristics and individual personality characteristics.

In addition, Iranian communication patterns are influenced by a hierarchy of relationships and depend on the social status of the other person in relation to oneself. For example, communication may be supportive of lower-status persons or competitive with those of equal status or may be characterized by currying the favor of those of higher status. The influence of intimate versus public spheres and hierarchical social relationships is seen clearly in the practice of **ta'arof** (ritual expressed courtesy), which is not practiced with intimates. In this system, there is a constant flow of offers of hospitality and compliments, which may sound very insincere to non-Iranians, particularly when they learn that taking these seriously is a social gaffe. However, such offers are sincere because they depend on the restraint of the respondent. The host has the pleasure of saying, "My house is your house" to a guest who enjoys this welcome but knows when to go home (Bateson et al., 1977). In essence, *ta'arof* expresses the public face, with its respectful forms of speech and behavior, and is used when dealing with persons whose status is unequal to one's own.

Social behavior is influenced by the constant awareness of the external judgment of others regarding whether a person is conforming to the ideal of "selflessness." It limits spontaneity and creates rules for approaching people of different ages and members of the opposite gender. What one says or feels is held back if it is believed to be outside of the prescribed social script. An example of *ta'arof* is when a guest is offered tea; the guest initially refuses it, so as not to put the host to any trouble. The host offers again, the guest again declines, the host offers again, and the guest finally accepts. The whole interaction is a ritual: The guest knows from the beginning that to refuse the tea or food would be an insult, but immediate acceptance would be seen as an act of egoism.

Communication in personal relationships varies according to **baten** and **zaher** and occurs on a continuum anchored at one end by the *baten* (inner self) in personal and intimate relationships and at the other end by the *zaher* (public persona) in the public sphere, which is structured by social hierarchy. A strong boundary exists between the internal world of family and close friends and the external world of acquaintances and everyone else. The *baten* is the true vulnerable self, a collection of freely expressed personal feelings. In contrast, *zaher* is proper and controlled behavior—a public face to protect and buffer the vulnerable world of the *baten* within. At the beginning of a new interaction, an Iranian is neither totally "outside" or "inside." If the exchange is oriented toward the *zaher* (outside), it is a sign of an unequal relationship where expressions become restricted. The Persian language and its nonverbal accompaniments have evolved to express and structure this exchange. Neither participant discloses the world of the *baten*; the relationship appears superficial, refined, and flawless, with social distance or aloofness to protect one's private self. Silence is used with regard to confidential matters and to manage impressions.

In contrast to hierarchical public relationships, in communication among intimate friends and family—the *baten* or **andarun**—is shared. Overwhelmingly emotional or intense feelings can be expressed freely, are understood, and not judged (Beeman, 1988). Privacy is important in family affairs; family matters remain within the family and are not for others' ears (Samiezade-Yazd, 1989). However, anger directed at people of higher status, like parents or superiors, is condemned. In addition, most Iranians refrain from showing anger or other strong emotions to outsiders. In Iranian society, where self-control is valued, showing anger can produce embarrassment, shame the family, or damage someone's reputation (Pliskin, 1992). To save face, Iranians may agree or say that they understand an outsider (whether they do or not) to avoid embarrassment.

In other words, there is a distinction between expressed emotion and felt emotion; a non-Iranian may view Iranians as highly emotional, but expressed emotion is based on the context of the situation in which it is appropriate to show emotions (Beeman, 1976), for example, weeping and crying loudly in a public context such as a funeral. Inner feelings may not match their outer expression because of the importance placed on being polite, pleasant, and keeping social relationships smooth.

Health-care providers should be aware of the manner in which Iranians handle potentially disturbing information. In general, at the beginning of any health-care encounter, the provider should take time to "warm up" with social conversation before "getting down to business." Any kind of "bad news" must be handled carefully by revealing it gently and gradually, in several meetings if possible, or only to the family spokesperson. A person should never be given bad news alone, for example, informed of a death or serious diagnosis.

Among more traditional Iranians, men and women do not hold hands or show affection towards each other in public. However, women often show affection for women, and men for men, for example, by walking hand in hand or greeting each other with a kiss on each cheek. In greeting acquaintances, some Iranians stand with the right hand on the chest and make a slight bow or extend a handshake. Strangers and health-care providers are greeted with both hands at the sides or a handshake. A slight bow or nod while shaking hands shows respect. Iranians generally stand when someone enters a room for the first time and takes leave (David M. Kennedy Center, 1984). It is appropriate to offer something with both hands, which shows respect. Crossing one's legs when sitting is acceptable, but slouching in a chair or stretching one's legs toward another is considered offensive; it is considered rude to show the sole of one's foot. Beckoning is done by waving the fingers with the palm down. Tilting the head up quickly means "no." Tilting the head to the side means "what?" and tilting it down means "yes." Extending the thumb (like "thumbs up") is considered a vulgar sign. Health-care providers should refrain from using nonverbal behaviors that may be offensive to Iranians. Nonverbal communication among acculturated immigrants resembles that of European-Americans.

As in Mediterranean cultures, personal distance is generally closer than that of North Americans or northern Europeans. The strength of the relationship does not alter communication distance, but it does affect how freely participants touch each other. For example, frequently touching one's sister and expressing emotions in conversation is acceptable, but this would not be done with a stranger. However, the greater the degree of acculturation, the more Iranians' behavior resembles that of European-Americans; although with health-care providers, respect for role and education might be demonstrated by keeping a wide distance.

Iranians maintain intense eye contact between intimates and equals of the same gender, but traditional Iranians tend to avoid eye contact with each other. Younger people and those of lower status do not sustain eye contact with those they perceive as being older or of higher status. When Irans speak, smiling and using the arms and hands help to convey the message, and conversation appears expressive.

## Temporal Relationships

Temporal relationships are a combination of present and future orientations. The ideal is to maintain a balance between enjoying life to the fullest on a daily basis while saving enough money to ensure a comfortable future life. Signs of daily gratification include intense family relationships and frequent visits, small trips, fashionable clothing, and proper meals. Financial planning, savings, and the importance of education demonstrate looking ahead.

With respect to health promotion, the future orientation enhances the effectiveness of health education. At the same time, a fatalistic theme in many Iranians' beliefs may hinder their understanding of teaching about risk reduction and health promotion.

Economic and social factors in Iran, especially scarce resources and virtually nonexistent competition, make the theme of "time is money" meaningless in business. Iranians are not clock watchers; rather, they are mood and feeling oriented. However, acculturation to American society brings with it timeliness and intense competition to sell goods and services.

Guests may arrive one to several hours after a social engagement. Thus, a party may last far into the night with guests arriving throughout the evening. While social time is flexible, Iranians meet the social expectations for timeliness in work and appointments.

## Format for Names

Iranians refrain from calling older persons by their first names. In highly traditional families, privacy demands that husbands do not mention their wives' first names to other men. Close friends and children may be called by their first names by family members, but others should not do so. Shaking hands with a child shows respect to the parents, but a man should wait for a woman to extend her hand first. One is expected to greet every member of the family with a handshake. Health-care providers should heed nonverbal cues and greet Iranians in culturally congruent ways.

## FAMILY ROLES AND ORGANIZATION

### Head of Household and Gender Roles

Iranian culture is patriarchal and hierarchical. The father rules the family and expects obedience and submission from family members. In the father's absence, the oldest son has authority. Families traditionally were large in Iran, with male children being highly desirable, but today more resemble the American norm. As a father ages, he may give property, the business, and control to the oldest son. In more traditional families, older male siblings have the authority to make decisions about younger siblings, even in the father's presence. However, this hierarchy is more flexible in cosmopolitan families. Siblings are taught from an early age to rely on each other for support, and sibling relationships are deep, trusting, and lively. Health-care providers should never underestimate the power of this hierarchy or the family in general in decision making. The individual usually cannot or will not make decisions.

Iranian men see their role as protecting and providing for the family, managing the finances, and dealing with matters outside the home. Women are expected to maintain the home; even working women may place their priorities on the family and home and do the cooking, cleaning, and laundry. Until the 1960s social reforms in Iran, women were legally expected to be obedient and submissive to their husbands, who had the right to correct them and used it frequently.

Women were traditionally expected to marry and bear sons as quickly as possible, although this is now changing. In traditional families, both daughters and sons stay at home until married, and marriages are arranged in the rural areas. In urban families in Iran and the United States, young people are free to select their own marriage partners, but families usually want to approve because of the importance of marriage alliances between families. Husbands are often five or more years older than their wives.

In the United States, stress occurs in Iranian families when men perceive that they have lost their power, particularly when they cannot regain their former social status. Many men complain that because of retirement, unemployment, or low-prestige jobs, their families no longer respect or obey them.

## Prescriptive, Restrictive, and Taboo Behaviors for Children and Adolescents

In Iran, children in rural areas are just as responsible for the family economy as adults, but their rights as children are not well delineated. In urban families, Iranian children have the same rights as children in the Western world.

In general, immigrant Iranian families are child oriented. Parents pay a lot of attention to their children and are willing to sacrifice for their welfare, especially for their higher education. Children are expected to be loyal to their families and behave respectfully toward their elders. Manners are considered important even outside the home, where children are expected to be clean and well-behaved and to refrain from rowdiness. Children are taught from an early age to avoid eating if no one else has food and never to speak rudely to elders. Girls are expected to behave and dress more modestly than boys, especially as they approach adolescence. Children and teens are usually included in adult gatherings. Young children are rarely left with babysitters.

Taboo behaviors for teens in Iran and in the United States differ only in degree and intensity. In Iran, parents are concerned about smoking, drugs, alcohol, and sex in that order. Young women are expected to remain virgins until they marry, but sexual activity outside marriage is tolerated among men. Dating is not allowed in the most traditional families, but this varies depending on ethnic group, length of time in the United States, and location.

While many adolescents in the United States resemble their non-Iranian peers in dress and outward behavior, they often behave more respectfully with family members, particularly the elderly and other highly respected persons. The fear of shaming the family and losing face in public act as strong social constraints. For example, adolescents are unlikely to express their anger to parents or teachers, preferring instead to be silent, because showing respect is more important than acting on the aggressive impulse; however, anger is expressed toward peers (Makaremi, 1990).

Adolescents are often caught in a dilemma, pulled between parents' attempts to maintain control and instill Iranian heritage and values and their own desire to be like their American peers. Some who came to the United States at a younger age tend to become more American than American teens, retaining only faint remnants of popular Iranian culture, whereas those who came at an older age—and are therefore likely to have developed a well-formed ego and personality—adjust more effectively to a bicultural identity.

## Family Roles and Priorities

The family is the most important institution in Iranian culture. Family members often live close to each other so they can visit whenever possible. Most do not like to be isolated and therefore maintain strong intergenerational involvement with grandmothers, mothers, and children in the domestic sphere and with male family members often employed in the family business. Families are child oriented and a childless couple is considered incomplete. Iranians share their daily life difficulties; the elderly often function like counselors, because many Iranians are uncomfortable discussing their problems with someone outside the family circle.

The primary goal of family life is to ensure the well-being and continuation of the family. Upholding the family's name is of great importance. Families desire good and well-educated children, safe and secure jobs, economic security, and social acceptance. If they are able, parents help to support their children financially throughout their lives, providing assistance with educational expenses, home buying, or business start-up.

Both Iranian and Iranian families who live far from the support of extended family members may experience a great deal of stress. Some Iranians complain about lack of close social ties in the United States, stating that they miss their families and old friends. Some socialize mainly or only with family members, stating that they have no "real" friends in the United States. They complain that Americans do not relate to and care for each other as Iranians do, giving as examples the "lack of closeness in families" and "lack of respect for old people" in Amerian families (Lipson, 1992). In other cases where many family members remain in Iran, relationships other than blood relationships, such as a network of friends, may define the extended family. The family gathers for any important event, such as visiting a sick person, funerals, mourning days, *Norooz*, births, weddings, or **Eid** (celebration or commemoration of one of several religious holidays). The power of the family is based on supportive relationships among its members, and relationships among kin and kinlike friends are more important than any other social alignment.

Some Iranians have clothing that is only worn inside the home, and they change into these clothes when they get home. Often they remove their shoes at the door and wear slippers. Outside the home, they tend to dress conservatively, but more traditional or religious women in the United States may choose to avoid bright colors, cover arms and legs, and conceal their heads with head covers or scarves **(hejab)**. In Iran, these coverings are mandatory, not a matter of choice. However, there is great variety in dress, depending on the age and tradition. Many Iranians dress stylishly, valuing a good personal appearance in clothing, household furnishings, and decorations.

Age is a sign of experience, worldliness, and knowledge. Thus, regardless of kinship or relationship, an elder is treated with respect. When grandparents reach an age where they can no longer care for themselves, they live with and are cared for by the famiy. Few nursing homes are in Iran, and they are viewed negatively. Caring for an elder is an obligation.

Respect for elders may be shown in various ways, including giving them attention, asking for their advice, or even agreeing (or being silent) when elders voice an opinion with which younger persons disagree. In essence, although one may not appreciate the older person's wisdom, one is bound to respect them because of their age. Respect for age is shown not only to grandparents but also to aunts, uncles, older siblings, and neighbors.

Despite their esteemed role within the Iranian family, elders in the United States who do not speak English may feel lonely and isolated from adults working and children at school. Loneliness and isolation among elderly persons are particularly common in neighborhoods where transportation is unavailable or walking is unsafe.

While social status in Iran is inherited, there is no caste system. One is usually born into the upper class, but one can ascend the class hierarchy through higher education and attainment of professional status. In addition, such valued individual characteristics as nobility, generosity, and courage are sources of social status. Parents often try to arrange marriages for their children with the children of families of higher status. Sometimes marriages are arranged within the kin group (cousins) to maintain marital harmony or to cement family relationships.

While growth of the middle class in Iran was rapid in the 1970s, the enormous expense of getting out of Iran since the revolution prohibited all but the wealthy or professional middle class from immigrating to the United States. Rural persons and those with limited financial resources could not afford plane tickets or lacked bribe money.

## Alternative Lifestyles

Iranians are conservative about male-female relationships and may discourage dating. Older and more traditional Iranians may be uncomfortable with unrelated members of the opposite sex. Most Iranians strongly disapprove of the American practice of living together before marriage. While divorce is viewed negatively, its rate has been increasing among Iranians in the United States, partly due to the increase in intercultural marriages. Rezaian (1989) found that intraculturally married Iranians reported more marital satisfaction than Iranians married to Americans or intraculturally married Americans. This may be due to Iranians' greater emotional expressiveness and shared frame of reference, which can improve communication. It may also be due to cultural mores that advocate ignoring or denying minor marital discord because of the importance of family stability, which encourages acceptance of suffering for the sake of maintaining family stability.

Out-of-wedlock teen pregnancy is neither talked about nor sufficiently prevalent to warrant public attention. In Iran, teen pregnancy can have a devastating outcome. If it happens in the United States, it may be taken care of quietly to preserve the face of the family.

While homosexuality undoubtedly occurs in Iranians as frequently as in any other group, it is highly stigmatized and not discussed; gays or lesbians remain in the closet. Since 1979, when the legal and religious systems became synonymous, homosexuality, which is considered unnatural and sacrilegious, has been a capital offense punishable by death (Clark, 1995). Members of an Iranian gay support group in the San Francisco Bay area use anonymity and pseudonyms to protect themselves from potential physical harm by fundamentalist groups. However, in certain areas of the United States, younger Iranians are increasingly tolerant of alternative lifestyles. While there is considerable social and family pressure to marry, more people feel free to remain single, celibate, or both.

## WORKFORCE ISSUES

### Culture in the Workplace

The greatest difficulty faced by Iranian immigrant health-care providers is acquiring legal residency. This is followed by finding a position that is not too damaging to the person's self-esteem. Often, to satisfy the need for financial stability, employment of any sort may be accepted, which can lead to the person experiencing continual bitterness or sadness.

Iranians perceive ethnic bias toward them from many people in the United States, including clients and coworkers. This varies with location; for example, bias is much less evident in such highly multicultural areas as the San Francisco Bay area and more evident in culturally homogenous areas. Common reactions include overt or subtle hostility, condescension, total lack of acknowledgment, or sarcasm. For example, one of the authors (Hafizi) encountered a physician who asked about her national origin, then responded, "Is this one of those countries that we like these days?" More acculturated immigrant professionals are more able to respond flexibly in the workplace. For example, when this same author perceives that a client is uncomfortable with her background or overtly expresses dislike, she uses *ta'arof* and becomes "superefficient." Her speech becomes polite and formal, yet cool; she enters the room only to do clinically necessary tasks but performs them so well that the client cannot complain that she is a "bad" or "rude" nurse. However, while her technical care is excellent, she is not satisfied because this approach lacks interpersonal rapport.

Iranian health-care workers strive for a balance of work and family, and work and leisure. If one spouse has to work, the wife is always the one who stays home. In some immigrant families, the wife finding a job before the husband creates problems for the entire family, despite the understanding that her employment is vital to the family's financial stability.

## Issues Related to Autonomy

In the workplace, Iranians are competitive and strive for a sense of personal accomplishment. They appreciate the importance of punctuality. Graduates of Iranian high schools are well educated in a broad curriculum with a sound science base. In contrast to the practical application emphasized in American professional schools, professional education in Iran is formal, theory based, and rigid in nature, with an emphasis on memorization. Practice is obtained through on-the-job training.

Most Iranian health-care providers speak English, but newcomers may not be familiar with American slang. An ongoing stressor is the condescending attitudes directed at anyone who speaks English with a strong accent. For example, a nurse with a master's degree described her first year in the United States as follows:

> I was seen as an ignorant nurse's aide who couldn't even speak English. One nurse used to follow me around, checking everything I did. I resented being treated that way, and my own self-esteem suffered (Lipson, 1992, p. 16).

## BIOCULTURAL ECOLOGY

### Skin Color and Other Biologic Variations

Iranians are a mixture of foreigners who invaded the area throughout Persian history and ethnic groups currently inhabiting Iran. As white Indo-Europeans, their skin tones and facial features resemble other Mediterranean and Southern European groups. Their coloring ranges from blue or green eyes, light brown hair, and fair skin to nearly black eyes, black hair, and brown skin. Because of the variations in skin color, health-care professionals may need to assess jaundice and anemia in Iranians by examining the sclera and oral mucosa rather than by relying solely on skin assessments.

### Diseases and Health Conditions

In Iran, the 1994 birth rate was 42 per 1000 persons and the infant mortality rate was 60 per 1000 infants (*World Almanac,* 1995). Heat and humidity in some provinces provide fertile ground for the spread of cholera, including new and mutant strains. Malaria is widespread in Baluchistan (southeast), with serological test results sometimes showing more than one strain in a single client. In rural areas that lack standardized sanitary systems, viral and bacterial meningitis, hookworms, and gastrointestinal dysenteries due to parasites are prevalent. Hypertension is widespread with 2 million cases reported in Tehran, or one-sixth of its population. Ischemic heart disease is on the rise, and the rise is generally perceived as related to the stress of living with daily uncertainties. Health-care providers should screen newer immigrants for diseases and illnesses common in their home country.

The most common health problems in Iran are linked to underdevelopment and the recent poor economy; for example, protein and vitamin deficiencies (due to malnutrition), hepatitis A and B (due to poor sanitary conditions, such as poor aseptic technique, or public health measures), rising rates of tuberculosis and syphilis, genetic problems (due to interfamily marriages), and blood dyscrasias. Interfamily marriage used to be common; however, increasing urbanization and scientific data has increased awareness of potential genetic diseases or birth defects resulting from these marriages and has led to a decrease in this practice. Diseases and birth defects associated with marriages between cousins include epilepsy, blindness, several forms of anemia, and hemophilia. Thalassemia, prevalent in northern and eastern provinces, is now being addressed through premarital screening for carriers and genetic counseling. Persons are also tested for vitamin $B_{12}$ or folic acid deficiencies linked to an enzyme deficiency. Mediterranean glucose-6-phosphate dehydrogenase deficiency is common and can precipitate a hemolytic crisis when fava beans are eaten and affects drug metabolism, such as increasing sensitivity to primaquine.

Allergies to plant pollens and air pollution induce pulmonary distress and exacerbate ischemic heart disease. These problems are also experienced by Iranians in the United States. In the United States, many Iranians experience stress-related health problems from culture conflict and loss, homesickness for family and relatives, and the previous conditions of war. Although northern California Iranians in Lipson's (1992) study were generally healthy, many expressed their ongoing stress somatically, through intermittent general symptoms or physical discomfort. Several articulated a direct connection between their worries and illness; for example, three of the first seven people interviewed had suffered from ulcers and attributed their "stomach problems" to their "worries" and "troubles." Others complained of headaches, backaches, a racing heart, or other manifestations of anxiety or depression. Ardehali and Backer (1980) noted that Iranians often focus their acute generalized stress on the alimentary system, attributing illness or its severity to something that has been eaten.

## HIGH-RISK BEHAVIOR

Iranians' high-risk behaviors are similar to those in the general population; however, they occur less frequently in more traditional groups. In Iran, more men smoke than Iranians in the U.S. and more men smoke than women, whereas in the United States, the reverse is true. In general, health education, through the media and the influence of their children encourage many Iranian immigrants to quit smoking.

Some alcohol and street-drug abuse occurs in the Iranian immigrant population, but the rate is no higher than that of the population at large. Alcohol is prohibited by the Qu'ran (Holy Book), although many Iranians are not religious and drink socially, a few to excess. In Iran, the most popular street drug among the older generation is opium, traditionally used for medicinal purposes. In some people, years of opium use create both psychological and physical addiction. Younger Iranians, who prefer heroin in Iran, take drugs for the same variety of reasons that American young people do, with availability and felt need determining continuation of use. Family responses to drug use range from complete support of the family member to disownment.

In the United States, alcohol and cigarettes are encouraged by advertising and are more generally accepted than in Iran. In some Iranian immigrants, abuse is related to a low level of acculturation and a sense of helplessness often experienced by displaced persons. In other cases, Iranian men demonstrate their "masculinity" through being able to "hold" their liquor. This need to assert masculinity combined with poor self-esteem increases the risk of alcohol addiction.

## Health-care Practices

Iranian children and young adults are more physically active than their elders, exercising as frequently as their peers in nonimmigrant groups. Soccer remains popular in Iran; some men continue to play soccer in the United States and encourage their children to play. Soccer promotes family fun and closeness and helps counteract the negative effects of peer pressure on children. Depending on their traditionalism, women may confine their exercise to housework or walking or may jog, swim, or do aerobics.

In Iran, seat belts were previously of lower priority than road conditions, but legislation has been passed requiring seat belts on intercity highways. In the United States, Iranians generally comply with seat belt and child restraint laws, valuing the safety of their children. Diet is an important part of maintaining health and is described in the next section. Health-care providers need to encourage positive health-seeking behaviors among their Iranian clients by using culturally congruent approaches and carefully explaining the detrimental physical and psychological effects of smoking, recreational drug use, and excessive consumption of alcohol.

## NUTRITION

### Meaning of Food

Food is a symbol of hospitality for Iranians. They prepare their best food for guests and insist that guests eat several servings. More food is prepared and presented than is needed to actually feed their guests to demonstrate their lavish hospitality. Iranian hosts go all out to make guests comfortable, serving them first or giving them the most comfortable seats. If guests arrive at times other than mealtime, tea is offered, usually with such snacks as fruits and nuts. The courteous guest, however, should refuse "to trouble" the host by politely refusing tea or food at least once; when accepting food, guests should first offer it to other guests before taking any themselves.

### Common Foods and Food Rituals

Iranian food is flavorful and takes hours to prepare. Presentation is important. At any given table, there is usually a pleasing mixture of foods of different colors and ingredients, composed of a balance of **garmie** and **sardie** (see section on dietary practices for health promotion). Tea and fruits are served for dessert after each meal. Iranians prefer to use only the freshest foods, although, in some cases, cost is a factor in their using some dried herbs. Canned, frozen, and fast foods are perceived to have less nutritional value and contain preservatives that can affect health. Eating fast food is less common because of concern about nutritional value and cost.

Hot tea is the most popular drink among Iranians. The most common starchy foods are rice and wheat bread. The art of preparing rice is the measuring stick against which teens and young women are judged as they complete their training in the kitchen. Long-grained, fluffy, and white rice is preferred. Bread is usually baked flat like **lavash** or pita. Corn and potatoes are used but less favored. Beans and legumes make up a fairly high proportion of the dietary intake and are commonly used in rice mixtures, for example, lentils, pinto, mung, kidney, lima and green beans, and split and black-eyed peas.

Dairy products are dietary staples, particularly eggs, milk, yogurt, and feta cheese, as well as dairy by-products, such as **doog** (yogurt soda) and **kashk** (milk by-product). Favorite meats are beef, chicken, fish, and lamb. Shellfish is sometimes eaten. Fresh fruit is always found in Iranian houses. Green leafy vegetables are used in cooking, and herbs such as parsley, cilantro (coriander), dill, fenugreek, tarragon, mint, savory, and green onions are served fresh at a meal.

Islam has a strict set of dietary prescriptions, **halal**, and proscriptions, **haram**. Slaughter of poultry, beef, and lamb must be done ritually to make the meat *halal*. Strict Muslims avoid pork and alcoholic beverages, and a few avoid shellfish. Historically, pork was prohibited for hygienic reasons, but food habits are passed down through the generations. However, avoidance of pork and alcohol is a cultural and religious tradition; for example, Armenians or Baha'is probably do not use it.

Generally, food is eaten with the right hand, and food or objects are passed with the right hand alone or both hands. Traditional or older people may be most comfortable sitting on the floor, with food on large platters in the center of a large tablecloth. Health-care providers may need to make adjustments to accommodate traditional food practices of Iranians, making provisions for the family to bring food from home if the client prefers.

## Dietary Practices for Health Promotion

Based on humoral theory, Iranians classify foods into one of two categories, **garm**, hot, and **sard**, cold, which sometimes correspond to high-calorie and low-calorie foods. The key is balance. The belief is that too much of one category can cause symptoms of being "overheated" or "chilled." Such symptoms are treated by eating food from the opposite group. For example, overheatedness, sweating, itching, and rashes may result from eating too many hot foods, such as walnuts, onions, garlic, spices, honey, or candy. Or the stomach may become chilled, causing dizziness, weakness, and vomiting, after eating too many cold foods, such as grapes, rhubarb, plums, beer (Ardehali & Backer, 1980), cucumbers, or yogurt. One of the authors was served fish and green salad at a meal, after which her hosts strongly recommended that she eat some dates with tea to offset the possibility of developing *sardie,* a digestive problem from ingesting too much cold food. She was perceived to be susceptible related to her light complexion. Women are believed to be more susceptible to *sardie* than *garmie,* a digestive problem from too much hot food. Health-care providers may need to incorporate Iranian foods and dietary practices in health teaching to improve compliance with special dietary restrictions.

## Nutritional Deficiencies and Food Limitations

Today, because of economic problems in Iran, certain foods are unavailable and the incidence of protein and vitamin deficiencies is increasing. The emphasis of food has changed from socializing around food to satisfying hunger. Because the Iranian immigrant diet is balanced and healthy, nutritional deficiencies are not usually a problem for those who have been in the United States for some time.

Almost all ingredients used in Iranian cooking can be found in the United States. When the cost of certain vegetables and herbs is too high, some families grow them in their backyards. Most commonly used medicinal herbs are available in Iranian or other Middle Eastern grocery stores. Iranians are not restricted from any foods whose absence might cause nutritional problems.

## PREGNANCY AND CHILDBEARING PRACTICES

### Fertility Practices and Views toward Pregnancy

In rural areas of Iran, traditional beliefs and practices are influenced by Galenic or humoral medicine, particularly with regard to hot and cold temperament and the conditions of pregnancy and birth. Conception is explained as "the man contributes the seed and the woman provides the vessel in which the seed grows" (Good, 1980, p. 149). Menstrual blood is believed to be ritually unclean and physically polluting to the body and must be discharged monthly (Good, 1980). Menstruating women are not allowed to touch holy objects or have intercourse. Menstruation is also considered a time of great fragility when a woman should not exercise or shower excessively, because these activities might cause a hemorrhage (Ardehali & Backer, 1980). At the end of the menses, the woman must wash and purify herself thoroughly before any religious rituals.

Before the 1979 revolution, birth control was rarely used in rural areas of Iran because having many children assured the continued financial success of the family. Women were concerned about the health of their uteri, and home remedies for infertility focused on improving the state of the uterus as a "vessel" of conception (Good, 1980). Infertility was blamed on the woman. Baluch, Al-Shawaf, and Craft (1992) found that reasons for seeking infertility treatment differed for men and women: Whereas men sought reproduction to ensure future support, women were fulfilling the social expectation to have babies at an early stage in the marriage.

After the 1979 revolution, contraception was discouraged in light of the Islamic emphasis on children as the symbol of God's blessing. With the recent population explosion and associated public health and welfare problems, birth control has again been cautiously encouraged. The annual growth rate remains at 3.8 percent, with higher fertility in the rural areas among tribal groups who marry young and have large families (Sheykhi, 1995). Traditionally, prolonged breast-feeding was often used as a method of contraception (Good, 1980).

In cosmopolitan and educated Iranian families, fewer children are the norm; a desirable family size is often three or four children. In the United States, young couples limit families to fewer children, the desirable number being two or three. Current methods used by Iranians to limit conception include the pill, intrauterine device, and natural methods. Vasectomies are just beginning to gain acceptance. However, traditional beliefs discourage contraceptive methods that decrease menstrual blood flow, and some women believe that some methods cause such symptoms as heart palpitations.

Pregnancy after marriage is desirable among Iranian women for several reasons. Women believe that their bodies are in a less healthy state, polluted with excess menstrual blood until they have given birth to a child (Good, 1980). Women's prestige is at its height when she delivers her first child, particularly if it is a boy. Delivering the first child releases anxiety and gives the young wife a more respected and cherished position among her in-laws. Health-care providers should consider these traditional beliefs of some Iranians in health teaching. Providing factual information regarding family planning is one area where health-care professionals can improve family care.

## Prescriptive, Restrictive, and Taboo Practices in the Childbearing Family

Cravings during pregnancy are seen as resulting from the needs of the fetus for particular foods; thus, cravings must be satisfied lest a miscarriage occur from not meeting the fetus's needs (Ardehali & Backer, 1980). Women avoid fried foods and foods that cause gas; fruits and vegetables are recommended, with attention to the balance of hot and cold foods. Heavy work is thought to cause a miscarriage. Sexual intercourse is allowed until the last month. The pregnant woman receives considerable support from female kin beginning in the sixth month until after the birth, relieving the pregnant and postpartum woman of household tasks.

During the birthing process, the woman receives support from her mother, sister, or aunt. In more traditional Iranian families, the father is not usually present at the birth to provide assistance. In the United States, delivery is typical of the dominant society, with some women choosing natural childbirth and involving their husbands fully in the process, and others preferring medication.

The postpartum period for Iranian women is 30 to 40 days. In rural Iran, female kin take the primary responsibility for supporting the mother during the postpartum period. Because of the belief in the polluting nature of blood, postpartum women are required to take a ritual bath after they stop bleeding, so they can resume normal religious activities. To strengthen the postpartum woman, a *ghorse kamar* (brown, flat disk of dried herbs) is mixed with eggs and placed on her lower back a few hours before bathing.

In rural Iran, postpartum diet and care are influenced by the need to balance hot and cold. Such hot foods as pistachio nuts and eggs are given to postpartum women to strengthen their bodies and combat *sardie*. New mothers avoid cold water for bathing, ablutions, or cleaning, although they now bathe sooner than the traditional first 30 days (Good, 1980). Baby boys are considered "hotter" than baby girls, and mothers of sons are considered to have hotter bodies, hotter milk, and hotter temperaments than mothers of girls. Mothers of girls are given a mixture of honey and other nutrients, an herbal extract called *taranjebin*, to raise their bodily heat to ensure that the next child is a boy. Some families keep an infant home for the first 40 days; by that time, it is believed that the baby is strong enough to fight off environmental pathogens. The baby is given a ritual bath between the 10th and 40th days. Healthcare providers should ask the childbearing family about prescriptive, restrictive, and taboo cultural practices that they customarily follow and incorporate these in their care.

# DEATH RITUALS

## Death Rituals and Expectations

In discussing the withdrawal of life support of a terminal client, some families may demand that strenuous efforts be made to prolong life, so it is important to assess each family individually. To discuss termination of life support with a practicing Muslim, the health-care provider can begin the conversation by noting God's will for human beings and His power over our destiny. This discussion can be followed by a dialogue about life and death as steps toward immortal life in heaven. Muslims may only need a gentle reminder that death is not a termination of life, but rather the beginning of a new and better life. However, Iranians usually oppose stopping life support, viewing it as "playing God," even though they may have no objection to beginning life support, viewing it as the "gift" of medical technology (Klessig, 1992).

When an Iranian is dying, family members and friends come to be with the patient and family. Among religious Muslims, the deathbed should be turned to face Mecca, so family members can read prayers from the *Qu'ran* to assure that the dying person hears this last. Because few traditional Muslim cemeteries exist in the United States, some terminally ill traditional Muslims request to return to Iran to either die or be buried.

After the death, the body should be washed in a ritual manner and wrapped in a special white cotton shroud by another Muslim. Ritual bathing is done with soap and water, proceeding from head to toe and front to back. All body orifices must be closed and slightly packed with cotton to prevent leakage of bodily fluids (considered unclean). The final rinse is performed with water. Prayers and verses from the *Qu'ran* are read during the procedure. A non-Muslim health-care provider should only touch the body wearing gloves (Klessig, 1992). There are no specific religious rules against autopsy. However, the body of the dead is to be respected; therefore, the reason for the autopsy must be made clear, and many people may refuse. In Iran, embalming of the dead is not practiced; rather, they are buried directly into the earth to facilitate the transition from "dust to dust." The shroud is removed from the face, and one side of the face is turned to be in contact with the earth. Cremation is not practiced in Iran.

## Responses to Death and Grief

Iranians may express their grief over the death of a loved one by crying, wailing loudly, or even striking the wall or a table. While loss of a loved one is met with expressive and strong grieving and support from family and friends, death is seen as a beginning, not an end, in which the mortal life gives way to the spiritual existence, a cherished state of solidifying one's relationship with God. This "fatalistic" belief and the belief in the power of God over all His creation makes "letting go" easier for some families. In general, it seems that Iranians let their loved ones go more easily but grieve longer and more expressively than Americans, who let go less easily but grieve for a shorter period and more privately.

After a Muslim's death, relatives, friends, and acquaintances gather on the 3rd, 7th, and 40th days after the death. Prayers are read by clergy, family, relatives, and friends. Special foods are served, and grieving may be expressed loudly. Attending a funeral is essential for paying respect to the dead and for offering support to the survivors. All Iranians wear black, and women relatives wear no makeup. Some believe that the family must pay the deceased's debts or life after death will be less favorable. If the deceased is young, a more extensive ceremony is held. On the anniversary of the death, the family gathers again to pay respect to the dead. In Iran, money may be set aside to help the needy instead of holding an anniversary ceremony, but relatives visit anyway to pay their respects, especially on the first anniversary. Spouses or parents visit the grave of their loved ones weekly, generally on a Thursday or Friday.

## SPIRITUALITY

### Religious Practices and Use of Prayer

Islam exerted its influence on Iran and its culture in five domains: (1) the domain of temporal focus, (2) the fate of an individual, (3) humoral medicine, (4) dietary laws, and (5) family loyalty (Jalali, 1982; Pliskin, 1987). However, certain norms embedded in Iranian culture transcend religious and ethnic boundaries, such as family loyalty and respect for elderly persons.

Specific Muslim practices include prayers, read in the name of 1 of the 12 imams (predecessors of the Prophet Mohammed), to provide peace of mind or to plead for a miracle. Sometimes, when an important asset needs protection, for example, a house, a child, or a life, a healer is sought to help with a sacrifice to keep the evil eye away. Although most Iranian Muslims in the United States are not ritually strict, strict Muslims pray five times daily and need privacy and water for ritual washing. They may fast from sunup to sundown during Ramazan, although pregnant women and the ill are exempt from fasting. Jewish, Christian, and Baha'i Iranians have religious beliefs and practices similar to those of other ethnic groups. Health-care providers may need to make environmental adjustments that allow Iranian immigrant clients to practice their religious beliefs.

### Meaning of Life and Individual Sources of Strength

An Iranian's understanding of and outlook on the world is influenced by national history and social expectations, which gives every experience a rich context in which everything and everyone has significance. For religious Iranians of all faiths, faith and acceptance of God's will is a source of strength and comfort, particularly in times of illness or crisis.

Family relationships and friendships are sources of strength and meaning in life for many individuals. Iranians are highly affiliative and thrive on social relationships. Close and regular contact with family and friends is both a pleasure and a necessity. Lack of social support in the United States is an ongoing stressor among many Iranian immigrants (Lindholm & Shoaee, 1984). Given the importance of family for providing meaning and strength for Iranians, health-care providers may need to adjust visiting policies in health-care settings to accommodate family and friends.

Family rules and societal norms are another source of strength for Iranians; they provide internal control, rather than the external control of law enforcement, over behavior. Religious beliefs are also a source of strength for many Iranians, particularly for older people, who might consult a spiritual advisor and become more in tune with God as they come closer to death.

Iran has been called a "grief society," in which sadness, often associated with death, is a strong theme. This theme emerges in Iranian culture; expression of the tragedies in life are depicted in poetry, art, music, and mythology. A sad person is considered to be deep, thoughtful, and sensitive, which are valued personality characteristics (Good et al., 1985).

## Spiritual Beliefs and Health-care Practices

*Tagdir*, God's will and power over one's fate in life and death, is a common belief among Iranians, which fosters a sense of passivity and dependence on a superior force. This belief is weaker or less prevalent among better-educated Iranians (Rezaian, 1989). Religious beliefs affect health-care beliefs and are described more fully in the next section. Hafizi's (1990) research also illustrates clearly the integration of religion and health concepts. In the words of this highly educated, devout Muslim man:

> To ask me what health means is to ask me what my worldly outlook is. How I see myself in relation to God, my family, the society as a whole and my relation to my material body. Man is the embodiment of the unworldly spiritual being whereby the body and the spirit work in such a close connection that the two work as one unit. Life then becomes a passage through time. The mortal life represents only one stage of this passage. Death is not a finalization, rather a graduation to a higher level of being. I believe in God and *His* plan for the future. For example, being sick is not having a cold, rather it is not having the vision to deal with the cold.

## HEALTH-CARE PRACTICES

### Health-seeking Beliefs and Behaviors

Traditional Iranian health beliefs and therapeutic processes are a combination of three high traditions of medicine: Galenic (humoral), Islamic (sacred), and modern biomedicine (Good, 1977). In classic humoral theory, illness arises from an imbalance (excess or deficiency) in the basic qualities, for example, hot and cold, wet and dry. The purpose of treatment is to restore balance. The Galenic-Islamic tradition of humoral medicine is widely practiced throughout Iran and influences the beliefs of the immigrant population. In Galenic thought, every individual has a distinctive balance of four humors, or *mezaj*, resulting in a unique temperament, or *tabi'at*. Physical and emotional illness is caused by an imbalance in humors of the body and mind, which may coexist; thus, an emotional upset could include physical illness and vice versa. Even among immigrants, practices related to the qualities of hot and cold and moist and dry in relation to food and climate are believed to be significant in affecting health (Pliskin, 1987). For example, wetness and wind are avoided; thus, a child's ears are covered on a windy day because cool wind is believed to cause earache or infection. Sacred medicine is from the *Qu'ran* and *hadith,* and holy men are able to heal. The sacred tradition includes beliefs in the evil eye and **jinns** as disease agents, as well as healing by a means of manipulating impurity. For those who believe strongly in God's control over their fate, a holy man can heal by writing prayers on a piece of paper, which can be placed in water and drunk, or burned and the smoke inhaled to incorporate the prayers.

Health is a diffuse concept deeply rooted in Iranian culture, an idea central to the governing of daily chores and the routines of one's social and personal life. Illness is discussed and challenged, with advice solicited to remedy the ailment. For example, a balanced intake of hot and cold foods to maintain health is a daily consideration, although it may be practiced subconsciously and not articulated (Hafizi, 1990; Pliskin, 1987).

Hafizi's research (1990) found that Iranians' concepts of health represented two of Smith's (1983) four domains: the clinical view (health as absence of disease) and the adaptive view (health as the ability to cope successfully). These are integrated in a view of healthy human beings as physiochemical and sociopsychological systems able to cope successfully with the changing world. This health-illness paradigm is characterized by a dynamic relationship between the individual and the environment, a harmonious exchange between nature's available resources and a person's capability to use these sources. Thus, health is not achieved through a preplanned, regimented schedule of diet, exercise, and therapy but is a daily way of life marked by new demands and adaptations (Hafizi, 1990).

Iranians accept both biomedical diagnoses and cultural illness categories. The concept of the body is viewed in relation to its total environment—society, God, and the supernatural. When someone has a discomforting symptom, often they are first asked whether they ate something that did not agree with their *mezaj* (humoral temperament). If the answer is no, then other causes are suspected.

## Responsibility for Health Care

Iranians often seek immediate relief or cures from the health-care system and may "shop around" until they find a provider they like. At the same time, they may seek advice from an elder who can suggest herbal remedies. Herbal remedies are used primarily to relieve symptoms. For example, mint tea and cilantro seeds are used to promote relaxation and sleep. Thus, Iranians' conceptions of illness are a combination of Western biomedical categories and culturally shaped explanatory models and syndromes.

To promote health, many Iranians watch their diets, particularly food choices and preparation, for example, including fruit and avoiding excessive fat and canned, frozen, or otherwise processed foods. They may be careful not to eat incompatible foods at the same meal, with an emphasis on balancing hot and cold. Iranians also protect their health by getting enough rest and exercise, by taking vitamins, and by keeping warm or dressing adequately. To introduce preventive education, Iranians can be reminded that prevention has always been and still remains a focal part of humoral medicine in Iran, and that Iranians have always practiced prevention.

Iranians practice self-medication and use both prescription and over-the-counter medications and home-based herbal remedies. Antibiotics, codeine-based analgesics, mood-altering drugs in the benzodiazepine family (e.g., diazepam [Valium]), and intramuscular vitamins are available over-the-counter in Iran, and immigrants often bring these medications with them to the United States. Thus, they are less cautious with such medications than Americans, who live under Food and Drug Administration regulations; they sometimes adjust the dosage of prescribed medications in the United States, particularly when finances are a problem. American health-care providers should consider carefully the dosage or type of medication prescribed based on these self-medicating practices; for example, because of prior overuse, a first-generation antibiotic may not be strong enough for some Iranians.

When Iranians are ill, they are expected to be passive and taken care of by health-care providers and family members, who visit frequently or are expected to be present continuously until the client is discharged from the hospital or functioning again. Self-care is a foreign concept to Iranians because, in Iran, the authoritative doctor tells the client what to do, even prescribing what and what not to eat. Even among highly acculturated immigrants in the United States, there is potential for misunderstanding because people rely on their cultural styles of coping in threatening situations like illness and hospitalization. For example, nurses on a neurosurgery unit requested consultation regarding an older male Iranian client because his wife and adult children were in constant attendance and demanded that the nurses take care of his every need immediately. We explained to the nurses that the family's unceasing attention to the client and their constant demands on staff were culturally appropriate ways of showing their care and concern. If they did not insist on immediate care or left him alone, they would have been seen as neglectful and unloving (Lipson & Meleis, 1983). Thus, many Iranian clients do not seem motivated to do self-care; this does not mean, however, that they do not care about their recovery. Rather, because of strong family values among Iranians, self-care should be interpreted as encouraging family members to take care of the sick person (Lipson & Steiger, 1996).

## Health-care Beliefs and Practices

Among Iranians, **naharati** is a general term used to express a wide range of undifferentiated, unpleasant emotional or physical feelings, such as feeling depressed, uneasy, nervous, disappointed, or not fully well. *Narahati* is often expressed nonverbally in silence, sullenness, crying, or avoidance of food (Pliskin, 1992). Iranians often somatize in a subconscious effort to communicate *narahati* or distress that cannot be otherwise expressed verbally or nonverbally. By somatizing, they construct an illness that is culturally sanctioned and socially understood. The source can be personal, social, spiritual, or psychological. Somatization also allows the persons to distance themselves from the actual problem, while putting the responsibility and focus on the metaphoric body. Since Iranians generally shy away from overt expressions of personal *naharati*, the "somatic self" becomes a focal point in the health-care encounter. When *naharati* is seen as being caused by fright, the evil eye or *jinns*, it may be treated with religious cures. If it is seen as caused by problems of blood, nerves, or humoral imbalance, it is treated with herbs or biomedicine.

Another cultural syndrome is **ghalbam gerefteh** (*narahatiye qalb,* or distress of the heart). Heart distress may be expressed as a feeling that the heart is being squeezed and can range in severity from mild excitation of the heart or palpitations to fainting and heart attack (Good, 1977; Good & Good, 1982). Good's (1977) classic study in rural Iran found that women of all ages comprised two-thirds of those who reported experiencing heart distress, the same proportion found in Lipson's (1992) study of immigrants to the United States. Heart distress was attributed to great sadness, being homesick, or having problems that seem insoluble. One woman stated, "I get it when I read Persian newspapers about the situation in Iran."

A widespread belief among Iranians is that fright or being startled by bad news negatively affects health. Symptoms caused by fright include extreme fatigue, with chills and fever as more severe symptoms. A client might be given salt or a mixture of hard sugar candy and water, taken to a physician, or be given herbal medicines or a religious cure. In one rural area of Iran, the fright is driven "out of the body by having the client ingest something polluting" (Good & Good, 1982, p. 153).

In other instances, a sudden ailment or symptom of puzzling origin may be attributed to the evil eye, or ***cheshm-i-bad***, which is the belief that the eyes of another person can cause illness. *Cheshm-i-bad* can be unintentional (enthusiastically complimenting someone without saying "In the name of God") or intentional (cast out of jealousy or enmity). Some Iranians burn *esfand* (wild rue) in the fireplace to prevent it; more acculturated and younger people state that only their grandparents or rural people believe in "the eye."

*Cheshm-i-bad* and other folk syndromes are better understood by viewing the body in the context of its social and supernatural environment. Similar to somatizing, which distances an individual from the actual problem, *cheshm-i-bad* attributes illness to an outside person or force. In reality, the evil eye gives meaning to an occurrence of puzzling origin. It puts the blame on someone or something else other than the client (Good & Good 1982; Pliskin, 1987).

Herbal remedies are used in a complementary manner with medications. Iranians often take herbal remedies recommended by relatives or friends to prevent or treat symptoms. They became increasingly popular in postrevolutionary Iran because of the economic embargo and scarcity of biomedical supplies; pharmacies and ***atary*** (herb shops) stock packaged herbal medications in tea bags, capsules, and creams, and farm areas are dedicated to the cultivation of plants for medicinal use.

Depending on the person's orientation, both in the United States as in Iran, herbal remedies are used as either adjuncts to Western biomedicine or the first line of treatment for an illness. Therefore, American health-care providers should ask if herbal therapies are being used in addition to prescribed medications. Many Iranians believe that complementary treatment is more effective than a single treatment. The literature reports no research data that contraindicates combining Iranian herbal and Western medications.

Common herbal remedies include dried flowers, seeds, leaves, and berries, steeped in hot or cold water and drunk for a variety of purposes, such as digestive problems, "cleaning the blood or kidneys," coughs, aches and pains, fevers, or nerves or fear (Pliskin, 1992). Some common herbal medications include ***gol-i-gov zabon*** (dried foxglove flowers) for imbalance in the digestive system or nervous upsets, which is sometimes taken with ***nabat***, a concentrated sugar (Lipson, 1992). ***Khakshir*** (flat, brown rocket seed) is used for stomach problems and "dirty blood," *razianeh* is used for halitosis, quince seeds are sucked for sore throats, and *sedr* prevents and treats dandruff. ***Neshasteh*** (wheat starch) is combined with boiling water and drunk for sore throats or coughs and also used to stop diarrhea. Mint extracts are used to relieve excess stomach gas. Plant extracts are popular both in Iran and the United States; for example, a plant called *shatareh* is thought to cure fever.

Grandmothers, aunts, and mothers are often consulted for mild illness and may prepare home herbal remedies. Families decide to consult physicians for conditions that do not respond to other remedies or that appear serious. Fathers often have responsibility for making health-care decisions, with the input of other family members.

## Barriers to Health Care

Language and communication problems for some of the newest Iranian immigrants limit access to health care. For example, a man with severely bleeding hemorrhoids, who telephoned a doctor and attempted to describe his problem as "pain in my back" was told to come in the next day (Lipson, 1992). Lack of health insurance is a major barrier to health care. In Iran, health care is publically and privately financed, and the concept of insurance has no meaning. In the United States, the major reason for lack of health insurance is inability to pay for it, particularly among those who are self-employed.

## Cultural Responses to Health and Illness

On the whole, Iranians are more expressive about their pain than European-Americans, but men are more stoic than women. Some justify suffering in light of later rewards. For example, the grandmother of a young women with a slow-growing brain tumor consoled herself and her granddaughter with the statement that suffering in this world assures her a place in heaven after death.

Mental illness is highly stigmatized among Iranians and is thought to be genetic. Should a family member have mental illness, it is likely to be called a "neurological disorder" to avoid stigmatizing the family, which may result in daughters having a lesser chance of marrying. Psychotherapeutic help may be avoided either because of stigma or because it is perceived as irrelevant; moreover, Iranians prefer a medicine that might cure them. Bagheri (1992) stated that Iranians tend to pay more attention to somatic symptoms when under emotional stress and consider psychopharmacological treatment most effective; such treatment also results in a higher rate of compliance.

Other than major mental illness, Iranian immigrants experience numerous stressors related to resettlement in a foreign culture. Health-care providers often do not recognize the subtle and not-so-subtle stressors their immigrant clients experience, such as daily necessities made difficult by financial strain or by accented or inadequate English. As measured by the Health Opinion Survey, 44 percent of Lipson's (1992) newer immigrant interviewees experienced medium stress or high stress compared with 14 percent of the longer-settled group. With reference to mood, about 35 percent of the informants answered "yes" when asked if they considered themselves to be "nervous," and about the same percentage stated that they did not have "peace of mind." The reasons given were mainly problems with life in the United States, missing family members, or concerns about relatives back home.

Despite these problems, most Iranian immigrants, like other Middle Eastern immigrants (Lipson & Meleis, 1983), stated that they were not likely to seek counseling or psychiatric help, preferring to discuss their problems with family members or to solve their problems by themselves. However, psychotherapy and counseling are beginning to be better accepted and perceived as helpful, particularly with reference to dealing with children.

While mental disability is less tangible and understood, physical disability has received recent attention in Iran. Before 1979, the disabled were hidden away at home because they brought stigma on the family and because few treatment options were available. The World Health Organization's Year of the Disabled stimulated Iran to institute civil rights for the disabled, guaranteeing access to health-care services and facilities. Today rehabilitation such as physical therapy and music therapy is embraced as the way to bring the disabled into the mainstream. Attitudes toward the disabled among Iranian immigrants depend partly on when they left Iran and vary from negative and embarrassed to open and helpful.

## Blood Transfusion and Organ Donation

Blood transfusions, organ donations, and organ transplants are widely practiced among Iranians. In Iran, donation of organs is often a business transaction—if a kidney is needed, it is purchased.

# HEALTH-CARE PRACTITIONERS

## Traditional Versus Biomedical Care

When asked to compare American medical care with that offered in Iran, most Iranian immigrants consider it to be very good, although they may shop around before finding a doctor they like (Jalali, 1982). They most appreciate the facilities and equipment and the lack of corruption in the system. On the other hand, they complain about the expense of health care and health insurance. Others dislike waiting for appointments; as one woman noted, "The patient could die while waiting" (Lipson, 1992).

A frequent source of difficulties, even for immigrants with good English skills, is differing expectations regarding the proper roles of health-care providers and clients and difference in diagnostic styles between Iranian and American physicians. According to one woman, for example, "Doctors here are horrible. They don't listen to you, they are always careful of malpractice, they don't want to be specific" (Lipson, 1992). Jalali (1982) noted that Iranian clients request medication and expect quick results, visiting a new doctor if a cure is not imminent. In comparing American physicians with their counterparts in Iran, immigrants think that Iranian doctors make more authoritative and quicker diagnoses, using minimal technology, even if they are uncertain or wrong. Sometimes, American physicians who are tentative, who ask the client to describe the problem, or who order too many tests are viewed as incompetent (Lipson & Meleis, 1983).

The acceptance of a health-care provider of a different gender from that of the client depends to some extent on the acculturation level of the family. In general, women prefer to be cared for by female nurses and physicians, and men prefer to be cared for by men. Iranian women are modest in front of men and may object to a male health-care provider. If possible, male health-care providers should try not to require women to undress fully for an examination or procedure. In very traditional families, resistance to having a woman client cared for by a man may be strong enough to have the family consider taking the client elsewhere or avoid care until the situation is acute. Caregivers of the same gender as the client should be provided whenever possible when performing intimate examinations and providing care to Iranians.

## Status of Health-care Providers

Traditional religious and folk practitioners may be sought by extremely religious persons or those who are superstitious, but not by most Iranian immigrants. If a magicoreligious healer's services are sought, it is generally for *naharatis* of unexplainable origin or nonmedical concerns.

The most respected health-care provider is an experienced middle-aged to elderly male physician, with several degrees and preferably with a high position in the hospital or university. He is considered the authority and is expected to act like one, making diagnoses quickly and prescribing remedies that cure the client. In Iran, physicians rely more on physiological cues than technology. Equipment such as computed tomography scanners are scarce, and the waiting lists are long for such equipment. Recently, the government of Iran has supported medical school admissions based on influential kin; therefore, graduates are of mixed quality.

The least respected health-care providers are students; immigrant families sometimes refuse student caregivers. Nurses are accorded little respect in comparison with physicians; male nurses or women who are grey haired and have positions of authority are accorded more respect than young, single, female nurses. Nurses who encourage self-care may be perceived as being uncaring or even incompetent.

Iranian nurses complain that Iranian physicians respect only each other and look down on other health-care providers. Physicians are on top, and other providers just follow orders. Because of these status and power differences, Iranian immigrant physicians may have conflicts with assertive American nurses, and Iranian nurses may not be as assertive as they should be in the American health-care system.

## CASE STUDY

Mustafa E, 46 years old , brought his wife Mina, 39 years old, and his three children to the United States in 1983. Son Hamid was 12 years old, daughter Maryam was 11 years old, and son Ali was 7 years old. In addition to economic difficulties imposed by the Iran-Iraq war, they feared that Hamid would be drafted and sent to the front. Mustafa preferred not to leave Iran; he spoke no English and was afraid that he would feel isolated in the United States. Mina, on the other hand, was somewhat eager to leave the social constraints that were becoming permanent; she had always hoped that their children, especially their daughter, would have the opportunity for more than her own ninth grade education and for a successful professional life.

Mustafa graduated from high school and worked in Iran's Ministry of Education. He held a bookkeeping job on the side, which allowed him to save money for the journey. Mina's brother, who had immigrated to the United States in the early 1970s, encouraged the family to go to Turkey, and he had arranged for an attorney to obtain a visa for the E family. They were granted a tourist visa and flew to Dallas. Mustafa quickly repaid his brother-in-law $5000 for legal fees.

Mina's brother and his wife, an American, welcomed the family into their house, but language and cultural differences made Mustafa and Mina uncomfortable. After 2 months, they rented an apartment nearby. With the help of her brother's acquaintances, Mina enrolled the children in school and registered herself in an adult learning center. Because they had a tourist visa, neither parent could get a work permit. With no knowledge of English or the local economy, Mustafa relied on the advice of everyone around him, such as an Iranian businessman who helped him look into purchasing a business. Within a few months he had bought a gas station. Mina began sewing and doing alterations for their small circle of Iranian acquaintances.

While the children were adjusting well, Mina and Mustafa were beginning to feel the strains of social and cultural alienation. The news of war and family affairs in Iran was getting more intense. Mustafa still showed no desire to learn more English than he needed to do the bookkeeping for the gas station and deal with customers. Deep inside, he believed that he would return home as soon as the children started college.

By 1990, Mustafa's business had gone bankrupt and the family's savings had dwindled. Their only source of income was Mina's earnings and Hamid's part-time job while attending the local junior college. Relations at home were extremely tense, with emotions always on the edge. Mustafa had increased his smoking to three packs of cigarettes daily, and he had frequent bouts of bronchitis. Mina had lost nearly 20 pounds since their arrival in the United States, and her migraine headaches had increased to almost daily, particularly after having lost her mother without having been able to visit her in Iran.

Mustafa found a bookkeeping job in an accounting firm owned by an Iranian, but his excessive smoking and occasional shortness of breath and heartburn continued. Mina had made several visits to the local hospital emergency room with complaints of fatigue and sleeplessness. Mustafa and Mina had treated some of their symptoms with herbal remedies, but their problems persisted to the point where Mustafa was admitted to the hospital with chest pain to rule out myocardial infarction. The two older children were attending school and working, leaving the youngest son to act as cultural and language interpreter for their parents during this hospitalization.

## STUDY QUESTIONS

1. Identify three major emotional and physiological problems commonly seen among Iranian immigrants.

2. Identify significant socioeconomic factors that limit access to health care for Iranian immigrants.

3. Identify the family spokesperson and discuss salient issues in establishing effective communication with this family.

4. How should prevention be taught to this family; what would be appropriate goals?

5. Name three major risk factors that this family experienced.

6. What mechanisms for coping with stress were predominantly used in this household?

7. Identify the family's social support system.

8. What hospital policies and constraints might negatively or positively affect this family's dynamics?

9. Compare and contrast the three waves of Iranian immigration in terms of educational status, reasons for migration, and occupations in the United States.

10. Explore assertiveness tactics for female Iranians in the American workforce.

11. What are the most common health problems of Iranian immigrants? What are some implications for health-care providers?

12. Identify characteristics of a healthy Iranian diet.

13. Identify contraception methods among Iranians.

14. Identify bereavement practices among Iranians.

## References

Ardehali, P., & Backer, D. (1980). Stress and the Iranian patient. *Behavioral Medicine, 7,* 31–37.

Bagheri, A. (1992). Psychiatric problems among Iranian immigrants in Canada. *Canadian Journal of Psychiatry, 37,* 7–11.

Baluch, B., Al-Shawaf, T., & Craft, I. (1992). Prime factors for seeking infertility treatments amongst Iranian patients. *Psychological Reports, 71,* 265–266.

Bateson, M., Clinton, S., Kassarjian, J., Safavi, H. & Soraya, N. (1977). Safa-yi Batin: A study of the interrelationship of a set of Iranian ideal character dimensions. In C. Brown & N. Kizkowitz (Eds.), *Psychological dimensions of Near Eastern studies* (pp. 257–273). Princeton, NJ: Darwin Press.

Beauchamp, M. (1988). *Welcome to Teheran.* California: Forbes.

Beeman, W. (1988). Affectivity in Persian language use. *Culture, Medicine and Psychiatry, 12,* 9–30.

Bozorgmehr, M., Sabagh, G., & Der-Martirosian, C. (1993). Beyond nationality: Religio-ethnic diversity. In R. Kelly (Ed.), *Irangeles: Iranians in Los Angeles* (pp. 59–79). Berkeley: University of California Press.

Clark, D. (1995, January 27). Small Iranian group maintains anonymity. *The Washington Blade,* p. 14.

Connell, C. (1981, December 7). Iran leads foreign-student population in United States schools. *San Francisco Chronicle,* pp. B1, B12.

Dallalfar, A. (1994). Iranian women as immigrant entrepreneurs. *Gender and Society, 8*(4), 541–561.

David M. Kennedy Center for International Studies (1984). *Culturegram: The Islamic Republic of Iran.* Provo, UT: Brigham Young University.

Fischer, M. (1978). On changing the concept and position of Persian women. In L. Beck & N. Keddie (Eds.), *Women in the Muslim World* (pp. 189–215). Cambridge, MA: Harvard University Press.

Good, B. J. (1977). The heart of what's the matter. *Culture, Medicine and Psychiatry, 1,* 25–58.

Good, B. J., & Good, M. D. (1982). Toward a meaning-centered analysis of popular illness categories: "Fright illness" and "heart distress" in Iran. In A. Marsella & G. White (Eds.), *Cultural conceptions of mental health and therapy,* pp. 141–166. Dordrecht, Netherlands: D. Reidel.

Good, B. J., Good, M. D., & Moradi, R. (1985). The interpretation of dysphoria and depressive illness in Iranian Culture. In A. Kleinman & B. Good (Eds.), *Culture and depression: Studies in the anthropology and cross-cultural psychiatry of affect and disorder* (pp. 369–428). Berkeley: University of California Press.

Good, M. D. (1980). Of blood and babies: The relationship of popular Islamic physiology to fertility. *Social Science & Medicine, 14b,* 147–156.

Hafizi, H. (1990). *Health and wellness: An Iranian outlook.* Unpublished master's thesis, University of California, San Francisco.

Hanassab, S. (1991). Acculturation and young Iranian women: Attitudes toward sex roles and intimate relationships. *Journal of Multicultural Counseling and Development, 19*(1), 11–21.

Herman, M., & Hojat, M. (1984). Distribution of Iranian and Filipino physicians in the United States by region of residence and medical specialty. *Del Medical Journal, 56*(9), 553–558.

Jalali, B. (1982). Iranian families. In M. McGoldrick, J. Pearce, & J. Giordano (Eds.), *Ethnicity and family therapy* (pp. 289–309). New York: The Guilford Press.

Kashani, H. (1988). *Grief and psychological adjustment to forced migration: A study of recent Iranian migrants to the United States.* Unpublished doctoral dissertation, California School of Professional Psychology, Berkeley.

Kelly, M. (1973). Beliefs of Iranian nurses and nursing students about nursing and nursing education. *International Nursing Review, 20*(4), 108–111.

Kelly, R., Friedlander, J., & Colby, A. (1993). *Irangeles: Iranians in Los Angeles.* Berkeley: University of California Press.

Klessig, J. (1992). The effect of values and culture on life-support decisions. *Western Journal of Medicine, 157*(3), 316–322.

Lewis, F., & Stevens, P. (1986). *Iranian refugees in America: A cross-cultural perspective.* Wilmette, IL: Baha'i Distribution Service.

Lindholm, K., & Shoaee, R. (1984, May). Parenting stress in immigrant Iranian parents: Impact of acculturative stress, coping and social support. Paper presented at the annual meeting of the Middle Eastern Studies Association, San Francisco.

Lipson, J. (1992). Iranian immigrants: Health and adjustment. *Western Journal of Nursing Research 14,* 10–29.

Lipson, J., & Meleis, A. (1983). Issues in health care of Middle Eastern patients. *Western Journal of Medicine, 139,* 854–861.

Lipson, J., & Meleis, A. (1989). Research with Middle Eastern immigrants: Methodological issues. *Medical Anthropology, 12,* 103–115.

Lipson, J. G., & Steiger, N. J. (1996) *Self-care nursing in multi-cultural context.* Thousand Oaks, CA: Sage.

Lorentz, J. & Wertime, J. (1980). Iranians. In S. Thernstrom (Ed.), *Harvard Encyclopedia of American Ethnic Groups.* Cambridge. MA: Harvard University Press.

Makaremi, A. (1990). Anger reactions of Iranian adolescents. *Psychological Reports, 67,* 259–260.

Peterson, W. (1958). A general typology of migration. *American Sociological Review, 23,* 256–266.

Pliskin, K. (1987). *Silent boundaries: Cultural constraints on sickness and diagnosis of Iranians in Israel.* New Haven, CT: Yale University Press.

Pliskin, K. (1992). Dysphoria and somatization in Iranian culture. *Western Journal of Medicine, 157,* 295–300.

Rezaian, F. (1989). *A study of intra- and inter-cultural marriages between Iranians and Americans.* Unpublished doctoral dissertation, California Institute of Integral Studies, San Francisco.

Ronaghy, H., Zeighami, B., Agah, T., Rouhani, R., & Zimmer, S. (1975). Migration of Iranian nurses to the United States: A study of one school of nursing in Iran. *International Nursing Review 22,* 87–88.

Ronaghy, H., Zeighami, E., Farahmand, N., & Zeighami, B. (1976). Causes of physician immigration: Responses of Iranian physicians in the United States. *Journal of Medical Education, 51*(9), 553–558.

Sabagh, G., & Bozorgmehr, M. (1987). Are the characteristics of exiles different from immigrants? The case of Iranians in Los Angeles. *Sociology and Social Research 71*(2) 77–84.

Samiezade-Yazd, C. (1989). Middle Eastern culture. In R. Murray & J. Zenter (Eds.), *Nursing assessment and health promotion strategies through the lifespan* (pp. 15–22, 90–91). Norwalk, CT: Appleton & Lange.

Smith, J. A. (1983). *The idea of health: Implications for the nursing profession.* New York: Teachers College.

*Statistics Canada: Ethnic Origin.* (1993). Ottowa, Canada: Minister of Industry, Science and Technology.

Stein, B. (1981). The refugee experience: Defining the parameters of a field study. *International Migration Review, 15,* 320–360.

Tyler, P. (1989, March 16). Millions of Iranians are trying to get out of the country. *San Francisco Chronicle,* p. A30.

Vatan, M. (1991). *The relationship between traditional roles and marital satisfaction among Iranian couples residing in California.* Unpublished doctoral dissertation, California Institute of Integral Studies, San Francisco.

*World almanac and book of facts* (1995). Mahwah, NJ: Funk and Wagnalls.

# Irish-Americans

*Sarah A. Wilson*

---

• Key terms to become familiar with in this chapter are:

Celtic                           Lace-curtain Irish
Dulse                            Limerick
Eire                             Shanty Irish
Great Potato Famine              Wake

## OVERVIEW, INHABITED LOCALITIES, AND TOPOGRAPHY

### Overview

The Republic of Ireland, whose capital city is Dublin, is also known as **Eire** and the Emerald Isle and covers most of the island bearing its name. The remainder of the island, Northern Ireland, is part of Great Britain. Ireland is the land of the practical-joking, red-haired leprechaun with a pot of gold at the end of the rainbow, fairy tales, queens of the underworld banchees, and a land of superstitions. The country's patron saint is St. Patrick.

With a population of 3.6 million people, Ireland has a land mass of 27,000 square miles, or half the size of the state of Arkansas and slightly larger than the state of West Virginia (Espenshade, 1990). The Irish Sea and St. George's Channel separate Ireland from Great Britain. Ireland is divided politically into 26 counties that make up the Republic of Ireland and six counties that are part of Northern Ireland. Northern Ireland has a land mass of 5400 square miles and a population of 1.6 million (Espenshade, 1990).

Ireland is bowl shaped and covered with a central plain and low mountains. An agricultural country, its principal product is potatoes. Mining has become an important economic activity with the discovery of lead, copper, silver, and zinc. Surrounded by water, Ireland has a cool maritime climate with an average annual rainfall of 118 inches. The winters are mild, with temperatures of 40°F in January, and the summers are also mild, with temperatures of 60°F common in July. With this type of climate, the island cannot support a large variety of plant and animal species.

The history of Ireland is a chronicle of bloodshed, spirit, and pride. The Irish people have wit and a sense of humor and can laugh at themselves in the best possible way. One of every five persons living in the United States, approximately 38.7 million people (15.6 percent of the population), is of Irish descent (Malone, 1994). Because Irish-Americans have assimilated well into American culture, they are becoming an invisible ethnic group (Moynihan, 1981). However, because of their influence, the nation celebrates St. Patrick's Day. St Patrick introduced Christianity in Ireland in 432 B.C., and the country developed into a center of Gaelic and Latin learning (*Information Please Almanac,* 1995).

The history of the Irish in America has not been harmonious. Early immigrants in America were subjected to religious persecution and economic discrimination. Irish-Americans are a diverse group, and health-care providers must be careful to avoid generalizations or assumptions, such as the Irish being superstitious, heavy drinkers, and practical jokers, because these do not apply to all Irish. Factors that influence Irish-American's cultural beliefs include socioeconomic status, education, geographic heritage, religion, generation, and length of time away from their homeland.

## Heritage and Residence

Historically, Ireland has been a melting pot. The Celts came to Ireland from Europe approximately 10,000 years ago. The Gales, a subgroup of **Celtic** people, gave Ireland the name Eire. The ancient Gaelic stock mixed with English, Scots, Welsh, French, Flemish, Norse, and German colonists. The gene pool of the Irish was probably set about 5000 years ago and is closely related to the gene pools of highland Britain, northern England, Wales, western Scotland, and Cornwall (DePaor, 1988). England dominated Ireland in the 16th century, creating a division between English Protestants and Irish Catholics.

The Irish immigrated to America in large numbers for almost three centuries beginning in the 1600s. The earliest settlements of Irish Catholics in America were in the colonies of Virginia and Maryland. The Irish ship, St. Patrick, arrived in Boston harbor in 1636. Irish Catholics experienced legal, social, and political discrimination in the early American colonies, and by 1699, Irish Catholic immigration was restricted in Virginia, Maryland, and South Carolina. For most of the 18th century, immigration from Ireland was dominated by Presbyterians. In the 19th and 20th century, most of the Irish immigrants were Catholic (Griffin, 1981).

The majority of the Irish immigrants settled in industrial areas in the northeastern United States along the Atlantic coast. Over 8 million Irish immigrants settled in these urban areas between the 1700s and 1965 (Boatman, 1992). The cities of Philadelphia, New York, and Boston have the largest Irish settlements, followed by the commercial centers in Ohio, Illinois, and Michigan. By 1800, Philadelphia was the most Irish city in the United States (Boatman, 1992). After 1820, Irish immigration into the United States was exceeded only by that of Germans. Irish settlements continued to concentrate in urban areas. Early Irish towns have been described as models for latter-day ghettos occupied by other groups whose race, religion, and nationality set them apart (Griffin, 1981). The Irish had the highest proportion of poor of any European-American ethnic group by the early 20th century.

In 1920, 90 percent of all Irish-Americans were residing in urban areas. However, second-generation and third-generation Irish families began leaving these areas around that time and moving to the suburbs. Suburban Irish became known as **lace-curtain Irish**, and those left in the city became known as **shanty Irish.**

Over 1.7 million Irish came to America between 1840 and 1860 (Griffin, 1981). Between 1970 and 1980, 11.4 thousand immigrated to the United States; between 1980 and 1990, another 32.2 thousand immigrated; and in 1993 alone, 13.6 thousand new Irish immigrants settled in the United States (*Information Please Almanac,* 1995). The Irish heritage has been characterized as one of continuity and change. From initial experiences of bigotry and prejudice, Irish-Americans brought their values of education, a strong work ethic, and the importance of children. They have made significant contributions to their new homeland in politics, the labor movement, the Catholic church, the arts, and service to their country.

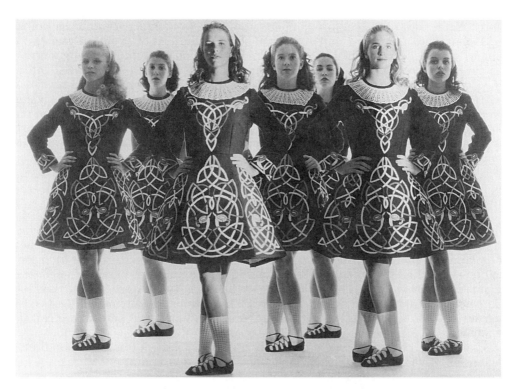

## TRINITY IRISH DANCERS

**Figure 14–1.** These Irish dancers in traditional costumes are helping to preserve and promote Irish culture in America. (Courtesy Trinity Dance Company, Chicago, IL. Photo by Dan Harris.)

## Reasons for Migration and Associated Economic Factors

The threat of famine was almost constant in early Ireland. Ireland had a population of 8.5 million until the **Great Potato Famine** of 1846 to 1848, when the population decreased to 3.4 million, where it has remained relatively steady since. During the potato famine, thousands of Irish died from malnutrition, typhus epidemics, dysentery, and scurvy, and millions immigrated to America. Mass burials were organized because the demand for coffins could not be met.

Religious persecution and deplorable economic conditions were primary reasons for early immigration to America. The first Irish immigrants to arrive in America in the 1600s were Catholics. They came because of discrimination from Protestant English and Scots moving into Ireland. Oliver Cromwell, a Protestant leader in the English Parliament, ordered English armies into Ireland, and Irish Catholics were forbidden from acquiring land from Protestants and leasing land for more than 31 years, were forced to learn English, and were not permitted to send their children to schools outside Ireland. Thus, early Irish immigrants who came to the United States had a history of oppression, violence, suffering, and misery (Greeley, 1972).

Most of the Irish-American experience was similar to other immigrant groups, except for three features. First, the period of immigration lasted longer for the Irish. For well over a century, many first-generation Irish-Americans saved money so other family members could come to America. Second, Irish women immigrated as single women rather than as part of a family group. This was in contrast to other immigrant groups and was without parallel in the history of European immigration (Rossiter,

1991). At the turn of the century, 88 percent of Irish women between the ages of 20 to 24 years were unmarried, and 53 percent between the ages of 25 and 34 years were unmarried. Third, established Catholic churches fulfilled a cultural and religious role for the Irish in America, became the center of their lives, and a symbol of identity. The Catholic parish was the cornerstone of the Irish community in America.

The Irish attained success in America because they spoke the same language, had the same physical appearance as other European-Americans, and mastered the political system. One-third of United States presidents trace their lineage to Irish descent. Three early presidents, Andrew Jackson, James Buchanan, and Chester Arthur were sons of Irish immigrants (Shannon, 1981).

## Educational Status and Occupations

Many Irish children went to work at a young age, often at the expense of their education, because they were needed to help provide for the family and to send money to Ireland for other family members. Educational attainment increased for each generation, with the descendants of Irish Catholic immigrants surpassing the general population in overall educational attainment (Blessing, 1980). According to the 1994 *Statistical Abstracts of the United States* (U.S. Department of Commerce, 1994), 63.9 percent of Irish-Americans are high school graduates, and 14.6 percent are college graduates.

Early Irish immigrants were primarily unskilled laborers from the agricultural regions of Ireland (Blessing, 1980). On arrival in America, conditions were not what they expected. These rural farmers were not well prepared for life in large urban areas, and this lack of preparation was reflected by their failure to secure employment in their prescribed occupational roles. They were the only group in the late 19th century whose occupational mobility was limited almost as much as Black-Americans (Blessing, 1980).

Early Irish male immigrants contributed to the growth of America by helping build the Erie Canal, the transcontinental railroad, and skyscrapers. They served their new country by fighting in major military conflicts. By the turn of the century, the Irish made up 11 percent of policemen and 18 percent of the country's coachmen. The priesthood was the leading career choice for second-generation Irish men in the early 1900s (Blessing, 1980).

## COMMUNICATIONS

### Dominant Language and Dialects

The major languages spoken in Ireland are English and Irish (Gaelic), the latter of which is the official language and is primarily spoken in the west. The Celts developed a written language late and relied on oral transmission of traditions, laws, customs, philosophy, and religion (Greeley, 1981). Language used in oral tradition is more descriptive and flexible than the written form, and poetry is a useful mnemonic device for oral tradition. Ancient Irish folk heroes, such as Finn MacCool and Cuchulin, were in love with their own voices and enjoyed telling long complicated tales. Greeley (1981) suggested that modern-day Irish priests, politicians, and others share the love of using many words and playing with language not only for communication, but also for enjoyment and entertainment. The Irish enjoy puns, riddles, **limericks**, and other storytelling. When one becomes accustomed to hearing the Irish-accented English used by the newer immigrants, there is little difficulty in understanding the accent. This Irish accent has a nasal quality and is spoken with a strong inflection on the first syllable of a word, resulting in a loss of weak syllables. Words ending in a vowel weaken the consonants following them.

The Irish, in love with their own voices, use low-context English, which uses many words to express a thought. This low contextual use of the English language has its roots in the Celtic folk tradition of storytelling. The writings of famous Irish authors, such as Johnathan Swift (although of English heritage, he was educated and wrote in Ireland), who wrote *Gulliver's Travels;* Lady Morgan, who wrote *The Wild Irish Girl;* and Joseph Sheridan, who wrote *Le Fanu Uncle Silas* and *In A Glass Darkly;* and James Joyce, who wrote *Dubliners, Odyssey,* and *Finnegan's Wake,* illustrate the low contextual use of the language. Some common Gaelic words with their meanings are *shamrock* for "emblem," *limer* for "folklore character," *colleen* or *lassie* for "girl," *sonsie* or *sonsy* for "handsome," *cess* for "luck," *brogue* for "shoe," *dudeen* for "pipe tobacco," and *pady* for "Irishman."

## Cultural Communication Patterns

Even though most Irish delight in telling long stories, when discussing personal matters they are much less expressive unless they are talking with close friends and family. Even then, many are still reluctant to express their innermost thoughts and feelings. Display of emotions and affections in public is avoided and often difficult in private. Family members are expected to know that they are loved without being told. To many, caring actions are more important than verbal expression.

The Irish use direct eye contact when speaking with each other. Not maintaining eye contact may be interpreted as a sign of disrespect or guilt or evidence that the other person cannot be trusted.

Personal space is important to Irish-Americans, who may require greater distance in spatial relationships. When speaking, they stand farther apart than other European-Americans (Greeley, 1981). Although the Irish may be less physically expressive with hand and body gesturing, facial expressions are readily displayed, with frequent smiling in the face of adversity (Fallows, 1979). However, the health-care provider must remember that responses vary from person to person.

## Temporal Relationships

Irish-Americans, with their strong sense of tradition, are typically past oriented. They have an allegiance to the past, their ancestors, and their history. The past is often the focus of Irish stories. Many, however, are past, present, and future oriented. While respecting the past, they balance "being" with "doing" and plan for the future by investing in education and saving money. Many Irish-Americans see time as being elastic and flexible. Therefore, Irish-Americans may have to be encouraged to arrive early for appointments.

## Format for Names

*Mac* before a family name means "son of," whereas the letter *O* in front of a name means "descended from." Gaelic names such as Brian, Maureen, Sheila, Sean, and Moria have become popular as first names for American children. Otherwise, names are written with the surname, and the person is called by their first name in informal situations.

## FAMILY ROLES AND ORGANIZATION

### Head of Household and Gender Roles

Irish-American family life is described as having a strong continuity over generations (Griffin, 1981). Families in western and southern Ireland were farmers who married young and had large families. The family structure was patrilineal, with land divided among the sons. The father ruled the family, but the mother had a significant influence over management of the household and education of children. The Irish have a strong sense of family obligation, and this pattern continued when they immigrated to America after the famine years. As the Irish settled in urban areas, the roles of women increased. Irish women have more power in family life than women in most other ethnic groups (Greeley, 1981). Traditional Irish women were expected to do "women's work," and men were supposed to do "men's work," with little role sharing. The family lived with rigid rules maintained by social and moral pressures of the society. Traditionally, the husband did not want the wife exposed to outside values and gave commands, which the wife was expected to follow unquestioningly. Women were reluctant to express their desires, and if they did, either their concerns were not validated or their importance minimized (Friedman, 1986). Many times, women were expected to do their work without male assistance, in addition to working outside the home when economic circumstances dictated. The roles for Irish-American family members are changing with a move toward more egalitarian relationships in which men assist with household duties and child care.

## Prescriptive, Restrictive, and Taboo Behaviors for Children and Adolescents

Kinship and sibling loyalty are important to the Irish. Irish families emphasize independence and self-reliance in children. Boys are allowed and expected to be more aggressive than girls. Children are expected to have self-restraint, self-discipline, and respect and obedience for their parents and elders.

In addition to having self-restraint and self-discipline, adolescents are expected to obey and show respect for their parents as well as church and community figures. Adolescent years are a time for experiencing emotional autonomy, independence, and attachment outside the family, while remaining loyal to the family and maintaining the traditional Irish belief in the importance of family. Peer group pressures at school may have a significant influence and often are incongruent with the belief systems of Irish Americans. While this rebellion is seen negatively by parents, it can provide a functional benefit for teenagers by helping them become autonomous individuals of which the family can be proud. During this time, close family relationships contain mixed motivations of love and hatred. Because it is difficult for many Irish-Americans to express their feelings, health-care providers can encourage openness between parents and teenagers.

## Family Roles and Priorities

The traditional Irish family is nuclear with parents and children living in the same household. Children are cherished, and primary socialization is aimed at making them productive members of society, providing necessary educational experiences, and conferring status on the family. Greeley and McCready (1975), in a study of female college graduates, found that Irish-American women are most likely to view the role of wife-mother as their dominant marital role.

Whereas marriage in ancient Ireland was delayed until age 30 years, in America, Irish-American Catholics marry at an age comparable to the rest of the population. Men typically marry at age 25 years and women at age 22 years (Greeley, 1977). Early immigrants were under pressure to marry within the Irish community; the pressure was especially strong for Irish Catholics to marry other Irish Catholics. Today, marriage with other groups is more common; however, it is still more socially acceptable to marry within one's group, thereby continuing the transmission of culture within the Irish-American community.

Irish women may consider sexual relationships as a matter of "duty" to their husbands (Greeley, 1981). This belief may have its roots in tradition, where men and women had different roles and lived in separate worlds and the sexes never learned to communicate with each other (Friedman, 1986). This attitude is diminishing as gender roles become more egalitarian.

Irish respect the experience of elderly persons and seek their counsel for decision making. Provisions are made in Irish homes for care of elderly persons, a task that becomes increasingly difficult when both parents work outside the home. The extended family is important to Irish-Americans. Although many Irish families have infrequent contact with extended family members and sentimental emotions are not expressed freely, they are available to assist when needed. Early Irish immigrants provided assistance to elderly Irish through immigrant aid societies, which were fraternal or religious in nature (Metress, 1985). However, since the Great Depression and passage of the Social Security Act, assistance for elderly care is provided through social security, private pensions, and private insurance. Newer immigrants continue the patterns of earlier immigrants and work long hours to earn a living and send money to their homeland, so that other family members can join them in America.

The Irish value physical strength, endurance, work, the ability to perform work, children, and the ability to provide their children with the education to attain respectable socioeconomic status and professional accomplishments. Members of the clergy in all religions are respected. Additional status can be gained by remaining in traditional ethnic Irish neighborhoods. Middle-aged and older family members voice pride in the ethnic neighborhoods in which they live.

The Irish contributed to the growth of the Catholic Church in America by providing it with leadership, money, and membership numbers. They built and established Catholic schools and colleges, health-care institutions, and social service agencies. John Carroll, a descendant of an Irish immigrant, was the first Catholic bishop in the United States and the founder of Georgetown College, now Georgetown University.

## Alternative Lifestyles

No information on alternative lifestyles specific to Irish-Americans was found in the literature. However, it has been reported that cases of acquired immunodeficiency syndrome (AIDS) related to homosexuality are low among the Irish. This may be related to the Catholic Church's teaching against homosexuality and the value placed on chastity among the Irish. Dignity USA, an organization for gay and lesbian Catholics, has denominations in several large cities in the United States. This organization provides emotional and financial support for those in need of services (*Washington Blade,* 1995). The choice not to marry and the choices of single parenthood and divorce do not carry the stigma that they did in the past.

## WORKFORCE ISSUES

### Culture in the Workplace

Most Irish immigrants came to America with a strong desire to work, survive, and send money to family back home. These early immigrants' competition for jobs exacerbated ethnic and religious animosities (Drudy, 1985). They experienced high mortality rates while working in industries and textile mills in New England and on the eastern seaboard. Irish immigrants were viewed as a cheap and willing source of hard labor.

Over time, the Irish have made a place for themselves in the workforce and are represented in all occupations and professional roles. By the late 1960s, Irish-Americans were overrepresented in law, medicine, and the sciences and slightly underrepresented in the social sciences and business. Second-generation and third-generation Irish women are widely represented in occupational and professional fields and, compared with other groups, are overrepresented in law, teaching, and clerical work. Often they moved from traditional service occupations to positions in education, health, and business (Blessing, 1980).

Because cultural differences between Ireland and the United States are minimal, Irish assimilate into the American workforce easily. Many endure short-term deprivations to achieve their long-term goal of improving family life. When change is necessary to improve the status quo, the Irish readily relinquish traditional beliefs and adjust to the workforce.

## Issues Related to Autonomy

Most past-oriented ethnic groups believe that the future is controlled by a higher power of fate and that humans must live in harmony with their surroundings and have respect for authority rather than question authority, and that group identity is more important than individual identity. Even though the Irish are typical of past-oriented groups in other ways, they tended to question the status quo of the American workforce. When individual efforts were unsuccessful in improving the work environment, the Irish joined forces and helped pave the way for change with early efforts of unionization and are one of the groups responsible for the current union culture in the American workforce.

Many Irish-Americans hold leadership positions and have made major contributions in their respective roles. Within the labor movement, Terrance Vincent Powderly, the son of Irish immigrants, became the head of the Knights of Labor, the most powerful labor union of its day. Joe Curran founded the National Maritime Union and was its first president. Mike Quill organized the Transport Workers of America. Mary Harris Jones, also known as "Mother Jones," an immigrant from County Cork, Ireland, was active in the labor movement into her 90s.

Most Irish-Americans speak English, and because Ireland has a 99 percent literacy rate (*Information Please Almanac,* 1995), newer Irish immigrants do not encounter language barriers in the workplace. The low contextual use of language, where most of the message is in the explicit mode rather than the implicit mode, enhances pragmatic communications in the workforce.

## BIOCULTURAL ECOLOGY

### Skin Color and Other Biologic Variations

Most Irish are either dark haired and fair skinned or have red hair, ruby cheeks, and fair skin; however, as with other ethnic groups, other variations exist in hair and skin color. The fair complexion of the Irish places them at risk for skin cancer. The Irish are taller and broader in build than the average European-American, Asian, or Pacific Islander. Hip width is greater and bone density less than in African-Americans but greater than in Chinese, Japanese, and Eskimos (Bowers & Thompson, 1994).

### Diseases and Health Conditions

Mining is an important economic activity in Ireland because many homes are heated with soft coal or peat. As a result, Irish miners are at an increased risk for respiratory diseases. In addition, the cool maritime climate of Ireland increases susceptible person's risk for respiratory diseases. Health-care providers should assess newer immigrants who worked in mining industries for respiratory health illnesses.

Northern Ireland has the second highest regional death rate for coronary heart disease in the United Kingdom, and for men, the highest death rate from ischemic heart disease in the world (Duddy & Parahoo, 1992; Davis, 1987). Irish-Americans had the highest mortality rates for coronary heart disease of all foreign-born Americans in the 1950s and 1960s (Blessing, 1980). Health providers can make a significant impact on the health of Irish-Americans by providing education and counseling regarding lifestyle and dietary changes to reduce risks associated with cardiovascular disease.

Cancer is second to coronary heart disease as a major cause of mortality in Northern Ireland (Barclay & Burnside, 1991), where more people die in one month from smoking than all forms of violence in one year (Burnside, 1985). Smoking cessation programs with group and one-to-one counseling are some important activities by which health providers can help Irish-Americans improve their health status.

Other conditions with a high incidence among the Irish are phenylketonuria (PKU), neural tubes defects, and alcoholism (Galanti, 1991; Geissler, 1995). Most states require screening all newborns for PKU, but the health-care provider may need to encourage women who give birth at home to seek PKU screening for their infants.

Newer immigrants from Ireland also have a higher incidence of mental illness than the rest of the population. Aroian (1993), in a study of undocumented Irish immigrants in the United States, reported that more stressors and mental heath problems are experienced by undocumented immigrants than their legal counterparts. In addition, second-generation Irish children lead all other second-generation European-Americans in rates of mental illness. Because many Irish have difficulty expressing emotions, health-care providers may need to encourage Irish-Americans to express their concerns.

## Variations in Drug Metabolism

Pharmacoanthropology (Kudzma, 1992), a relatively new field of theoretical inquiry, has reported no studies on drug responses specific to the Irish. Most studies of pharmacological responses that include people of Irish descent have used data aggregated under the category of whites. Because Irish diets are similar in carbohydrate, protein, and fat ratio to many other European-American diets, until further research is done, the health-care provider might expect that the pharmacodynamics of drug metabolism among Irish-Americans are similar to those of other white ethnic groups.

## HIGH-RISK BEHAVIORS

The use of alcohol, tobacco, and intravenous drugs are associated with major health problems among Irish and Irish-Americans. Immigrants are identified as high-risk populations for many health conditions because they are confronted with many challenges in their adaptation to a new environment and lifestyle (Aroian & Patsdaughter, 1989). Alcohol problems in Ireland are among the highest internationally, and Irish-Americans rank among the highest of all ethnic groups in heavy alcohol use (Estes & Heinemann, 1986). Greeley (1981) attributed problems with alcoholism to the Great Potato Famine in Ireland, which was a bleak period in Irish history when marriage was postponed until a person's 30s and when immigration to America was the only alternative for any person who would not inherit the family farm. Drinking became recreation and an escape. The village pub became the center of the community, and heavy drinking and alcoholism spread throughout postfamine Ireland. This legacy of socializing in taverns continues in America. Irish pubs are popular establishments synonymous with alcohol intake, lively music, and a vivacious time. This image of the Irish pub perpetuates the stereotype of Irish as being heavy drinkers, but health-care providers should be careful not to ascribe this label to all Irish-Americans.

Stivers (1976) believes the Irish drank in America because they were expected to be heavy drinkers. However, many factors, including family characteristics, social and economic conditions, and psychological orientation, influence alcoholism. Irish mothers who rule the family by strong will and manipulation may be a contributing factor to alcoholism in Irish males (Ablon & Cunningham, 1981; Greeley, 1972). In addition, alcohol allows one to release aggressions and relinquish responsibility for one's actions, and decreases stress. Because drinking may be a way of coping with problems, the health professional needs to assist the Irish-American clients in exploring more effective coping strategies and caution them against the dangers of mixing alcohol with medications.

Smoking, another high-risk behavior common among the Irish, is associated with the high incidence of lung cancer among men in Northern Ireland, where lung cancer accounts for 26 percent of premature deaths in males (Barclay & Burnside, 1991). Although smoking is declining in the male population, smoking is increasing among females. The incidence of lung cancer in the United States is similar to that of Northern Ireland with men having higher mortality rates associated with smoking than women. However, the women's rate for lung cancer is increasing as more women smoke. Health promotion efforts should be directed at decreasing the incidence of smoking among Irish-Americans.

The incidence of AIDS among the Irish is primarily related to the use of intravenous drugs. As mentioned earlier, the incidence of AIDS associated with homosexual behavior is low (Lewis, 1988; Melby, Boore, & Murray, 1992), suggesting that the Irish may observe the Catholic Church's prohibition against homosexual behavior. Health promotion should be directed at educating Irish-Americans about high-risk behaviors for the prevention of AIDS.

## Health-care Practices

Irish-Americans may ignore symptoms and delay seeking medical attention until symptoms interfere with the ability to carry out activities of daily living. Zola (1983), in a study of Irish and Italians, reported that Irish limit and understate problems as compared with Italians, who describe problems in detail. The Irish handle problems by using denial, which is culturally prescribed. The Irish view life as difficult and hard (Zola, 1983), which is understandable within the cultural context of a people who have experienced periods of deprivation and overindulgence.

Irish-Americans believe that having a strong religious faith, keeping one's feet warm and dry, dressing warmly, eating a balanced diet, getting enough sleep, and exercising are important for staying healthy.

## NUTRITION

### Meaning of Food

Food is an important part of health maintenance and celebrations for Irish-Americans. Within their religious framework, most Irish Catholics have a primary obligation to use food in moderation and in ways that are not injurious to their health. Traditional Catholic holidays that are celebrated with food include the Solemnity of Mary (Mother of God), January 1; Easter Sunday; Ascension Thursday, 40 days after Easter; the Feast of the Assumption, August 15; All Saints Day, November 1; the Feast of the Immaculate Conception, December 8; and Christmas, December 25. Many holidays and special events are celebrated with specific foods appropriate to the occasion. Irish food is unpretentious and wholesome if eaten in recommended proportions.

## Common Foods and Food Rituals

Meat, potatoes, and vegetables are the staples of both the Irish and Irish-American diet. Lamb, mutton, pork, and poultry are common meats. Seafoods include salmon, mussels, mackerel, oysters, and scallops. Popular Irish dishes include Irish stew made with lamb, potatoes, and onions. Potatoes are used in a variety of ways. Colcannon is made with hot potatoes, mashed with cabbage, butter and milk, and seasoned with nutmeg. This dish may be served at Halloween. Champ is a popular dish made with mashed potatoes and scallions. The scallions are cut in small pieces, including the green tops, boiled in milk until tender, and then added to the mashed potatoes and served with butter. **Dulse** (also known as "Irish moss"), an iodine-rich seaweed found in northern latitudes, may be used in place of scallions. Potato cakes made with mashed potatoes, flour, salt, and butter are shaped into a patty and fried in bacon grease. Potato cakes are served hot or cold with butter and sometimes molasses or maple syrup. Another popular dish is Dublin coddle, made with bacon, pork sausage, potatoes, and onions.

Oatmeal is popular in Ireland. During times of food shortages, oatmeal was a primary food. It was watered down to make it last longer. Soda bread, another popular food in Ireland and America, is made with flour, baking soda, salt, sugar, tartar, and sour milk. In Ireland, it is usually made fresh daily. Broths and pudding are served frequently in Ireland. Ale, instead of beer, is a common beverage. Contrary to the popular belief in America, corn beef and cabbage is not a traditional food in Ireland.

Because the Irish-American diet has the potential for being high in fats and cholesterol, the health-care provider may need to assist the client with balanced food selections and preparation practices to reduce their risks of cardiovascular disease.

Mealtime is an important occasion for the Irish family to socialize and discuss family concerns. Meals are eaten three times a day, with a large breakfast in rural areas, lunch around noon, and a late dinner. Some-Irish Americans continue the afternoon tradition of a light sandwich or biscuit with hot tea.

More devout Catholics fast and abstain from meat on Ash Wednesday, Good Friday, and all Fridays in Lent. Fasting is valued as a discipline. In addition, there are other times of the year when Irish Catholics have obligations to abstain from meat and meat products. Such dietary practices are not required in times of illness.

## Dietary Practices for Health Promotion

Eating balanced meals is considered important even if it means the individual is late for an appointment. Vitamins are commonly used as a dietary supplement. Generally, fast foods are considered less healthy than home-prepared foods.

## Nutritional Deficiencies and Food Limitations

No specific nutritional deficiencies or food intolerances were found in the literature specific to Irish-Americans. However, low-weight Irish women are at increased risk for osteoporosis and may need to increase the amount of calcium in their diet.

Most foods eaten in Ireland are available in America with the possible exception of dulse. Dulse is used in clarifying beer and some wines and as a suspension medium in pharmaceutical preparations. Irish-Americans have a greater variety of foods available in America than in their home country.

# PREGNANCY AND CHILDBEARING PRACTICES

## Fertility Practices and Views toward Pregnancy

Because fertility practices for many Irish are influenced by Catholic religious beliefs and the tendency to view sexual relationships as a "duty," the only acceptable methods of birth control are abstinence and the rhythm method. Women practice other means of birth control, but no statistics are available on their exact numbers. Abortion is considered morally wrong and is against the law in Ireland. Women's groups have been vocal in Ireland and in America about concerns over women's rights, especially reproductive rights. The mean number of children for Irish-American families is 2.6, which is comparable to the national mean of 2.4 (Martin, 1991).

## Prescriptive, Restrictive, and Taboo Practices in the Childbearing Family

Prescriptive beliefs for a healthy pregnancy include eating a well-balanced diet. The Irish believe that not eating a well-balanced diet or not eating the right kinds of food may cause the baby to be deformed. In addition, the Irish share the belief common to many other ethnic groups that the mother should not reach over her head during pregnancy because the baby's cord may wrap around its neck. A taboo behavior in the past, which some women still respect, is that if the pregnant woman sees or experiences a tragedy during pregnancy, a congenital anomaly may occur.

Eating a well-balanced diet after delivery continues to be a prescriptive practice for ensuring a healthy baby and maintaining the mother's health. Plenty of rest, fresh air, and sunshine are also important for maintaining the mother's health. The Irish believe that going to bed with wet hair or wet feet causes illness in the mother.

# DEATH RITUALS

## Death Rituals and Expectations

The Irish's reaction to death is a combination of their pagan past and current Christian faith. The Celts denied death and ridiculed it with humor. The Irish are fatalists and acknowledge the inevitability of death. However, American emphasis on technology and dying in the hospital may be incongruent with the Irish-American belief that family members should stay with the dying person. After death, family and friends make every effort to be present for the funeral.

## Responses to Death and Grief

A traditional practice in Ireland was for a deceased family member to be "laid out" in the home for a final farewell by the family. Ancient Gaelic women practiced "keening," or "loud wailing" at **wakes**, while men socialized with bottles and pipes. The wake continues as an important phenomenon in contemporary Irish families and is a time of melancholy, rejoicing, pain, and hopefulness. The wake represents the Irish's "stubborn refusal to believe death is the end" (Greeley, 1977). Cremation is an individual choice, and there are no proscriptions against autopsy if required.

# SPIRITUALITY

## Religious Practices and Use of Prayer

The predominant religion of most Irish is Catholicism, and the church is a source of strength and solace for many Irish-Americans. In times of illness, the Irish Catholics receive the Sacrament of the Sick, which includes anointing, communion, and a blessing by the priest. The Eucharist, a small wafer made from flour and water, is given to the sick as the food of healing and health. Family members can participate if they wish. The obligation to fast and abstain from meat on specified days is relinquished in times of illness. Other religions common among Irish-Americans include various Protestant dominations, such as the Church of Ireland, Presbyterian, Quaker, and Episcopalian.

Prayer is an individual and private matter. In the health-care setting, clients should be given privacy for prayer whether or not a clergy member is present. In times of illness, the clergy may offer prayers to the sick, as well as the family, because they too need support. Attending Mass daily is a common practice among many traditional Irish Catholic families. For those Irish Catholics who practice their religion regularly, Holy day worship begins at 4 P.M. the evening preceding the holy day; and all Sundays are holy days.

## Meaning of Life and Individual Sources of Strength

Many Irish are fatalistic and view man as being subjected to the harshness of nature. To help overcome stresses associated with the harshness of nature, many Irish view life in a comic sense and use their capacity for satire and self-burlesque, (Shannon, 1964) which helps them keep a sense of proportion about their problems. In addition, they gain meaning in their life through the home, religion, the church, and the saloon, which are centers of life in Irish communities (Shannon, 1964).

The Irish have a strong faith in life and a passion for freedom. Christianity existed in Ireland before the arrival of Ireland's patron saint, St. Patrick, in the fifth century. The theology and philosophy of Christianity was interwoven with the older Gaelic culture, creating a lasting identification between faith and the nation (Griffin, 1981).

## Spiritual Beliefs and Health-care Practices

Religion is important for many Irish-Americans in their daily life and in times of sickness. Irish Catholics continue to receive sacraments when sick. Health-care providers should inquire whether the sick persons want to see a member of the clergy, even if they have not been active in church. Some Irish-Americans may wear religious medals to maintain health. These emblems provide them with solace and should not be removed by the health-care provider.

# HEALTH-CARE PRACTICES

## Health-seeking Beliefs and Behaviors

The Irish's fatalistic outlook and external locus of control influences health-seeking behaviors. Irish-Americans use denial as a way of coping with physical and psychological problems. Zola (1983), in a study of Irish- and Italian-American's perceptions of symptoms, found that the Irish view of life is illustrated in the belief that "life was black and long suffering and the less said about it the better" (Zola, 1983, p. 104).

Many Irish limit and understate symptoms when ill. For some Irish-Americans, illness behavior does little to relieve suffering and perpetuates a self-fulfilling prophecy. Illness or injury may be linked to guilt and the result of having done something morally wrong. Restraint is a modus operandi in the Irish culture, and temptation is ever present and must be guarded against (Zola, 1983). Most Irish-Americans believe that one is obligated to use ordinary means to preserve life. Therefore, extraordinary means may be withheld to allow the person to die a natural death. The sick person and family define extraordinary means; the decision is usually influenced by finances, quality of life, and effects on the family.

## Responsibility for Health Care

Although good health is valued by Irish-Americans, they often delay seeking treatment for health problems, hoping the problems will go away. Because Irish-Americans may not be very descriptive about their symptoms, treatment may be more difficult. Early Irish-American immigrants depended on fraternal organizations and religious institutions for assistance with health care in times of need. Today, most Irish Americans have some type of coverage for health care such as private insurance, medicare, and medicaid. Those without coverage usually cannot afford it.

## Folk Practices

Recent studies show that the practice of traditional home remedies is increasing in the United States, and most patients do not discuss these home remedies with their health-care providers (Eisenburg et al., 1993). Irish-American folk medicine practices include traditional remedies passed down through generations and effective in health promotion. These include eating a balanced diet, getting a good night's sleep, exercising, dressing warmly, and not going out in the cold air with wet hair. Other folk practices include wearing religious medals to prevent illness, using cough syrup made from honey and whiskey, drinking hot tea for nausea, drinking tea and eating toast for a cold, and putting a damp cloth to the forehead for a headache (Spector, 1991). Some folk practices may be harmful, such as the use of senna to cleanse the bowels every 8 days, eating a lot of oily foods, and avoiding seeing a physician.

Common illnesses such as colds, stomachaches, and sore throats may be treated in the home. Honey and lemon is given for a sore throat. Hot tea with whiskey is used for treating a cold or upset stomach. The literature reports no data indicating that the Irish use over-the-counter medications more than any other group. The health-care provider should ask Irish-Americans about their perception of their illness, its cause, treatments used (including prescription and over-the-counter medications and home remedies) and their effectiveness, and whether they know anyone else with a similar problem (Kleinman, 1980).

## Barriers to Health Care

Most Irish-Americans have few barriers to health care. One self-imposed barrier is delaying treatment of symptoms. Irish-Americans in lower socioeconomic classes experience health-care barriers such as lack of transportation, money, insurance, and knowledge about the availability of health-care resources.

## Responses to Health and Illness

The relationship of ethnicity and pain experience has been demonstrated in a number of studies (Flannery, Sos, & McGovern, 1981; Lipton & Marbach, 1984; Neill, 1993; Zborowski, 1952; Zola, 1983). Zborowski (1969), in a classic study on pain and ethnicity, describes differences in the pain responses of Irish, Italian, Jewish, and Yankee subjects. The behavioral response of the Irish to pain is stoic, usually ignoring or minimizing it. Irish deny pain and delay seeking medical treatment longer than Italians (Zola, 1983).

Irish immigrants have high rates of mental illness. Although children of Irish immigrants have fewer psychological problems than their parents, they lead all other second-generation Americans in frequency of mental health problems (Blessing, 1980). One explanation for high rates of mental illness may be associated with the Irish having difficulty describing emotions and expressing feelings. The health-care provider can encourage the expression of emotions and feelings before symptoms become a problem. In the past, the mentally and physically ill were taken care of in the home, not because of the stigma associated with mental illness and the family's desire to shield them, but rather because of the Irish-American family preference for caring for each other whenever possible.

Although some Irish-Americans attribute illness to sin and guilt, they readily excuse sick persons from their obligations and become a source of support by assuming their normal roles until they regain their functioning.

## Blood Transfusion and Organ Donation

Blood transfusions are acceptable to most Irish-Americans. The literature does not reveal any information on organ donation and organ transplant specific to Irish-Americans. No religious or cultural proscriptions exist regarding this practice. Many Irish participate in organ harvest and indicate their willingness to do so on their driver's license. Health-care professionals should obtain this information on an individual basis, be sensitive to client and family concerns, explain procedures involved with organ donation and procurement, answer questions factually, and explain risks involved.

## HEALTH-CARE PRACTITIONERS

## Traditional Versus Biomedical Care

In most Irish families, nuclear family members are consulted first about health problems. Mothers and older women are usually the family members who possess the knowledge of folk practices to alleviate common problems such as colds. The Irish are one of the few ethnic groups that do not have a hierarchy of folk and traditional practitioners. When home remedies are not effective, the Irish seek out the care of biomedical practitioners.

Although Irish-Americans are not noted for being overly modest, many may prefer intimate care from someone of the same gender. In general, men and women may care for each other in the health-care setting as long as privacy and sensitivity are maintained.

## Status of Health-care Practitioners

Although the Irish do not readily seek health care for early symptoms, they do respect health-care professionals. Nursing in Ireland is considered a worthwhile occupation and is predominately a female occupation. Similar to the United States, in Ireland, nurses are not held in as high regard as physicians, which may be attributed to educational differences.

---

### CASE STUDY

The O'Rourke family lives on a small farm in Iowa and comprises David, age 30; his wife Mary, age 29; and two children, Bridget, age 7, and Michael, age 6. Both David and Mary are second-generation Irish-Americans. Before purchasing their farm 5 years ago, David sold farm equipment in Ohio. The O'Rourkes are Catholic; Mary converted to Catholicism when they married.

David, who works long hours outdoors, is concerned about profitability from his corn crop because income varies depending on the weather. Mary does not work outside the home because she wanted to be with their children until they started school. However, because both children are now school age, Mary has discussed with David the possibility of working part time to supplement the family income. He would prefer that she stay at home, but Mary is anxious to return to the workforce and believes the timing is right.

Both David and Mary are happy with just two children and do not desire more. They use the rhythm method for family planning.

Eating a healthy breakfast is important to the O'Rourkes. Because eggs are readily available on the farm, they have fried eggs with potato bread and juice at least four times a week. Their main meal in the evening usually includes meat, potatoes, and a vegetable. David enjoys a glass of beer with dinner.

David has been a little edgy lately because of his concerns about the corn crop. He admits to having some minor chest pain, which he attributes to indigestion. His last visit to a physician was before their marriage. Mary knows David is concerned about finances and believes if she had a job it would help.

Bridget and Michael spend a lot of time outside playing and doing some minor chores for their parents. Both children enjoy school and are looking forward to returning in the fall. Bridget is starting to show concern over her appearance. She does not like her red hair and all those freckles on her face. Her teacher has noted that Bridget has trouble reading and may need glasses. Michael wants to be a farmer like his Dad but worries about his Dad being tired at night.

The O'Rourke family has not taken a vacation since they were married. They go to the state fair in the summer, which is the extent of their trips away from home. They are active in the church and attend services every Sunday.

---

### STUDY QUESTIONS

1. Describe the O'Rourke family structure in terms of individual roles.

2. Identify two potential family problems related to the O'Rourke's dietary practices.

3. Identify potential health risk factors for the O'Rourkes as a family unit and for each family member.

4. Explain the relationship between risk factors and ethnicity specific to the O'Rouke family and their Irish heritage.

5. Describe culturally competent health promotion strategies for the identified risk factors for the O'Rourke family.

6. Describe the O'Rouke family's fertility practices. Are they congruent with their Irish background and religious beliefs?

7. Describe the O'Rourke family's communication patterns.

8. What are predominant health conditions among Irish immigrants?

9. Explain the significance of the Great Potato Famine for Irish-Americans.

10. Name two genetic diseases common among Irish-Americans.

11. Identify accepted fertility practices for Irish-American Catholics.

12. Identify three sources of strength for the Irish-American in times of illness.

13. Identify traditional home remedies commonly used by Irish-Americans.

## References

Ablon, J., & Cunningham, W. (1981). Implications of cultural patterning for the delivery of alcoholism services. *Journal of Studies on Alcohol, 42*(9), 185–206.

Aroian, K. J. (1993). Mental health risks and problems encountered by illegal immigrants. *Issues in Mental Health Nursing, 14*(4), 379–397.

Aroian, K. J., & Patsdaughter, C. A. (1989). Multi-method, cross-cultural assessment of psychological distress. *Image: Journal of Nursing Scholarship, 2*(21), 90–93.

Barclay, L., & Burnside, G. (1991). Cancer at the workplace: Health promotion and care programs. *AAOHN Journal, 39*(7), 328–332.

Blessing, P. (1980). Irish. In S. Thernstrom (Ed.), *Harvard encyclopedia of American ethnic groups* (pp.524–545). Cambridge, MA: Belknap Press.

Boatman, J. (1992). *A survey of the United States ethnic experience* (Vol. 1). Milwaukee, WI: University of Wisconsin-Milwaukee.

Bowers, A., & Thompson, J. (1994). *Clinical manual of health assessment.* St. Louis: C. V. Mosby.

Burnside, G. (1985). United against cancer: The Ulster cancer foundation. *Nursing Mirror, 161*(14), 33–35.

Davis, A. M. (1987). The heart campaigns: The basis for action. *Health Education Journal, 46*(1), 3–10.

DePoar, L. (1988). The people of Ireland. In P. Loughrey (Ed.) *The people of Ireland* (pp. 185–199). Dublin: Appletree Press.

Drudy, P. J. (Ed.) (1985). *Irish studies.* Cambridge: Cambridge University Press.

Duddy, I., & Parahoo, K. (1992). The evaluation of a community coronary specialist nursing service in Northern Ireland. *Journal of Advanced Nursing, 17,* 288–293.

Eisenburg, D. M., Kessler, R., Foster, C., Norlock, M., Calkins, D., & Delbanco, T. (1993). Unconventional medicine in the United States. *New England Journal of Medicine, 328*(4), 246–252.

Espenshade, E. (Ed.) (1990). *Goodes world atlas* (18th ed.). Chicago: Rand McNally.

Estes, N. & Heinemann, M. E. (1986). *Alcoholism.* St.Louis: C.V. Mosby.

Fallows, M. (1979). *Irish Americans.* Englewood Cliffs, NJ: Prentice Hall.

Flannery, R. B., Sos, J., & McGovern, P. (1981). Ethnicity as a factor in the expression of pain. *Psychosomatics, 22*(1), 39–50.

Friedman, M. (1986). *Family nursing: Theory and assessment,* (2nd. ed.). East Norwalk, CT: Appleton-Century-Crofts.

Galanti, G. A. (1991). *Caring for patients from different cultures.* Philadelphia: University of Pennsylvania Press.

Geissler, E. M. (1995). *Pocket guide to cultural assessment.* St. Louis: Mosby-Year Book.

Greeley, A. (1972). *That most distressful nation: The tanning of the American Irish.* Chicago: Quadrangle Books.

Greeley, A. (1977). *The American Catholic: A social portrait.* New York: Basic Books.

Greeley, A. (1981). *The Irish Americans.* New York: Harper & Row.

Greeley, A., & McCready, W. (1975). The transmission of cultural heritages: The case of the Irish and Italians. In N. Glazer, & D. P. Moynihan (Ed.), *Ethnicity: Theory and experience* (pp. 209–235). Cambridge, MA: Harvard University Press.

Griffin, W. (1981). *A portrait of the Irish in America.* New York: Charles Scribner's Sons.

*Information please almanac.* (1995). Boston: Houghton Mifflin.

Kleinman, A. M. (1980). *Patients and healers in the context of culture.* Berkeley: University of California Press.

Kudzma, E. (1992). Drug response: All bodies are not created equal. *American Journal of Nursing, 92*(12), 48–50.

Lipton, J. A., & Marbach, J. J. (1984). Ethnicity and the pain experience. *Social science and medicine, 19*(12), 1279–1298.

Malone, R. (1994). *Guide to Irish America.* New York: Hippocrene Books.

Martin, C. (1991). Irish Americans. In J. N. Giger, & R. E. Davidhizar (Eds.), *Transcultural nursing: Assessment and Intervention* (pp. 315–334). St. Louis: Mosby-Year Book.

Melby, V., Boore, J. R. P., & Murray, M. (1992). Acquired immunodeficiency syndrome: Knowledge and attitudes of nurses in Northern Ireland. *Journal of Advanced Nursing, 17,* 1068–1077.

Metress, S. P. (1985). The history of Irish-American care of the aged. *Social Service Review, 59*(1), 18–31.

Moynihan, D. P. (1981). Introduction. In W. D. Griffin (Ed.), *A portrait of the Irish in America* (pp. ix–xi). New York: Charles Scribner's Sons.

Neill, K. (1993). Ethnic pain styles in acute myocardial infarction. *Western Journal of Nursing Research, 15*(5), 531–547.

Rossiter, A. (1991). Bringing the margins into the center: A review of aspects of Irish women's emigration. In S. Hutton & P. Stewart (Eds.), *Ireland's histories: Aspects of state, society, and ideology* (pp. 223–242). Routledge, London: Chapman and Hall.

Shannon, W. V. (1964). *The American Irish.* New York: MacMillan.

Shannon, W. V. (1981). Foreword, in W. D. Griffin, *A Portrait of the Irish in America.* New York: Charles Scribner's Sons.

Spector, R. E. (1991). *Cultural diversity in health and illness* (3rd ed.). Norwalk, CT: Appleton & Lange.

Stivers, R. (1976). *A hair of the dog: Irish drinking and American stereotype.* University Park: Pennsylvania State University Press.

U. S. Department of Commerce. (1994). *Statistical Abstract of the United States, 1994.* Washington, DC: U. S. Government Printing Office.

*Washington Blade* (1995, January 27), p. 73.

Zborowski, M. (1969). *People in pain.* San Francisco: Jossey-Bass.

Zola, I. K. (1983). *Socio-medical inquiries: Recollections, reflections, and reconsideration.* Philadelphia, PA: Temple University Press.

# Jewish-Americans

*Janice Selekman*

• Key terms to become familiar with in this chapter are:

| | |
|---|---|
| Ashkenazi | Orthodox |
| *Bris* or *brit milah* | Pogrom |
| Conservative | Rabbi |
| Halakhah | Reconstructionism |
| Hasidic or Chasidic | Reform |
| Hebrew | Sephardic |
| Kaddish | Synagogue, temple, or shul |
| Kashrut or Kashrus | Torah |
| Kosher | *Treyf* |
| Mezuzah | *Tzedakah* |
| Mikveh | Yarmulka or *kippah* |
| Minyan | Yiddish |
| *Mohel* | |

## OVERVIEW, INHABITED LOCALITIES, AND TOPOGRAPHY

### Overview

Being Jewish refers to both a people and a religion; it is not a race. Throughout history, the terms *Hebrew, Israelite,* and *Jew* have been used interchangeably. In the Bible, Abraham's grandson, Jacob, was also called Israel. His twelve sons and their descendants became known as the children of Israel. The term *Jew* is derived from Judah, one of Jacob's sons. **Hebrew** is the official language of the state of Israel and is used for religious prayers by all Jews wherever they live. "Thus today, the people are called Jewish, their faith Judaism, their language Hebrew, and their land Israel" (Donin, 1972, p. 7). Judaism is both a religion and a culture. The religion is practiced along a wide continuum that ranges from liberal Reform to strict Orthodox. Although Reform Jews might not engage in any special daily practices, they may still observe holidays, religious rites, and selected dietary or cultural customs. The traditional Orthodox Jew attempts to adhere to most of the religious laws. There are also ultra-Orthodox groups. No caste system or social hierarchy exists within the Jewish-American community. There are, however, instances within the ultra-Orthodox communities when individuals cannot make decisions without consulting their rabbis.

One of the issues that rages within Orthodox communities in Israel and frequently seeps into America is "Who is a Jew?" It is recognized that a child born to a Jewish mother is Jewish. As mixed marriages have increased in number, the debate has ensued over patrilineal descent. A child born from the union of a Jewish father and a non-Jewish mother is recognized as Jewish by those in the Reform movement, but is not recognized as Jewish by those in the Orthodox movement.

While the goal of this chapter is to provide an understanding of all Jewish-Americans, the focus is on the needs of the more traditional religious individuals and their families.

## Heritage and Residence

There are 5.798 million Jews throughout the United States (Singer, 1992). They can be found in every large city with a greater prevalence in the states of California, New York, Texas, Florida, Pennsylvania, Illinois, and Ohio. The states with the highest percentages of Jewish populations are New York (9.1%), New Jersey (5.5%), Florida (4.6%), Massachusetts (4.6%), and Maryland (4.4%) (Singer, 1992). Forty-nine percent of the American-Jewish population lives in the Northeast.

There has been a Jewish presence in the New World since the earliest days of American history. A group of 23 Sephardic Jewish settlers came to New Amsterdam (New York) in America from Brazil around 1654 (Glazer, 1957). By 1776, there were approximately 2000 Jews in the 13 colonies (Fischel & Pinsker, 1992). Many fought in the colonial army during the Revolutionary War.

## Reasons for Migration and Associated Economic Factors

Migration of Jews from Europe began to increase in the mid-1800s, often due to the fear of religious persecution. However, the greatest influx of immigrants occurred between 1880 and 1920. Many of these immigrants came from Russia and eastern Europe after a wave of **pogroms** (anti-Jewish riots and murders) and anti-Jewish decrees (Glazer, 1957). Once in America, assimilation became their motivation to live in safety and practice their Judaism.

Most Jewish families in America today are descendants of these eastern European and Russian immigrants. They are referred to as Ashkenazi Jews; **Ashkenazi** is the Yiddish word for Germany. Ashkenazi Jews make up 82 percent of the world's Jewish population (Fischel & Pinsker, 1992). Many American Jews of Ashkenazi descent have stories of only parts of their families escaping to America, with millions killed in the pogroms and the holocaust. **Sephardic** Jews, on the other hand, are from Spain, Portugal, the Mediterranean area, Africa, and South and Central America. They represent a more diverse group. A Sabra is a Jew who was born in Israel.

In the 1980s and 1990s, a significant increase occurred in the number of Jewish immigrants from Russia. Because the practice of religion was illegal there for over half a century, these Jews often have different practices and a different understanding of their religion than the previous generation.

## Educational Status and Occupations

Despite bias against Jews in every century, they have made major contributions to society, especially in the sciences and health care. Throughout their history, they have placed a major emphasis on education and social justice through social action.

Continued learning is one of the most respected values of the Jewish people. They reinforce the concept by one generation teaching the next (Waxman, 1960).

Formal education is promoted and advanced degrees are respected. In general, this is a well-educated population. For all Jewish adults over the age of 25 years, only 27.7 percent have a high school education or less, compared with 62.2 percent of the United States white population. Over 19 percent have some college education, 26.7 percent have completed college, and 26.4 percent have completed graduate studies. This last figure compares to only 8.7 percent of the total United States white population (Goldstein, 1992). Jews have won 39 percent of the Nobel prizes in the life sciences, 11 percent in chemistry, and 41 percent in physics (Fischel & Pinsker, 1992).

Because of the emphasis on continued education, there is a high percentage of Jewish-Americans who have succeeded in science, medicine, law, and dentistry. Thirty-nine percent of Jewish males and over 36 percent of Jewish females list their occupation as professionals, compared with only 15 percent of the U.S. white population (Goldstein, 1992). With respect to higher education, over 10 percent of professors in American colleges and universities are Jewish (Fischel & Pinsker, 1992).

Because throughout their history, Jews were repeatedly forbidden to own land, and the Church barred Christians from money lending, Jews frequently became money lenders, peddlers, and tailors, as these were the only options available to them. The early Jews in America were businessmen and craftsmen (Fischel & Pinsker, 1992). They became well respected for their expertise in trade and commerce. Today, one-quarter of Jewish males are in retail sales.

Because of the emphasis on social action, volunteerism and involvement in helping others are common vocations or avocations. *Tzedakah* (a term that means righteousness and sharing and is a central concept to Judaism) is commonly used to indicate charity. Jewish children are raised with the concept of giving *tzedakah*, sharing with others who have less than they have.

## COMMUNICATIONS

### Dominant Language and Dialects

English is the primary language of Jewish-Americans. Although Hebrew is the official language of Israel and is used for prayers, it is generally not the language used for conversation. Hebrew is read from right to left, and books are opened from the opposite side compared with English books.

Many elderly Ashkenazi Jews who immigrated early in the 20th century or who are first-generation Americans speak **Yiddish,** a Judeo-German dialect (Fischel & Pinsker, 1992). Many Yiddish terms have worked their way into the English language, including the following: kvetch (someone who complains a lot); chutzpah (clever audacity); bagel (a circular roll); challah (braided white bread); knish (dumpling with filling); nosh (snack); zoftic (plump); tush, tushie, or tuchus (buttocks); ghetto; shlep (drag or carry); kosher (legal or okay); and oy, oy vey (oh my), and oy veys mier (woe is me).

Common expressions include *lechayim* (to life), which is said during a toast of wine; *shalom alechem* (peace be with you) as a traditional salutation; *mazal tov* (congratulations), and *shabbat shalom* (a good and peaceful Sabbath) said every Friday evening and Saturday morning.

### Cultural Communication Patterns

No religious ban or ethnic characteristic prevents Jews from sharing their feelings. This practice is more related to their American upbringing rather than to their religious practices.

Humor is frequently used by Jews as a way to cope and a way to communicate with others. However, jokes are considered to be insensitive when they reinforce mainstream stereotypes about Jews, such as implying that Jews are cheap or pampered (Jewish-American princess). Any jokes that refer to the holocaust or concentration camps are also inappropriate. However, Jewish self-criticism through humor is acceptable.

The philosophy that actions speak louder than words is prominent throughout Jewish teachings. It is believed that people are judged by their actions, not by what they say and feel, because only the actions can last beyond the persons themselves (Amsel, 1994).

Modesty is a primary value in Orthodox Judaism. It is not only seen in the Orthodox style of dress but it is also seen in one's actions. Modesty involves humility. Jews are encouraged not to "show off" or constantly try to impress others.

Hasidic Jewish males are not permitted to touch a woman other than their wives. They often keep their hands in their pockets to avoid touch. They do not shake hands with women, and their failure to do so when one's hand is extended should not be interpreted as a sign of rudeness. Because women are considered seductive, Hasidic males may not engage in idle talk with them nor look directly on their face (Latner, 1981). Non-Hasidic Jews may be much more informal and may use touch and short spatial distance when communicating.

## Temporal Relationships

While Jews live for today and plan for and worry about tomorrow, they are raised with the stories of their past, especially the holocaust. They are warned to "never forget," lest history be repeated. Therefore, their time orientation is to the past, the present, and the future simultaneously.

The Jewish Calendar is based on both a lunar and solar year, with each month beginning with the birth of the new moon. The festivals and holidays are based on the phases of the moon, whereas the seasons are based on the solar year. The lunar year is 11 days shorter than the solar year. Therefore, an extra month is periodically added (Siegel & Rheins, 1980).

All Jewish holidays, including the weekly Sabbath, begin at sunset. When the Bible describes creation, it indicates "and there was evening and there was morning." Consequently, when using Americanized calendars that indicate a Jewish holiday, the holiday always begins the evening before.

## Format for Names

The Jewish format for names follows the Western tradition. The given name comes first and is followed by the family surname. Only the given name is used with friends and in informal situations. In more formal situations, the surname is preceded by the appropriate title of Mr., Miss, or Mrs.

Babies may be named after someone who has died to keep the person's name alive. They may also be named after a living person for the same reason. The format chosen depends on whether the family is of Ashkenazi or Sephardic heritage. In ultra-Orthodox circles, a child is not referred to by his name until after the **bris** or **brit milah** (Latner, 1981). Infants are also given a Hebrew first name that is used when they are older and called to read from the torah. An example would be Efriam ben Reuven (Frank son of Robert).

# FAMILY ROLES AND ORGANIZATION

## Head of Household and Gender Roles

The family is the core of Jewish society, and the needs of all family members are respected. While the male is considered the breadwinner for the household, the woman is recognized for running the home and being responsible for the children. According to Jewish law, the father must provide for an education for his sons and must teach them a trade; he must also give his daughters away in marriage (Waxman, 1960). With assimilation, there is little difference seen today between Jewish and non-Jewish white families with regard to gender roles. In most Jewish families, the responsibilities of supporting the home and raising the children are shared by both parents.

Although traditional Jewish law is plainly male oriented, Jewish women have been at the forefront of activities to demand and protect the rights of all humans, especially women. They were prominent in movements to gain voting rights for women, reproductive health-care rights, and equal rights for all segments of society. Women are now expected to achieve their maximal level of education and to seek gainful employment if they so desire. Both sexes are expected to give service to their community.

## Prescriptive, Restrictive, and Taboo Behaviors for Children and Adolescents

Children are the most valued treasure of the Jewish people (Amsel, 1994). They are considered a blessing and are to be treated with respect and provided with love. Jewish children are to be afforded an education, not only in studies that help them progress in society, but also in studies that transmit their Jewish heritage and the laws. Jewish school-age children typically attend Hebrew school as least two afternoons a week after public school throughout the school year. The child plays a role in most of the holiday celebrations and services.

Respecting and honoring one's parents is one of the Ten Commandments. Children should be forever grateful to their parents for giving them the gift of life. Jewish parents are expected to be consistent and fair to all their children. Favoritism is not a positive quality. In addition, parents should not promise something to their children that they cannot deliver. They must be flexible and be both caring and attentive to discipline. The individuality of each child's special traits should be recognized (Amsel, 1994).

In Judaism, the age of majority is 13 years for a male and 12 years for a female. At this age, children are deemed capable of differentiating right from wrong and capable of committing themselves to performing the commandments (Amsel, 1994). Recognition of adulthood occurs during a religious ceremony called a *bar* or *bat mitzvah* (son or daughter of the commandment). In America, this rite of passage is usually accompanied by a family celebration. However, because the son or daughter is still a teenager living at home, it is recognized that they are still the responsibility of their parents.

## Family Priorities and Goals

The goal of the Orthodox family is to live their lives as prescribed in the *halakhah*, which emphasizes maintaining health, promoting education, and helping others. In addition, "each person must find those qualities and characteristics that make him or her unique and then he or she must attempt to maximize potential by fully developing those qualities" (Amsel, 1994, p. 234). The family is central to Jewish life and is essential to the continuation of Judaism from one generation to the next.

Marriage is considered the ideal human state for adults. The Bible stated that man should not be alone. The two goals of this union are to propagate the race and companionship (Klein, 1992). It allows an individual to focus on another person. Marriages are monogamous and there are multiple restrictions as to whom one may marry. Sibling, parent-child, aunt-nephew, or uncle-niece combinations are prohibited (Klein, 1992).

Sexuality is a right of both men and women. In addition to procreation requirements, there exists the conjugal rights for women. Nonprocreative intercourse is required for married women who may be pregnant, too young to conceive, barren, postmenopausal, or posthysterectomy (Rosner, 1972). Sexual intercourse is viewed as a pure and holy act when performed mutually within the relationship of marriage. With some exceptions, "refusal of sexual relationship by either is grounds for a divorce" (Latner, 1981, p. 10). However, the act of sex, if performed in the wrong context, is considered disgusting and against Jewish values (Amsel, 1994). Premarital sex is not condoned. Domestic violence affects Jewish families just slightly less than it is seen in non-Jewish families (Vorspan, 1992).

Among the ultraobservant, women must physically separate themselves from all men during their menstrual periods. No man may touch her nor sit where she sat until she has been to the **mikveh**, a ritual bath, after her period is over. Sexual contact for this group may only occur during 2 weeks of each month (Amsel, 1994).

Judaism supports the need for sex education. The Jewish community sees this as their responsibility. This belief has been recently re-emphasized during the acquired immunodeficiency syndrome (AIDS) epidemic, where the goal is to protect the next generation and provide them with accurate information so that they can make informed choices.

The median age of Jewish-Americans is 37.3 years, 4 years higher than for white non-Jewish Americans (Goldstein, 1992). The fact that 17.2 percent of the Jewish population is 65 years old and older reflects both a healthy aging population and a large number of aging immigrants. Just over 13 percent of the non-Jewish white population is over age 65 (Goldstein, 1992). One-third of Jewish elderly persons are older than 74, and 10 percent are 85 years old and older (Fischel & Pinsker, 1992).

While it is recognized that the later years are a time of physical decline, the elderly are to receive respect, especially for the wisdom they have to share. "Learning from the elderly is preferred over learning from a younger person" (Amsel, 1994, p. 80). It is believed that old age is a state of mind rather than a chronological age. One may never "retire" from practicing the commandments.

Honoring one's parents is a lifelong endeavor and it includes maintaining their dignity by feeding, clothing, and sheltering them, even if they suffer from senility. Giving elderly persons respect is essential even when their action is irrational (Amsel, 1994). The care of an elderly family member is the responsibility of the family; when the family is unable to provide care; owing to physical, psychological, or financial reasons, the responsibility falls to the community (Fischel & Pinsker, 1992). Large numbers of Jewish elderly adults move to Florida after retirement because the weather there is more conducive to maintaining health and safety. Of noninstitutionalized elderly persons, one-third live alone.

Only 7 percent of Jewish-American families have three generations living together (Fischel & Pinsker, 1992). It should be noted that a number of elderly immigrants who experienced imprisonment in concentration camps during the holocaust in the 1940s, or those more recently incarcerated in Russia, may refuse to enter a nursing home for fear of returning to an institutional environment that robs them of their freedoms (Fischel & Pinsker, 1992).

## Alternative Lifestyles

The Jewish view on homosexuality varies with the branch of Judaism. The "Bible prohibits homosexual intercourse and labels it as an abomination" (Lamm, 1978, p. 379). Within the ancient writings, lesbians were not treated as harshly as male homosexuals. Some of the objections to this lifestyle include the inability of this union to fulfill the commandment of procreation and the possibility that acting on the recognition of one's homosexuality could ruin a marriage. The liberal movements within Judaism have fully accepted gay and lesbian Jews, citing the "inherent dignity and equality of all God's children" (Vorspan, 1992, p. 201).

# WORKFORCE ISSUES

## Culture in the Workplace

Specific workforce issues may occur when staff are Jewish, especially when they are observant of the Sabbath. Jews who observe the Sabbath must have Friday evening and Saturday off. They may work on Sundays. Supervisors must be sensitive to the needs of Jewish staff and recognize the holiness of the Sabbath. It is also important for Jewish staff to be allowed to request the major Jewish holidays off. Remembering that all holidays begin the evening before, they must have off the evening shift and the following day. Staff should not be penalized by having to use this time-off as unpaid holidays or vacation time, but rather they should have the opportunity to use them in exchange for Christmas and Easter holiday time usually afforded to Christian staff.

Jewish health-care providers are fully acculturated into the American workforce. Judaism's beliefs are congruent with the values that American society places on the individual and family, and because English is the primary language for Jewish-Americans, there are no language barriers for communicating in the workplace.

## Issues Related to Autonomy

Jewish nurses have begun to speak out on their needs in the workplace. With the recent emphasis on cultural competence, including cultural sensitivity, many are now addressing this long-ignored area. In 1990, a National Nurses Council was established through Hadassah, the Zionist women's organization (Benson, 1994). This group promotes solidarity and empowerment to enhance sensitivity within the health-care community.

# BIOCULTURAL ECOLOGY

## Skin Color and Other Biologic Variations

Ashkenazi Jews have the same skin coloring as white Americans. They may range from fair skin and blonde hair to darker skin and brunette hair. Sephardic Jews have a slightly darker skin tone and hair coloring, similar to those from the Mediterranean area. There are also Jewish groups throughout Africa who are black. Most notably are the Jews from Ethiopia, known as *Falashas,* who recently made a mass exodus to Israel.

## Diseases and Health Conditions

Genetic risk factors vary based on whether the family immigrated from Ashkenazi or Sephardic areas. Most genetic conditions are seen in those who immigrated from Eastern Europe (see subsequent discussion of genetic disorders). Because Jews are integrated throughout the United States, there are no specific risk factors based on topography. There is a greater incidence of some genetic disorders among individuals of Jewish descent, especially those who are Ashkenazi. The majority of these disorders are autosomal recessive, meaning the affected gene is carried by both parents. "Most [of the resulting conditions] are severely incapacitating and often debilitating, leading to early death in infancy or childhood" (Fischel & Pinsker, 1992, p. 204). Perhaps the best known is Tay-Sachs disease. Others include familial dysautonomia, torsion dystonia, Gaucher's disease, mucolipidosis IV, Niemann-Pick disease, and Bloom's syndrome (Fischel & Pinsker, 1992).

Gaucher's disease is most prevalent among Jews, with 1 in 2500 Ashkenazi Jews having the disease (Fischel & Pinsker, 1992) and 1 in 25 Jews being a recessive carrier. In Gaucher's disease, a deficiency of the $\beta$-galactosidase degrades glucosylceramide, resulting in decreased brain size, neuronal degeneration, and loss of neurons in the spinal cord. Hepatosplenomegaly is common with varying other symptoms, degrees of severity, and prognoses, depending on the type of Gaucher's disease (Behrman & Vaughan, 1987).

The gene for Tay-Sachs disease (also called infantile, cerebromacular degeneration) is carried by 1 in 30 to 40 Ashkenazi Jews as compared with 1 in 300 non-Jews. This autosomal recessive condition is a lysosomal sphingolipid storage disorder characterized by an absence of hexosaminidase A. The condition results in the onset of mental and developmental retardation beginning in the middle of the first year of life, with progressive deterioration, increasing seizure activity, and death by approximately age 5 years (Behrman & Vaughan, 1987). Because of the ease of testing for carriers as well as of providing prenatal testing, and because of a concerted effort among the Jewish-American community to provide testing, the incidence of Tay-Sachs disease has decreased from 70 new cases a year in 1970 to only 3 per year in 1993 (Kaback et al., 1993). Because the ultra-Orthodox are opposed to abortion, this group only recommends the testing before marriage (Baskin, 1983).

Familial dysautonomia, or Riley-Day syndrome, is also genetic in etiology, causing dysfunction of the autonomic and peripheral sensory nervous systems. Affected children have decreased myelinated fibers on nerves that carry pain, temperature, and taste as well as other afferent impulses. The disease leads to the absence or a decrease in the number of taste buds; altered pain sensation; increased salivation and sweating; swallowing difficulties; decreased tears, resulting in increased risk of corneal ulceration; and blood pressure alterations (Behrman & Vaughan, 1987). Death often occurs by late childhood. One in 30 Ashkenazi Jews are carriers (Fischel & Pinsker, 1992).

The gene for torsion dystonia is carried by 1 in 70 Ashkenazi Jews in the United States. The disease leads to rapid progression in loss of motor control. Niemann-Pick disease, Bloom syndrome, and mucolipidosis IV are also autosomal recessive conditions. Niemann-Pick disease involves an abnormal storage of sphingomyelin and cholesterol in organs, with the possibility of central nervous system degeneration. Bloom's syndrome involves erythema, telangiectasia, photosensitivity, and dwarfism. While the intelligence is usually normal, there is increased risk of later malignancy (Jones, 1988). Bilateral corneal opacities, strabismus, hypotonia, and psychomotor retardation develop in the first year. Death usually occurs during childhood (Behrman & Vaughan, 1987).

Other conditions are found to occur with increased incidence in the Jewish population. Inflammatory bowel disease (ulcerative colitis and Crohn's disease) is seen four to five times more often in white Jews than in other white groups (Cooke, 1991).

Familial mediterranean fever, an autosomal recessive condition characterized by fever, abdominal pain, and arthritis, occurs with increased frequency in Jews of non-Ashkenazi descent (Pras et al., 1992). Phenylketonuria (PKU), a metabolic condition due to the absence of the enzyme phenylalanine hydroxylase, can result in the development of mental retardation unless dietary restrictions are implemented shortly after birth. A higher incidence than expected is seen in Yemenite Jews (Avigad et al., 1990). Health-care providers need to respect and support Jewish clients' decisions for genetic testing and counseling for selected conditions. Nutritional education congruent with the religious practices of the selected denomination must be provided for PKU.

One of the few nonpediatric conditions is Kaposi's sarcoma, most commonly seen in men of Ashkenazi descent who are over 50 years of age. This condition involves malignant tumors of the endothelium that are usually very slow growing and limited to the skin, particularly on the legs. The tumors are different from those seen in persons with AIDS, which are aggressive and affects multiple internal organs (Thompson et al., 1993).

## Variations in Drug Metabolism

One of the few drugs found to have a higher rate of side effects in persons of Ashkenazi ancestry is clozapine, used to treat schizophrenia. Twenty percent of Jewish clients taking this drug developed agranulocytosis, as compared with about 1 percent of non-Jewish clients. A specific genetic haplotype has been identified to account for this finding (Levy, 1993). Thus, the health-care provider must institute testing for agranulocytosis when Jewish clients are prescribed clozapine.

## HIGH-RISK BEHAVIORS

According to Jewish law, persons may not intentionally damage their bodies or place themselves in danger. The basic philosophy is that the body must be protected from harm. To the religious, the body is viewed as belonging to God; therefore, it must be returned to him intact when death occurs. Consequently, any substance or act that harms the body is not allowed. This includes smoking, suicide, or taking nonprescription or illegal medications (Amsel, 1994; Rosner, 1972).

Alcohol, especially wine, is an essential part of religious holidays and festive occasions and is a traditional symbol of joy. The Jewish attitude toward wine is ambivalent. The Bible speaks of the undesirable effects of wine on the person as well as on its use as medicine (Amsel, 1994). Consequently, wine is appropriate and acceptable as long as it is used in moderation. Throughout the first half of the 20th century, it was assumed that alcoholism was not a condition affecting Jews. This trend appears to be changing. According to Amsel (1994), "alcoholism among Jews is rising fastest in homes that no longer keep the traditions" (p. 60). In addition, there is an increasing incidence of cross-addiction with other substances (Steinhardt, 1988).

## Health-care Practices

Because of the respect afforded physicians and the emphasis on keeping the body and mind healthy, Jewish-Americans are health conscious. In general, they practice preventive health care, with routine physical, dental, and vision screening. This is also a well-immunized population. Health-care providers need to encourage these positive health promotion and disease prevention practices among Jewish-American clients.

## NUTRITION

## Meaning of Food

Eating is an important function among Jews. Besides satisfying hunger and sustaining life, it also teaches discipline and reverence for life (Klein, 1992). For those Jews who follow the dietary laws, a tremendous amount of attention is given to the slaughter, preparation, and consumption of food. In addition, the dinner table is often the site for numerous religious holiday celebrations and services, especially the Sabbath, Passover, Rosh Hashana (the Jewish New Year), and breaking the fast for Yom Kippur (the Day of Atonement). The dietary practices of Jews serve as a spiritually refining act of self-discipline and a unifying factor as an instrument of ethnic identity (Kolatch, 1981; Latner, 1981; Wouk, 1986).

## Common Foods and Food Rituals

Perhaps the food identified as "Jewish" that receives the most attention is chicken soup. This has frequently been referred to as "Jewish penicillin." It is often served with knaidle balls in it (dumplings made of matzah meal). Though having no intrinsic meaning or religious value, it is a staple in religious homes, especially on Friday evenings to usher in the Sabbath and during times of illness. It is frequently associated with the mother's warmth and love.

Other common foods include gefilte fish (ground freshwater fish molded into oblong balls and served cold with horseradish); challah (braided white bread); kugel (noodle pudding); blintzes (crepes filled with a sweet cottage cheese); chopped liver; hamentashen (a triangular pastry with different types of filling); and lox and bagel sandwich. Lox is cold smoked salmon, served with cream cheese and salad vegetables, on a round roll (bagel) with a hole in it.

The laws regarding food are in Leviticus and Deuteronomy. They are commonly referred to as the laws of **kashrut,** or the laws that dictate which foods are permissible under religious law. The term **kosher** means "properly preserved" or "fit for eating"; it is not a brand or form of cooking. Whereas some believe that the mandatory statues were developed and implemented for health reasons, religious scholars dispute this view, claiming that the only reason for following the laws is that they are mandatory commandments of God. The "purpose of the dietary laws was to bring holiness and unity to the Jewish people, not good health" (Kolatch, 1981, p. 87). Thus, the laws' promotion of health was only a secondary gain.

Foods are divided into those considered kosher (permitted or clean) and those considered *treyf* (forbidden or unclean). A permitted animal may be rendered *treyf,* or forbidden, if it is not slaughtered properly or if it is cooked or served improperly. Because life is sacred and animal cruelty is forbidden, kosher slaughter of animals must be done in a way that prevents undue cruelty to the animal and ensures the animal's health for the consumer. The jugular vein, carotid artery, and vagus nerve must be severed in a single quick stroke with a sharp, smooth knife, causing the animal to die instantaneously. No sawing motion and no second stroke is permitted (Wouk, 1986). This also allows the maximal amount of blood to leave the body. Care must be taken that all blood is drained from the animal before eating it. Drinking of blood is prohibited.

In accordance with Jewish dietary laws, hunting is not permitted because the animal would have suffered from its wound. It is, however, appropriate to trap animals and then to kill them ritually (Kolatch, 1981). An animal that dies from old age or disease may not be eaten, nor may it be eaten if it meets a violent death or is killed by another animal (Wouk, 1986). In addition, flesh cut from a live creature may not be eaten.

Milk and meat may not be mixed together in cooking, serving, or eating. To avoid mixing foods, utensils used to prepare foods and the plates used to serve them are separated. Religious Jews following the dietary laws also have two sets of dishes, pots, and utensils: one set for milk products (*milchig* in Yiddish) and the other for meat (*fleishig*). Because glass is not absorbent, it can be used for either meat or milk products, although religious households still usually have two sets (Kolatch, 1981). Therefore, cheeseburgers, lasagna made with meat, and grated cheese on meatballs and spaghetti is unacceptable. Milk cannot be used in coffee if served with a meat meal. Nondairy creamers can be used instead, as long as they do not contain sodium caseinate, which is derived from milk.

### Table 15–1 • Allowable and Nonallowable Foods According to Kashrut Laws

#### MAMMALS

| Allowable: | Nonallowable: | |
| --- | --- | --- |
| Antelope | Ape | Horse |
| Buffalo | Ass | Hyena |
| Cattle | Bat | Jackal |
| Deer | Bear | Leopard |
| Gazelle | Boar | Lion |
| Goat | Camel | Llama |
| Ibex | Cat | Mouse/rat |
| Ox | Dog | Mule |
| Sheep | Elephant | Pig |
| | Fox | Whale |
| | Hare | Wolf |
| | Hippo | Zebra |

#### BIRDS

| Allowable: | Nonallowable: |
| --- | --- |
| Hen/chicken | Buzzard |
| Duck | Hawk |
| Goose | Ostrich |
| Partridge | Pelican |
| Pheasant | |
| Quail | |
| Turkey | |

#### SEAFOOD

| Allowable: | Nonallowable: |
| --- | --- |
| All fish except: | Catfish |
| | Porpoise |
| | Shark |
| | Shellfish (crab, clam, lobster, oyster) |

#### OTHER

| Nonallowable: |
| --- |
| Crocodile |
| Frog |
| Snail |
| Snake |
| Tortoise |

*Source:* Adapted from Siegel, R., & Rheins, C. (1980). *The Jewish almanac.* New York: Bantam Books.

A number of foods are considered *parve,* or "neutral," and may be used with either dairy or meat dishes. These include fish, eggs, vegetables, and fruits (Latner, 1981). A "U" with a circle around it is the seal of the Union of Orthodox Jewish Congregations of America used on food products to indicate that they are kosher. A circled "K" and other symbols may also be found on packaging to indicate that a product is kosher.

When working in a Jewish person's home, the health-care provider should not bring food into the house without knowing whether or not the client is kosher. If the client is kosher, do not use any cooking items, dishes, or silverware without knowing which are used for meat and which are used for dairy. It is important for health-care providers to fully understand the dietary laws so that they do not offend the client, can advocate for kosher meals if they are requested, and can plan medication times accordingly.

Mammals are considered clean if they meet the other requirements for their slaughter and consumption and have both split (cloven) hooves and chew their cud. These animals include buffalo, cattle, goat, and sheep (Table 15–1). The pig is an example of an animals that does not meet these criteria (see Table 15–1 for a list of others). Although liberal Jews decide for themselves which dietary laws they will follow, many still avoid pork and pork products out of a sense of tradition and symbolism. It would be insensitive to serve pork products to a Jewish client unless they specifically request it.

Birds are acceptable unless they are birds of prey and grab their food with their claws; then they are considered "unclean." Chicken is one of the most frequently consumed meats by Jews. Fish can be eaten if it has both fins and scales. Nothing that crawls on its belly is allowed, including clams, lobster and other shellfish, tortoise, and frogs.

In religious homes, meat is prepared for cooking by soaking and salting it to drain all the blood from the flesh (Latner, 1981). Broiling is acceptable, especially for liver, because it drains the blood (Kolatch, 1981). Care must be taken in serving cheese to ensure that no animal substances are included. Breads and cakes made with lard are *treyf,* and breads made with milk or milk by-products (for example, casein) cannot be served with meat meals. Eggs from nonkosher birds, milk from nonkosher animals, and oil from nonkosher fish are not permitted. Butter substitutes are used with meat meals. Honey from bees is allowed because it is produced from the nectar of flowers.

Kosher meals are available in hospitals. They arrive on paper plates and with plastic utensils sealed. Health-care providers should not unwrap the utensils or change the foodstuffs to another serving dish. Determining a client's dietary preferences and practices regarding dietary laws should be done during the admission assessment.

## Dietary Practices for Health Promotion

As mentioned previously, although many of the Jewish dietary practices afford the secondary gain of preventing disease, their intention is not for health promotion, but rather for observance of a commandment. This is also true of the practice of washing one's hands before eating. Religious Jews wash their hands while reciting a prayer.

## Nutritional Deficiencies and Food Limitations

There are no nutritional deficiencies common to individuals of Jewish descent. As with any ethnic groups, nutritional deficiencies may occur with individuals in lower socioeconomic groups because of the unaffordability of certain foods.

In addition to the dietary laws discussed previously, there are certain times when additional dietary laws are followed. For example, during the week of Passover, no bread or product with yeast may be eaten. Matzah (unleavened bread) is eaten instead. Any product that is fermented or can cause fermentation (souring) may not be eaten (Kolatch, 1981). Rather than attend synagogue, the service (seder) is held  around the dinner table during the first two nights and incorporates dinner into a service that includes all participants and retells the story of Moses and the Exodus from Egypt.

There are a number of fast days within the Jewish calendar. The most observed is the holiest day of the Jewish calendar, Yom Kippur. On this day of atonement, Jews abstain from food and drink as they pray to God for forgiveness for the sins they have committed during the past year. They eat an early dinner on the evening the holiday begins and then fast until after sunset the following day. It should be noted that ill persons are absolved from fasting and may need to be reminded of this exception to Jewish law. Maintaining an ill person's health supersedes the act of fasting. If concerns arise, a consultation with the client's rabbi may be necessary.

## PREGNANCY AND CHILDBEARING PRACTICES

### Fertility Practices and Views toward Pregnancies

God's first commandment to man is, "Be fruitful and multiply." Children are considered a gift and a duty, with males being considered more important to the ultra-Orthodox, as they can say **kaddish** (the prayer for the dead) for their parents. In other branches of Judaism, both sexes may recite the kaddish (Bial, 1971).

Because children are considered a blessing, sterility is regarded as a curse. A marriage is deemed a failure in ultrareligious circles if it did not result in the birth of an offspring (Klein, 1992). According to traditional Jewish law, a man may not abstain from procreation until he has children. Masturbation, or "improper emission of seed," and coitus interruptus are forbidden among the Orthodox (Rosner, 1972).

The lower number of pregnancies occurring among Jewish-Americans and the high intermarriage rate is resulting in a decreased Jewish population. By age 45 years, Jewish women averaged 1.6 children compared to 2.1 children born to non-Jewish white women in the same age range. Data from 1970 indicated that Jewish women had an average of 2.4 children (Goldstein, 1992). Because one-third of all Jews were killed during the holocaust, some believe that today's Jews "have a special moral obligation to bring one more child into the world than they would have normally" (Amsel, 1994, p. 314).

Prevention of pregnancy in the more Orthodox view implies deferring the commandment to be fruitful and multiply. Unless pregnancy jeopardizes the life or health of the mother, contraception is not looked on favorably among the ultra-Orthodox Klein, 1992). Liberal Judaism recognizes that children have the right to be wanted and that they should be born into homes where their needs can be met. Therefore, the use of temporary birth control may be acceptable (Bial, 1971). Reform Judaism supports the access of minors to reproductive health services, including contraceptives, that are unrestricted by parental notification or permission (Vorspan, 1992).

To the Orthodox, it is important to know the mechanism of action of the birth control. Coitus interruptus and masturbation are not acceptable because they result in the needless expenditure of semen. Barrier techniques are not acceptable because they interfere with the full mobility of the sperm in its natural course (Rosner, 1972). The birth control pill does not result in any permanent sterilization, nor does it prevent semen from traveling its normal route. Therefore, use of this method is the least objectionable to most branches. Sterilization implies permanence, and Orthodox Jews would probably oppose this practice, unless the life of the mother is in danger. Reform Jews leave the choice up to the woman.

There has been a great deal of discussion whether artificial insemination is allowable. Most religious denominations within Judaism accept the practice if the donor is the husband of the woman being impregnated. If the sperm donor is other than that of the husband, many oppose it because of the possibility of incest and a lack of genealogy in later generations. Those who favor it indicate that since no sexual intercourse occurs, there can be no charge of adultery and it does allow the couple to fulfill the commandment of procreation (Rosner, 1972).

Recognizing that Judaism's primary focus is the sanctity of life, it is important to identify when life begins. The fetus is not considered to be a living soul or person until it has been born. Birth is determined when the head or "greater part" is born (Klein, 1992). Until that time, it is merely part of the mother's body and has no independent identity.

Before 40 days after conception, the fertilized egg is only considered to be "fluid." After that time, it is referred to as a fetus. The act of birth changes the fetus's status from a nonperson to a person and infanticide is condemned. However, the newborn in traditional Judaism still does not have all the rights of a person and is not considered fully viable until 30 days after birth (Rosner, 1972).

The mother and her health are paramount. If her life is in danger or if her health is seriously imperiled by the fetus, all branches of Judaism see the fetus as an aggressor and require an abortion (Bial, 1971). While saving the mother's life is certainly grounds for abortion, random abortion is not permitted by the Orthodox branch because the fetus is a potential human being and abortion would be considered "expending semen for naught" (Rosner, 1972). Abortion would also be denied because it entails wounding oneself, which is not permitted, and it would place the mother in some danger.

If the mother's mental health is in question, whether abortion is permissible would probably be debatable. The Orthodox would tend to disapprove of the abortion, and the Reform would tend to allow it. Reform Jews believe that a woman maintains control over her own body and it is up to her as to whether she needs to abort. Although no connotation of sin is attached to abortion, the decision is not to be made without serious deliberation. Eighty-seven percent of Jews favor a woman's right to choose regarding abortion (Vorspan, 1992).

## Prescriptive, Restrictive, and Taboo Practices in the Childbearing Family

A Hasidic husband may not touch his wife during labor and may choose not to attend the delivery, because he is not permitted by Jewish law to view his wife's genitals. These behaviors should never be interpreted as insensitivity on the part of the husband. During the delivery of a child to an ultra-Orthodox family, the following interventions should be initiated. The mother should be given hospital gowns that cover her in the front and back to the extent as possible. She may prefer to wear a surgical cap so that her head remains covered (because the hair is considered a private part of her body). The father should be given the opportunity to leave during procedures and during the birth, or if he chooses to stay, the mother can be draped so that the husband may sit by his wife without viewing her perineum, including by way of mirrors, in order to protect her dignity. Because he is not permitted to touch his wife, he may offer only verbal support. The female nurse may need to provide all of the physical care (Lutwak, Ney, & White, 1988).

For male infants, a ritual is planned that dates back to Abraham and Isaac in the Book of Genesis. A circumcision, which is both a medical procedure and a religious rite, is performed. A **bris milah** means a covenant and it is symbolized through the circumcision (Amsel, 1994). The procedure and the ceremony are performed on the eighth day of life by a person called a **mohel,** an individual trained in the circumcision procedure, asepsis, and the religious ceremony. Although a rabbi is not necessary, it is also possible to have the procedure done by a physician with a rabbi present to say the blessings.

Attending a *bris milah* is the only mitzvah for which religious Jews must violate the Sabbath, so that the *bris* can be completed at the proper time (Amsel, 1994). The *bris* is a family festivity with many relatives invited. In most cases today, the *bris* is performed in the home; however, if the child is still in the hospital, it is important for the hospital to provide a room for a small private party to celebrate.

A circumcision may be delayed for medical reasons. These may include unstable condition due to prematurity, life-threatening concerns during the early weeks after birth, bleeding problems, or a defect of the penis, which may require surgery. At birth, a child is free of all sin, failure to circumcise carries no eternal consequences should the child die.

Although there is no opposition to designating godparents for a new child, there is no role for them in Judaism.

# DEATH RITUALS

## Death Rituals and Expectations

Traditional Judaism believes in an afterlife where the soul continues to flourish, although it is not mentioned specifically in the Torah (Amsel, 1994). It is believed that whatever is not understood in this life becomes clear in the world to come. In that world, persons are judged on their actions in life and it is believed that the righteous persons are rewarded (Amsel, 1994). Most Jews do not give much thought to life after death and are unconcerned about it; their focus is on how one conducts one's present life.

Active euthanasia, where something is given or done to result in death, is forbidden for the religious Jew. One of the Ten Commandments is "Thou shalt not kill," and euthanasia is considered murder. A dying person is considered a living person in all respects. The withholding of food from a deformed child to speed its death is considered active euthanasia and is forbidden.

Passive euthanasia may be allowed depending on its interpretation. Nothing may be used or initiated that prevents a person from dying naturally or that prolongs the dying process. Therefore, anything that artificially prevents death (cardiopulmonary resuscitation, ventilators, and so forth) may possibly be withheld, depending on the wishes of the patient and his or her religious views (Rosner, 1972). "One is not required to begin treatment if death is imminent" (Vorspan, 1992, p. 276).

Taking one's own life is prohibited and is viewed as a criminal act and morally wrong because it is forbidden to harm any human being. Suicide removes all possibility of repentance. Adult Jews who commit suicide and who belong to ultrareligious factions of Judaism are not afforded full burial honors (Vorspan, 1992). They are buried on the periphery of the Jewish cemetery and mourning rites are not observed, unless the individual was not mentally competent. However, the more liberal view is to emphasize the needs of the survivors, and all burial and mourning activities proceed according to the usual traditional rites and wishes of the family. Children are never considered to have intentionally killed themselves and are afforded all burial rights.

Death is an expected part of the life cycle. Yet each day is to be appreciated and lived as if it was one's last day (Amsel, 1994). Religious Jews start each day with a prayer of appreciation for having lived another day. The goal is to appreciate things and people while one still has them.

The dying person should not be left alone. It is considered respectful to stay with a dying person, unless the visitor is physically ill or their emotions are uncontrollable (Lamm, 1972). Judaism does not have any ceremony similar to Last Rites. Any Jew may ask God's forgiveness for their sins; no confessor is needed (Rabinowicz, 1994).

Some Jews feel solace in saying the *Shema* in Hebrew or English. This prayer just confirms one's belief in one God.

According to the Orthodox, "death coincides with the cessation of both heart and respiratory functions" (Rabinowicz, 1994, p.8). Liberal Jews recognize death as a process, the end of which is the absence of all electrical activity in the brain. This difference is critical if organ transplant is involved. At the time of death, the eyes and mouth can be gently closed by the nearest relative and the face is covered with a sheet. The body is treated with respect and revered for the function it once filled (Lamm, 1972).

Ultra-Orthodox Jews follow a protocol that is not conducive to hospital protocols. After the body is wrapped, it is briefly placed on the floor with the feet pointing toward the door. A candle may be placed near the head. However, this does not occur on the Sabbath or holy days. The dead body is not left alone until the funeral, so as not to leave the body defenseless.

Autopsy is usually not permitted among religious Jews. On one hand, it results in desecration of the body, and it is important that the body be interred whole. Allowing an autopsy might also delay the burial, something that is not recommended. On the other hand, however, autopsy is allowed if its results would save the life of another patient who is immediately at hand. Many branches of Judaism currently allow an autopsy under the following conditions: (1) It is required by law; (2) the deceased person has willed it; (3) it saves the life of another, especially an offspring (Rosner, 1972).

Any attempt to hasten or retard decomposition of the body is discouraged. Cremation is prohibited because it unnaturally speeds the disposal of the dead. Embalming is prohibited because it preserves the dead (Lamm, 1972). However, in circumstances where the funeral must be delayed, some embalming may be approved. Cosmetic restoration for the funeral is discouraged.

The Jewish funeral and burial follow certain practices. The service is directed at honoring the departed by only speaking well of him. It is not customary to have flowers either at the funeral or at the cemetery because this was a Christian custom to offset the odor of decaying bodies (Kolatch, 1981). The casket is frequently made of wood with no ornamentation. The body may only be wrapped in a shroud to ensure that the body and casket decay at the same rate. No wake and no viewing are part of a Jewish funeral. The prayer said for the dead, the *kaddish,* it is usually not said alone. Actually, the prayer says nothing about death, but rather it praises God and reaffirms one's own faith.

After the funeral, mourners are welcomed to the home of the closest relative. Outside the front door is water to wash one's hands before entering, which is symbolic of cleansing the impurities associated with contact with the dead. The water is not passed from person to person, just as it is hoped that the tragedy is not passed. At the home, a meal is served to all the guests. This "meal of condolence" is traditionally provided by the neighbors.

*Shiva* (Hebrew for "seven") is the 7-day period that begins with the burial. It helps the individual face the actuality of the death of the loved one. During this period when the mourners are "sitting shiva," they do not work. In some homes, mirrors are covered, no activity is permitted to divert attention from thinking about the deceased, and evening services may be conducted in the closest relative's home. Condolence calls and the giving of consolation are appropriate during this time.

After shiva, the mourning period varies based on who has died. Mourning for a relative lasts 30 days, and for a parent, 1 year. Judaism does not support prolonged mourning (Amsel, 1994). A tombstone is erected within 1 year of the death, at which time a graveside service is held. This is called an "unveiling." The anniversary of the death according to the Jewish calendar is called *yahrzeit,* and at this time, candles are lit and the Kaddish is said.

When a limb is amputated before death, within Orthodoxy, the amputated limb and/or blood-soaked clothing are buried in the person's future gravesite (Lamm,

1972). Because the blood and limb were part of the person, they are buried with the person. No mourning rites are required.

The health-care provider may need to ask the closest relative of the deceased specifically about the practices to follow after death. In the case of an amputation, the health-care provider may need to assist with arrangement for burial of the body part.

## Responses to Death and Grief

The period following a death has discrete segments to assist the mourners in their adjustment to the loss. The period of time from the death to the burial is short. The burial may only be delayed if required by law, if relatives must travel great distances, or if it is the Sabbath or a holy day. The period from the death to the burial is the time for the emotional reaction to the death. Mourners are absolved from praying during this time. Crying, anger, and talking about the deceased person's life are acceptable. A common sign of grief is the tearing of the garment that one is wearing before the funeral service. In liberal congregations, a black ribbon with a tear in it is a symbolic representation of mourning. During shiva, the mourner sets the tone and initiates the conversation. Because there are such discrete periods of mourning, Judaism tells the mourner that it is wrong to mourn past 30 days for a relative and a year for parents.

## SPIRITUALITY

### Religious Practices and Use of Prayer

Judaism is over 3000 years old. Its early history and laws are chronicled in the Old Testament. Jews consider only the Old Testament as their Bible. They have a history of being singled out as a people and often persecuted; expelled from countries; "black-balled" from jobs, housing, and admission to college; rounded up and killed; and mass-exterminated.

Many Jews in America have immediate family who were killed in the pogroms in Russia in the early 1900s and in the holocaust in eastern Europe. Yet throughout this persecution, Judaism has lived and flourished. The spiritual leader is the **rabbi,** which means "teacher." He or she is the interpreter of Jewish law. Rabbis are not any closer to God than the common man. All Jews pray directly to God. They do not need the rabbi to intercede, to hear confession, or to grant atonement. Some of the major principles that guide Judaic bioethics are as follows:

1. Man's purpose on earth is to live according to certain God-given guidelines;

2. life possesses enormous intrinsic value, and its preservation is of great moral significance;

3. all human lives are equal;

4. our lives are not our own exclusive private possessions (Glick, 1994, p. 19).

Judaism is a monotheistic faith that believes in one God as the creator of the universe. The watchword of the faith is found in Deuteronomy (6:4), "Hear O Israel, the Lord is our God, the Lord is One." No physical qualities are attributed to God, and making and praying to statues or graven images are forbidden in the second commandment. "The Jewish conception of God is of a moral God who demands moral, ethical living and justice for all mankind. He is a universal God, whose sovereignty is over all the world" (Donin, 1972, p. 22).

The first five books of the Bible, also known as the five books of Moses, are handwritten in Hebrew on parchment scrolls called **Torah.** These scrolls are kept in the "Holy Ark" within each synagogue under an "eternal light." The Torah directs Jews regarding how they should live their lives; it provides guidance on every aspect of human life. The rest of the Bible includes sacred writings and teachings of the prophets.

The 613 commandments within the Torah (also called Mitzvot) and the oral law derived from the biblical statutes determine Jewish law, or **halakhah.** It asks for a commitment in behavior and also addresses ethical concerns. Thus, the commandments reflect the will of God, and a religious Jew feels it his duty to carry them out to fulfill his covenant with God. This makes Judaism not only a religion but a way of life (Amsel, 1994).

Current practice of Judaism in America spans a wide spectrum. While there is only one religion, there are three main branches or denominations of Judaism. The **Orthodox** are the most traditional. They adhere most strictly to the halakhah (Code of Jewish Law) of traditional Judaism and try to follow as many of the laws as possible while fitting into American society. They observe the Sabbath by attending the synagogue on Friday evening and Saturday morning and by abstaining from work, spending money, and driving on the Sabbath. Orthodox Jews observe the Jewish dietary laws; males wear a **yarmulka,** or *kippah* (head covering), at all times in reverence to God, whereas women usually wear long sleeves and modest dress (Siegel & Rheins, 1980). In many Orthodox synagogues, the services are primarily in Hebrew and men and women sit separately. In America, 6.1 percent of the Jewish population consider themselves Orthodox (Singer, 1992).

The **Conservative** denomination (35.1 percent of American Jewry) is not quite as strict in its tradition (Singer, 1992). While Conservative Jews observe most of the halakhah, they do make concessions to modern America. Many drive to the synagogue on the Sabbath, and men and women sit together. Many keep a kosher home, but they may or may not follow all of the dietary laws outside the home. Women are ordained as rabbis and are counted as a minyan (the minimum number of ten required) for prayer. These practices are unacceptable to the Orthodox. While a yarmulke is required in the synagogue, it is optional outside of that environment.

The liberal or progressive movement is called **Reform** (38 percent of Jewish-Americans). Reform Jews claim that postbiblical law was only for the people of that time, and only the moral laws of the Torah are binding (Fischel & Pinsker, 1992). They practice fewer rituals, although they frequently have a **mezuzah** (parchment with a religious passage within a small receptacle) posted on the doorpost of their homes, celebrate the holidays, and have a strong ethnic identity. They consider education and ethics of paramount importance in one's personal life and try to link Jewish religious values with American political liberalism (Fischel & Pinsker, 1992). They do not usually follow the Jewish dietary laws, but they may have specific unacceptable foods (for example, pork), which they abstain from eating. There is full equality for men and women, and they engage in many social action activities. Reform Jews do not celebrate the extra day added to many Jewish holidays.

There are multiple small groups of ultra-Orthodox fundamentalists; the **Hasidic** (or **Chasidic**) Jews are perhaps the most recognizable to Americans. They usually live, work, and study within a segregated area. They are usually easy to identify by their full beards, uncut hair around the ears *(pais),* black hats or fur *streimels,* dark clothing, and no exposed extremities. Women, especially those who are married, also keep their extremities covered and may have shaved heads covered by a wig and often a hat as well.

A relatively new denomination, **Reconstructionism** (1.3 percent of American Jewry), is a mosaic of the three main branches. It views Judaism as an evolving religion of the Jewish people and seeks to adapt Jewish belief and practice to the needs of the contemporary world (Fischel & Pinsker, 1992). In addition to these groups, many Jews do not indicate an affiliation (Singer, 1992).

The Jewish house of prayer is called a **synagogue, temple,** or **shul.** It is never referred to as a church. However, Jews may pray anywhere alone or may pray as a group anywhere that 10 Jews over age 13 years who have had their bar mitzvah are together for prayer. This group is called a **minyan.** The Orthodox Jew prays three times a day: morning, late afternoon, and evening. They wash their hands and say a prayer on awakening in the morning and before meals.

Religious clients in hospitals may want their prayer items (yarmulke, *tallit, tefillin*) and may request a *minyan* (10 males older than 13 who have had their bar mitzvah). Hospital policies regarding the number of visitors in the sick person's room may have to be ignored in such instances. The *tefillin,* or "phylacteries," are used by Orthodox men during morning prayer services. They contain two small black boxes with parchment containing biblical passages on them that are connected to long leather straps. These are wrapped around the arms and forehead as reminders of the laws of the Torah. The *tallis* (or *tallit*) is a rectangular prayer shawl with fringes *(tzitzit* or *tsitsis).* This is also only used during prayer but is frequently used by both Conservative and Orthodox Jews. Ultra-Orthodox men wear a special garment under their shirts year-round; it has long fringes, also called *tsitsis,* that are worn hanging from the belt as a reminder of the laws of the Torah.

A **mezuzah** is a small container with scripture included inside. It serves as a reminder of the presence of God, His commandments, and a Jew's duties to Him. Jewish homes have a mezuzah on the doorpost of the house. Its origin was as a sign insuring God's protection. A number of individuals also wear a mezuzah as a necklace. Other religious symbols include the Star of David, a six-pointed star that has been a symbol of the Jewish community since the 1350s, and the menorah (candelabrum).

One of the most common religious practices related to patients involves "visiting the sick" *(bikkur cholim).* This is one of the social obligations of Judaism (Rabinowicz, 1994). One is to consider the patient's welfare. This means not staying too long or tiring the patient, nor should one come to satisfy one's own needs.

## Meaning of Life and Individual Sources of Strength

The preservation of life is one of Judaism's greatest priorities. "When a person's life is in danger, it is a duty to do whatever is necessary to save the life" (Donin, 1972, p. 96). While the Sabbath is the holiest day of each week, the laws that govern it may be broken if one can help save a life. Each individual is considered special. The individuality of the human experience is one of the precepts of the faith. "Good health is prized above almost all other considerations" (Charnes & Moore, 1992, p. 66).

## Spiritual Beliefs and Health-care Practices

The Sabbath is the holiest day. One of the Ten Commandments is to remember the Sabbath day and keep it holy. It begins 18 minutes before sunset on Friday and ends 42 minutes after sunset or when three stars can be seen on Saturday. It serves as a release from weekday concerns and pressures. This weekly holy day is ushered in by lighting candles, saying prayers over challah and wine, and participating in a festive Sabbath meal. It ends on Saturday with a service called *Havdalah.* During this time, religious Jews do no manner of work, including answering the telephone, operating any electrical appliance, driving, or operating a call bell from a hospital bed.

If an Orthodox client's condition is not life-threatening, medical and surgical procedures should not occur on the Sabbath or holy days. However, "illness, extremely foul weather, or great distance from the synagogue are legitimate reasons for

**Table 15–2 • Jewish Holidays for Calendar Years 1997–2000***

| Holiday | 1997 | 1998 | 1999 | 2000 |
|---|---|---|---|---|
| Purim | March 23 | March 12 | April 2 | March 21 |
| Passover | April 22–29 | April 11–18 | May 1–8 | April 20–27 |
| Shavuot | June 11–12 | May 31 to June 1 | June 21–22 | June 9–10 |
| Rosh Hashana (Jewish New Year) | October 2–3 | September 21–22 | September 11–12 | September 30 to October 1 |
| Yom Kippur | October 11 | September 30 | September 20 | October 9 |
| Succot | October 16–24 | October 5–13 | September 25 to October 3 | October 14–22 |
| Chanukah | December 24–31 | December 14–21 | December 4–11 | December 22–29 |

*Jewish holidays always begin at sundown the evening before the date recorded on this type of calendar; holidays end at sundown on the date shown.

not attending the services" (Donin, 1972, p. 75). Although the Sabbath is holy, matters involving human life take precedence over it (Waxman, 1960). Therefore, a gravely ill person and the work of those who need to save him are exempted from following the commandments regarding the Sabbath.

In addition to the Sabbath, there are a number of Jewish holidays that are celebrated with special traditions. Rosh Hashana (the Jewish New Year) and Yom Kippur (the Day of Atonement) are called the high holy days and are usually in September. They mark a 10-day period of self-examination and repentance. Rosh Hashana is started by eating apples and honey to wish for a sweet year, and on Yom Kippur, one fasts for a day to cleanse and purify oneself. Fasting for Yom Kippur may be broken for reasons of critical illness, labor and delivery, or for children under age 12 years.

Other holidays include Passover, the Feast of the Unleavened Bread, which lasts 7 days and celebrates the Jews' Exodus from Egypt and slavery; Sukkot, a festival of the harvest where individuals may live in temporary huts built outside their homes or synagogues for a week; Chanukah, an 8-day holiday that celebrates religious freedom; Purim, which also commemorates religious freedom; and Shavuot, which celebrates the giving of the Ten Commandments. Table 15–2 provides a listing of Jewish holidays for 1997 through the year 2001.

## HEALTH-CARE PRACTICES

### Health-seeking Beliefs and Behaviors

According to those who interpret Jewish law, each person has a duty to keep themselves in good health (Latner, 1981). This encompasses physical and mental well-being and includes not only early treatment for illness but also prevention. "Judaism does not permit refusing medication and treatment if there is any chance that it will make the patient well" (Latner, 1982, p. 313). All denominations recognize that religious requirements may be laid aside if a life is at stake or if an individual has a life-threatening illness. However, halakhah also differentiates a non–life-threatening illness from a "slight illness" or "mere discomfort." For the non–life-threatening illness, the commandments may be modified (Schwartz & Spero, 1983). "Hospice care is fully consonant with Jewish ethics, Jewish customs, and Jewish law" (Rosner, 1993, p. 9).

In ultra-Orthodox denominations of Judaism, the taking of medication on the Sabbath that is not necessary to preserve life may be viewed as "work" (i.e., an action performed with the intention of bringing about a change in existing conditions), and would therefore be unacceptable. Some persons with conditions such as asthma may not recognize the severity of their condition nor be aware of the laws that allow them to take their necessary medications (Schwartz & Spero, 1983). These patients need to be taught about the potential life-threatening sequelae of their condition as well as the exceptions to Jewish law that permit them to take their medications.

All individuals are considered to have value regardless of their condition. This includes individuals with developmental disabilities and AIDS. Judaism opposes discrimination against persons with AIDS (Vorspan, 1992).

## Responsibility for Health Care

While it is the responsibility of the physician to heal, the person must seek the services of the physician to ensure a healthy body (Rosner, 1972). Once persons have the knowledge to heal, it is their obligation to do so. To abstain from healing would be equivalent to murder (Amsel, 1994).

Jews believe that God provides humans with wisdom, and it is up to them to use that wisdom to create a better world. This includes the discovery of new medications and treatments to eliminate or modify disease and suffering. Jews also believe that God gives humans freedom of choice (Vorspan, 1992).

Because the preservation of life is paramount, all ritual commandments are waived when danger to life exists. Physical and mental illnesses are legitimate reasons for not fulfilling some of the commandments (Schwartz & Spero, 1983).

Because adult Jews are often well read, they may try many of the treatment modalities about which they have read. This could have both positive and negative consequences. The literature reveals no studies regarding Jews' self-medicating practices.

## Folk Practices

Jewish folklore practices are historically and biblically based. Specific practices are explained under Nutrition and Spiritual Beliefs and Health-care Practices sections.

## Barriers to Health Care

Except for the unavailability of health insurance for some persons, there are no major barriers to health care for Jews in contemporary America. In early colonial America, Jews were only allowed to stay on the condition that they support their own poor and care for their own sick (Fischel & Pinsker, 1992). The Jewish community helped those in need, including new immigrants, and assisted fellow Jews to become self-sufficient. This practice continued so that "the 230,000 Jews in the United States in 1880 absorbed 3 million immigrants in the next 50 years" (Fischel & Pinsker, 1992, p. 106).

## Cultural Responses to Health and Illness

The verbalization of pain is acceptable and common (Fischel & Pinsker, 1992). Zborowski's study (1969) revealed that Jews were more vocal than the Irish in their response to pain; they also wanted to know the reason for the pain, which they considered just as important as obtaining relief from pain.

A high proportion of Jews became psychoanalysts, psychiatrists, and psychologists. In addition, a high number of their clients are Jewish (Fischel & Pinsher, 1992). The maintenance of one's mental health is considered just as important as the maintenance of one's physical health.

A number of Russian Jews who have immigrated since 1973 have a different view towards seeking mental health services than their predecessors. They are often overwhelmed by the "freedom of choice" available, having lived in a society that offered so few choices. They also experience guilt and anxiety from having left relatives behind in Russia, who may have been punished during the emigree's exodus. They do not always comprehend the difference between government officials, whom they fear and mistrust, and social service agencies offering them help. They seek medical care and view health-care practitioners as less threatening than those treating mental health (Brodsky, 1988). Thus, the health-care provider may need to reorient the client to the role of social service agencies.

Mental incapacity has always been recognized as grounds for exemption from all obligations under Jewish law (Amsel, 1994). This designation includes psychiatric conditions. However, requirements for those who are rational but have cognitive deficiencies are decided on an individual basis. Regardless of the age or developmental level of a developmentally disabled person, according to Jewish law, they must be taught the Torah. This speaks to the unique value of each individual.

The sick role for Jews is highly individualized and may vary among individuals according to symptom severity. As prescribed in the halakhah, the family is central to Jewish life; therefore, the emphasis on maintaining health and assisting with individual responsibilities are shared by family members during times of illness.

## Organ Transplant and Organ Donation

Jewish law views organ transplants from four perspectives: the recipient, the living donor, the cadaver donor, and the dying donor (Abraham, 1994). Because life is sacred, if the recipient's life can be prolonged without considerable risk, then transplant is ordained. For a living donor to be approved, the risk to the life of the donor must be considered. One is not obligated to donate a bodily part unless the risk is small. This would include kidney and bone marrow donations.

The use of a cadaver for transplant is usually approved if it is saving a life. No one may derive economic benefit from the corpse (Vorspan, 1992). Although desecration of the dead body is considered purposeless mutilation, this does not apply to the removal of organs for transplant. Use of skin for burns is also acceptable, although no agreement has been reached on the use of cadaver corneas (Abraham, 1994).

Taking potential organs for donation from a dying individual is still being hotly debated. These individuals are still alive, and their deaths cannot be delayed nor speeded up. In liberal Judaism, if the donor has consented, then organ transplant is acceptable. The health-care provider may need to assist the Jewish client to obtain a rabbi when making a decision regarding organ donation or transplant.

## HEALTH-CARE PRACTITIONERS

### Traditional Versus Biomedical Care

The ancient Hebrews are credited with promoting hygiene and sanitation practices and basic principles for public health care. From the practice of visiting the sick and the desire to initiate measures to prevent the spread of disease, Lillian Wald, a Jewish nurse, developed the Henry Street Settlement as a prototype of public health nursing for those in need (Benson, 1993).

Health-care providers should only touch Hasidic males when providing direct care. "Therapeutic touch" is not appropriate with these clients.

## Status of Health-care Providers

Physicians are held in high regard (Rabinowicz, 1994). While physicians must do everything in their power to prolong life, they are prohibited from initiating measures that prolong the act of dying (Rosner, 1993). Once standard therapy has failed or if additional treatments are unavailable, "the physician's role changes from that of curer to that of carer. Only supportive care is required at that state and includes care such as food and water, good nursing care and maximal psychosocial support" (Rosner, 1993, p. 10).

### CASE STUDY

Selecting a "typical" Jewish client is difficult. An ultra-Orthodox Jew has a particular set of special needs. Yet, it is more common to see a Jew who is a middle-of-the-road Conservative.

Sonia is an 80-year-old woman who was born near Kiev, Russia. Most of her family was killed in the pogroms, and she escaped to the United States at the age of 10. She married and raised a family in a Conservative traditional home. As she aged, she became less committed to keeping kosher outside her home, although her home is kosher.

At age 62, she was diagnosed with type I diabetes. She expressed some concern initially about her use of pork-based insulin. Currently, she is admitted for amputation of her right leg due to the complications of diabetes. Her hospital room is always filled with visitors.

### STUDY QUESTIONS

1. What questions will you specifically ask Sonia about her dietary preferences?

2. How would you have responded to her initial concern about using insulin made from pork?

3. What questions do you need to ask in the initial patient interview to assess her degree of religious practice, and how will you determine her spirituality needs?

4. What must you anticipate discussing with her about her surgery as relates to the disposition of her leg?

5. What is your understanding of the reason she has so many visitors in her room?

6. How might your care be altered if the client in this case study were a Hasidic male? (Your answers will vary depending on whether you are a male or a female health-care provider.)

*continued on page 394*

7. Describe three genetic or hereditary diseases common with Ashkenazi Jews.

8. Describe the Jewish ritual of circumcision.

9. Discuss the laws of Kashrut in regard to food practices for observant Jewish clients.

10. What should the health-care provider keep in mind when entering a Jewish home to provide care?

11. Distinguish between the terms Sephardic and Ashkenazi.

12. How might a non-Jewish and Jewish coworker share holidays in the workforce.

13. What is the official language the Jewish people use for prayer?

14. Identify fertility practices for Jewish-Americans from all three denominations.

## References

Abraham, A. (1994). Organ Transplantation and Jewish Law. In H. Branover & I. Attia (Eds.), *Science in the light of Torah.* Northvale, NJ: Jason Aronson.

Amsel, N. (1994). *The Jewish encyclopedia of moral and ethical issues.* Northvale, NJ: Jason Aronson.

Avigad, S., Cohen, B., Bauer, S., Schwartz, G., Frydman, M., Woo, S., Niny, Y., & Shiloh, Y. (1990). A single origin of phenylketonuria in Yemenite Jews. *Nature, 344,* 168–170.

Baskin, J. (1983). Prenatal testing for Tay-Sachs disease in the light of Jewish views regarding abortion. *Issues in Health Care of Women, 4,* 41–56.

Behrman, R., & Vaughan, V. (1987). *Nelson textbook of pediatrics.* Philadelphia: W. B. Saunders.

Benson, E. (1994). Jewish nurses: A multicultural perspective. *Journal of the New York State Nurses Association, 25*(2), 8–10.

Benson, E. (1993). Public health nursing and the Jewish contribution. *Public Health Nursing, 10*(1), 55–57.

Brodsky, B. (1988, Spring). Mental health attitudes and practices of Soviet Jewish Immigrants. *Health and Social Work,* 130–136.

Charnes, L., & Moore, P. (1992). Meeting patients' spiritual needs: The Jewish perspective. *Holistic Nursing Practice, 6*(3), 64–72.

Cooke, D. (1991). Inflammatory bowel disease: Primary health care management of ulcerative colitis and Crohn's disease. *Nurse Practitioner, 16*(8), 27–39.

Donin, H. (1972). *To be a Jew: A guide to Jewish observance in contemporary life.* New York: Basic Books.

Fischel, J., & Pinsker, S. (1992). *Jewish-American history and culture: An encyclopedia.* New York: Garland Publishing.

Glazer, N. (1957). *American Judaism.* Chicago: University of Chicago Press.

Glick, S. (1994). *Trends in medical ethics in a pluralistic society: A Jewish perspective.* University of Cincinnati, Judaic Studies Program, Cincinnati, Ohio.

Jones, K. (1988). *Smith's recognizable patterns of human malformation.* Philadelphia: W. B. Saunders.

Kaback, M., Lim-Steel, J., Dabholkar, D., Brown, D., Levy, N., & Zeiger, K. (1993). Tay-Sachs Disease: Carrier screening, prenatal diagnosis, and the molecular era. *Journal of the American Medical Association, 270*(19), 2307–2315.

Klein, I. (1992). *A guide to Jewish religious practice.* New York: The Jewish Theological Seminary of America.

Kolatch, A. (1981). *The Jewish book of why.* Middle Village, New York: Jonathan David.

Lamm, M. (1972). *The Jewish way in death and in mourning.* Middle Village, NY: Jonathan David.

Lamm, N. (1978). Judaism and the modern attitude to homosexuality (pp. 375—399). In M. Kellner (Ed.), *Contemporary Jewish ethics.* New York: Sanhedron Jewish Studies.

Latner, H. (1981). *The book of modern Jewish etiquette.* New York: Schocken Books.

Levy, R. (1993). Ethnic and racial differences in response to medicines: Preserving individualized therapy in managed pharmaceutical programmes. *Pharmaceutical Medicine, 7,* 139–165.

Pras, E., Aksentijevich, I., Gruberg, L., Balow, J., Prosen, L., Dean, M., Steinberg, A., Pras, M., &

Kastner, D., (1992). Mapping of a gene causing Familial Mediterranean Fever to the short arm of Chromosome 16. *New England Journal of Medicine, 326*(23), 1509–1513.

Rabinowicz, T. (1994). *A guide to life: Jewish laws and customs of mourning.* Northvale, NJ: Jason Aronson.

Rosner, F. (1993, July/August). Hospice, medical ethics and Jewish customs. *American Journal of Hospice and Palliative Care,* 6–10.

Rosner, F. (1972). *Studies in Torah Judaism: Modern medicine and Jewish law.* New York: Yeshiva University.

Schwartz, H., & Spero, M. (1983). Management of the asthmatic, Sabbath-Observant Jewish patient: Some guidelines in the light of Jewish law. *Chest, 84*(6), 762–765.

Siegel, R., & Rheins, C. (1980). *The Jewish almanac.* New York: Bantam Books.

Singer, D. (1992). *American Jewish year book 1992.* Philadelphia: The Jewish Publication Society.

Steinhardt, D. (1988). Alcoholism: The myth of Jewish immunity. *Psychology Today, 22*(2), 10.

Thompson, J., McFarland, G., Hirsch, J., & Tucker, S. (1993). *Mosby's clinical nursing.* St. Louis: Mosby.

Vorspan, A. (1992). *Tough choices: Jewish perspectives on social justice.* New York: UAHC Press.

Waxman, M. (1960). *Judaism: Religion and ethics.* New York: Thomas Yoseloff.

Wouk, H. (1986). *This is my God.* New York: Simon & Shuster.

Zborowski, M. (1969). *People in pain.* San Francisco: Jossey-Bass.

# Mexican-Americans

*Larry D. Purnell*

---

• Key terms to become familiar with in this chapter are:

| | |
|---|---|
| *Ataque de nervios* | *Latino* |
| *Caida de la mollera* | Machismo |
| Chicano | *Mal ojo (mal de ojo)* |
| *Curandero* | Mestizo |
| *El ataque* | *Personalismo* |
| *Empacho* | *Respeto* |
| *Espirituista* | *Sobador* |
| Familism | *Susto* |
| Hispanic | *Velorio* |
| *La gente de la raza* | Wetback |
| *Ladino* | *Yerbero* (or *jerbero*) |

## OVERVIEW, INHABITED LOCALITIES, AND TOPOGRAPHY

### Overview

Mexican-Americans are not easy to group or describe. Although no specific set of characteristics can describe Mexican-Americans, some commonalities distinguish them as an ethnic group, with multiple regional variations reflective of selective subcultures in Mexico. A common term used to describe Spanish-speaking Americans, including Mexican-Americans, is **Hispanic.** However, many Hispanic people prefer to be identified by descriptors more specific to their cultural heritage, such as Mexican, Mexican-American, Latin American, Spanish-American, **Chicano,** *Latino,* or *Ladino.* As a broad ethnic group, they often refer to themselves as *la gente de la raza*, which means "the people of the race." The Spanish word race has a different meaning from the American interpretation of race. *La raza* is a genetic determination to which all Spanish-speaking people belong, regardless of class differences or country of origin (Monrroy, 1983). This chapter uses the term *Mexican-American* to refer to persons who identify themselves as Americans of Mexican origin.

"Few other ethnic minority groups have been as persistent in maintaining their language, cultural beliefs, and traditions as have the Mexican-Americans" (Reinert, 1986, p. 23). As with other large ethnic populations, the Mexican-American population is characterized by great diversity. Factors that influence acculturation and maintenance of traditional practices and beliefs are race, age, generation, length of time away from the home country, socioeconomic status, educational attainment, religious beliefs, rural versus urban residence, reasons for immigration, and immigration status. Individual subgroups include educated urban dwellers, remote village peasants, and groups emigrating from diverse areas such as international Cancun, port cities, and mountain villages populated predominantly by indigenous Indian groups. These indigenous Indian groups include Mayan, Aztec, Zapotec, Yaqui, and Mixtec. With 50 different ethnic groups in Mexico (Heusinkveld, 1993), the health-care provider must be careful not to ascribe characteristics that are not a part of the individual's belief system.

## Heritage and Residence

Mexico, with a population of 81 million, is 60 percent **mestizo,** a blend of Spanish white and Indian; 30 percent Native-American; 9 percent white; and 1 percent other (Heusinkveld, 1993). Mexican-Americans are descendants of Spanish and other European whites; Aztec, Mayan, and other Central American Indians; and Inca and other South American Indians. Some individuals can trace their heritage to North American Indian tribes in the Southwest. In the 1500s and 1600s, a significant number of intermarriages occurred between Spanish and native Indian populations. Since the 1800s, this practice is less common. Mexico City, the largest city in the world, has a population of over 21 million. Mexico is undergoing rapid changes in business and health-care practices. Undoubtedly, these changes will accelerate with the passage of the North American Free Trade Agreement (NAFTA) as people are more able to move across the border to seek employment and educational opportunities.

Hispanics, the fastest growing minority population in the United States, include 22.3 million people, or 9.6 percent of the population. Sixty-two percent are of Mexican ancestry (*Statistical Abstracts,* 1995). The Hispanic population will contribute 33 percent to the national population growth from 1992 to 2000 and 57 percent by 2050 (Rojas, 1994). Mexican-Americans reside predominantly in California, Texas, New York, Florida, Illinois, Arizona, New Jersey, New Mexico, and Colorado. In addition, significant numbers reside in Canada. Texas and Mexico are intertwined in many ways, including through intermarriage of powerful Texan and Mexican families; many Texans have relatives across the border in Mexico (Hudson, 1995). Ninety percent of Mexican-Americans live in urban areas such as San Diego, Los Angeles, New York City, and Chicago, whereas only 10 percent reside in rural areas. Many second-generation and third-generation Mexican-Americans are well educated and represented in all professions and occupations. However, some have not acculturated, do not speak English, and adhere to their traditional ethnic beliefs.

## Reasons for Migration and Associated Economic Factors

Limited employment and job opportunities in Mexico, especially in rural areas, encourage Mexicans to migrate to the United States as sojourners, immigrants, or undocumented aliens, often derogatorily referred to as **wetbacks** *(majodos).* Of the 3.4 million undocumented aliens in the United States, over one-third are from Mexico (Hudson, 1995). Before the Immigration Reform and Control Act of 1986, hundreds of thousands of Mexicans crossed the border, found jobs, and settled in the United States. Although the numbers have decreased since 1986 (Gelfand & Bialik-Gilad, 1989), border towns in Texas and California still experience a large influx of Mexicans to the United States for improved job and educational opportunities (Burk, Weiser, & Keegan, 1995). Many individuals from lower socioeconomic backgrounds live in substandard housing, are employed in low-paying jobs, and live in neighborhoods with overcrowded living conditions (Ginsberg, 1992). Twenty-nine percent of Hispanics live in poverty as compared with a poverty rate of 11.6 percent for non-Hispanics (Nickens, 1995). More recent Mexican immigrants are more likely to live in poverty, are more pessimistic about their future, and are less educated than previous immigrants (Chapa & Valencia, 1993).

## Educational Status and Occupations

Many second-generation and third-generation Mexicans have significant job skills and education. In Texas, Hispanics (primarily Mexican-Americans) make up 17 percent of the state's senate and 33 percent of the state's house of representatives. The speaker of New Mexico's house of representatives is a Mexican-American (Hudson, 1995).

By contrast, many, especially newer immigrants from rural areas, have poor educational backgrounds and may place little value on education because it is not needed to obtain jobs in Mexico (Marshall, 1992). Once in the United States, they initially find work similar to that which they did in their native land, including farming, ranching, mining, oil production, construction, landscaping, and domestic jobs in homes, restaurants, and hotels and motels. Many Mexicans and Mexican-Americans work as seasonal migrant workers, who may relocate several times each year as they "follow the sun." Sometimes their unwillingness to learn English is related to their intent to return to Mexico; however, this hinders their ability to obtain better-paying jobs.

The mean educational level in Mexico is 5 years. The primary method of learning focuses on rote learning of abstract concepts rather than on the development of critical thinking skills. Student work is sometimes more valued for the attractiveness of the presentation than for the quality of the content (Kras, 1989). Until 1992, Mexican children were required to attend school through the sixth grade, but since the Mexican School Reform Act of 1992, a ninth-grade education is required. A common practice among parents in poor rural villages is to educate their children in what they need to know. This group often finds immigration to the United States to be their most attractive option. For many Mexicans, high school education is unavailable, and sometimes a good education is interpreted as having good manners (Heusinkveld, 1993).

Hispanics are the most undereducated ethnic group in the United States, with only 43.6 percent of Mexican-Americans aged 25 years or older having a high school education compared with 80.5 percent for non-Hispanics. Some migrant worker camps have free or low-cost bilingual educational programs to assist Mexican-Americans to learn to read and write in both languages. Only 6.2 percent of Mexican-Americans aged 25 years or older have a college degree. The educational levels of Mexican-Americans are also below those of all other Hispanics (Trevino, 1994). In an effort to improve educational levels, Mexican students can attend American border colleges and pay the same tuition fees as state residents (Hudson, 1995).

## COMMUNICATION

## Dominant Language and Dialects

Second to Spain, Mexico is the largest Spanish-speaking country in the world (*Statistical Abstracts,* 1992). The dominant language of Mexicans and Mexican-Americans is Spanish. However, The National Institute of Anthropology and History reports 54 indigenous languages and more than 500 different dialects in Mexico. Knowing the region from which a Mexican-American originates may help to identify the language or dialect the individual speaks. For example, major indigenous languages besides Spanish include Nahuatl and Otami, spoken in central Mexico; Mayan, spoken in the Yucatan peninsula; Maya-Quiche, spoken in the state of Chiapas; Zapotec and Mixtec, spoken in the valley of Oaxaca; Tarascan, spoken in the state of Michoacan; and Totonaco, spoken in the state of Veracruz. Many of the Spanish dialects spoken by Mexican-Americans have word meanings that are similar. However, the dialects of Spanish spoken by other groups may not have the same word meanings. Because of the rural isolationist nature of many ethnic groups and the influence of native Indian languages, the dialects may be so diverse in selected regions that it may be difficult to understand the language, regardless of the degree of fluency in Spanish.

Radio and television programs broadcast in Spanish in both the United States and Mexico have helped to standardize Spanish. For the most part, public broadcast communication is primarily derived from Castilian Spanish. This standardization reduces the difficulties experienced by subcultures with multiple dialects. When speaking in a non-native language, health-care providers must select words that have relatively pure meanings in the language and avoid the use of regional slang.

Contextual speech patterns among Mexican-Americans may include a high-pitched, loud voice and a rate that seems extremely fast to the untrained ear. The language uses apocopations, which account for this rapid speech pattern. An apocopation occurs when one word ends with a vowel and the next word begins with a vowel. This creates a tendency to drop the vowel ending of the first word and results in the abbreviated rapid-sounding form. For example, in the Spanish phrase for How are you?, ¿Cómo está usted? may become ¿Comestusted?. The last word, usted, is frequently dropped. Some may find this fast speech difficult to understand. However, if one asks the individual to enunciate slowly, the effect of the apocopation or truncation is less pronounced.

To help bridge potential communication gaps, health-care providers need to watch the client for cues, paraphrase words with multiple meanings, use simple sentences, repeat phrases for clarity, avoid the use of regional idiomatic phrases and expressions, and ask the client to repeat instructions to ensure accuracy. Approaching the Mexican-American client with respect and personalism and directing questions to the dominant member of a group (usually the male) may help to facilitate more open communication.

## Cultural Communication Patterns

While some topics such as one's income, salary, or investments are taboo, Mexican-Americans generally like to express their inner beliefs, feelings, and emotions once they get to know and trust a person (Heusinkveld, 1993). Meaningful conversations are important, often become loud, and seem disorganized. To the outsider, the situation may seem stressful or hostile, but this intense emotion means that the conversants are having a good time. Within the context of **personalismo,** personalism, and **respeto,** respect, health-care providers can encourage open communication and sharing and develop the client's sense of trust by inquiring about family members before proceeding with the usual business.

Mexican-Americans place great value on closeness and togetherness, including when they are in the hospital or a long-term care facility. They frequently touch and embrace and like to see relatives and significant others. Touch between men and women, between men, and between women is acceptable.

Mexican-Americans consider sustained eye contact when speaking directly to someone rude. Direct eye contact with teachers or superiors may be interpreted as insolence. Avoiding direct eye contact with superiors is a sign of respect. The condition **mal ojo**, "evil eye," a culture bound syndrome is discussed under the Health-care Practices section.

To demonstrate respect, compassion, and understanding, health-care providers should greet Mexican-Americans clients with a handshake. On establishing rapport, providers may further demonstrate approval and respect through backslapping, smiling, and affirmative nods of the head. Given the diversity of dialects and the nuances of language, culturally congruent use of humor is difficult to accomplish and therefore should be avoided unless the health-care provider is absolutely sure that there is no chance of misinterpretation. Otherwise, inappropriate humor may jeopardize the therapeutic relationship and opportunities for health teaching and health promotion.

## Temporal Relationships

Mexican-Americans, especially in the lower socioeconomic groups, are necessarily present oriented. Many individuals do not consider it important nor have the income to plan ahead financially. The trend is to live in the "more important" here and now, because *mañana* (tomorrow) cannot be predicted. With this emphasis on living in the present, preventive health care and immunizations may not be a priority. *Mañana* may or may not really mean tomorrow, but rather it often means "not today."

Mexicans perceive time as relative rather than categorically imperative. Deadlines and commitments are flexible, not firm. Punctuality is generally relaxed, especially in social situations. This concept of time is innate in the Spanish language. For example, one cannot be late for an appointment, one can only arrive late! In addition, newer immigrants who come from a rural environment where adhering to a strict time clock is unimportant may not own a clock or be able to tell time.

Because of their more relaxed concept of time, Mexican-Americans may arrive late for appointments, although the current trend is toward greater punctuality. Health-care facilities that use an appointment system for clients may need to make special provisions to see clients whenever they arrive.

## Format for Names

Names in most Spanish-speaking populations seem complex to those unfamiliar with the culture. A typical name is La Señorita Olga Gaborra de Rodriguez. Gaborra is the name of her father, and Rodriguez is her mother's surname. When she marries a man with the surname name of Guiterrez, she becomes La Señora (denotes a married woman) Olga Guiterrez de Gaborra y Rodriguez. The word *de* is used to express possession, and the father's name, which is considered more important than the mother's name, comes first. However, this full name is rarely used except on formal documents and for recording the name in the family bible. Out of respect, most Mexican-Americans are more formal when addressing non-family members. Thus, the best way to address Olga is not by her first name but rather as Señora Guiterrez.

## FAMILY ROLES AND ORGANIZATION

### Head of Household and Gender Roles

The typical family dominance pattern in traditional Mexican-American families is patriarchal, with only slight evidence of slow change toward a more egalitarian pattern in recent years (Burk, Wieser, & Keegan, 1995; De Leon Siantz, 1994). Change to a more egalitarian decision-making pattern is primarily identified with more educated and higher socioeconomic families. The **machismo** of the Mexican culture sees men as having strength, valor, and self-confidence. Men are seen as being wiser, braver, stronger, and more knowledgable regarding sexual matters. The female takes responsibility for decisions within the home and for maintenance of the family's health (Burk, Wieser, & Keegan, 1995). Women are expected to be devoted mothers and receive great respect from their husbands and children (Kras, 1989). Male opinions dominate decision making in most other aspects of life (Condon, 1985), including health-care, where decisions are usually made after considering others' opinions. In addition, women are taught not to criticize men, especially in public (Heusinkveld, 1993).

## Prescriptive, Restrictive, and Taboo Practices for Children and Adolescents

Children are highly valued (Smith & Weinman, 1995) because they ensure the continuation of the family and cultural values. They are closely protected and not encouraged to leave home. Even godparents (*compadres*) are included in the care of the young. It is essential for each child to have godparents in case something interferes with the parents' ability to fulfill their childrearing responsibilities. Children are taught at an early age to respect parents and older family members, especially grandparents. Physical punishment is often used as a way of maintaining discipline and is sometimes considered child abuse in the United States.

Many young men and women become independent from their families, especially in the urban setting, but independence is more difficult for women than for men. Large families are desirable and the United States birth rate for Hispanic-American households is 106.7 births per 1000 compared with 42.7 for non-Hispanic households (Smith & Weinman, 1995).

## Family Roles and Priorities

The concept of familism is an all-encompassing value in the Mexican-American culture, where the traditional family is still the foundation of society. Family takes precedence over work and all other aspects of life. The North American health-care culture stresses including the client and family in the plan of care. Mexican-Americans are strong proponents of this family-care concept, which includes the extended family. By including all family members in care, the health-care provider can build greater client trust and in turn increase compliance with health-care regimens and prescriptions.

Within the context of a patriarchal heritage, the family on the male side of the household is considered more important (Murillo, 1978). Blended communal families are almost the norm in lower socioeconomic groups and in migrant worker camps. Single, divorced, and never-married male and female children usually live with their parents or extended families. Even when economics do not dictate, this practice is still common. Godparents are considered coparents, and close friends are usually considered family members. Thus, the words brother, sister, aunt, and uncle do not necessarily mean that they are blood related. For many men, having children is evidence of their virility and is a sign of machismo, a valued trait among many.

Grandparents and elderly parents, when unable to live on their own, generally move in with their children. The extended family structure and the Mexican-American's obligation to visit sick friends and relatives encourages large numbers to visit hospitalized family members and friends. This practice may necessitate that health-care providers relax strict visiting policies in health-care facilities.

Social status is highly valued among Mexican-Americans, and a person who holds an academic degree or position with an impressive title commands great respect and admiration from family, friends, and the community. Good manners, a family, and family lineage, as indicated by extensive family names (Condon, 1985; Heusinkveld, 1993; & Kras, 1989), also confer high status for Mexican-Americans.

## Alternative Lifestyles

Thirty percent of Latino families live in poverty and are headed by a single female parent. This percentage is lower than that for other minority groups in the United States (Romer & Kim, 1995). Because the Hispanic cultural norm is for a pregnant female to marry, Mexican-Americans are more likely to marry at a young age when pregnancy occurs. For example, 50 percent of non–English-speaking Mexican-American females aged 13 to 17 years who become pregnant marry in comparison with 23 percent of English-speaking Mexican-Americans in the same age group, and 85 percent of non–English-speaking Mexican-American females aged 18 to 20 years married compared with 62 percent of English-speaking Mexican-Americans (Smith & Weinman, 1995). Yet, common law marriages *(unidos)* are frequently practiced and readily accepted, with many couples living together their entire lives.

Homosexual behavior occurs in every society, despite its denial (Brink, 1987). No information has been found in the medical literature regarding same-sex Mexican-American couples living together as a family unit. Newspapers from Houston, Texas; Washington, D.C.; and Chicago, Illinois, report on the efforts of Hispanic lesbian and gay organizations in the areas of human immunodeficiency virus (HIV) and acquired immunodeficiency syndrome (AIDS, *La SIDA* in Spanish) and life partner benefits. Larger cities may have *Ellas,* a support group for Latina Lesbians; El Hotline of Hola Gay, which provides referrals and information in Spanish; or Dignity, for gay Catholics. Such agencies may be used by health-care providers who wish to refer gay and lesbian clients to a support group.

If celibacy is discussed among Mexican-Americans outside the religious context, it is mentioned only with close friends.

> . . . Mothers encourage their daughters to go to college, they also want them to be traditional—to marry and have babies. For that reason daughters who leave home and don't get married have a real struggle; they are viewed as having failed to meet the expectations of their culture. (Miller, 1989, p. 198)

# WORKFORCE ISSUES

## Culture in the Workplace

In Mexico, 57 percent of health-care workers are female and 23.3 percent of physicians are female (Harrison, 1994). However, in the United States, Hispanics are the most underrepresented major minority group in the health-care workforce. Although almost 10 percent of the United States population is of Hispanic origin, only 4.2 percent of physicians and 2.4 percent of registered nurses are from Hispanic heritage (Trevino, 1994). In Texas, the overall population is 30 percent Hispanic, but only 3 percent of nurses are Hispanic (Bond & Jones, 1994). Cultural differences that influence workforce issues include values regarding family, pedagogical approach to education, emotional sensitivity, views toward status, aesthetics, ethics, balance of work and leisure, attitudes toward direction and delegation, sense of control, views about competition, and time.

Persons educated in Mexico are likely to have been exposed to pedagogical approaches that include rote memorization and emphasis on theory, with little practical application, within a rigid, broad curriculum. American educational systems usually emphasize an analytical approach, practical applications, and a narrow, in-depth specialization (Kras, 1989). Thus, additional training may be needed for some Mexicans when they come to the United States.

Mexican-Americans' emphasis on presentation extends into the workplace. A good presentation is judged to be as important as the content (Heusinkveld, 1993).

Mexican-Americans are a product of their childrearing practices, which discourage independence and may not value competition in the workforce. Most Mex-ican-Americans favor harmony and avoid personal competition in the workforce (Kras, 1989), discouraging the development of personal leadership skills and achieve-ment among many Mexicans-Americans.

Because family is a first priority for most Mexican Americans, activities that involve family members usually take priority over work issues. Putting up a tough business front may be seen as a weakness in the Mexican-American culture. Because of this separation of work from emotions in American culture, most Mexican-Americans tend to shun confrontation for fear of losing face. Many are very sensitive to differences of opinion, which are perceived as disrupting harmony in the workplace.

For many Mexican-Americans, truth is tempered by diplomacy. When a service is promised for tomorrow, even when they know the service will not be completed tomorrow, it is promised to please, not to deceive. Thus, for many Mexican-Americans, truth is seen as a relative concept (Condon, 1985; Kras, 1989), whereas for most European-Americans, truth is an absolute value, and people are expected to give direct yes and no answers. These conflicting perspectives about truth can complicate treatment regimens and commitment to the completion of work assign-ments. Intentions must be clarified.

Work to most Mexican-Americans is viewed as a necessity for survival and may not be highly valued in itself, and money is for enjoying life (Kras, 1989; Murillo, 1978). Most Mexican-Americans place a much higher value on other life activities. Material objects are usually necessities and not ends in themselves. The concept of responsibility is based on values related to attending to the immediate needs of fam-ily and friends (Kras, 1989; Murillo, 1978) rather than on the work ethic. For most Mexican-Americans, titles and positions may be more important than money.

Many Mexican-Americans believe that time is relative and elastic, with flexible deadlines, rather than stressing punctuality and timeliness. In Mexico, shop hours may be posted but not rigidly respected. A business that is supposed to open at 8 A.M. opens when the owner arrives; a posted time of 8 A.M. may mean the business will open at 8:30 A.M., later, or not at all. The same attitude toward time is evidenced in reporting to work and in keeping social engagements and medical appointments. If persons believe that an exact time is truly important, such as the time an airplane leaves, then they may keep to schedule. The real challenge for employers is to stress the importance and necessity of work schedules and punctuality in the American workforce.

Acculturated Mexican-Americans are more likely to adhere to work schedules, but even then, punctuality can remain an overriding concern for the employer. The Mexican-American is considered a good, hard worker and may willingly stay late to complete work or to take on unexpected assignments without regard to a set quitting time.

## Issues Related to Autonomy

Many Mexican-Americans respond to direction and delegation differently from Eu-ropean-Americans. Many newer immigrants are used to having traditional autocratic managers, who assign tasks, but not authority, although this practice is beginning to change with more American-managed companies relocating in Mexico. A Mexican-American not accustomed to responsibility may have difficulty assuming account-ability for decisions. The individual may be sensitive to the American practice of checking employees' work.

Mexican-Americans born and educated in the United States usually have no difficulty communicating with others in the workplace. When better-educated Mex-ican immigrants arrive in the United States, they usually speak some English. Newer immigrants from lower socioeconomic groups have the most difficulty acculturating in the workplace and may have great difficulty with the English. While no one knows the extent of literacy for this group, estimates of illiteracy in their own language are as high as 80 percent (Delmarva Rural Ministries, personal communication, March 1994).

## BIOCULTURAL ECOLOGY

### Skin Color and Other Biologic Variations

Because Mexican-Americans draw their heritage from Spanish peoples and various North American and Central American Indian tribes, few physical characteristics give this group a distinct identity. Some persons with a predominant Spanish background might have light-colored skin, blond hair, and blue eyes, whereas persons from indigenous Indian backgrounds may have black hair, dark eyes, and cinnamon-colored skin. Intermarriages among these groups have created a diverse gene pool and have not produced a typical-appearing Mexican-American.

Cyanosis and decreased hemoglobin levels are more difficult to detect in dark-skinned persons, whose skin appears ashen instead of the bluish color seen in light-skinned persons. To observe for these conditions in dark-skinned Mexican-Americans, the practitioner must examine the sclera, conjunctiva, buccal mucosa, tongue, lips, nailbeds, palms, and soles. Jaundice, likewise, is more difficult to detect in darker-skinned persons. Thus, the practitioner needs to observe the conjunctiva and the buccal mucosa for patches of bilirubin pigment in dark-skinned Mexican-Americans.

### Diseases and Health Conditions

In 1993, the common health problems in Mexico were cancer, alcoholism, drug abuse, obesity, hypertension, diabetes, adolescent pregnancy, dental disease, and HIV and AIDS (Torres, 1994). Child mortality due to diarrheal disease in Mexico in 1990 was 14,000. Researchers believe that there are many more cases than reported because communities with populations of fewer than 500 do not benefit from medical practice and do not report many of these deaths (Larrauri, Larrauri, & Carreras, 1994).

In Mexican-American migrant worker populations, infectious, communicable, and parasitic diseases continue to be major health risks (Torres, 1994). Substandard housing conditions and employment in low-paying jobs have perpetuated higher rates of tuberculosis in Mexican-Americans. Intestinal parasitosis, amoebic dysentery, and bacterial diarrhea (shigella) are common diseases among Mexican immigrants (Sumaya, 1992). Mexican-Americans have a higher rate of syphilis; four times the incidence of gonorrhea; three times the incidence of chlamydia; and an increased incidence of HIV infection, tuberculosis, and hepatitis B than the rates for European-Americans.

Research has revealed an increase in the incidence of malaria in the border towns of the Southwest (Sumaya, 1992). Newer Mexican immigrants from coastal lowland swamp areas, where mosquitoes are more prevalent, may also have a higher incidence of malaria. Persons from high mountain terrains may have increased red blood cell counts on immigration to the United States. Health-care providers must take these topographic factors into consideration when performing health screening for such symptoms as anemia, lassitude, failure to thrive, and weight loss among Mexican-Americans.

Higher rates of hypertension and ischemic heart disease are also reported among Mexican-Americans (Ailinger, 1982; Becker et al., 1993). High rates of malnutrition and anemia are common because of poverty and lower educational levels (Mendoza et al., 1993).

Mexican-Americans have five times the rate of diabetes mellitus, with an increased incidence of related complications, when compared with their European-Americans counterparts (Stern & Haffner, 1992). In 1991, in Cameron County, Texas, the rate of anencephaly was 20 per 10,000 live births as compared with the overall rate for the United States of 3 to 4 per 10,000 live births (Burk, Wieser, & Keegan, 1995). In addition, Hispanics have a higher death rate from suicide (Becker et al., 1993), unintentional injury, homicide, and chemical dependency than non-Hispanic whites (Nickens, 1995). Health-care professionals working with Mexican immigrants and Mexican-Americans should offer screening and teach clients preventive measures regarding pesticides and communicable and infectious diseases.

## Variations in Drug Metabolism

Because of the mixed heritage of many Mexican-Americans, it may be more difficult to determine a therapeutic dosage of selected drugs. Several studies report differences in absorption, distribution, metabolism, and excretion of drugs, including alcohol in some Hispanic populations. The mixed heritage of Mexican-Americans makes it more difficult to generalize drug metabolism. Few studies include only one subgroup of Hispanics, and, therefore, health-care providers need to consider some notable differences when prescribing medications. Hispanics require lower doses of antidepressants and experience greater side effects than non-Hispanic whites. Spanish white subpopulations are poor metabolizers of debrisoquine as compared with other groups of European-Americans (Levy, 1993).

## HIGH-RISK BEHAVIORS

Alcohol plays an important part in the Mexican culture. Many of this group's colorful lifestyle celebrations include alcohol consumption. Males drink in greater proportion than females, but both sexes begin drinking at early ages and consume large quantities of alcoholic beverages (Chavez et al., 1993).

Because of these drinking patterns, alcoholism represents a crucial health problem for many Mexican-Americans. It is the number one admitting diagnosis for Mexican-Americans in the psychiatric setting (Monroy, 1983). There is evidence to support that low acculturation and distorted application of the chivalric norm of machismo influences the high alcoholism rates in this group (Fernandez-Pol et al., 1985; Marin, Posner, & Kenyon, 1993). In a study by Marin, Posner, & Kenyon (1993), less acculturated Hispanics were more likely to consume alcoholic beverages than more acculturated Hispanics. Even the more acculturated Hispanics consume more alcoholic beverages than non-Hispanic whites, expecting alcohol to make them more emotional and socially extroverted. Low acculturation and distorted self-image problems have special implications for counseling (Zimmerman & Sodowsky, 1993). Many deny the physiological problems of alcoholism. Hispanics suffer higher rates of automobile accidents and other types of injuries associated with alcohol consumption (Marin, Posner, & Kenyon, 1993). In another study contrasting the drinking patterns of Latinos and non-Latino whites in San Francisco, Perez-Stable, Marin, and Marin (1994) reported that Latinos of both sexes consume less alcohol than non-Latino whites, but Latino men are more likely to drink to excess and engage in binge drinking.

Marijuana is the number two drug used by Mexican-Americans because it is readily available in their native land and easily accessible from people who work in farming and ranching occupations. Cocaine and heroin are used by some adults who can afford them, and inhalants are used by the younger population (Eden & Aguilar, 1989).

The trend toward decreasing cigarette smoking in the United States may not extend to the Mexican-American culture, where cigarette smoking rates remain steady (Escobebe & Remington, 1989; Fiore et al., 1989). However, Perez-Stable, Marin, and Marin (1994), in their San Francisco study, reported that Latino smokers of both sexes smoke fewer than half as many cigarettes per day as non-Latino whites. The differing results from these two studies attest to the fact that health-care providers should not generalize high-risk behaviors.

## Health-care Practices

Responsibility for health promotion and safety may be a major threat (Burk, Wieser, & Keegan, 1995) for those of Mexican heritage accustomed to depending on the family unit and traditional means of providing health care. Continuing disparities in health and health-seeking behaviors have been reported in several studies. Lower socioeconomic conditions are responsible for Latina women being overweight, exhibiting hypertension, experiencing high cholesterol levels, and having increased smoking behaviors (Blantan et al., 1993). In addition, Latina women are less likely to have Pap smears, medical examinations, or clinical breast examinations as compared with non-Latino whites (Perez-Stable, Marin, & Marin, 1994). Latino men are less likely to have cancer screening or physical examinations than their non-Latino white counterparts. High-risk health behaviors such as drinking and driving, cigarette smoking, sedentary lifestyle, and nonuse of seat belts increase with fewer years of educational attainment. Through educational programs and enforcement of state laws, more Mexican-Americans are beginning to use seat belts; however, it is still common to see children traveling unrestrained in automobiles.

Both Mexican and Puerto Rican women in the lower socioeconomic levels have lower physical activity levels and increased body fat, but their nutritional status improves when they receive welfare or food stamps (Lopez, 1993). Some evidence suggests that positive health-seeking behaviors increase among Mexican-Americans who are married (Kuster & Fong, 1993).

## NUTRITION

### Meaning of Food

Like many other ethnic groups, Mexicans and Mexican-Americans celebrate with food. Mexican foods are rich in color, flavor, texture, and spiciness. Any occasion—births, birthdays, religious holidays, official and unofficial holidays, and anniversaries of deaths—is seen as a time to celebrate with food and enjoy the companionship of family and friends. Because food is a primary form of socialization in the Mexican culture, Mexican-Americans may have difficulties adhering to a prescribed diet for illnesses such as diabetes mellitus and cardiovascular disease (Monrroy, 1983).

### Common Foods and Food Rituals

The Mexican-American's diet is extremely varied and may depend on the individual's region of origin in Mexico. Thus, one needs to ask the individual specifically about his or her dietary habits.

The staples of the Mexican-American diet are rice (*arroz*), beans, and tortillas, which are made from corn (*maíz*) treated with calcium carbonate, although, in many parts of the United States, only flour tortillas are available. Even though the diet is low in calcium derived from milk and milk products, tortillas treated with calcium carbonate provide essential dietary calcium. Popular Mexican-American foods are eggs (*huevos*); pork (*puerco*), chicken (*pollo*), sausage (*salchicha*); lard (*lardo*); mint (*menta*); chili peppers (*chile),* onions (*cebollas*), tomatoes (*tomates*), squash (*calabaza*); canned fruit (*fruta de lata*); mint tea (*hierbabuena*), chamomile tea (*té de camomile or manzanilla*); carbonated beverages (*bebidas de gaseosa*), beer (*cerveza*), coca cola, sweetened packaged drink mixes (*agua fresa)* that are high in sugar (*azucar*); sweetened breakfast cereals (*cereales de desayuno*); potatoes (*papas*), bread (*pan*), corn (*maíz*); gelatin (*gelatina*), custard (*flan*), and other sweets (*dulces*). Other common dishes include chile, chile con carne, enchiladas, tamales, tostadas, chicken molé, arroz con pollo, refried beans, and tacos. (Nachos are American!)

Mealtimes may vary among different subgroups of Mexican-Americans. Whereas many individuals adopt North American schedules and eating habits, many continue their native practices, especially those in rural settings and migrant worker camps. For these groups, breakfast is usually fruit, perhaps cheese, or bread alone or in some combination. A snack may be taken in midmorning before the main meal of the day, which is eaten anytime from 2 to 3 P.M., and in rural areas especially, may last for 2 hours or more. Mealtime is an occasion for socialization and keeping family members informed about each other. The evening meal is usually late and is taken between 9 and 9:30 P.M. The health-care provider must consider Mexican-Americans' mealtimes when teaching clients about medication and dietary regimens related to diabetes mellitus and other illnesses.

## Table 16–1 • Table of Mexican Foods

| Common Name | Description | Ingredients |
|---|---|---|
| Arroz con pollo | Chicken with rice | Chicken baked, boiled, or fried and served over boiled or fried rice |
| Chili | Chili | Same as the United States but tends to be more spicy |
| Chili con carne | Chili with meat | Chili with beef or pork |
| *Chili con salsa* | Chili with sauce | Chili with a sauce that contains no meat |
| *Dulces* | Sweets | Candy and desserts usually high in sugar, lard, and eggs |
| Enchiladas | Enchiladas | Tortilla rolled and stuffed with meat or cheese and a spicy sauce |
| *Papas fritas* | Fried potatoes | Potatoes usually fried in lard |
| Flan | Flan | Popular dessert made of egg custard and may be filled with fruit or cheese |
| *Gelatína* | Gelatin | Popular dessert made with sugar, eggs, and jelly |
| *Pollo con molé* | Chicken molé | Chicken with a sauce made of hot spices, chocolate, and chili |
| *Salchica* or *chorizo* | Sausage | Sausage almost always made with pork and spices |
| Tacos | Tacos | Tortilla folded around meat or cheese |
| Tamales | Tamales | Fried or boiled chopped meat, peppers, cormeal, and hot spices |
| Tortilla | Tortilla | A thin unleavened bread made with cornmeal and treated with lime (calcium carbonate) |
| Tostadas | Tostadas | Toast that may have a spicy sauce |

## Dietary Practices for Health Promotion

A dominant health-care practice for Mexicans and many Mexican-Americans is the hot and cold theory of food selection. This theory is a major aspect of health promotion and illness prevention and treatment. According to this theory, illness or trauma may require adjustments in the hot and cold balance of foods to restore body equilibrium. The hot and cold theory of foods is described under the section Health-Care Practices later in this chapter.

## Nutritional Deficiencies and Food Limitations

In lower socioeconomic groups, wide-scale vitamin A deficiency and iron deficiency anemia exist (Mendoza et al., 1992). Some data suggest a tendency to lactose intolerance among some Mexican-Americans (Monrroy, 1983), which may cause problems for schools and health-care organizations that provide milk in the diet for its high calcium content.

Because major Mexican foods and their ingredients are available throughout the United States, native food practices may not change much when Mexicans come to America. Of course, Mexican foods are extremely popular throughout the United States and are eaten by many Americans because of the strong flavors, spiciness, and color. Table 16–1 lists the Mexican names of popular foods, their description, and ingredients. Individual adaptations to these preparations commonly occur.

## PREGNANCY AND CHILDBEARING PRACTICES

### Fertility Practices and Views toward Pregnancy

Mexican-American birth rates are 3.45 per household in comparison with 2.6 per household among other minority groups (Chapa & Valencia, 1993). Multiple births are common, especially in the economically disadvantaged groups. Men see a large number of children as proof of their virility. Optimal childbearing age for Mexican women is between 19 and 24 years. If a woman has not had babies by 24 years old, she may be considered too old to conceive (Carbonell, 1992). Fertility practices of Mexican-Americans are connected with their predominant Catholic religious beliefs and their tendency to be modest. The only acceptable methods of birth control are abstinence and the rhythm method. Some women practice the belief that prolonged infant breast-feeding is a method of birth control. Theoretically, most other types of birth control, on the surface, are unacceptable. Abortion is considered morally wrong and is practiced (theoretically) only in extreme circumstances to keep life intact. However, legal and illegal abortions are common in some parts of Mexico and the United States (Heusinkveld, 1993). Despite the strong influence of the Catholic Church over fertility practices, Catholicism does not prevent some Mexican-American women from using contraceptives, sterilization, or abortion for unwanted pregnancies (Amaro, 1988).

Diaphragms, foams, and creams are not commonly used for birth control practice, mostly because they are not approved by the Catholic doctrine and partly because of the belief that women are not supposed to touch their genitals. Birth control pills are unacceptable because they are an artificial means of birth control. Physicians' offices and clinics that see large numbers of migrant workers on the Delmarva Peninsula on the east coast report that many younger female clients are using Norplant for birth control. Men are reluctant to use prophylactics because they are associated with prostitutes and because of the belief that they should be used only for disease control. Family planning is one area in which the health-care provider can help the family to identify more realistic outcomes consistent with current economic resources and family goals.

Because pregnancy among Mexican-Americans is viewed as a natural and desirable condition, many women do not seek prenatal evaluations. In addition, because prenatal care is not available to every woman in Mexico, some women do not know about the need for prenatal care. With the extended family network and the woman's role of maintaining the health status of family members, many pregnant women seek family advice before seeking medical care. Thus, **familism** may deter and hinder early prenatal checkups. To encourage prenatal checkups, the health-care provider can encourage female relatives and husbands to accompany the pregnant woman for health screening and incorporate advice from family members into health teaching and preventive care services. Using videos with Spanish-speaking Hispanics is one culturally effective way for incorporating health education, especially for those who have a limited understanding of English. In addition, incorporating cultural brokers known to the Mexican-American family may help to empower clients and reduce conflict for Mexican-Americans using the health-care system (Jezewski, 1993).

## Prescriptive, Restrictive and Taboo Practices in the Childbearing Family

Beliefs related to the hot and cold theory of disease prevention and health maintenance influence conception, pregnancy, and postpartum rituals. For instance, during pregnancy, a woman is more likely to favor hot foods, which are believed to provide warmth for the fetus and enable the baby to be born into a warm and loving environment. Cold foods and environments are preferred during the menstrual cycle and in the immediate postdelivery period. Many pregnant woman sleep on their backs to protect the infant from harm, keep the vaginal canal well lubricated by having frequent intercourse to facilitate an easier birth, and keep active to ensure a smaller baby and to prevent a decrease in the amount of amniotic fluid (Burk, Wieser, & Keegan, 1995). An important activity restriction is that pregnant women should not walk in the moonlight because it might cause a birth deformity. To prevent birth deformities, pregnant women may wear a safety pin, metal key, or some other metal object on their abdomen (Villarruel & Montellano, 1992). Other beliefs include avoiding cold air, not reaching over the head to prevent the baby's cord from wrapping around its neck, and avoiding lunar eclipses because they may result in deformities.

The father in the more traditional Mexican-American family is not included in the delivery experience and should not see the mother or baby until after both have been cleaned and dressed. This practice is based on the fear that harm may come to the mother, baby, or both (Baca, 1978). Integrating men into the birthing of a child is a process of changing social habits in relation to cultural aspects of life and gender roles. The presence of men during delivery is considered an uninvited intrusion in the Mexican-American culture (Aliaga, 1992).

Among less traditional and more acculturated Mexican-Americans, men participate in prenatal classes and assist in the delivery room. However, in the author's personal experience, men who provide support during delivery may receive friendly gibing from their male counterparts for taking the role of the wife's mother.

During labor, traditional Mexican-American women are quite vocal and are taught to avoid breathing air in through the mouth because it can cause the uterus to rise up. Immediately after birth, they may place their legs together to prevent air from entering the womb (Olds, Landon, & Ladewig, 1992). Health-care providers can help the Mexican pregnant woman have a better delivery by encouraging attendance at prenatal classes.

The postpartum preference for a warm environment may restrict bathing or hair washing for up to 40 days in postpartum women (Reinert, 1986). Although postpartum women may not take showers or sit in a bath tub, this does not mean that they do not bathe. They take sitz baths, wash their hair with a washcloth, and take sponge baths. Other postpartum practices include wearing a heavy cotton abdominal binder, cord, or girdle to prevent air from entering the uterus; covering one's ears, head, shoulders, and feet to prevent blindness, mastitis, frigidity, or sterility; and avoiding acidic foods to protect the baby from harm (Olds, Landon, & Ladewig, 1992).

When the baby is born, special attention is given to the umbilicus; the mother wears a stomach belt *(ombliguero)* to prevent the naval from popping out when the child cries. Cutting the baby's nails in the first 3 months is thought to cause blindness and deafness (Rosa M. Solórzano, M.D., personal communication, Sept., 1995).

Health-care providers need to make special provisions to provide culturally congruent health teaching for lactating women who work with or are exposed to pesticides, such as dichlorodiphenyldichlorothene (DDE), the most stable derivative from the pesticide DDT. High DDE levels among lactating women have a direct correlation with a decrease in lactation and increase in breast cancer, especially in women who have had more that one pregnancy and previous lactation (Gladen & Rogan, 1995). Education level and degree of acculturation are key issues when developing health education and interventions for risk reduction (Balcazar, Castro, & Krall, 1995).

# DEATH RITUALS

## Death Rituals and Expectations

Mexican-Americans often may have a stoic acceptance of the way things are and view death as a natural part of life (Heusinkveld, 1993). Death practices are primarily an adaptation of their religion. Family members may arrive in large numbers at the hospital or home in times of illness or an approaching death. In more traditional families, family members may take turns sitting vigil over the sick or dying person. Autopsy is acceptable as long as the body is treated with respect. Burial is the common practice; cremation is an individual choice.

## Responses to Death and Grief

When a person dies, the word travels rapidly, and family and friends travel from long distances to get to the funeral. They may gather for a **velorio**, a festive watch over the body of the deceased person before burial. Some Mexican-Americans bury the body within 24 hours, which is required by law in Mexico.

More traditional grieving families may engage in **ataque de nervios,** a culture-bound syndrome characterized by hyperkinetic shaking and seizurelike activity that releases strong emotions of grief. No treatment is necessary; the person recovers at their own will and pace (Bullough & Bullough, 1972). American health-care providers must not confuse *el ataque* with a seizure. The author has observed cases in which grieving family members experiencing *el ataque* have been taken to emergency rooms by those who did not understand the culture. In these cases, the health-care provider can assist the person by discussing the circumstances surrounding the death and by contacting family members or friends who can provide bereavement support.

More traditional Mexican-Americans may continue their native practice of erecting altars in their homes to honor deceased relatives on the anniversary of their death. The dead are honored, sometimes annually, with candles, decorations, and bringing the deceased's favorite meal to a picnic at the grave site (Heusinkveld, 1993).

# SPIRITUALITY

## Religious Practices and Use of Prayer

The predominant religion of most Mexicans and of most Mexican-Americans is Catholicism. Over the last several years, other religious groups such as Mormons, Jehovah's, Witnesses, Seventh Day Adventists, Presbyterians, and Baptists have been gaining in popularity in Mexico (Heusinkveld, 1993). Although many Mexicans and Mexican-Americans may not appear to be practicing their faith on a daily basis, they may still consider themselves devoted Catholics, and their religion has a major influence on health-care practices and beliefs. For many, Catholic religious practices are influenced by indigenous Indian practices.

Newer immigrant Mexican-Americans may continue their traditional practice of having two marriage ceremonies, especially in lower socioeconomic groups. A civil ceremony is performed whenever the two people decide to make a union. When the family gets enough money for a religious ceremony, they schedule an elaborate celebration within the church. Common practice, especially in rural Mexican villages and rural villages in the southwestern United States, is to post a handwritten sign on the local church announcing the marriage, with an invitation for all to attend.

Frequency of prayer is highly individualized for most Mexican-Americans. Even though some do not attend church on a regular basis, they may have an altar in their home and say prayers several times each day, a practice which is more common among rural isolationists.

## Meaning of Life and Individual Sources of Strength

The family is foremost to most Mexican-Americans, and individuals get strength from family ties and relationships. Individuals may speak in terms of a person's soul or spirit (*alma or espiritu*) when they refer to one's inner qualities. These inner qualities represent the person's dignity and must be protected at all costs (Condon, 1985) in times of both wellness and illness. In addition, Mexicans-Americans derive great pride and strength from their nationality, which embraces a long and rich history of traditions (Kras, 1989).

Leisure is considered essential for a full life, and work is a necessity to make money for enjoying life. Mexican-Americans pride themselves on good manners, etiquette, and grooming (Condon, 1985; Heusinkveld, 1993; Kras, 1989) as signs of respect. Because the overall outlook for many Mexican-Americans is one of fatalism, pride may be taken in stoic acceptance of life's adversities.

## Spiritual Beliefs and Health-care Practices

Most Mexican-Americans enjoy talking about their soul or spirit, especially in times of illness. Many health-care providers may feel uncomfortable talking about spirituality. This tendency may communicate to Mexican-Americans that the health-care provider has suspect intentions, is insensitive, and not really interested in them as an individual (Condon, 1985). Additional spiritual beliefs are covered under Folk Practices.

# HEALTH-CARE PRACTICES

## Health-seeking Beliefs and Behaviors

The family is viewed as the most credible source of health information and the most significant impediment to positive health-seeking behaviors (Sandoval, 1994). Mexican-Americans' fatalistic worldview and external locus of control are closely tied to health-seeking behaviors. Because expressions of negative feelings are considered impolite, Mexican-American may be reluctant to complain about health problems or to place blame on the individual for poor health. If a person becomes seriously ill, that is just the way things are (Heusinkveld, 1993)—all events are acts of God (Condon, 1985). This belief system may impair communications and hinder health teaching, health promotion, and disease prevention.

## Responsibility for Health Care

Good health to many Mexican-Americans means being free of pain (Cavallo & Flaskerud, 1991). The hospital may be seen as a place to die. Many Mexican-Americans may elect to see health professionals as a last resort, often when they are in the terminal stages of disease. As a result, many do die in the hospital. Many Mexican-Americans in higher socioeconomic groups take responsibility for their own health care, whereas many uneducated immigrant populations may not know what constitutes good health (Cassetta, 1994). For example, many migrant workers do not protect themselves against pesticides and herbicide poisoning because they do not understand the health hazards posed by working with these chemicals. (Miralles, 1989). This resistance to taking responsibility for one's health is supported by studies showing that Mexican-Americans are less likely to have medical checkups or engage in health-promoting behaviors than other minority groups (Kuster & Fong, 1993; Perez-Stable, Marin & Marin, 1994).

The use of over-the-counter medicine may pose a significant safety problem related to self-care for many Mexican-Americans. In part, this is a carryover from Mexico's practice of allowing over-the-counter purchases of antibiotics, intramuscular injections, intravenous fluids, birth control pills, and other medications that require a prescription in the United States. Often Mexican immigrants bring these medications across the border and share them with friends; in addition, friends and relatives in Mexico send drugs through the mail. To protect clients from contradictory or potentiating effects of prescribed treatments, the health-care provider needs to ask clients about prescription and nonprescription medications that they may be taking.

## Folk Practices

Mexican-Americans engage in folk medicine practices and use a variety of prayers, herbal teas, and poultices to treat illnesses. Many of these practices are regionally specific and vary between and among families. The Mexican *Ministerio de Salud Publica y Asistencia Social* (Ministry of Public Health and Social Assistance) publishes an extensive manual on herbal medicines that are readily available in Mexico. Although traditional and folk medicine are practiced more often by lower socioeconomic groups, well-educated upper-class and middle-class Mexicans to some degree seek out and practice these beliefs (Heusinkveld, 1993; Keefe, 1981). Many of these practices are harmless in and of themselves but may contradict or potentiate therapeutic interventions. Thus, as with the use of other prescription and nonprescription drugs discussed earlier, it is essential for the health provider to be aware of these practices and to take them into consideration when providing treatments. The provider must ask the Mexican-American client specifically whether they are using folk medicine practices.

Mexicans believe that good health, which is largely God's will (Monrroy, 1983), can be maintained by dietary practices that keep the body in balance. To provide culturally competent care, the health-care practitioner must be aware of the hot and cold theory of disease when prescribing treatment modalities and when providing health teaching. According to this theory, many diseases are thought to be caused by a disruption in the hot and cold balance of the body. Thus, eating foods of the opposite variety may either cure or prevent specific hot and cold illnesses and conditions.

Examples of hot diseases and conditions include infection, diarrhea, sore throats, stomach ulcers, liver conditions, kidney problems, gastrointestinal upsets, and fever. Common cold foods used to treat hot diseases and conditions include fresh fruits and vegetables, dairy products (even though fresh fruits and dairy products may cause diarrhea), barley water, fish, chicken, goat meat, and dried fruits (Harwood, 1981).

Examples of cold diseases and conditions include cancer, malaria, earaches, arthritis and related conditions, pneumonia and other pulmonary conditions, headaches, menstrual cramping, and musculoskeletal conditions. Common hot foods used to treat cold diseases and conditions include cheeses, liquor, beef, pork, spicy foods, eggs, grains other than barley, vitamins, tobacco, and onions (Harwood, 1981).

Folk practitioners are consulted for several notable conditions. *Mal ojo,* (bad eye or evil eye) is a folklore illness that occurs when one person (usually older) looks at another (usually a child) in an admiring fashion. Such eye contact can be either voluntary or involuntary. Symptoms are numerous, ranging from fever, anorexia, and vomiting to irritability. The spell can be broken if the person doing the admiring touches the person while they are admiring them. Children are more susceptible to this condition than women, and women are more susceptible than men. To prevent *mal (de) ojo,* the child wears a bracelet with a seed (*ojo de venado*) or a bag of seeds pinned to the clothes (Rosa M. Solorzano, M.D., personal communication, Sept., 1995).

Another condition of children treated by folk practitioners is **caida de la mollera** (fallen fontanel). The condition has numerous causes, which may include removing the nursing infant too harshly from the nipple or handling an infant too roughly. Symptoms range from irritability to failure to thrive. To cure the condition, the child is held upside down by the legs.

**Susto** (magical fright or soul loss) is associated with epilepsy, tuberculosis, and other infectious diseases and is caused by the loss of spirit from the body. This culture-bound disorder may be psychological, physical, or physiological in nature. There are no specific symptoms, and symptoms may or may not be fabricated. Treatment sometimes includes elaborate ceremonies with herbs to return the spirit to the body. Developing the symptoms associated with *susto* releases the person from work and life's responsibilities and allows them to enter the sick role (Martaus & Hentges, 1986).

**Empacho,** blocked intestines, may result from an incorrect balance of hot and cold foods, causing a lump of food to stick in the gastrointestinal track. Older women usually treat the condition in children by massaging their stomach and back to dislodge the food bolus and to promote its continued passage through the body.

Health-care practitioners are cautioned against diagnosing psychiatric illnesses too readily in the Hispanic population. The syndromes *mal ojo, susto,* and *ataque de nervios* are culture bound and are potential sources of diagnostic bias.

## Barriers to Health Care

Thirty-five percent of Mexican-Americans, as compared with 10 percent of the U.S. population in general, do not have health insurance (Perez-Stable, Marin, & Marin, 1994; Torres, 1994). A number of factors may account for this high percentage of uninsured. First, many Mexican-Americans constitute the working poor and are unable to purchase insurance. Second, many are migratory and do not qualify for Medicaid. Third, many are undocumented aliens and are afraid to apply for health insurance. Fourth, even though insurance is available in their native homeland, it is very expensive and not part of the culture.

Whereas wealthier Mexican-Americans have little difficulty accessing health care in the United States, lower socioeconomic groups may experience significant barriers, including inadequate financial resources, lack of insurance and transportation, limited knowledge regarding available services, language difficulties, and the culture of health-care organizations (Cassetta, 1994; Larrauri, Larraui, & Carraras, 1994; Torres, 1994). In addition, many lack a primary health-care provider and underuse health services when they are available (Sandoval, 1994). Like many other immigrant groups who lack a primary provider, they may use the emergency room for minor illnesses. Research evidence shows that Mexican-American clients in ethnically specific mental health programs are 11 times more likely to return after a first session than those in mainstream programs (Takeuchi, Sue, & Yeh, 1995). Health-care providers have the opportunity to improve the care of Mexican-Americans by explaining the health-care system, incorporating a primary care provider whenever possible, using an interpreter of the same gender, securing a cultural broker, and assisting clients in locating culturally specific mental health programs (Jezewski, 1993).

## Cultural Responses to Health and Illness

Good health to many Mexican-Americans is to be free of pain, not knowing the cause of the pain, and bearing pain stoically because it is God's will (Condon, 1985). These attitudes toward pain delay seeking treatment; many hope that the pain will simply go away. Research has shown that many Mexican-Americans experience more pain than other ethnic groups, but that they report the occurrence of pain less frequently and endure pain longer (Villarruel & Montellano, 1992). Six themes have emerged that describe culturally specific attributes of Mexican-Americans experiencing pain. They are as follows:

1. Mexicans accept and anticipate pain as a necessary part of life.

2. They are obligated to endure pain in the performance of duties.

3. The ability to endure pain and to suffer stoically is valued.

4. The type and amount of pain a person experiences is divinely predetermined.

5. Pain and suffering are a consequence of immoral behavior.

6. Methods to alleviate pain are directed toward maintaining balance within the person and the surrounding environment (Villarruel & Montellano (1992).

By using these themes, the health-care provider can evaluate Mexican-Americans experiencing pain within their cultural framework and provide culturally specific interventions.

Because long-term care facilities in Mexico are rare and tend to be crowded, understaffed, and expensive, many Mexican-Americans may not consider long-term care as a viable option for a family member. In addition, because of the importance of extended family, Mexican-Americans may prefer to care for their family members with mental illness, physical handicaps, and extended physical illnesses at home. In Mexican-American culture, someone with a mental illness is not looked on with scorn or blamed for their condition because mental illness, like physical illness, is viewed as God's will (Condon, 1985; Kras, 1989; Heusinkveld, 1993).

Mexican-Americans can readily enter the sick role without personal feelings of inadequacy or blame. A person can enter the sick role with any acceptable excuse and be relieved of life's responsibilities. Other family members willingly take over the sick person's obligations during his or her time of illness.

## Blood Transfusion, Organ Donation, and Organ Transplant

Extraordinary means to preserve life are frowned on in the Mexican and Mexican-American cultures, and ordinary means are commonly used to preserve life (Miralles, 1989). Extraordinary means are defined and determined by the individual, taking into account such factors as finances, education, and availability of services.

Blood transfusions are acceptable if the individual and the family agree that the transfusion is necessary. Organ donation, although not deemed morally wrong, is not a common practice and is usually restricted to cadaver donations, because donating an organ while the person is still alive means that the body is not whole. Acceptance of organ transplant as a treatment option is seen primarily among more educated persons. One reason that organ transplant is unacceptable with some groups is the belief that *mal aire* (bad air) enters the body if it is left open too long during surgery and increases the potential for the development of cancer.

## HEALTH-CARE PRACTITIONERS

### Traditional Versus Biomedical Health Care

Educated physicians and nurses are often seen as outsiders, especially among newer immigrants. To overcome this initial awkwardness, the health-care provider should attempt to get to know the client on a more personal level before initiating treatment regimens. Engaging in small talk unrelated to the health-care encounter before obtaining a health history or providing health education is advised. It is important for the health-care provider to respect this cultural practice to achieve an optimal outcome from the encounter.

Folklore practitioners, who are usually well known by the family, are usually consulted before and during biomedical treatment. Numerous illnesses and conditions are thought to be caused by voodoo or witchcraft. Specific rituals are carried out to eliminate the evils from the body. Lower socioeconomic and newer immigrants are more likely to use folk practitioners, but well-educated upper-class and middle-class persons also visit folk practitioners on a regular basis (Heusinkveld, 1993). Although as mentioned earlier, often no contradictions or contraindications to folk remedies exist, the health-care provider must always consider the client's use of this practice to prevent conflicting treatment regimens.

Even though the Catholic church preaches against some types of folk practitioners, they are common and meet yearly for several days in Catemaco, Veracruz. Folk practitioners include the **curandero,** who may receive their talents from God or serve an apprenticeship with an established practitioner. The *curandero* has great respect from the community, accepts no monetary payment, is usually a member of the extended family, and treats many traditional illnesses. A *curandero* does not usually treat illnesses believed to be caused by witchcraft.

Another practitioner, the **espirituista,** may receive his or her talents from God or serve an apprenticeship. An *espirituista* uses medals or amulets to prevent illnesses or to treat conditions believed to be caused by witchcraft. Prayer is a large part of their treatment.

The **yerbero** (also spelled *jerbero*) is a folk healer without specialized training in growing herbs, teas, and roots and who prescribes these remedies for prevention and cure of illnesses. A *yerbero* may suggest that the person go to a botanica (herb shop) for specific herbs. In addition, these folk practitioners frequently prescribe the use of laxatives.

A **sobador** subscribes to treatment methods similar to those of a Western chiropractor. The *sobador* treats illnesses, primarily those affecting the joints and musculoskeletal system, with massage and manipulation.

Even though Mexican-Americans like closeness and touch within the context of family, most tend to be modest in other settings. Women are not supposed to expose their bodies to men or even to other women. Female clients may experience embarrassment when it is necessary to touch their genitals or may refuse to have pelvic examinations as a routine part of a health assessment. Men may have strong feelings about modesty as well, especially in front of women, and may be reluctant to disrobe completely for an examination. Mexican-Americans often desire that intimate care be delivered only by members of the same gender (Burk, Wieser, & Keegan, 1995). The health-care provider must keep in mind these clients' need for modesty when disrobing or being examined. Thus, only the body part being examined should be exposed, and direct care should be provided in private. Whenever possible, a same gender caregiver should be assigned to care for Mexican-Americans.

## Status of Health-care Providers

Mexican-American clients have great respect for health-care providers because of their training and experience. They expect health-care providers to project a professional image and be well groomed and dressed in attire reflective of their professional status (Rosa M. Solorzano, M.D., personal communication, Sept., 1995).

While having great respect for health-care providers, some Mexican-Americans may distrust them out of fear that they will disclose their undocumented status. Health-care practitioners who incorporate folk practitioners, the concept of personalism, and respect into their approaches to care of Mexican-American clients will gain their clients' confidence and be able to obtain more thorough assessments.

Health-care providers can demonstrate respect for Mexican-American clients by greeting the client with a handshake, touching the client, or holding the client's hand, all of which help to build trust in the therapeutic relationship. Providing information and involving the family in decisions regarding health; listening to the individual's concerns; and treating the individual with *personalismo,* which stresses warmth and personal relationships, also fosters trust.

---

**CASE STUDY**

Pablo Gaborra, aged 32 years, and his wife Olga, aged 24 years, live in a migrant worker camp on the eastern shore of Maryland (Fig. 16–1). They have two children: Roberto, aged 7 years, and Linda, aged 18 months. Olga's two younger sisters, Florencia aged 16 years, and Rosa, aged 12 years, live with them. Another distant relative, Rodolpho, aged 28 years, comes and goes several times each year and seems to have no fixed address.

Pablo and Olga, born in Mexico, have lived in the United States for 13 years, first in Texas for 6 years and then in Delaware for 1 year, before moving to the eastern shore of Maryland 5 years ago. Neither of them have their citizenship, but both children were born in the United States.

Pablo completed the sixth grade and Olga the third grade in Mexico. Pablo can read and write enough English to function at a satisfactory level. Olga knows a few English words but sees no reason for learning English, even though free classes are available in the community. Olga's sisters have attended school in the United States and can speak English with varying degrees of fluency. Roberto attends school in the local community but is having great difficulty with his educational endeavors. The family speaks only Spanish at home. Not much is known about the distant relative Rodolpho, except that he is from Mexico, speaks minimal English, drinks beer heavily, and occasionally works picking vegetables.

*continued on page 418*

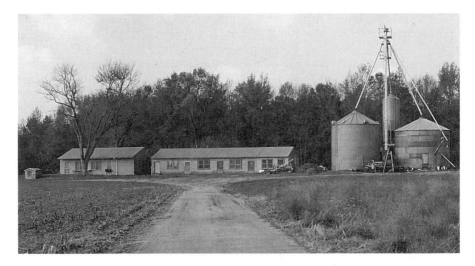

**Figure 16–1.** A migrant worker camp on Maryland's eastern shore. The Gaborra family lives in such a camp, as do many Mexican-American farm workers in the United States.

The Gaborra family lives in a trailer house on a large vegetable farm. The house has cold running water but no hot water, an indoor bathroom without a shower or bathtub, and is heated with a wood-burning stove. The trailer park has an outside shower, which the family uses in the summer.

The entire family picks asparagus, squash, peppers, cabbage, and spinach at various times during the year. Olga takes the infant, Linda, with her to the field where her sisters take turns watching the baby and picking vegetables. When the vegetable-picking season is over, Pablo helps the farmer to maintain machinery and to make repairs on the property. Their income last year was $30,000.

From the middle of April until the end of May, the children attend school sporadically because they are needed to help pick vegetables. During December and January, the entire Gaborra family travels to Texas where they visit relatives and friends, taking them many presents. They return home in early February with numerous pills and herbal medicines.

Olga was diagnosed with anemia when she had an obscure health problem with her last pregnancy. Because she frequently complains of feeling tired and weak, the farmer gave her the job of handing out "chits" to the vegetable pickers so that she did not have to do the more strenuous work of picking vegetables.

Pablo has had tuberculosis for years and sporadically takes medication from a local clinic. When he is not traveling or is too busy picking vegetables to make the trip to the clinic for refills, he generally takes his medicine. Twice last year, the family had to take Linda to the local emergency room because she had diarrhea, was listless, and was unable to take liquids. The Gaborra family subscribes to the hot and cold theory of disease and health prevention maintenance.

## STUDY QUESTIONS

1. Identify three socioeconomic factors that influence the health of the Gaborra family.

2. Name three health-teaching interventions the health-care provider might use to encourage Olga to seek treatment for her anemia.

3. Identify strategies to help improve communications in English for the Gaborra family.

4. Identify three health-teaching goals for the Gaborra family.

5. Name three interventions Olga must learn regarding fluid balance for the infant, Linda.

6. Discuss three preventive maintenance teaching activities that respect the Gaborra family's belief in the hot and cold theory of disease management.

7. Identify strategies for obtaining health data for the Gaborra family.

8. Identify four major health problems of Mexican-Americans that affect the Gaborra family.

9. If Olga were to see a folk practitioner, which one(s) would she seek?

10. Explain the importance of familism in the Mexican-American culture.

11. Distinguish between the two culture-bound syndromes *el ataque* and *susto*.

12. Discuss culturally conscious health-care advice consistent with the health belief practices of the pregnant Mexican-American woman.

13. Discuss two interventions to encourage Mexican-American clients with tuberculosis to keep clinic appointments and to comply with the prescribed medication regimen.

14. Identify where the majority of Mexican-Americans have settled in the United States.

## References

Ailinger, R. (1982). Hypertension knowledge in a Hispanic community. *Nursing Research, 31*(4), 207–210.

Aliaga, E. M. (1992). Hagamos en lugar al padre [We make room for the parent]. *EPAS, 2*(4), 26–30.

Amaro, H. (1988). Women in the Mexican American community: Religion, culture, and reproductive attitudes and experiences. *Journal of Community Psychology, 16*(1), 16–20.

Baca, J. E. (1978). Some health beliefs of the Spanish speaking. In R. A. Martínez (Ed.), *Hispanic culture and health care: Fact, fiction, folklore* (pp. 92–98). St. Louis: C. V. Mosby.

Balcazar, H., Castro, F., & Krall, J. (1995). Acculturation and education: Key factors for cancer risk reduction. *Health Education Quarterly, 22*(1), 61–84.

Becker, T. M., Wiggins, C. M., Key, C. R., & Samet, J. M. (1993). Ischemic heart disease and mortality. In T. M. Becker, C. L. Wiggins, R. S. Elliott, C. R. Key, & A. M. Samet (Eds.), *Racial and ethnic patterns of mortality in New Mexico* (pp. 83–97). Albuquerque: University of New Mexico Press.

Blantan, M. L., Martinez, R. M., Taylor, A. K., & Robinson, B. G. (1993). Latin and African women: Continuing disparities in health. *International Journal of Health Services, 23*,(2), 555–584.

Bond, M. L., & Jones, M. E. (1994). Short-term cultural immersion in Mexico. *Nursing Health Review, 15*(5), 248–254.

Brink, P. (1987). Cultural aspects of sexuality. *Holistic Nursing Practice, 1*(4), 12–20.

Bullough, B., & Bullough V. (1972). *Poverty, ethnic identity and health care.* New York: Appleton-Century Crofts.

Burk, M., Wieser, P., & Keegan, L. (1995). Cultural beliefs and health behaviors of pregnant Mexican-American women: Implications for primary care. *Advances in Nursing Science, 17*,(4). 37-52.

Calvillo, E. R., & Flaskerud, J. H., (1991). Review of literature on culture and pain of adults with focus on Mexican-Americans. *Journal of Transcultural Nursing, 2,*(2), pp. 16–23.

Cassetta, R. A. (1994, June). Needs of migrant workers challenge RNs. *American Nurse.* Washington, DC: American Nurses Association.

Chapa, J., & Valencia, R. R. (1993). Latino population growth, demographics, characteristics, and educational stagnation: An examination of recent trends. *Hispanic Journal of Behavioral Science, 15*(2), 165–187. London: Sage Publications.

Chavez, L. S., Becker, T. M., Wiggins, C. L., Key, C. R., & Samet, J. M. (1993). Alcohol-related mortality. In T. M. Becker, C. L. Wiggins, E. S. Elliott, C. R. Key, & J. M. Samet (Eds.), *Racial and ethnic patterns of mortality in New Mexico* (pp. 108–117). Albuquerque: University of New Mexico Press.

Condon, J. C. (1985). *Good neighbors.* Yarmouth, ME: Intercultural Press.

De Leon Siantz, M. (1994). The Mexican-American migrant farmworker family: Mental health issues. *Nursing Clinics of North America, 29*(1), 65–72.

Eden, S., & Aguilar, R. (1989). The Hispanic chemically dependent client: Considerations for diagnosis and treatment. In G. Lawson & A. Lawson (Eds.), *Alcoholism and substance abuse in special populations.* Rockville, MD: Aspen.

Escobebe, L. G., & Remington, P. L. (1989). Birth cohort analysis of prevalence of cigarette smoking among Hispanics in the United States. *Journal of the American Medical Association, 261*(1), 66–69.

Fernandez-Pol, J. E., Bluestone, H., Morales, G., & Mirzurchi, M. (1985). Cultural influences and alcoholism: A study of Puerto Rican Alcoholism. *Clinical and Experiential Research, 9*(5), 443–446.

Fiore, M. C., Novolny, T. T., Pierce, J. P., Hatziandrew, E. J., Patel, K. M. & Davis, R. M. (1989). Trends in cigarette smoking in the United States: The changing influence of gender and race. *Journal of American Medical Association, 261*(1), 49–55.

Gelfand D., & Bialik-Gilad (1989). Immigration reform and social work. *Social Work, 34*(1), 23–27.

Ginsberg, E. (1992). Access to health care for Hispanics. In A. Furino (Ed.), *Health policy and the Hispanic* (pp. 22–31). Boulder, CO: Westview Press.

Gladen, B., & Rogan, W. (1995). DDE and shortened duration of lactation in a northern Mexican town. *American Journal of Public Health, 85*(4), 504–508.

Harrison, M. (1994). Hobby or job: Mexican female health workers. *Health care for Women International, 15*(5), 379–412.

Harwood, A. (1981). *Ethnicity and medical care.* Cambridge: Harvard University Press.

Heusinkveld, P.(1993). *The Mexicans: An inside view of a changing society.* Worthington, OH: Renaissance Press.

Hudson, T. (1995). Cutting of care. *Hospitals and Health Networks, 69*(12), 36–40.

Jezewski, M. (1993). Culture brokering as a model for advocacy. *Nursing and Health Care, 14*(2), 78–85.

Kras, E. S. (1989). *Management in two cultures: Bridging the gap between U.S. and Mexican managers.* Yarmouth, ME: Intercultural Press.

Kuster, A. E., & Fong, C. M. (1993). Further psychometric evaluation of the Spanish language health-promoting lifestyles inventory. *Nursing Research, 42*(5), 266–269.

Larrauri, A. A., Larrauri, A. C., & Carreras, J. J. (1994). Aprendido a provenir la deshidration en comunidades alejadas y mercados [Learning to prevent dehydration in distant communities and markets]. *Social Science and Medicine, 38*(11), 1499–1507.

Levy, R. A. (1993). Ethnic and racial differences in response to medicines: Preserving individualized therapy in managed pharmaceutical programmes. *Pharmaceutical Medicine, 7,* 139–165.

Lopez, M. L. (1993). Body fatness, socioeconomic status and food stamps. *Health Values, 17*(4), 3-10.

Marin, G., Posner, S. F., & Kenyon, J. B. (1993). Role of drinking status and acculturation. *Hispanic Journal of Behavioral Science, 15*(3), 343–354.

Marshall, R. (1992). Education, productivity, and the nation's future. In A. Furino (Ed.), *Health policy and the Hispanic* (pp. 48-56). Boulder, CO: Westview Press.

Martaus, W., & Hentges, K. (1986). Mexican folk remedies and conventional medical care. *American Family Physician, 37,* 257–262.

Mendoza, F. S., Ventura, S. J., Saldivar, L., Baisden, K., & Martello, R. (1992). In A. Furino (Ed.), *Health policy and the Hispanic* (pp. 97–115). Boulder, CO: Westview Press.

Miller, N. (1989). *Women and men in a time of change: In search of gay America.* New York: Harper and Row.

Miralles, M. A. (1989). *A matter of life and death: Health seeking behaviors of Guatemalan refugees in South Florida.* New York: AMS Press.

Monrroy, L. S. (1983). Nursing care of Raza/Latino patients. In M. S. Block & L. S. A. Monrroy (Eds.), *Ethnic nursing care: A multicultural approach* (pp. 115–145). St. Louis: Mosby.

Murillo, N. (1978). The Mexican American family. In R. A. Martínez (Ed.), *Hispanic culture and health care: Fact, fiction, folklore* (pp. 3–18). St. Louis: C. V. Mosby.

Nickens, H. (1995). Role of ethnicity and social class in minority health status. *Health Services Research, 31*(1), 11–29.

Olds, S., Landon, M., & Ladewig, P. (1992). *Maternal newborn nursing: A family-centered approach* (4th ed). Redwood City, CA: Addison Wesley.

Perez-Stable, E. J., Marin, G., & Marin, B. V. (1994). Behavioral risk factors: A comparison of Latinos and non-Latino Whites in San Francisco. *American Journal of Public Health, 84*(6), 971–976.

Reinert, B. (1986). The health care beliefs and

practices of Mexican-Americans. *Home Healthcare Nurse, 4*(5), 23–31.

Rojas, S. (1994). Leadership in a multicultural society: A case in role development. *Nursing and Health Care, 15*(5), 258–261.

Romer, D., & Kim, S. (1995). Health interventions for African American and Latino youth: The potential role of mass media. *Health Education Quarterly, 22*(2), 172–189.

Sandoval, V. A. (1994). Smoking and Hispanics: Issues of identity, culture, economics, prevalence, and prevention. *Health Values, 18*(1), 44–53.

Smith, P., & Weinman, M. (1995). Cultural implications for public health policy for pregnant Hispanic adolescents. *Health Values, 19*(1), 3–9.

*Statistical Abstracts of the United States* (1995). U. S. Department of Commerce, Bureau of the Census. Washington, DC: U. S. Government Printing Office.

*Statistical Abstracts of the United States* (1992). U. S. Department of Commerce, Bureau of the Census. Washington, DC: U. S. Government Printing Office.

Stern, M. P., & Haffner, S. (1992). Type II diabetes in Mexican Americans: A public

health challenge. In A. Furino (Ed.), *Health policy and the Hispanic* (pp. 57–75). Boulder, CO: Westview Press.

Sumaya, C. V. (1992). Major infectious diseases causing excess morbidity in the Hispanic population. In A. Furino (Ed.), *Health policy and the Hispanic* (pp. 76-96). Boulder, CO: Westview Press.

Takeuchi, D., Sue, S., & Yeh, M. (1995). Ethnic mental health programs. *Journal of Public Health, 85*(5), 638–643.

Torres, S. (1994). A challenge to nursing education: Meeting the health needs of the Hispanic community. *Dean's Notes, 15*(4), 1–3.

Trevino, F. (1994). The representation of Hispanics in the health professions. *Journal of Allied Health, 23*(2), 65–77.

Villarruel, A., & Montellano B. (1992). Culture and pain: A Mesoamerican experience. *Advances in Nursing Science, 15*(1), 32–38.

Zimmerman, J. E., & Sodowsky, G. R. (1993). Influences of acculturation on Mexican-American drinking practices: Implications for counseling. *Journal of Multicultural Counseling and Development, 21*(1), 22–35.

# Navajo Indians

*Olivia Still and David Hodgins*

---

• Key terms to become familiar with in this chapter are:

Bureau of Indian Affairs
  (BIA)
Clan
Cosmology
Crystal gazers
Hand tremblers
Hogan

Indian Health Service (IHS)
Navajo neuropathy
Sand painting
Severe combined immunodeficiency
  syndrome (SCIDS)
Tribe

## OVERVIEW, INHABITED LOCALITIES, AND TOPOGRAPHY

### Overview

American Indians are the original inhabitants of North America. Although these groups are referred to as Native Americans and Alaskan Natives, many prefer to be called American Indians or names more specific to their cultural heritage. The amount of Indian blood necessary to be considered a tribal member or American Indian varies with each tribe. Navajo Indians claim the distinction of being the largest tribe that requires at least one-fourth Navajo blood to be considered a member of the tribe. Even among themselves, there is controversy concerning what constitutes an American Indian. This chapter primarily describes the cultural attributes, values, beliefs, and health-care practices of the Navajo.

The **Bureau of Indian Affairs (BIA)** recognizes over 500 different American Indian tribes that extend throughout Alaska and Canada, from Maine to Florida, and from the East Coast to the West Coast. Subdivisions of American Indians include the Plains Indians, the Pueblos, and the five civilized tribes. These five civilized tribes are further subdivided into eastern and western bands. The Pueblo, Navajo, and Apache are located in New Mexico and Arizona, whereas the Pima and Papago tribes are located in southern Arizona. Each of these American Indian cultures is unique unto itself; however, some share similar views regarding cosmology, medicine, and family organization. (See Table 17–1 for a comparison of Indian and non-Indian cultural value systems.)

The Navajo reservation is located on a high desert plateau with sparse grazing

## Table 17–1 • Comparison of Cultural Value Systems

In comparing patterns of behavior between Indian culture and non-Indian culture, one should recognize that the differences are relative and not absolute. Some of these differences are as follows:

| Tribal Traditional Cultural Values | Middle-Class, Urban Values |
| --- | --- |
| Group, clan, or tribal emphasis | Individual emphasis |
| Present oriented | Future oriented |
| Time, always with us | Time, use every minute |
| Age | Youth |
| Cooperation | Competition |
| Harmony with nature | Conquest of nature |
| Giving, sharing | Saving |
| Pragmatic | Theoretical |
| Mythology | Scientific |
| Patience | Impatience |
| Mystical | Skeptical |
| Shame | Guilt |
| Permissiveness | Social coercion |
| Extended family and clan | Immediate family |
| Nonaggressive | Aggressive |
| Modest | Overconfident |
| Silence | Noise |
| Respect others' religion | Convert others to religion |
| Religion, way of life | Religion, a segment of life |
| Land, water, forest belong to all | Land, etc., a private domain |
| Beneficial, reasonable use of resource | Avarice, greedy use of resource |

*Source:* Sando, Joe S. (1976). *Pueblo Indians.* San Francisco: Indian Historian Press, with permission.

due to very poor soil. Water, often scarce, is a valuable commodity. Sometimes, individuals have to haul water obtained from natural springs or windmills for long distances.

## Heritage and Residence

The Navajo, the largest American Indian **tribe,** consists of approximately 200,000 persons and has one of the largest reservations in the United States, covering portions of Arizona, Utah, and New Mexico (Rose, 1993). In New Mexico, the Navajo are scattered in settlements intermingled with the Zuni Indians and Mormon settlers. The Navajo Indians are nomadic and wander great distances searching for adequate grazing grounds for their sheep. Their **cosmology** states that they came from the lower world, the black world full of demons, and entered the fourth world, the present turquoise world. Thus, the value of the turquoise stone is established as an important reminder of their beliefs (Spector, 1991). In addition, animals play a vital role in Navajo mythology. For example, the coyote is considered a trickster who plays pranks on other animals and humans.

## Reasons for Migration and Associated Economic Factors

In the early 1800s, many American Indian tribes were forced to migrate or were contained in forts by the military (Irwin, 1992). Many Navajo were gathered and contained in Fort Sill in Oklahoma. Because of the proximity of the eastern reservation to major cities, these Navajos had earlier contact with Western civilizations. The earliest governmental agencies, trading centers, schools, and roads were in the eastern reservation. The western reservation remained isolated until the last 15 to 20 years. When the Navajos were released from Fort Sill, they returned to the eastern reservation, where many remained, but others returned to the western location.

Because of severe economic conditions and high unemployment, significant migration occurs into and out of the reservations. Commercial activities on reservations are limited to businesses owned by American Indians or partnerships in which an American Indian must own the controlling interest. On some reservations, the business owner must be from the same tribe, whereas on other reservations, other groups may not own any interest in a business. Such restrictions severely limit employment. Occasionally big businesses contract with the reservation for mining, timbering, and electrical power services. These companies usually employ Navajo residents to the maximum extent possible.

Most Indians from the western and northern tribes tend to remain on the reservation. Many of those who leave the reservation experience culture shock resulting from a rapid and drastic change in their environment. They usually return because of lack of social support systems and loss of identity and self-esteem (Wilson, 1987). Many Indians return to their reservation on a regular basis to refresh and renew themselves.

In contrast to the poor economic environment of some tribes, an unusual example is the Osage tribe in Oklahoma, who have oil leases. Each tribal member has head rights and receives an income from these leases. More recently, to increase revenues on reservations, many tribes have instituted gaming in the form of bingo, poker, black jack, video poker, and slot machines. The Navajo are reluctant to participate in these activities and have vetoed gaming. While gaming brings revenue, the problems associated with gaming have caused the Navajo to reject it.

## Educational Status and Occupations

Educational levels for American Indians are lower than those of similar populations, creating another barrier to employment. American Indians have consistently been identified as the most underrepresented of all minority groups in colleges and universities. Before the 1970s, an increase occurred in educational achievement among American Indians; however, since then there has been a downward curve (Preito, 1989). Overall, 55.3 percent of American Indians have completed high school (Discharry, 1986.)

Traditional educational values for most American Indians are reflected in learning the tribal culture and clarifying their roles in the **clan** and the community. Competitiveness is generally discouraged among American Indian populations. In contrast to some other cultures, the American Indian culture views group activities as more important than individual accomplishments. With few support systems from American society, many American Indians quit school and return to the reservation, even in the face of severe economic difficulties. An additional practice that influenced poor educational achievement was the past practice of the BIA that took children from their parents and placed them in boarding schools where many were forbidden to speak their native language.

Occupations selected by American Indians vary, and the health-care field severely lacks Navajos. Nursing is perceived as an undesirable profession because Navajo beliefs consider it inadvisable to be around sick people. Additionally, since the culture of nursing is based on middle-class values related to competition, it is difficult for American Indian students to adjust in the nursing environment (Crow, 1993). As a result, the need for American Indian workers to staff hospitals and other health-care facilities remains high. Navajos choosing to work in a hospital must sometimes have a special cleansing ceremony to protect themselves (Wilson, 1987). Many American Indian students choose careers as social workers, laborers, artists, and weavers.

Art is an important occupation and takes such forms as rug weaving, basket weaving, pottery making, and bead work. Rug weaving and jewelry making are the most common forms of art among the Navajo. They are also noted for **sand painting,** and many of their sand paintings have been available on the market for years. Traditionally, sand paintings were used in healing ceremonies by medicine persons and not intended for sale. Original sand paintings, created on the hogan floor, were gathered and returned to the earth (Personal communication with Medicine Man, Coho, August 1994).

## COMMUNICATIONS

### Dominant Language and Dialects

The dominant language varies with each American Indian tribe. The Navajo language was not reduced to writing until the 1970s; consequently, most elderly Navajo speak only their native language and few are literate. The few elderly Navajo who are bilingual, speak limited Spanish or English. The younger populations are usually bilingual, with their native tongue being spoken primarily in the home. Both the Navajo and Zuni tribes had assistance from non–American Indians in developing the written form of their language.

Dialects also differ among tribes. The Navajo and the Apache have similar dialects and are able to understand one another to a limited extent. These dialects are similar to variations in English found among the northern and southern regions in the United States. Even though a common language is spoken, the tribes have difficulty understanding one another related to regional accents and the use of slang expressions. The health-care provider must be extremely careful when attempting to use an American Indian dialect, because minor variations in pronunciation may change the entire meaning of a word or phrase. Differences in pronunciation, particularly while speaking with an elderly Navajo, may cause a misunderstanding. Such misunderstandings make subsequent caring for the individual difficult. Thus, it is often safer to use an interpreter.

Talking loudly among Navajo Indians is considered rude. When American Indians talk outside their group, voice tones are quiet, but not monotone. Their language is full of inflections with different meanings, making the language melodious with a quiet volume.

### Cultural Communication Patterns

Nonverbal communication styles have different connotations within each tribe. For example, the willingness of Indians to share their thoughts and feelings varies from group to group and from individual to individual. In addition, there is no set pattern regarding their willingness to share tribal ceremonies. However, suspicion always exists because earlier governments and church groups banned tribal ceremonies and events. Navajos generally do not share inner thoughts and feelings with anyone outside their clan. It sometimes takes nontribal health-care providers a long time to build trust with American Indians.

Navajo Indians are comfortable with long periods of silence. Interest in what an individual says is shown through attentive listening skills. Chisolm (1983) reported that to establish a positive social relationship, the rule of silence is considered a serious matter that calls for caution, careful judgment, and plenty of time. It is important to allow time for elderly Navajo to respond to questions. Failing to allow adequate time for information processing may result in an inaccurate response or no response (Wilson, 1987). One may be considered immature if answers are given quickly or one interrupts another who is forming a response.

The elderly Navajo are more somber and less likely to laugh aloud except in family settings. For example, a nurse complained, "I don't know why the family comes in here for they only sit there. They don't even say a word to the person and then they get up and walk out." What this nurse failed to realize was that they were supporting the individual, not through talking, but just by being present. The nurse's view reflects her cultural bias that saying something is essential for demonstrating support, but in reality, for American Indians, silence is being supportive. An awareness of nonverbal communication is extremely helpful for the health-care provider who wishes to establish a mutually satisfying relationship.

Touch among the Navajo is unacceptable unless one knows the person very well. In some tribes, touch is very important because many forms of traditional medicine involve massaging and rubbing by the traditional healer, a family member, or both. However, if a Western health-care provider were to do this within the context of treatment, it would not be permissible. If contact is made, it is in the form of a handshake. Close observation of body language is very important for determining cues and the permissibility of touch.

In the Navajo tribe, shaking hands is the traditional greeting. However, their handshake is different from that of other populations where a firm handshake is expected. In the Navajo world, the handshake is light, more of a passing of the hands. This type of handshake in the European-American society is known as a "dead fish handshake." Traditionally, Navajo's greet by saying *Yay ta hey*, literally translated as "all is well" or "it is well," and by shaking hands.

Among the Navajo, it is considered rude for people to point with their fingers. Rather than pointing a finger to indicate a direction, individuals shift their lips toward the desired direction. Seeing this nonverbal behavior for the first time can be puzzling for non–American Indian health-care providers.

Physical distance between conversants differs among friends and strangers. One quickly learns that the acceptable personal space for American Indians is much greater than that of most European-American cultures.

Direct eye contact is considered rude and possibly confrontational for Navajo. Even close friends do not maintain eye contact, and this rule does not change with socioeconomic status. This is in direct opposition to some other populations where maintaining direct eye contact is essential to trust.

The American Indian is often referred to as having a deadpan expression. This is only true with strangers and not among their own group, where smiling and laughing are quite common. However, in unfamiliar settings, behaviors may be different.

## Temporal Relationships

The time sequences of importance for American Indians are present, past, and future in comparison with the time sequences important to most European-Americans, which are present, future, and past (Burke, Kisilevsky, & Maloney, 1989). Most American Indian tribes are not future oriented. Very little planning is done for the future because their view is that many things are outside of the individual's control and may affect or change the future. In fact, the Navajo language does not include a future tense verb. Time is not viewed as a constant or something that one can control, but rather as something that is always with the individual. Thus, to plan for the future is sometimes viewed as foolish. Past events are an important part of the American Indian's heritage as evidenced in verbal histories passed down from generation to generation. The present is addressed as a here-and-now issue.

The term *Indian time* has little meaning in a European-American worldview, but it assumes particular importance for those who supervise an American Indian workforce, where time has no meaning or importance. Events do not always start on time, but rather time starts when the group gathers. To help prevent frustration in scheduling events, time factors need to be taken into consideration and the speaker made aware of these unique time perceptions. Appointments may not always be kept, especially if someone else in the clan needs help.

## Format for Names

Elderly persons are addressed as grandmother or grandfather, or mother or father by members in their clan. Otherwise, they are called by a nickname. A health-care provider can call an older Navajo client "grandmother" or "grandfather" as a sign of respect.

## FAMILY ROLES AND ORGANIZATION

### Head of Household and Gender Roles

The Navajo society and most other American Indian tribes are matrilineal in nature. The land is not owned, but grazing rights are passed from mothers to daughters. While men are seen as important, the grandmothers and mothers are at the center of Indian society. In Navajo tradition, the relationship between brother and sister is often more important than the relationship between husband and wife. These defined roles have been maintained over centuries. Some tribes are bilineal and share equally in the decision making. When providing family care, it is important to note that no decision is made until the appropriate elderly woman is present. If the health-care provider does not find the appropriate gatekeeper, time is lost and the problem must be addressed again at a later time.

Traditionally, Navajo men are expected to care for the livestock, the corral, and the fields. Men move with their sheep grazing over large areas. Women care for and stay close to the hogan, are independent, and often weave. In recent times, changes from traditional roles have created stress and cultural disintegration as some family members have migrated off the reservation.

## Prescriptive, Restrictive, and Taboo Behaviors for Children and Adolescents

Children are looked on with joy and proudly welcomed into the family. Ritual ceremonies and practices occur at various stages for both children and adolescents. Even though children may be named at birth, their names are not revealed until their first laugh, when they are considered to officially have a soul and self-identity. This protects the children and keeps them in tune with the Holy People. The "first laugh ceremony" is celebrated with food, which encourages the child to be a generous individual. Anthropologists believe that the tradition of not naming the infant until this time came about because of high infant mortality in the past.

During the cradleboard phase of childrearing, infants are kept in the cradleboard (Box 17–1) until they begin walking (Arthur, 1976). The cradleboard protects them when they start to crawl and is introduced to siblings and inattentive adults. How-

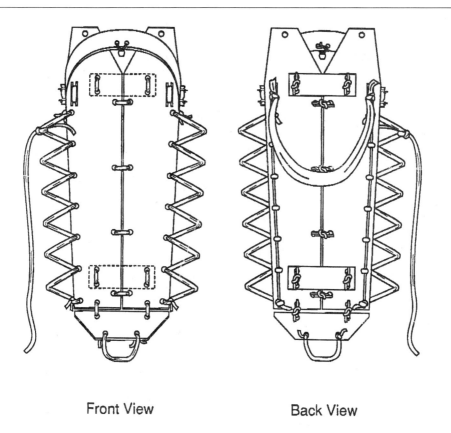

**Front View**        **Back View**

**Box 17–1.** Navajo Cradleboard, *Awee Ts'aal*

Each tribe has its own name for a cradleboard; the Navajo name is *awee ts'aal*. It is still used extensively as a baby carrier and protects the infant from falls and from exposure to the elements. Most Navajo infants like the secure feeling it provides and fuss when they are not laced into their cradleboard.

Years ago, when infant mortality was much higher, cradleboards were improvised and thrown away if the infant died. If the child survived and grew, a second and better cradleboard was made and then a third and even better one. This indicated that the child had survived for a long time. The fourth and final cradleboard was used until the baby outgrew it.

Today, not all Navajos use cradleboards, and if they do, they use only one—the fourth type—from birth onward. The father of the infant is supposed to construct it, selecting cottonwood or pine for the two back boards. These are laced together and cut into a V shape. A piece of the same wood is added at the bottom for a footrest to symbolize that the infant is resting its feet on Mother Earth. The baby's head is protected by a piece of oak, which is bent into a bow to form the headpiece. This represents a rainbow, and when the baby is placed in the cradleboard, it is said to be "under the rainbow."

The carrier is arranged in the following way: The infant is laid on a blanket on top $of the cradleboard; the blanket is then folded around the child, with its arms at its sides. There are loops along the sides of the cradleboard through which a lacing strip of buckskin is drawn to fasten the infant into the carrier. The lacings represent lightning, another element in the world surrounding the child. Finally, a cloth is draped over the top of the board to shield the baby while it is sleeping. The cradleboard represents the maleness and femaleness inside all of us as well as the elements of the universe that surround us.

ever, hip dysplasia may be exacerbated by the cradleboards. In recent years, the use of diapers has decreased the incidence of hip dysplasia because diapers bind the hips in a slightly abducted position.

The postcradleboard period consists of weaning, toilet training, and disciplining, which is frequently left to the grandmother. Thus, the language and culture are well entrenched as traditions are passed to grandchildren (Arthur, 1976). If the grandmother is unavailable, an aunt or a sister assumes this role. Weaning is started during this phase if the mother is pregnant. However, if the mother is not pregnant, weaning is more gradual.

Navajo women in the past almost exclusively practiced breast-feeding, but within the last 15 to 20 years, the use of formula has become popular. As a result, an increased incidence of bottle caries has been observed among Navajo children, because many babies go to bed with a bottle of juice or soda pop. This practice causes children to lose their teeth by the age of 4 years. One health promotion priority is to educate parents about this early cause of dental caries and to encourage a return to breast-feeding.

A primary social premise is that no person has the right to speak for another (Phillips & Lobar, 1990). Thus, Navajo children are frequently allowed to make decisions that other cultures might consider irresponsible. For example, children may be allowed to decide if they want to take their medicine. This practice may present an ethical concern for some health-care providers. Such practices support perceptions among health-care providers that children are undisciplined. Children who do not listen to their parents or elders accept the consequences regardless of their age. As clients, Navajo children are usually shy and wary of strangers.

An important ceremonial ritual in Navajo society for teenage girls is the onset of menarche, which is celebrated with special foods that symbolize passage into adulthood. Men are usually excluded from this celebration, with only aunts and grandmothers participating. Some tribes have a specific rite of passage for males, but the Navajo do not. Older children may be more comfortable with physical closeness rather than actual contact. In addition, older children are taught to be stoic and uncomplaining.

## Family Roles and Priorities

Family goals are a priority in the American Indian culture. Family bonds remain strong, even after marriage joins the couple with another family. When a couple marries in the Zuni tribe, it is the man who goes to live in the female's house. In Navajo tradition, families have separate dwellings but are grouped together by familial relationships. The Navajo family unit consists of the nuclear family and relatives such as sisters, aunts, and their female descendants. Family goals do not center on wealth or the attainment of possessions. In fact, if one person has more wealth than other relatives, the member who has more has a responsibility to assist relatives who have less.

The elderly Navajo are looked on with clear deference. A man with many dependents, though poor, is listened to with respect (Phillips & Lobar, 1990). The elderly Navajo play an important role in the keeping of rituals and in instructing children and grandchildren. Even though the elderly are respected, elder neglect is on the rise, possibly due to the increased survival of individuals with chronic disease and improved longevity. Younger adults are faced with the responsibility of caring for relatives over a longer period of time. In addition, there are few nursing homes, and hospitals are forced to keep patients until a nursing home placement is found (Hobus, 1990). When nursing home placement is found, it may be at a great distance from the family, making it difficult for family visits. Hence, elders are often taken from the nursing home, even though the family is not in a position to care for their needs. Patients end up being readmitted to the hospital and a revolving door syndrome develops.

Extended family members are important in Navajo society, particularly the mother's family. A sister's children are considered the same as her own children. If a mother dies or for some other reason cannot care for her children, it is assumed that the grandmother or sister will raise the children as her own.

Social status is determined by age and life experiences. Generally, individuals are discouraged from having more than their peers, and those who display more material wealth are ignored. Status derives from not standing out in the clan or tribe.

## Alternative Lifestyles

Alternative lifestyles are not discussed among the Navajo. However, special individuals exist who are not looked on with disfavor, but rather are accepted as being different. In Zuni society and some northern tribes, some men take on women's roles. There are no pressures for them to change. Single-parent households are becoming more prevalent and are an accepted practice, with family members providing assistance with childrearing. It is common for a mother to have children from different fathers.

## WORKFORCE ISSUES

### Culture in the Workplace

Many American Indians remain traditional in their practice of religious activities. Navajo are compelled to attend these ceremonies and often must take time from work to do so. For example, the burial ceremony of the Zuni requires individuals to take off 3 days from work. During this time, they should not have contact with small children or bathe. The needs of the individual must be weighed against organizational requirements in the development of a reasonable solution. Many persons in the community function informally as cultural brokers and assist by helping non–American Indian staff to understand important cultural issues. Sensitivity on the part of the employer is of utmost importance. The Indian Health Service (IHS) has developed a method for addressing these needs. Besides allowing employees to use annual leave, employees may earn religious compensatory time. Respected non-Indian staff on the reservation are those persons who are sensitive to American Indian cultural issues. The American Indian staff reciprocate this respect during traditional European-American holidays.

European-Americans who are upset or in conflict often want to talk through the issue that has caused the conflict. This may not be the case with the American Indian. Many American Indians avoid persons with whom they are in conflict. A persistence to deal immediately with the conflict causes additional ill feelings. This may continue to the point that the American Indian loses his temper and expresses anger toward the other person. The European-American, in the eyes of the American Indian, exhibits rude behavior by continuing to press for resolution. The American Indian method of resolving anger and conflict among themselves is much different. If one tribal member has a disagreement with another, that member does not address the second party face to face. Rather the member tells a third person, who then relays the information to the second party. The conflict is resolved through a third-party compromise.

## Issues Related to Autonomy

Group activities are an important norm in the Navajo culture. One individual should not be singled out for answering a question because one's mistakes are generally not forgotten by the group. For example, if an individual is quick to answer and is wrong, the entire group laughs. Later, the group talks about the mistake and again laughs about it. Conversely, when remarks are made concerning an individual without group participation, revenge may be sought in a passive-aggressive manner. The transgression is not forgotten. Conversely, in American society, mistakes may be forgiven as an acceptable method of learning as long as the mistakes are not repeated. Administrators who respect these differences are more effective.

This concept is also true in the classroom. The instructor who allows adequate time for observation has a greater chance of success with American Indian students. Improved success is achieved if the American Indian is allowed to observe the task several times before being asked to demonstrate it. Their first effort at completing the task in front of a group should occur without error. This is especially true when delivering care to their own people. Mistakes made are discussed in the community. Because educational levels may be low, work assignments should be made in clear concrete terms.

Issues of superior-subordinate roles exist related to age. Younger supervisors may not be respected because they are not perceived as possessing the life experiences necessary to lead. In like situations, major decisions are made by the group with the assistance of the group leader, who is generally the senior female. Thus, a young male manager on the reservation may face resistance when attempting to direct a work group.

Because English is not their primary language, one must often allow extra time for a verbal response from most Navajo. This extra time is required to think about a response and translate it into their language. When translating from the native Indian language into English, adjectives and adverbs sometimes follow the noun or verb, making it appear that the person is speaking backwards.

Most American Indian students are not good test takers, which poses a special problem. Although the individual may have the knowledge necessary to complete an examination, the translation of the knowledge into written form is especially difficult. When tested verbally on the same material, students pass the examination. To the extent possible, examinations that consist of return demonstration and that do not use abstract terminology are preferred. Thus, in the ethnocultural context of teaching Navajo students and staff, actions should be directed toward assisting, supporting, or enabling the individual or group to improve a human condition or way of life (Leininger, 1988).

# BIOCULTURAL ECOLOGY

## Skin Color and Biologic Variations

Skin color among American Indians varies from light brown to very dark brown depending on the tribe. To assess for oxygenation in darker-skinned people, the health-care professional must examine the client's mucous membranes and nailbeds for capillary refill. Anemia is detected by examining the mucous membranes for pallor and the skin for a grayish hue. To assess for jaundice, it is necessary to examine the sclera rather than to rely on skin hue. Newborns and infants commonly have Mongolian spots on the sacral area. Health-care professionals unfamiliar with this trait may mistake these spots for bruises and suspect child abuse.

Each of the American Indian tribes has varying degrees of Asian traits. In facial appearance, the Athabascan tribes such as the Navajo are Asian appearing with epithelial folds over the eyes. The Navajo are generally taller and thinner than other American Indian tribes. The Navajo have traditionally been good runners and excel in relay races and long-distance running. The health-care provider must remember that these characteristics are not seen with everyone; variations in this population do exist.

# Diseases and Health Conditions

The water on the Navajo reservation is often impure and unchlorinated, making those who drink it susceptible to water-borne bacteria such as shigella. Some notable risk factors are related to the topography of the Navajo reservation: *Salmonella* is common because of the lack of refrigeration, and hypothermia because of frequent snow storms and conditions that limit their ability to gather wood. For example, most of the dirt roads quickly become impassable with rain or snow.

Common diseases related to living in close contact with others include upper respiratory illnesses and acute otitis media (U.S. Department of Health, 1995). In the 1950s, many families suffered from tuberculosis, but more recent cases are related to isolated family groups. Other health problems include the plague, tick fever, and recently the Muerto Canyon Hanta virus. Many of these illnesses are due to the area's rodent population, consisting of prairie dogs and deer mice.

Type I diabetes mellitus is almost nonexistent in American Indians; however, type II diabetes mellitus is the third most prevalent disease affecting all American Indian tribes. In 1993, the IHS and tribal clinics recorded almost 280,000 outpatient visits for diabetes (U.S. Department of Health, 1995). The incidence of diabetes varies among tribes. The Zuni have the highest rate, approaching 25 percent, with the Papago and Navajo following closely behind. Poor control and dietary compliance is associated with major long-term complications such as blindness and kidney failure (Huse et al., 1989). These complications in American Indians occur at a greater rate than in European-American populations.

Because of the prevalence of diabetes among Indians, Congress has delegated funds exclusively for diabetes research and education in this population. The National Institute for Health and the diabetes team at Zuni is presently engaged in research with high school students to determine the age of onset of type II diabetes (Stracqualursi et al, 1993). Thus far, the youngest one is aged 13 years; however, controversy exists over whether this case is type I or type II diabetes.

Historically, most diseases affecting American Indians were infectious diseases. In the past, contact with settlers who had communicable diseases wiped out entire tribes because they had no acquired immunity for some infectious diseases common among other American populations.

Cardiovascular diseases are on the increase among the Navajo. The incidence of myocardial infarction, nearly nonexistent until recent times, is increasing as is the incidence of renal disease and gallbladder disease.

Studies with the Navajo have identified a high incidence of **severe combined immunodeficiency syndrome (SCIDS),** an immunodeficiency syndrome unrelated to AIDS, that results in a failure of the antibody response and cell-mediated immunity (World Health Organization Scientific Group, 1986). An epidemiological study is underway to determine the prevalence of SCIDS in the Navajo population (Jones et al., 1991). Factors being examined include space, time, pedigree, and immunologic status. Affected infants who survive initially are sent to tertiary care facilities. Survivors must receive gamma globulin on a regular basis until a bone marrow transplant can be performed. Thus far, studies indicate that SCIDS is unique to this Navajo population.

**Navajo neuropathy,** researched on two separate occasions since 1974, is also unique to this population. Characteristics of this disease include poor weight gain, short stature, sexual infantilism, serious systemic infections, and liver derangement. Manifestations include weakness, hypotonia, areflexia, loss of sensation in the extremities, corneal ulcerations, acral mutilation, and painless fractures (Singleton et al., 1990). Sural nerve biopsies show a nearly complete absence of myelinated fibers, which is different from other neuropathies that present a gradual demyelination process. Individuals who survive have many complications and are generally ventilator dependent. None have been known to survive past the age of 24 years.

Albinism occurs in the Navajo and Pueblo tribes. An additional disease that affects Navajos who live in the Rainbow Grand Canyon area is genetically prone blindness that develops in individuals during their late teens to early 20s. Many of these hereditary and genetic diseases are believed to result from a limited gene pool. As a result of the increased availability of Western medicines, improved sanitary conditions, increased community surveillance, early case finding, and improved education (Mail, Mckay, & Katz, 1989), survival has increased and chronic diseases related to lifestyle are surfacing.

## Variations in Drug Metabolism

Research has documented adverse reactions to medication in Navajo populations (Hodgins & Still, 1989). Lidocaine reactions occur in 29 percent of the Navajo population as compared with 11 to 15 percent of European-Americans. Little research has been completed that distinguishes absorption differences of specific medications in American Indian populations.

## HIGH-RISK BEHAVIORS

Most American Indian tribes exhibit high-risk behaviors related to alcohol abuse, along with its subsequent morbidity and mortality (Mail, Mckay, & Katz, 1989). Alcohol use is more prevalent than any other form of chemical abuse. Health problems related to alcoholism include motor vehicle accidents, homicides, suicides, and cirrhosis (U.S. Department of Health, Education, and Welfare, 1991). Many accidents are attributed to drinking while driving. Although alcohol is illegal on most reservations, alcohol is purchased off the reservation by many, and bootleggers make money selling alcohol on reservations at grossly inflated prices. The northern tribes living on the Rosebud Sioux reservation have a higher alcoholism rate than most other American Indian tribes. This is often attributed to an unemployment rate of 50 percent among these tribes.

Spouse abuse is common and is frequently related to alcohol use. The wife is the usual recipient of the abuse, but occasionally the husband is abused. Emergency rooms have documented cases of husbands being beaten by their wives with baseball bats in response to their drinking. The effects of alcohol abuse are also evidenced in newborns as fetal alcohol syndrome, in teenagers as pregnancies and sexually transmitted diseases, and in adults as liver failure.

Although smoking is not as prevalent as in some other cultures, the use of smokeless tobacco has steadily increased among teenagers and those in their early 20s. Cocaine is rarely used by Navajo Indians because of its high cost and limited accessibility.

Suicide is becoming more prevalent among the adolescent population. Attempted drug overdoses occur in an effort to get even with or back at someone. In Tuba City, two sisters decided to commit suicide together because they felt there was no alternative to their present life.

Acquired immunodeficiency syndrome, thus far, has not presented a major problem on the Navajo reservation. However, health officials believe that when it does occur, it will spread rapidly because there are high rates of other sexually transmitted diseases in Navajo communities. To help combat these diseases, an increased emphasis on community-based programs has been initiated to provide improved education for adults and teenagers (Mail, Mckay, & Katz, 1989).

## Health-care Practices

A number of programs among the Navajo promote public awareness and encouragement for positive health-seeking behaviors. These include programs encouraging seat belt and helmet use for those who bicycle or ride motorcycles. Unfortunately, the success of these programs has been limited. Seat belts are required by state law as well as by tribal law enforcement agencies. Although many adults comply with these laws, noncompliance is high among younger Indians. Unfortunately, children are often permitted to ride in the back of open trucks, resulting in serious and sometimes fatal injuries when they fall off or are thrown from the vehicle.

The Zuni have a model wellness program that encourages healthy behaviors. This program also promotes runs, relay races, and aerobic classes (Heath et al., 1987). The Navajo have visited this program in an attempt to develop a similar program. The younger generation has responded well to wellness programs. However, promoting these programs among the elderly tribal members has met with limited success.

# NUTRITION
## Meaning of Food

Food has major significance beyond nourishment in American Indian populations; it is offered to family and friends or may be burned to feed higher powers and those who have died (Discharry, 1986). Life events are celebrated with food. Food is the center of all dances and many healing and religious ceremonies.

The importance of food is evident when a family sponsors a dance. Sponsors of this event are expected to feed the participants and their entire families. Food preparation takes several days. Women cook large amounts of food, which may include green chili stew, mutton, and fry bread, cooked over an outdoor fireplace.

## Common Foods and Food Rituals

Sheep are a major source of meat, and sheep brains are considered a delicacy by the Navajo. Traditionally, in sheep camps where the herds are tended, food is limited to what can be cooked outside. Fry bread and mutton are cooked in lard. Access to fresh fruits or vegetables is minimal except during the fall. Squash is common at harvest time.

In years past, it was taboo for the Navajo to eat chicken. This is no longer the case, and now chicken is an integral part of their diet. In fact, chicken is so popular that commercial fast-food chicken establishments have emerged on the Navajo reservation. A concurrent increased incidence of gallbladder disease is attributed to this dietary practice. Clients as young as 11 years old are having cholecystectomies.

Corn is an important staple in the diet of Navajo and other American Indian tribes. Rituals such as the green corn dance of the Cherokees and harvest time rituals for the Zuni surround the use of corn. Corn pollen is used in the Blessingway and many other ceremonies by the Navajo.

## Dietary Practices for Health Promotion

Food is not generally associated with promoting health or illness among the Navajo. The establishment of diabetic projects in all American Indian service units has prompted teaching that integrates the optimal selection, preparation, and quantities of native foods to encourage good health habits. This is especially important for elderly tribal members, who are less likely to change their diets but may be willing to change methods of preparation or amounts eaten. Herbs are used in the treatment of many illness to cleanse the body of ill spirits or poisons.

## Nutritional Deficiencies and Food Limitations

American Indian diets may be deficient in vitamin D because many individuals suffer from lactose intolerance or do not drink milk. Many individuals in the Navajo tribe and some other isolated tribes lack electricity for refrigeration. Therefore, they have difficulty storing fresh vegetables or milk. Malnutrition, such as kwashiorkor and marasmus, occurred in the Navajo as late as the 1960s and 1970s (Schaefer, 1977). After some ceremonies, individuals may not eat salt or particular foods. For example, during initiation into some American Indian societies, young boys have a restricted diet. It is important for the health-care provider to assess whether a ceremony has been recently performed and ask if there are specific food restrictions.

## PREGNANCY AND CHILDBEARING PRACTICES

### Fertility Practices and Views toward Pregnancy

Traditional American Indians do not practice birth control and, thus, do not limit the size of their families. The birth rate among American Indians is 96 percent higher than the birth rate in the overall U.S. population. Large families are looked on favorably because, in times past, many children died at an early age. Survival rates of American Indian children have greatly improved within the last few years.

In the past, many traditional Navajo women did not seek prenatal care because pregnancy was not considered an illness. Today, more pregnant women seek prenatal care at IHS facilities. Health-care providers can improve the health of Navajo women and children by encouraging prenatal care. (See Table 17–2 for a cultural nursing intervention assessment tool for expectant Navajo women.)

Twins are not looked on favorably and are frequently believed to be the work of a witch, in which case one of the babies must die. Recent observations reveal that this no longer happens, but sometimes the mother may have difficulty caring for two infants. For example, twins may be readmitted to the hospital for neglect and failure to thrive. In such instances, culturally sensitive counseling assists adoption. Despite a social worker's assistance, some mothers may not be able to cope with twins, and eventually tribal members adopt the children.

### Prescriptive, Restrictive, and Taboo Practices in the Childbearing Family

Arthur (1976) described Navajo pregnancy ceremonies, taboos, and herbal medicine practices in the prebirth phase of pregnancy recognition. In this phase, the extended family and community assists the mother in recognizing the pregnancy as a reality. During the precradleboard phase, a **hogan** is designated for the birth and a religious practitioner ties to the hogan a red sash for a girl and a buckskin rope for a boy. These are used to give the mother support during delivery. At this time, the pregnant woman becomes one with Mother Earth, Father Sky, and the Universe with the Holy People; therefore, she is actually reliving the creation plan of humankind (Arthur, 1976). It is especially important to adhere to the many prescriptive and restrictive taboo practices related to pregnancy, which involve both husband and wife. See Table 17–3, Navajo Taboos Regarding Expectant Women, and Table 17–4, Taking Care of Yourself during Pregnancy: Navajo Rules for Expectant Couples, which were developed by Urusla Wilson in 1987.

Many Navajo women are reluctant to deliver their babies in a hospital setting. They know that people have died in hospitals and thus perceive that pregnant women should not be around the dead or in a place where people have died. To provide culturally competent care, many facilities, with the assistance of individuals

## Table 17–2 • Nursing Care and Beliefs of Expectant Navajo Women: Cultural Nursing Intervention Assessment Tool

1. Do you want blood, urine, or other specimens returned?
   __ Yes __ No  Comments:

2. Do you wish to use herbs during labor and after delivery?
   __ Yes __ No  Comments:

3. According to your beliefs, what foods are you not allowed to eat?

4. During labor, would you like a medicine woman present to perform a ceremony if necessary?
   __ Yes __ No  Comments:

5. During labor, do you want your long hair braided?
   __ Yes __ No  Comments:

6. During labor, what position do you want to deliver in?
   __ Squatting position    __ Lying-down position
   __ Side-lying position   __ Use stirrups
   __ Any position that is comfortable for me
   Comments:

7. During labor, do you want to use the sash belt to hold onto for delivery?
   __ Yes __ No  Comments:

8. Who will be with you during labor and delivery?

9. After delivery, do you or someone in your family want to massage the baby?
   __ Yes __ No  Comments:

10. Do you want to save the afterbirth (placenta)?
    __ Yes __ No  Comments:

11. Do you want to save the baby's umbilical cord?
    __ Yes __ No  Comments:

12. After delivery, do you want to save the baby's first stool?
    __ Yes __ No  Comments:

13. Do you want to __ breast-feed or __ formula feed your baby? If you want to do both ways of feeding, please tell us the reason?

14. What kinds of things do you expect nurses to do for you during labor and delivery?

*Source:* Ursula Wilson, *July 1987.* IHS inservice seminar, Tuba City Indian Health Center, Tuba City, AZ, with permission.

like Ursula Wilson, are reinstituting more traditional American Indian methods of birthing into the hospital setting. These adaptations include birthing rooms that are more acceptable to Navajo women. The blending of Western traditional methods with American Indian practices has greatly improved the health care of American Indian women.

During the labor process, birthing necklaces made of juniper seeds and beads

### Table 17–3 • Navajo Taboos Regarding Expectant Women

1. Don't wear two hats at once; you'll have twins (or two wives).
2. Don't hit babies in the mouth; they'll be stubborn and slow to talk.
3. Don't have a weaving comb (rug) with more than five points; your baby will have extra fingers.
4. Don't have a baby cross its fingers; its mother will have another one right away.
5. Don't swallow gum while you are pregnant; the baby will have a birthmark.
6. Don't kill animals while your wife is pregnant; the baby will look like a bird.
7. Don't stand in the doorway when a pregnant woman is present.
8. Don't make a sling shot while you are pregnant; the baby will be crippled.
9. Don't go to ceremonies while pregnant; it will have a bad effect on the baby.
10. Don't eat a lot of sweet stuff while you are pregnant; the baby won't be strong.
11. Don't sleep too much when you are about to have a baby; the baby will mark your face with dark spots.
12. Don't look at a dead person or animal while you are pregnant; the baby will be sickly because of bad luck.
13. Don't jump around if you are pregnant or ride a horse; it will induce labor.
14. Don't cut gloves off at the knuckles, the baby will have short round fingers.
15. Don't cut a baby's hair when it is small; it won't think right when it gets older.
16. Don't put on a Yei mask while your wife is pregnant; the baby will have a big head and look strange.
17. Don't let a baby's head stay to one side in the cradle board; it will have a wide head.
18. Don't watch or look at an accident while your wife is present; it will affect the baby.
19. Don't sew on a saddle while your wife is pregnant; it will ruin the baby's mouth.

*Source: Ursula Wilson, July 1987. IHS inservice seminar, Tuba City Indian Health Center, Tuba City, AZ, with permission.*

are worn by the mother to assist with a safe birth. Woven belts or sashes are used to help push the baby out (see Table 17–4). This practice is also used by Navajo midwives in caring for their clients.

A taboo practice among the Navajo is purchasing clothes for an infant before birth. Outsiders may interpret this practice as the mother not wanting the baby. In reality, preparing for the baby before birth is forbidden by Indian tradition.

Many different rituals related to postpartum care exist for each tribe. Table 17–4 lists some Navajo taboos during the postpartum period. The cultural assessment tool (see Table 17–2) developed by Ursula Wilson can be adapted to the practices of other tribes to acknowledge general American Indian beliefs and values regarding labor and delivery.

Immediately after birth, the placenta is buried as a symbol of the child being tied to the land. Sometimes it is buried by a fire. This is considered a safe place because fire is sacred and protects the baby against evil spirits. After birth, the baby is given a mixture with juniper bark to cleanse its insides and rid it of mucus. In addition, a ceremonial food of corn pollen and boiled water is given. Corn symbolizes healthy nutrients and an enduring nature.

## DEATH RITUALS

### Death Rituals and Expectations

Death rituals vary among tribes. The body must go into the afterlife as whole as possible. In some tribes, amputated limbs are given to the family for a separate burial. These limbs are later exhumed and buried with the body. The Navajo do not bury the body for approximately 4 days after death. A cleansing ceremony must be performed after an individual dies or the spirit of the dead person may try to assume control of someone else's spirit. Frequently, family members are reluctant to deal

**Table 17–4 • Taking Care of Yourself during Pregnancy: Navajo Rules for Expectant Couples**

### DURING PRENATAL PERIOD

**Mind/Soul**

**Do's**
· Keep the peace
· Keep thoughts good
· Talk with "corn pollen sprinkled" words
· Say morning (dawn prayers)
· Have shielding prayers done if you have nightmares

**Don'ts**
· Argue with partner or others
· Scold children
· Allow bad thoughts to occupy mind for long period of time
· Talk negatively or with criticism

**Body**

**Do's**
· Eat foods good for baby
· Get up early and walk around
· Have a Blessingway ceremony for a safe delivery

**Don'ts**
· Drink milk or eat salt or foods taken away by Navajo ceremonies
· Lay around too much
· Tie knots
· Attend funerals or look at body of deceased person
· Be with sick people for long or go to crowded place
· Attend healing ceremonies for sick people like "Yei Bei Chai Dance"
· Look at dead animals or taxidermic trophies
· Look at eclipse of moon or sun
· Make plans for baby or prepare layette sets until after birth
· Don't lift heavy things
· Don't kill living things or cut a sheep's throat
· Don't weave rugs or make pottery

### DURING LABOR

**Mind/Soul**

**Do's**
· Think about a good delivery
· Have medicine people do "Singing Out Baby" Chants
· Have medicine person perform "Unraveling" songs if necessary

**Don'ts**
· Let too many people observe labor; only people who are helping you in some way

**Body**

**Do's**
· Loosen your hair
· Drink corn meal mush
· Wear juniper seed beads
· Burn cedar
· Hold onto sash belt when ready to push
· Have someone apply gentle fundal pressure during pushing effort

**Don'ts**
· Braid or tie hair in a knot
· Tie knots

*continued on page 440*

Table 17–4 • **Taking Care of Yourself during Pregnancy: Navajo Rules for Expectant Couples** (*Continued*)

**DURING LABOR**

**Body**

| Do's | Don'ts |
|---|---|
| · Get in squatting position for pushing | |
| · Drink herbal tea to relax if necessary | |
| · Drink herbal tea to strengthen contractions if necessary | |

**AFTER BIRTH OF BABY (POSTPARTUM PERIOD)**

| Do's | Don'ts |
|---|---|
| · Bury the placenta | · Drink cold liquids or be in cold draft |
| · Drink juniper/ash tea to cleanse your insides | · Smell afterbirth blood for too long |
| · Drink blue cornmeal mush | · Show signs of displeasure if baby soils on you or during diaper change |
| · Smear baby's first stool on your face | · Burn placenta or afterbirth blood fluids |
| · Breast-feed your baby | · Have sexual intercourse for 3 months after delivery |
| · Wrap sash belt around waist for 4 days after delivery | |

*Source:* Ursula Wilson, July 1987. IHS inservice seminar, Tuba City Indian Health Center, Tuba City, AZ, with permission.

with the body because those who work with the dead must have a ceremony to protect themselves from the deceased's spirit. If the person dies at home, the hogan must be abandoned or a ceremony must be held to cleanse it. The dead are buried with their shoes on the wrong feet and rings on their index fingers. Individuals who choose embalming as a profession are rare, and people tend to avoid the area where the dead lived.

One death taboo involves talking with clients concerning a fatal disease or illness. Effective discussions require that the issue be presented in the third person. The health-care provider must never suggest that the client is dying. To do so would imply that the provider wishes the client dead. If the client does die, it would imply that the provider may have evil powers.

## Responses to Death and Grief

Because their fear of the power of the dead is very real, excessive displays of emotion are not looked on favorably among some tribes. However, the Navajo are not generally open in their expression of grief and touching the body. Grief among the Pueblo is expressed openly and involves much crying among extended family members. Even if the deceased is a distant relative and has not been seen in years, much grief is expressed. The health-care provider must support survivors and permit family bereavement and grieving in a culturally congruent and sensitive manner that respects the beliefs of each tribe.

## SPIRITUALITY

### Religious Practices and Use of Prayer

American-Indian religion predominates in many tribes. Missionaries continue their efforts to convert American Indians to Christian religions, such as the Church of Jesus

Christ of Latter Day Saints, Jehovah's Witnesses, and to a lesser extent, Evangelical groups. When illnesses are severe, consultations with appropriate religious organizations are sought. Sometimes hospital admissions are accompanied by traditional ceremonies and consultation with a pastor. Even if persons are strong in their adopted beliefs, they honor their parents and families by having a traditional healing ceremony. The current director of the IHS has issued a memorandum that reaffirms the rights of American Indians to conduct ceremonies in health-care facilities. This memorandum also directs IHS health-care providers to be attuned to the total needs of the client to provide culturally competent and congruent care.

Navajos start the day with prayer, meditation, corn pollen, and running in the direction of the sun (Goldstein, 1987). Prayers ask for harmony with nature and for health and invite blessings to help the person exist in harmony with the earth and sky. Along with certain ceremonies, prayer helps the Navajo to attain fulfillment and inner peace with themselves and their environment.

## Meaning of Life and Individual Sources of Strength

Spirituality for most American Indians is based on harmony with nature. The meaning of life for the Navajo is derived from being in harmony with nature. The individual's source of strength comes from the inner self and also depends on being in harmony with one's surrounding.

Many tribes are concerned about outsiders from New Age movements attempting to participate in native medicine practices without an appropriate background, knowledge, and true inner source of peace. These persons often seek to be spiritual healers using traditional Indian medicines.

## Spiritual Beliefs and Health-care Practices

Spirituality cannot be separated from the healing process in ceremonies that are holistic in nature. Illness results from not being in harmony with nature, the spirits of evil persons such as a witch, or violation of taboos. Healing ceremonies restore mental, physical, and spiritual balance.

## HEALTH-CARE PRACTICES

## Health-seeking Beliefs and Behaviors

Traditional American Indian beliefs influence biomedical health-care decisions. For example, for many elderly persons, the germ theory is nearly impossible to comprehend. In addition, asking the client questions to make a diagnosis fosters mistrust. This approach is in conflict with the practice of traditional medicine men, who tell persons what is wrong without their having to say anything.

## Responsibility for Health Care

Through existing treaties (U.S. Department of Health and Human Services, 1991), the federal government assumes responsibility for the health-care needs of American Indians. Government services respect a blending of both worlds. Some tribes have contracted for monies to operate their own health-care systems. Few American Indians on reservations have traditional health insurance, and recent efforts at health-care reform have caused many tribes to fear that the government will not continue to honor its obligations under existing treaties.

The **Indian Health Service (IHS),** a federal agency providing health services to American Indians, has shifted its focus over the last 20 years from acute care to programs directed at health promotion, disease prevention, and chronic health. The tribes and the IHS have specific mandates to meet certain health goals and objectives for a healthy population by the year 2000. While health promotion and disease prevention is a major focus of the IHS, these programs are often in conflict with American Indian values. Projects promoting community involvement and culturally sensitive client education are effective strategies for implementing these goals and objectives. In the last 20 years, an increase has occurred in wellness promotion activities and a return to past traditions such as running for health, avoiding alcohol, and using purification ceremonies. Mental health programs are not well funded within the IHS and are thus traditionally understaffed.

The focus of acute care is curative and is based on promoting harmony with Mother Earth. Before the U.S. government assumed responsibility for health care to American Indians, health care was provided by medicine men and other traditional healers.

The use of traditional healing practices is explained to physicians practicing on the reservations, but if clients perceive reluctance to accept these practices, they do not reveal their use. This is especially true among the elderly population who seek hospital or clinic treatments only when their conditions becomes life-threatening. Younger generations seek treatment sooner and use the health-care system more readily than do elderly persons. However, if their parents are traditional, they may combine native traditional medicine with Western medicine.

Self-medication with over-the-counter drugs does not present a major health concern because there are no pharmacies on the Navajo reservation. Medications are available at IHS facilities at no cost.

## Folk Practices

The Navajo believe wellness is a state of harmony with one's surrounding. When persons are ill or out of harmony, the medicine man or, in some cases, a diagnostician, tells them what they have done to disrupt their harmony. They are returned to harmony through the use of a healing ceremony. The medicine man is expected to diagnose the illness and prescribe necessary treatments for regaining health. In Western health care, the practitioner asks the client what he or she thinks is wrong and then prescribes a treatment. This practice is sometimes interpreted by the American Indian as ignorance on the part of the white healer.

## Barriers to Health Care

On the Navajo reservation, great distances must be traveled to reach a hospital or health-care facility. Many families do not have adequate transportation and must wait for others to transport them into town. Some urban dwellers have a car but live in an area where access to an IHS facility is limited. Even when a car is available, many do not have the money for gasoline. There has been a recent increase in the number of urban facilities, and some tribes have established outreach clinics that help to cope with health problems.

Immunizations may be missed because parents do not have transportation. Close attention should be paid to the immunization status of a client on arrival to the emergency department or clinic. If the client is not current with immunizations, scheduling an appointment may be a waste of time because they may not be able to return until a ride is found. The health-care providers might have better success by taking the time to administer the immunization on the spot or by making a referral to the public health nursing office.

## Cultural Responses to Health and Illness

Obtaining adequate pain control is of concern for American Indians who receive care within the context of Western medicine. Frequently, pain control is ineffective because the actual intensity of their pain is not obvious to the health-care provider and because clients do not request pain medication. The Navajo views pain as something that is to be endured, and thus, they do not ask for analgesics and may not understand that pain medication is available. Other times, herbal medicines are preferred and used without the knowledge of the health-care provider. Not sharing the use of herbal medicine is a carryover from times when individuals were not allowed to practice their native medicine.

Mental illness is perceived as resulting from witches or witching (placing a curse) on a person. In these instances, a healer who deals with dreams or a crystal gazer is consulted. Persons may wear turquoise to ward off evil; however, a person who wears too much turquoise is sometimes thought to be an evil person and thus someone to avoid. In some tribes, mental illness may mean that the affected person has special powers.

The concept of rehabilitation is relatively new to American Indians because, in years past, they did not survive to an age where chronic diseases became an issue. Because life expectancy is increasing, an additional stress is placed on families who are expected to care for elderly relatives. Many families do not have the resources to assume this responsibility. Home health care is occasionally available, but this is a recent development that tribes are just beginning to accept. Federal public health nursing is also available to assist with home care. Those with physical or mental handicaps are not seen as different; rather, the limitation is accepted and a role is found for them within the society.

Cultural perceptions of the sick role for the American Indian are based on the ideal of maintaining harmony with nature and with others. Ill persons have obviously done something to place themselves out of harmony or have had a curse placed on them. In either case, support of the sick role is not generally accepted, but rather support is directed at assisting the person with regaining harmony. Elderly persons frequently work even when seriously ill and often must be encouraged to rest.

## Blood Transfusion and Organ Donation

Autopsy and organ donation are unacceptable practices to traditional American Indians. The concepts of organ transplant and organ donation may result in a major cultural dilemma. For example, in one case, a woman needing a kidney transplant consulted a medicine man who advised against having the transplant performed. She elected to have the transplant done against the medicine man's advice, which created a cultural dilemma for her family. As more American Indians accept biomedical care from Western medical practitioners, medicine men and traditional healing practices may be lost. Increasing Western medical practices on the reservations must be accompanied by attempting to incorporate culturally congruent traditional care into Western practices.

## HEALTH-CARE PRACTITIONERS

## Traditional Versus Biomedical Care

Native healers are divided primarily into three categories: those working with the power of good or evil or both. Generally, they are divinely chosen and promote activities that encourage self-discipline and self-control and that involve acute body awareness (Bean, 1976).

Within these three categories are several types of practitioners. Some practitioners are endowed with supernatural powers, whereas others only have knowledge of herbs and specific manipulations. The first type are persons who can only use their power for good, can transform themselves into other forms of life, and can maintain cultural integration in times of stress. The second group can use their powers for both evil and good and are expected to do evil against someone's enemies. Persons in this group have knowledge of witchcraft, poisons, and ceremonies designed to afflict the enemy. The third type is the diviner diagnostician, such as a **crystal gazer,** who can see what caused the problem but not implement a treatment. Another example of this type is a **hand trembler.** These persons, instead of using crystals, practice hand trembling over the sick person to determine the cause of an illness. A fourth group are the specialist medicine persons. They treat the disease after it has been diagnosed and specialize in the use of herbs, massage, or midwifery. A fifth group are those who care for the soul and send guardian spirits to restore a lost soul. A sixth group are singers, who are considered to be the most special. They cure through the power of their song. These healers are involved in the laying on of hands and usually remove objects or draw disease-causing objects from the body while singing.

Navajo tribal practitioners divide their knowledge into preventive measures, treatment regimens, and health maintenance (Wilson, 1987). An example of a preventive measure is carrying an object or a pouch filled with objects, prescribed by a medicine man that wards off the evil of a witch. Health-care providers must not remove these objects or pouches from the client. These objects contribute to the client's mental well-being, and their removal creates undue stress. Treatment regimens prescribed by a medicine man not only cure the body but also restore the mind. An example of a health maintenance practice among the Navajo is the Blessingway ceremony. Prayers and songs are offered during this ceremony. Individuals who live off reservations frequently return to participate in this ceremony, which returns them to harmony and restores a sense of well-being.

Acceptance of Western medicine is variable with a blending of traditional health-care beliefs. Experienced IHS providers understand the concepts of holistic health for American Indians, and a few are beginning to make referrals to the medicine man. Few physicians possess this level of cultural experience, and there are even fewer American Indian physicians. This is also true of the nursing profession. The majority of registered nurses in the IHS are not American Indians. American Indians who seek careers in the health field often go against traditional beliefs.

Male health-care providers are generally limited in the care they provide to women, especially during their menses. Women are generally modest and wear several layers of slips. This practice is very common among elderly women.

## Status of Health-care Providers

It is frequently said that if an American Indian becomes a physician, the physician must not be traditional. Therefore, many Navajo are suspicious of American Indian physicians. The factors that influence acceptance of American Indian health-care providers have not been adequately researched, but the lack of respect by some Western health-care providers for Indian beliefs has contributed to the Navajo's inability to trust them. Many health concerns of American Indians can be treated by both traditional and Western healers in a culturally competent manner when these practitioners are willing to work together and respect each other's differences.

Western practitioners, traditional medicine men, and herbal healers receive respect on the reservation. However, not all American Indians accord equal respect to these groups, and many prefer one group over the other or use all three.

Mr. Yassie, aged 78, lives with his wife in a traditional Navajo hogan. He has lived in the same area all his life and has worked as a farmer herding sheep. His hogan has neither electricity nor running water. Heat is provided by a fire, which is also used for cooking. Lighting is obtained from propane lanterns. Water is hauled from a windmill site 20 miles away and is stored in 50-gallon steel drums. Because the windmill freezes and the roads are often too muddy to travel in the winter, sometimes he must travel an additional 10 miles to the trading post to obtain water. Because Mr. Yassie does not own a car, he must depend on transportation from extended family members who live in the same vicinity.

Mr. Yassie was hospitalized 1 year ago for tuberculosis and severe dehydration secondary to diarrhea caused by shigella. He had a cholecystectomy at age 62 years. His diet is traditional and is supplemented by canned foods, which are obtained at the trading post.

All health care is obtained at the Public Health Service Hospital in Tuba City. Neither Mr. Yassie nor his wife obtains routine preventive health care. Mr. Yassie has been in relatively good health until 1 week ago when he began experiencing shortness of breath, a productive cough, and a fever. He was admitted from the clinic to the hospital with a diagnosis of pneumonia.

Mr. Yassie shows clinical improvement after initial intravenous antibiotic therapy. However, his mental status continues to decline. His family feels that he should see a traditional medicine man and discusses this with his physician. The physician agrees and allows Mr. Yassie to go to see the medicine man. Several members of the nursing staff disagree with the physician's decision and have requested a patient care conference with the physician. The physician agrees to the conference.

## STUDY QUESTIONS

1. Identify three physical barriers Mr. Yassie must overcome to obtain health care.

2. Discuss the benefits of Mr. Yassie seeing the traditional medicine man.

3. Identify some potential negative outcomes of Mr. Yassie seeing the traditional medicine man.

4. Identify interventions to reduce Mr. Yassie's potential for the recurrence of shigella.

5. Identify at least two major health risks that face the Yassies based on their current lifestyle.

6. Discuss potential outcomes for negotiation during the conference.

7. Mr. Yassie's diet is described as traditional Navajo. What foods are included in this diet?

8. What services do you anticipate for Mr. Yassie when he returns home?

9. What might the nurse do to encourage preventive health measures for the Yassie family?

*continued on page 446*

10. Identify at least three types of traditional Navajo healers.

11. Identify contextual speech patterns of the Navajo Indians.

12. Distinguish differences in gender roles among Navajo Indians.

13. Identify two culturally congruent teaching methods for the Navajo client.

14. Discuss the meaning of the First Laugh Ceremony for the Navajo?

15. Identify two culturally congruent approaches for discussing a fatal illness with a Navajo client.

16. Identify traditional practices used by the Navajo to start their day in regard to spirituality.

## References

Arthur, B. J., (1976). *Traditional Navajo childbearing practices: A survey of the traditional childbearing practices among elderly Navajo parents.* Unpublished master's thesis, University of Utah, Salt Lake City.

Bean, L. J. (1976). California Indian shamanism and folk curing. In W. D. Hand (Ed.), *American folk medicine: A symposium* (pp. 109–123). Berkeley: University of California Press.

Burke, S., Kisilevsky, B., & Maloney, R. (1989). Time orientations of Indian mothers and white nurses. *Canadian Journal of Nursing Research, 21,*(4), 14–20.

Chislom, J. S. (1983). *Navajo infancy: An ethnological study of child development.* New York: Aldine.

Crow, K. (1993). Multiculturalism and pluralistic thought in nursing education: American Indian world view and the nursing academic view. *Journal of Nursing Education, 32,*(5), 198–204.

Discharry, E. K. (1986). Delivering home health care to the elderly in Zuni Pueblo. *Journal of Gerontological Nursing, 12,*(7), 25–29.

Goldstein, D. (1987). A traditional Navajo medicine woman: A modern nurse midwife: Healing in harmony. *Frontier Nursing Service Quarterly Bulletin, 62*(3), 6–13.

Heath G., Leonard, B., Wilson, R., Kendrick, J., & Powell, K. (1987). Community-based exercise intervention: Zuni diabetes project. *Diabetes Care, 10,*(5), 579–583.

Hobus, R. (1990). Living in two worlds: A Lakota transcultural nursing experience. *Journal of Transcultural Nursing, 2,*(1), 33–36.

Hodgins, D., & Still, O. (1989). *Lidocaine reactions in the American Indian population* [quality assurance study]. Unpublished research, Tuba City Indian Health Center, Tuba City, Arizona.

Huse, D. M., Oster, G., Kildeen, A. R., Lurey, M. T., & Coldez, G.A. (1989). The economic costs of non-insulin dependent diabetes mellitus. *Journal of the American Medical Association, 8,* 391–406.

Irwin, L. (1992, Spring). Cherokee healing: Myth, dreams, and medicine. *American Indian Quarterly,* 237–257.

Jones, J., Ritenbaugh, C., Spence, M., & Hayward, A. (1991). Severe combined immunodeficiency among the Navajo: Characterization of phenotypes, epidemiology, and population genetics. *Human Biology, 63,*(5), 669–682.

Leininger, M. M. (1988). Leininger's theory of nursing: Cultural diversity and universality. *Nursing Science Quarterly, 1,*(4), 152–160.

Mail, P., Mckay, R., & Katz, M. (1989). Expanding practice horizons: Learning from American Indian patients. *Patient Education and Counseling 13,* 91–104.

Phillips, S., & Lobar, S. (1990). Literature summary of some Navajo child health beliefs and childbearing practices within a transcultural nursing framework. *Journal of Transcultural Nursing, 1,*(2), 13–20.

Preito, D. O. (1989). American Indians in medicine: The need for Indian healers. *Academic Medicine, 64,* 388.

Rose, V. (1993, April). Mother earth: American Indian beliefs and practices in childbearing. *Midwives Chronicle and Nursing Notes,* 104–107.

Schaefer A. E. (1977). Nutritional needs of a special population at risk. *Annals of the New York Academy of Science, 300,* 419–427.

Singleton, R., Helgerson, S., Snyder, R., O'Conner, P., Nelson, B., Johnsen, S., & Allanson, J. (1990). Neuropathy in Navajo children: Clinical and epidemiologic features. *Neurology, 40,*(2), 363–367.

Spector, R. E. (1991). *Cultural diversity in health and illness,* (3rd ed.). New York: Appleton & Lange.

Stracqualursi, F., Gohdes, D., Najarian, S.,

Hosey, G., & Lundgren, P. (1993) Assessing and implementing diabetes patient education programs for American Indian communities. *Diabetes Educator, 19,*(1) 31–34.

U.S. Department of Health and Human Services (1995). *Trends in Indian Health.* Public Health Service: Indian Health Services, Office of Planning and Evaluation. Rockville, MD.

World Health Organization Scientific Group.

(1986). Primary immunodeficiency diseases. In M. M. Eibl & F. S. Rosen (Eds.) *Primary immunodeficiency diseases* (pp. 341–375). Amsterdam: Exerpta Medica.

Wilson, U. (1983). Nursing care of the American Indian patient. In M. S. Orque, B. Block, & L. S. A. Monrroy, *Ethnic nursing care: A multicultural approach.* St. Louis: C. V. Mosby Co.

# Vietnamese-Americans

*Thu T. Nowak**

---

• Key terms to become familiar with in this chapter are:

| | |
|---|---|
| *Am* | *Mien* |
| *Be bao (Bat gio)* | Moxibustion |
| *Cao gio* | Pseudofamilies |
| *Duong* | *Tet* |
| *Giac* | Wind |
| Indochinese | *Xong* |
| *Lien* | |

## OVERVIEW, INHABITED LOCALITIES, AND TOPOGRAPHY

### Overview

Vietnam is located at the extreme southeastern corner of the Asian mainland along the South China Sea. Bordered by China on the north and Laos and Cambodia (Kampuchea) on the west, it has a land mass of 127,330 square miles, which is about the size of New Mexico. Although relatively narrow in width, its north-south length equals the distance from Minneapolis to New Orleans, and its rapidly growing population of 73 million is the 13th largest in the world. Vietnam consists largely of a remarkable blend of rugged mountains and the broad, flat Mekong and Red River deltas. There are other riverine lowlands and a long, narrow coastal plain. The deltas mainly produce rice. Much of the rest of the country is covered with tropical forests. The ethnic Vietnamese live mainly in the lowlands.

### Heritage and Residence

Vietnamese, a Mongolian racial group closely related to the Chinese, make up approximately 85 percent of the population in Vietnam. The terms *Southeast Asian*

---

*The author thanks her husband, Ron Nowak, for his assistance in the preparation of this chapter.

*refugee, Indochinese,* and *Vietnamese* are not synonymous. Indochina is a supra-national region that includes Vietnam, Laos, and Cambodia. Muecke (1983a) distinguished 11 different **Indochinese** groups based on ethnicity, habitat, and differences in language and religion. Included among these are Laotian, Cambodian, Thai, and Hmong and Tai Dam mountain people in Laos and in northern Vietnam. One factor in providing proper health care to Vietnamese-Americans is understanding that they differ substantially between and among themselves, depending on age, generation, length of time away from Viet Nam, education, and language skills. Chung and Kagawa-Singer (1993) found clear differences between Vietnamese, Cambodians, and Laotians with respect to premigration experiences influencing subsequent manifestations of psychological distress.

More than 655,000 Vietnamese live in the United States (*Information Please: Almanac,* 1995), and 84,005 live in Canada (*Canadian Abstracts: Ethnic Origins,* 1993). Gold (1992) puts the total Vietnamese population in the United States at more than 700,000 and estimates that by the century's end, the Vietnamese will be the third largest Asian-American group, outnumbered only by the Chinese and Filipinos. Asian-Americans in general are considered to be the fastest growing minority in the United States, followed by Hispanics (Yu, 1991). From 1980 to 1990, Vietnamese in the United States increased by 135 percent, compared to 108 percent for all other Asians (U.S. Bureau of the Census, 1992). The majority settle in the West, followed by the South, the Northeast, and the Midwest. California has the largest Vietnamese population followed by Texas.

The influx of Vietnamese and other Southeast Asians during the past 20 years is perhaps the most complex and unusual phase of immigration ever experienced by the United States. Although the movement of refugees from Cuba to the United States is comparable in scope, Vietnamese immigrants confronted a unique set of problems, including dissimilarity of culture, no family or relatives here to offer initial support, and a negative identification with the unpopular Vietnam War (Nguyen, 1985). Many Vietnamese are involuntary immigrants. Their expatriation was unexpected and unplanned, and their departure precipitous and often tragic. Escape attempts were long, harrowing, and for many fatal (Muecke, 1983b). Survivors were often placed in squalid refugee camps for years.

The first wave of Vietnamese immigration began in April 1975 when South Vietnam fell into the communist control of North Vietnam and the Viet Cong. At that time, many South Vietnamese businessmen, military officers, professionals, and others closely involved with America feared persecution by the new regime and sought to escape. Some were rescued by U.S. ships and aircraft. The 130,000 Vietnamese refugees who arrived in the United States in 1975 came mainly from urban areas, especially Saigon, and consequently had some prior orientation to Western culture. Many spoke English or soon learned English in relocation centers. More than half were Christian. Sixty-two percent consisted of family units of at least five persons, and nearly half were female. They were dispersed over much of the United States, often in the care of sponsoring American families. One year after arrival, 90 percent were employed, and by the mid-1980s their average income matched that of the overall U.S. population. These first-wave immigrants adjusted well in comparison to the subsequent wave of refugees.

Over the next few years, many Vietnamese grew disenchanted with communism, their living standard had declined, great numbers had been forced into labor in new countryside settlements, and young men were often fearful of being called to fight against China or in the new war with Cambodia. More than 100,000 Vietnamese left their homeland in 1978, and more than 150,000 in 1979. Some left by land across Cambodia or Laos, commonly joining refugees from those countries in an effort to reach Thailand. For more than a decade, many others, known as the "boat people," departed Vietnam in small, often unseaworthy and overcrowded vessels in hopes of reaching Malaysia, Hong Kong, the Philippines, or another noncommunist port. Half died during their journey. Many were forcibly repatriated to Vietnam or eventually returned voluntarily; others continue to languish in camps.

Most of the second-wave refugees represented lower socioeconomic groups and had less education and little exposure to Western cultures. Most did not speak English. This wave of Vietnamese included far more young men than women, children, or older people, which disrupted intact families and normal gender ratios. Many spent months or years in refugee camps under deplorable and regimented conditions. When they finally arrived in the United States and Canada, many did not fit into American communities, did not learn English effectively, and remained unemployed or obtained menial jobs. These hardships contributed to physical problems, psychological stress, and depression. Some exceptions were found among the ethnic Chinese refugees, who often came from the established business community and could afford to keep extended families together.

A third wave of immigration started in 1979 with creation of the Orderly Departure Program, which provided safe and legal exit for Vietnamese seeking to reunite with family members already in America. Initially small in scope, this program eventually supported the annual air travel of tens of thousand of ethnic Vietnamese and Chinese-Vietnamese to the United States (D'Avanzo, 1992a; Hinton et al., 1993; McKelvey, Webb & Mao, 1993).

In 1987, a fourth wave of immigration began with passage of the Amerasian Homecoming Act, which provided for the entry of former South Vietnamese military officers, other political detainees, children of American servicemen and Vietnamese women, and their close relatives.

## Reasons for Migration and Associated Economic Factors

Vietnamese, whether as immigrants or sojourners, have fled their country to escape war, persecution, or possible loss of life (D'Avanzo, 1992b). Better-educated first-wave immigrants from urban areas had professional, technical, or managerial backgrounds. Less-educated second-wave immigrants from less urbanized areas were fishermen, farmers, and soldiers and had only minimal exposure to Western culture. Factors influencing the ability of displaced Vietnamese to obtain employment include higher education and the ability to speak English on arrival (Calhoon, 1986). Thus, the second-wave immigrants are significantly more disadvantaged.

Because the majority of refugee heads of households worked, families were not totally dependent on welfare for financial assistance. Many worked for comparatively low wages, and their families often required some supplemental aid. However, "like other Indochinese groups, the Vietnamese are becoming independent of the welfare system at a relatively fast rate. Pride, a tradition of hard work, and the pooling together of family resources account for their aversion to relying on outside assistance" (Calhoon, 1986, p. 16).

## Educational Status and Occupations

Vietnamese place a high value on education and accord scholars an honored place in society. The teacher is highly respected as a symbol of learning and culture. In contrast to American schools' emphasis on experimentation and critical thinking, Vietnamese schools emphasize observation, memorization, and repetitive learning (Calhoon, 1986).

Approximately 62.2 percent of all Vietnamese-Americans 25 years of age or older have a high school education, and 54 percent of Vietnamese-American women aged 25 or older and about 71 percent of Vietnamese men in this age group have at least a high school education. This compares favorably with 66 percent of women and 67 percent of men in the same age group in the general U.S. population. Eight percent of all Vietnamese women 25 years old or older and at least 18 percent of Vietnamese men in this age group have a college education. This compares with 13 percent of women and 20 percent of men in the same age group in the general U.S. population (Stauffer, 1991).

Gold (1992) reported that 78 percent of the refugees who arrived between 1975 and 1977 had been in white-collar occupations in Vietnam, as compared with 49 percent of those coming since 1978. The latter group experienced greater difficulty in adapting economically and suffered higher levels of unemployment and welfare dependency (64 percent). Professionals, mostly men, and unskilled laborers are often unable to find work in their former fields, with the recent reduction in professional, technical, and managerial positions in the United States and an increased concentration of craft, operative, and service employment (Takaki, 1991). Some Vietnamese fishermen on the Gulf Coast of Texas have been able to maintain their traditional occupation, but experience hostility from American fishermen who consider them competitors.

## COMMUNICATION

### Dominant Language and Dialects

Ethnic Vietnamese speak a single distinctive language, with northern, central, and southern dialects, all of which can be understood by anyone speaking any one of these dialects. The language differs from those spoken in the neighboring countries of Laos and Cambodia and from those spoken by highland tribal groups of Southeast Asia. The Vietnamese language resembles Chinese and contains many borrowed words, but someone speaking one of these languages cannot necessarily understand the other. All words in Vietnamese consist of a single syllable, although two words are commonly joined with a hyphen to form a new word. Contextually, the Vietnamese language is musical and flowing. It is polytonal, with each tone of a vowel conveying a different meaning to the word. The language is spoken softly and its monosyllabic structure lends itself to rapidity, but spoken pace varies according to the situation. Whereas grammar is mostly simple, pronunciation can be difficult for westerners, mainly because each vowel can be spoken in five or six tones that may completely change the meaning of the word. Vietnamese is the only language of the Asian mainland that, like English, is regularly written in the Roman alphabet. Although the letters are the same, pronunciation of vowels may vary radically depending on associated marks indicating tone and accent, and certain consonant combinations take on unusual sounds.

Even if someone learns how to pronounce and translate Vietnamese, problems may remain with respect to intended meaning of various words. One minor but perennial stumbling point with potential medical connotations is that the word for "blue" and "green" is the same (Felice, 1986). More important, the word for "yes," rather than expressing a positive answer or agreement, may simply reflect an avoidance of confrontation or a desire to please the other person (Hoang & Erickson, 1982; Nguyen, 1985). The terms *hot* and *cold,* rather than expressing physical feelings associated with fever and chills, may actually relate to other conditions associated with perceived bodily imbalances (Eyton & Neuwirth, 1984). Various medical problems might be described differently than a westerner might expect; for example, a "weak heart" may refer to palpitations or dizziness, a "weak kidney" to sexual dysfunction, a "weak nervous system" to headaches, and a "weak stomach or liver" to indigestion (Muecke, 1983b).

Most Vietnamese refugees, even those who have been in the United States for many years, do not feel competent in English (D'Avanzo, 1992a). Although many refugees eventually learn English, their skills may not be sufficient to communicate in psychiatric interviews, which are usually carried out at a highly abstract level (Lin & Shen, 1991).

The health-care provider may need to watch the client for behavioral cues, use simple sentences, paraphrase words with multiple meanings, avoid metaphors and idiomatic expressions, ask for correction of understanding, and explain all points carefully. Approaching Vietnamese clients in a quiet, unhurried manner, opening discussions with small talk, and directing the initial conversation to the oldest member of the group facilitates communication (Calhoun, 1986).

## Cultural Communication Patterns

Traditional Vietnamese religious beliefs transmitted through generations produce an attitude towards life that may be perceived as passive. For example, whenever confronted with a direct but delicate question, many Vietnamese cannot easily give a blunt "no" as an answer because they feel that such an answer may create disharmony. Self-control, another traditional value, encourages keeping to oneself, whereas expressions of disagreement that may irritate or offend another person are avoided. One may be in pain, distraught, or unhappy, yet one rarely complains except perhaps to friends or relatives. Expression of emotions is considered a weakness and interferes with self-control (Nguyen, 1985). Vietnamese are unaccustomed to discussing their personal feelings openly with others. Instead, at times of distress or loss, they often complain of physical discomforts, such as headaches, backaches, or insomnia (Kinzie et al., 1982).

The strong influence of the Confucian code of ethics means that proper form and appearance are important to Vietnamese and form the foundation for nonverbal communication patterns. For example, the head is a sacred part of the body and should not be touched. Similarly, the feet are the lowest part of the body, and to place one's feet on a desk is considered offensive to a Vietnamese. To signal for someone to come by using an upturned finger is a provocation, usually done to a dog; waving the hand is considered more proper (Nguyen, 1985).

Hugging and kissing are not seen outside the privacy of the home. Men greet each other with a handshake but do not shake hands with a woman unless she offers her hand first (Calhoun, 1986). Women do not usually shake hands. It is acceptable practice for two men or two women to walk hand in hand and does not carry sexual connotations. However, for a man to touch a woman in the presence of others is insulting.

Looking another person directly in the eyes may be deemed disrespectful. Women may be reluctant to discuss sex, childbearing, or contraception when men are present and demonstrate this by giggling, shrugging their shoulders, or averting their eyes (Calhoun, 1986).

Negative emotions and expressions may be conveyed by silence or a reluctant smile. A smile may express joy, convey stoicism in the face of difficulty, indicate an apology for a minor social offense, or be a response to a scolding to show sincere acknowledgment for the wrongdoing or to convey the absence of ill feelings (Stauffer, 1991). Vietnamese prefer more distance during personal and social relationships than other cultures, but extended Vietnamese families of many persons live comfortably together in close quarters (Stauffer, 1991).

## Temporal Relationships

Vietnamese religion and tradition place emphasis on continuity, cycles, and worship of ancestors. Traditional Vietnamese may be less concerned about the present and precise schedules than are European-Americans. To cope with their changed situation, many Southeast Asian refugees concentrate on the present and to some extent on the future (Beiser, 1988).

Asians frequently arrive late for appointments. Noncompliance in keeping appointments may relate to not understanding oral or written instructions, or not knowing how to use the telephone. On the other hand, many Vietnamese-Americans fully understand the significance of punctuality (Stauffer, 1991).

One other aspect of time involves the treatment of age. Vietnamese pay much less attention to people's precise ages than Americans. Actual dates of birth may pass unnoticed, with everyone celebrating their birthdays together during the Lunar New Year **(Tet)** in January or February. In addition, a person's age is calculated roughly from the time of conception; most children are considered to already be a year old at birth and gain a year each Tet. A child born just before Tet could be regarded as 2 years old when only a few days old by American standards (Nguyen, 1985). Because the practice of determining age is so different in Vietnam than in America, many immigrants may have difficulty determining their exact birth date and are often given January 1 as a date of birth for official records.

## Format for Names

Most Vietnamese names consist of a family name, a middle name, and a given name of one or two words, always written in that order. There are relatively few family names, with Nguyen (pronounced "nwin") and Tran accounting for more than half of all Vietnamese names. Other common family names are Cao, Dinh, Hoang, Le, Ly, Ngo, Phan, and Pho. There are relatively few middle names, with Van being used regularly for males and Thi (pronounced "tee") for females. Given names frequently have a direct meaning, such as a season of year or object of admiration. Family members often refer to offspring by a numerical nickname indicating order of birth.

This practice may increase the difficulty of modern record keeping and identification of specific individuals. It is therefore advantageous to use the family name in combination with the given name. Indeed, Vietnamese refer to each other by given name both in formal and informal situations. For example, a typical woman's name is Tran Thi Thu. That is how she would write or give her name if requested. She would expect to be called simply "Thu" or sometimes "*Chi* (sister) Thu" by friends and family. In other situations she would expect to be addressed as *Cô* (Miss) or *Ba* (Mrs.) Thu. If married to a man named Nguyen Van Kha, the proper way to address her would be as Mrs. Kha, but she would retain her full three-part maiden name for formal purposes. The man would always be known as Kha or *Ong* (Mr.) Kha. Some Vietnamese-American women have adopted their husband's family name. Children always take the father's family name.

## FAMILY ROLES AND ORGANIZATION

### Head of Household and Gender Roles

The traditional Vietnamese family is strictly patriarchal and is almost always an extended family structure, with the male having the duty of carrying on the family name through his progeny (Hoang & Erickson, 1982). Some families not accustomed to female authority figures may have difficulty relating to women as professional health-care providers (Felice, 1986). With the move into Western society, the father may no longer be the undisputed head of the household, and the parents' authority may be undermined (Kinzie, 1986). Immigrant Vietnamese families frequently experience role reversals, with wives or children adapting more easily than men to the Western workplace, becoming the primary providers, and thus gaining increased authority. Some families adapt well to this situation, whereas others experience resentment and hostility, which may erupt into child or wife abuse, depression, and alcoholism (Gold, 1992).

A Vietnamese woman lives with her husband's family after marriage but retains her own identity. Within the family, the division of labor is gender related: the husband deals with matters outside of the home, and the wife is responsible for the actual care of the home. Although her role in family affairs increases with time, a Vietnamese wife is expected to be dutiful and respectful toward her husband and his parents throughout the marriage (Calhoun, 1985). Vietnamese women often make family health-care decisions (D'Avanzo, 1992a).

Vietnamese refugees of all subgroups have various degrees of reversal of the provider and recipient roles that existed among family members in Vietnam. "Women's jobs," such as hotel maid, sewing machine operator, and food service worker, are more readily available than male-oriented unskilled occupations. Role reversals between parents and children are also common because children often learn the English language and American customs more rapidly than their parents and may be able to find employment more quickly than their parents (Gold, 1992).

Vietnamese families in the United States experience a tendency towards nuclearization, a growth in spousal interaction and interdependency, more egalitarian spousal relations, and shared decision making (Fox, 1991).

## Prescriptive, Restrictive, and Taboo Behaviors for Children and Adolescents

Traditionally, children are expected to be obedient and devoted to their parents, their identity being an extension of the parents. Children are obliged to do everything possible to please their parents while they are alive and to worship their memory after death. The eldest son is usually responsible for rituals honoring the memory and invoking the blessings of departed ancestors. This pattern of respect is ingrained from early childhood and is tantamount to a natural law (Leininger, 1970).

Vietnamese children are prized and valued because they carry the family lineage. For the first 2 years, they are cared for primarily by their mothers; thereafter, their grandmothers and others take on much of the responsibility. Parents usually do not discipline or place extensive limits on their children at a young age. Generally, Vietnamese do not use corporal punishment such as spanking; rather, they speak to the children in a quiet, controlled manner (Calhoun, 1986).

Young people are expected to continue to respect their elders and to avoid behavior that might dishonor the family. As a result of the effects of their exposure to Western cultures, a disproportionate share of young people in the refugee population, which has a median age of 18 years, have difficulty adapting to this expectation. A conflict often develops between the traditional notion of filial piety, with its requisite subordination of self and unquestioning obedience to parental authority, and the pressures and needs associated with adaptation to American life. Ironically, successful relationships with Americans at school have placed Vietnamese adolescents at risk for conflicts with their parents. Conversely, failure to form such relationships has sometimes appeared to be a precursor of emotional distress. Parents do, however, show relative approval for adolescent freedom of choice regarding dating, marriage, and career (Nguyen & Williams, 1989).

The extreme bipolarities of the adaptation of Vietnamese youth is sometimes overemphasized (Gold, 1992). One group, usually the children of the first-wave refugees, are often portrayed as academic superstars. At the other end of the social spectrum are the criminal and gang elements, who often direct their activities against other Asian immigrants. Most Vietnamese adolescents, however, fall between these two extremes and have the same pressures and concerns as other youths.

## Family Roles and Priorities

The traditional Vietnamese family is perhaps the most basic, enduring, and self-consciously acknowledged form of national culture among refugees, providing life-long protection and guidance to the individual. It is customarily a large, patriarchal, and extended family unit, including minor children, married sons, daughters-in-law, unmarried grown daughters, and grandchildren under the same roof. Other close relatives may be included within the extended family structure (Stauffer, 1991). The family is explicitly structured and assigned priorities, with parental ties being paramount. A son's obligations and duties to his parents may assume a higher value than those to his wife, children, or siblings. Sibling relationships are considered permanent. Vietnamese self is defined more along the lines of family roles and responsibilities and less along individual lines. These mutual family tasks provide a framework for individual behavior, promoting a sense of interdependence, belonging, and support (Timberlake & Cook, 1984). The traditional family has been altered as a consequence of Western influence, urbanization, and the war-induced absence of men. Nevertheless, many Vietnamese continue to uphold this social form as the preferable basis of social organization in the United States (Gold, 1992). As mentioned in the previous section, exposure of the younger generation to the American culture can become a source of conflict with considerable family strain as adolescents are influenced by the perceived American values of individuality, independence, self-assertion, and egalitarian relationships (Nguyen, 1985).

Traditionally, elders are honored and have a key role in most family activities for transmitting guidelines related to social behavior, preparing younger people for handling stressful life events, and serving as sources of support in coping with life crises (Timberlake & Cook, 1984). Elders are usually consulted for important decisions. Addressing a client in the presence of an elder, whether they speak English or not, may be interpreted as disrespectful to the family (D'Avanzo, 1992b).

Homesickness and bewilderment are especially acute in older refugees when

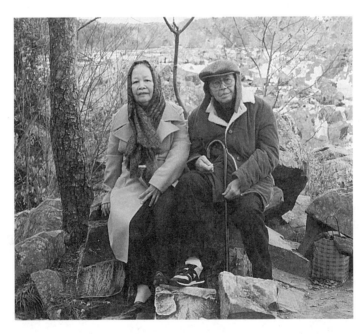

**Figure 18–1.** Elders are honored in traditional Vietnamese culture, but the effects of American culture on immigrant families may sometimes be troubling to elderly Vietnamese-Americans.

confronted with the strange Western culture and despair about the future (Fig. 18–1). Accustomed to considerable respect and esteem in their homeland, they may feel increasingly alienated and alone as the younger generations adopt new values and ignore the counsel and values of the elders (Robinson, 1980). Living within the family unit facilitates the social adjustment of elderly refugees into American society (Tran, 1991). However, those who live in overcrowded households and in households with children under the age of 16 years experience a poorer adjustment.

Traditional Vietnamese are class conscious and rarely associate with persons at different levels of society. Traditional respect is accorded to persons in authoritative positions, who are well educated or otherwise successful, or who have professional titles. However, class distinctions are sometimes blurred in the turmoil of war and resettlement. Two concepts govern the gain and loss of prestige and power, thereby maintaining face: *mien,* based on wealth and power, and *lien,* based on demonstration of control over and responsibility for moral character. For example, to smile in the face of adversity is to maintain *lien* and is considered of great importance (Eyton & Neuwirth, 1984).

## Alternative Lifestyles

The complex extended Vietnamese family in America is extremely vulnerable to change. Many young people, frequently unmarried couples, seek their own living accommodations away from the control of older generations. Unattached male refugees may join **pseudofamilies,** households made up of close and distant relatives and friends that share accommodations, finances, and companionship (Gold, 1992). These families form an important source of social support in the refugee communities. Because of the high regard for chastity placed on Vietnamese adolescents, the number of single-parent households is low.

## WORKFORCE ISSUES

### Culture in the Workplace

First-wave immigrants adjusted well to the American workplace, and within a decade, their average income equaled that of the general U.S. population. Many later immigrants who had less education and did not know English work in lower-paying jobs. However, some learned English and opened their own businesses and prospered.

Traditionally, priority is given to the concerns of the family, rather than to those of the employer. However, this emphasis is not a detriment to productivity in work habits, because a good work record and steady pay brings honor and prosperity to the family. The Vietnamese are highly adaptable and adjust their work habits to meet requirements for successful employment.

Most Vietnamese respect authority figures with impressive titles, achievement, education, and a harmonious work environment. They may be less concerned about such factors as punctuality, adherence to deadlines, and competition. Other traditions include a willingness to work hard, sacrificing current comforts, and saving for the future to ensure that they assimilate well into the workforce. Many seek the same material, financial, and status rewards that beckon native-born Americans.

### Issues Related to Autonomy

The Vietnamese outlook has been heavily influenced by Confucianism and its stress on the maintenance of formal hierarchies within governmental, religious, and educational institutions; commercial establishments; and families. This cultural background results in conformity and reluctance to undertake independent action. At the same time, the cultural outlook of company and family values superseding personal values creates a cohesive work group.

Vietnamese quickly learn vocabulary for pragmatic communication but may have difficulty with complex verbal skills. Values related to their own culture discourage disclosure of inner thoughts and feelings. These barriers adversely affect employment opportunities and limit their ability to communicate needs relative to social, psychological, and economic matters. Despite extensive English instruction programs, many Vietnamese may still lack transcultural communication skills; thus, "the critical ingredient of helping the traumatized refugees to cope and function in the mainstream society and world of work is not there" (August, 1987, p. 829). Employers may need to allow extra time, provide visually oriented instructions, and provide programs that enhance communications to promote increased harmony in the workplace.

## BIOCULTURAL ECOLOGY

### Skin Color and Other Biologic Variations

Vietnamese are members of the Mongolian or Asian race. Although their skin is often referred to as "yellow," it varies considerably in color, ranging from pale ivory to dark brown. Mongolian spots, bluish discolorations on the lower back of a newborn child, are normal hyperpigmented areas in many Asians (Overfield, 1977).

To assess for oxygenation and cyanosis in dark-skinned Vietnamese, the healthcare provider must examine the sclera, conjunctiva, buccal mucosa, tongue, lips, nailbeds, palms, and soles. These same areas should be observed for signs of reactions during blood transfusions, giving special attention to diaphoresis on the forehead, upper lip, and palms, which may signify impending shock.

One of the first signs of iron deficiency anemia is pallor, which varies with skin tones. Dark skin loses the normal underlying red tones so that Vietnamese clients with brown skin will appear yellow-brown. Petechiae and rashes may be hidden in dark-skinned persons as well, but they can be detected by observing for patches of melanin in the buccal mucosa and on the conjunctiva. Jaundice can be observed in dark-skinned Vietnamese by a yellow discoloration of the conjunctiva. Because many dark-skinned persons have carotene deposits in the subconjunctival fat and sclera, the hard palate should also be assessed.

The Vietnamese are usually small in physical stature and light in build relative to most European-Americans. Adult women average 5 feet tall and weigh 80 to 100 pounds. Men average a few inches taller and weigh 110 to 130 pounds. Although Roberts et al. (1985) reported no significant difference in birth weight between refugee babies and those of other parents, Vietnamese children are small by American standards, not fitting the published growth curves (Felice, 1986). Barry et al. (1983) found that 47 percent of the refugee children are below the fifth percentile in height for age, and 22 percent are below the fifth percentile in weight for age on standard American growth curves. However, no clinical evidence shows that such development is the result of disease or malnutrition. According to Pickwell (1982), 72 percent of refugee children examined fall below the 10th percentile for weight, stature, or both in relation to age. However, when these are plotted on the weight-for-stature graphs, they fall within the normal range. Thus, growth charts commonly used in America cannot provide adequate assessments for evaluating the physical development of Vietnamese children. Other parameters, such as parental height and weight, apparent state of health, the energy level of the child, and progressive development over time, need to be considered. The development of standing, walking, and language skills begin at a slightly later age in Vietnamese children, but they rapidly catch up with American norms by the age of 1.5 to 2 years (Sokoloff et al. 1984).

Typical physical features of the Vietnamese include inner eye folds that make the eyes look almond-shaped, sparse body hair, and coarse head hair (Calhoun, 1986). According to Overfield (1977), Vietnamese also have dry ear wax, which is gray and brittle. Persons with dry ear wax have few apocrine glands, especially in the underarm area and thus produce less sweat and associated body odor. Asians generally have larger teeth than European-Americans, creating a normal tendency towards a prognathic profile, the mouth area coming out farther than the upper part of the face. In addition, there may be a torus, bony protuberance, on the midline of the palate or on the inner side of the mandible near the second premolar. Mandibular tori occur in about 40 percent of Asians as compared with only 7 percent of European-Americans.

Betel nut pigmentation may be found in some Vietnamese adults, resulting from the practice of chewing betel leaves (*chau*). This practice is common among older women and has a narcotic effect on diseased gums. Some elderly women lacquer their teeth, believing that it strengthens the teeth and symbolizes beauty and wealth (Calhoun, 1986).

## Diseases and Health Conditions

Mental health research has indicated that Vietnamese refugees have disturbingly high rates of depression, generalized anxiety disorders, and post-traumatic stress associated with military combat, political imprisonment, harrowing events during escapes by sea (Hinton et al., 1993), and brutal pirate attacks. Chronic personal and emotional problems often stem from post-traumatic stress experiences in this population.

Of immediate concern to health-care providers working with Vietnamese refugees is the treatment of infectious conditions that jeopardize both the refugee and the resident population. Some refugees suffer from malaria, parasites, and other problems associated with the tropics. Catanzaro and Moser (1982) reported that Vietnamese have a lower incidence of intestinal parasites, anemia, and hepatitis B antigenemia than other refugee groups. However, 69 percent of tuberculin tests return positive in the Vietnamese, and this high rate of positive results correlates with their origins from crowded, poorly ventilated cities. Screening of second-wave refugees reveals a higher incidence of tuberculosis, intestinal parasitism, anemia, malaria, and hepatitis B (Catanzaro & Moser, 1982; Hoang & Erickson, 1982; Muecke, 1983b). Sutter and Haefliger (1990) reported an estimated annual risk for tuberculosis of 2.2 percent in Vietnamese and that the disease was present before arrival in refugee camps. Franks et al. (1988) reported that the hepatitis B virus is hyperendemic in Indochina, with most people being infected during childhood and spreading the infection to others. HBV vaccination is recommended for all newborn refugee children.

Other endemic diseases include leprosy (a rate of about 20 to 30 cases per 1000 population as compared with a U.S. rate of fewer than 0.25 per 1000 population; high levels of parasitism, particularly the intestinal nematodes *Ascaris* (roundworm) and *Trichuris* (whipworm), which are associated with contaminated or poorly cooked foods, and the liver fluke *Clonorchis,* which is introduced in raw, pickled, or dried fish (Dao, Gregory, & McKee, 1984), hookworm (Necator) (Calhoun, 1986), and malaria with the arrival of refugees (Guerrero, Chin, & Collins, 1982).

To determine the presence of parasites, the health-care provider must assess for symptoms of anemia, lassitude, failure to thrive, abdominal pain, weight loss, and skin rashes. In the first two waves of refugees, major health problems also include skin infections, including those caused by fungus, impetigo, scabies, and lice (7 to 15 percent); infections of the upper respiratory tract and otitis media (20 percent); anemia including parasitic iron deficiency (16 to 40 percent), with a higher occurrence in young children; hemoglobin disorders (30 percent); chronic diseases (10 percent); and malnutrition and poor immunization status (Ross, 1982).

Two clinical illnesses that may mimic tuberculosis, melioidosis and paragonimiasis, are also reported among refugees. Sutherland et al. (1983) reported that 14 percent of the Vietnamese refugees in their Mayo Clinic study exhibited microcytosis, which can lead to an incorrect diagnosis of iron deficiency and inappropriate treatment with iron. Erythrocytic microcytosis in Southeast Asians is most likely a reflection of the presence of thalassemia or of hemoglobin E trait, conditions which are usually harmless and necessitate no treatment. These disorders should be suspected in persons with findings consistent with tuberculosis but with a negative purified protein derivative response (Ross, 1982).

Screening of immigrants for syphilis demonstrates an incidence as low as 1 to 5 percent. Sporadic cases and limited outbreaks of cholera, measles, diphtheria, epidemic conjunctivitis, and typhoid fever fail to show notable secondary spread (Ross, 1982). Observations at the Mayo Clinic (Sutherland et al., 1983) reported that refugee populations are young and generally healthy, despite a prevalence rate of 82 percent for intestinal parasites. Hoang and Erickson (1982) reported that moderate to severe dental problems occur in 90 percent of children, whereas Pickwell (1982) reported that 51 percent had such severe decay or periodontal disease or both that emergency referral was needed.

## Variations in Drug Metabolism

Little pertinent drug research exists specifically on the Vietnamese. Clinical studies comparing other Asians with European-Americans provide some idea of what might be expected. For example, the Chinese are twice as sensitive to the effects of propranolol on blood pressure and heart rate; experience a greater increase in heart rate from atropine; require lower doses of benzodiazepines, diazepam, and alprazolam owing to their increased sensitivity to the sedative effects of these drugs; require lower doses of imipramine, desipramine, amitriptyline, and clomipramine; and are less sensitive to cardiovascular and respiratory side effects of analgesics (for example, morphine) but more sensitive to their gastrointestinal side effects. Asians require lower doses of neuroleptics (for example, haloperidol) (Levy, 1993).

Lin and Shen (1991) expressed concern about the lack of research on pharmacotherapy specifically with regard to major depressive and post-traumatic stress disorders in Southeast Asian refugees. They suggested that drug metabolism is comparable to that of other Asian groups with important common traits such as genetic, cultural, and environmental influences. Asian diets, for example, are similar in carbohydrate-to-protein ratio, which significantly influences the metabolism of some commonly prescribed drugs. Also, as most Asians come from areas with similar degrees of socioeconomic development, exposure to various enzyme-inducing agents, such as drugs and industrial toxins, is likely to be similar. On the other hand, the exposure of the refugees to war, trauma, starvation, and other adverse conditions could have an effect on the enzyme systems governing psychotropic medications. One precaution involves the continued extensive use of traditional herbal medicines by the refugees. Some of these herbal drugs have active pharmacologic properties that may interact with psychotropic drugs. For example, some may cause atropine psychosis when ingested concomitantly with tricyclic antidepressants or low-potency neuroleptics.

Significantly lower dosages of psychotropic medications are prescribed in Asian countries than are common in Western countries (Rosenblat & Tang, 1987). Low doses of antidepressant medications are often effective. Weight standards for neuroleptic dose ranges are significantly lower in Asians than in European-Americans (Lin & Finder, 1983). Because Vietnamese are considerably smaller than most European-Americans, medication dosages may need to be reduced. Vietnamese generally consider American medicines to be more concentrated than Asian medicines; thus, they may take only half of the dosage prescribed (Stauffer, 1991).

Genetic factors result in 25 to 50 percent of Asians being slow metabolizers of alcohol (Levy, 1993). Thus, Asians are more sensitive than European-Americans to the adverse effects of alcohol as expressed by facial flushing, palpitation, and tachycardia.

## HIGH-RISK BEHAVIORS

Alcohol and tobacco use by Vietnamese has been reported to be relatively low (Calhoun, 1985, 1986; Stauffer, 1991). However, some adolescents have turned to alcohol, often drinking alone and claiming that it helps them forget what they experienced in their homeland (Felice, 1986). Fitzpatrick et al. (1987) cautioned that peer pressure to drink and experiment with drugs might be greater than realized for Indochinese teenagers. Yu (1991) reported a substantial increase in smoking among Asian-American women in general. Jenkins et al. (1992) found the incidence of smoking among California men is higher in Vietnamese than in Chinese or Hispanics.

Data suggest a possible high mortality from cancer at certain sites among Vietnamese (Jenkins et al., 1990). Cigarette smoking, excessive dietary intake of fat, low dietary intake of fiber, and consumption of alcohol have been linked epidemiologically to an increased risk of cancer. In a survey of Vietnamese adults in the San Francisco area, 13 percent had never heard of cancer, 27 percent did not know that cigarette smoking can cause cancer, and 28 percent believed that cancer is contagious. Although hepatitis B–related liver cancer is endemic among Vietnamese, 48 percent never heard of hepatitis B. Among men, 56 percent are smokers versus 32 percent in the general population. Of those, 88 percent report smoking high-tar, high-nicotine brands. Most wanted to quit and said that their physicians had advised them to quit or reduce smoking. Cigarette smoking in males is strongly associated with incomes below the poverty level, residence in the United States of 9 years or less, not knowing that smoking causes cancer, and limited English proficiency. Only 9 percent of Vietnamese women are smokers versus 27 percent of women in general.

The prevalence of alcohol consumption is 67 percent among Vietnamese men and only 18 percent among women versus 66 percent and 47 percent in the general population. Binge drinking is reported by 35 percent of men. Among women, 89 percent say they had never heard of the Pap test; after this procedure is explained, 32 percent say they never had one (versus 9 percent of U.S. women). In addition, 28 percent of women never had a breast examination and 83 percent never had a mammogram.

Lung cancer is 18 percent higher among Southeast Asian men than among European-American men, and liver cancer is more than 12 times higher among Southeast Asian men and women. The high rate of liver cancer is associated with the prevalence of hepatitis B in Southeast Asian immigrants (Olsen & Frank-Stromborg, 1993). High rates of gastrointestinal cancer indicate this may be due to asbestos in some parts of the world that is used in the process of "polishing" rice. Thus, imported rice should always be washed (Paxton, Ramirez, & Walloch, 1976).

Asians are less likely to be aware of hypertension than are persons of other races (Stavig, Igra, & Leonard, 1988). In one study, 85 percent of Southeast Asians did not know what to do to prevent heart disease (Chen et al., 1991).

Young Asians are less sexually active than other groups and have a lower risk of acquired immunodeficiency syndrome (AIDS), and Vietnamese have a lower incidence of AIDS than the Japanese (Cochran, Mays, & Leung, 1991). Indochinese teenagers may have a high rate of certain hemoglobinopathies, and their pairing poses an increased risk of passing these conditions to offspring (Fitzpatrick et al., 1987).

Trichinosis risk is 25 times greater in Southeast Asian refugees than in the general population. This increased risk is related to undercooking pork and direct farm purchases of pigs (Stehr-Green & Schantz, 1986).

Depression is the greatest threat to refugee health (Muecke, 1983a, 1983b). Half or more Vietnamese clients are diagnosed with depression, anxiety, or both. The risk of developing depression is moderated by social support from the established ethnic community and by having an intact marriage. However, sponsorship by groups with a different religion than that of the refugees can act as an additional source of stress (Beiser, Turner, & Ganeson, 1989).

Possibly related to psychological pressures on refugees is the occurrence of sudden unexplained death syndrome (SUDS), a phenomenon reported mainly for the Hmong, but also affecting Vietnamese and other Asian groups. Nearly all deaths involve physically healthy, young adult men who die at night or during sleep (Baron et al., 1983). The Centers for Disease Control (1990) reported 117 cases from 1981 to 1988 and suggested that a structural abnormality of the cardiac conduction system and stress may be risk factors for SUDS. The exact cause of the deaths remains unknown. These deaths may be a form of unconscious suicide associated with nightmares brought on by intensive feelings of depression and survivor guilt (Tobin & Friedman (1983).

## Health-care Practices

The Vietnamese approach to health care is one of ambivalence. Many Vietnamese immigrants are accustomed to dependence on the family unit and traditional means of providing for health needs. They may be distrustful of outsiders and Western methods. Most are familiar with immunizations and diagnostic tests. They want to avoid health problems and are anxious to follow reasonable procedures. Newly arrived refugees are less likely to seek Western health care, but Vietnamese are the most likely of the Southeast Asians to seek care and to do so earlier (Strand & Jones, 1983). Most Southeast Asian refugees want to go to a physician for an illness, but they rarely seek care when they are asymptomatic and few are familiar with the appointment system. Some regard the most convenient physician as the closest one not requiring an appointment and accepting medical coupons, which usually translates into a hospital emergency room (Muecke, 1983a).

The Vietnamese family may not seek outside assistance for illness until it has exhausted its own resources (Calhoun, 1986). The family may try various home remedies, allowing the condition to become serious before seeking professional assistance. Once a physician or nurse has been consulted, the Vietnamese are usually quite cooperative and respect the wisdom and experience of health-care professionals. Hospitalization is viewed as a last resort and is acceptable only in case of emergency when everything else has failed. With respect to mental health, Vietnamese do not easily trust authority figures, including treatment staff, because of their refugee experiences (Gold, 1992).

## NUTRITION

### Meaning of Food

Meals are an important time to the Vietnamese, allowing the entire family to come together and share a common activity. Preparation is precise and may occupy much of the day. Celebrations and holidays involve elaborately prepared meals, often of a type traditionally associated with the occasion.

## Common Foods and Food Rituals

Because of their size, the normal daily caloric intake of Vietnamese is approximately two-thirds that of average Americans. Rice is the main staple in the diet, providing up to 80 percent of daily calories. Other common foods are fish (including shellfish), pork, chicken, soybean curd (tofu), noodles, various soups, and green vegetables. Preferred fruits are bananas, mangoes, papayas, oranges, coconuts, pineapples, and grapefruits. Soy sauce, garlic, onions, ginger root, lemon, and chili peppers are used as seasoning (Calhoun, 1985, 1986).

The Vietnamese eat almost exclusively white or polished rice, disdaining the more nutritious brown or unpolished variety. Rice and other foods are commonly served with *nuoc mam*, a salty, marinated fish sauce. A meal typically consists of rice, *nuoc mam*, a variety of other seasonings, green vegetables, and sometimes meat cut into slivers. Chicken and duck eggs may be used. The Vietnamese prefer white bread, particularly French loaves and rolls, and pastry. A regular dish is *pho*, a soup containing rice noodles, thinly sliced beef or chicken, and scallions (Stauffer, 1991).

Other Vietnamese dishes resemble Chinese foods commonly seen in the United States. Such include *com chien* (fried rice) and *thit bo xau ca chua* (beef fried with tomatoes). Perhaps the favorite of Americans is *cha gio* (pronounced "cha-yuh"), a combination of finely chopped vegetables, mushrooms, meat or bean curd, rolled into delicate rice paper and deep fried. It is served as part of elaborate meals or during celebrations; proper preparation may require many hours.

Vietnamese eat three meals a day: a light breakfast, a large lunch, and dinner with optional snacks. Meals are served communal style, with food being placed in the center of the table or passed around with everyone taking what they wish. Children wait for their elders to pass each dish. Chopsticks and sometimes spoons are used for eating. Knives are seldom necessary at the table, since meat and vegetables are usually cut into small pieces before serving. Stir frying, steaming, roasting, and boiling are the preferred methods of cooking. Hot tea is the usual beverage.

## Dietary Practices for Health Promotion

A predominant aspect of the traditional Asian system of health maintenance is the principle of balance between two opposing natural forces, known as *am* and *duong* in Vietnamese. These forces are represented by foods that are considered hot (*duong*) or cold (*am*). The terms have nothing to do with temperature and are only partly associated with seasoning. Rice, flour, potatoes, most fruits and vegetables, fish, duck, and other things that grow in water are considered cold. Most other meats, fish sauce, eggs, spices, peppers, onions, candies, and sweets are hot. Tea is cold, coffee is hot, water is cold, and ice is hot.

Illness or trauma may require therapeutic adjustment of hot-cold balance to restore equilibrium. Hot foods and beverages, used to replace and strengthen the blood, are preferred after surgery or childbirth. During illness, certain foods are consumed in greater quantity, such as a light rice gruel (*chao*) mixed with sugar or sweetened condensed milk, and a few pieces of salty pork cooked with fish sauce. Fresh fruits and vegetables are usually avoided, being considered too cold. Water, juices, and other cold drinks are restricted (Calhoun, 1985, 1986; Muecke, 1983a). Nutritional counseling should take into consideration these factors and other aspects of the usual Vietnamese diet, because advice to simply eat certain kinds of American foods may be ignored (Uba, 1992).

## Nutritional Deficiencies and Food Limitations

The traditional Vietnamese diet is basically nutritious, comparing favorably with U.S. federal guidelines for a diet low in fat and sugar, high in complex carbohydrates, and moderate in fiber (Stauffer, 1991). However, the prevalence of anemia in children may be associated with an iron deficiency (Goldenring, Davis, & McChesney, 1982). The Vietnamese diet may also be deficient in calcium and zinc, but exceedingly high in sodium, with implications relevant to hypertension (Calhoun, 1986).

Most Vietnamese adults and many children have lactose intolerance, which may cause problems in schools, other institutional settings, and adoptive families. The health-care provider may need to encourage the use of substitute milk products that use soybeans (Calhoun, 1986; Overfield, 1977; Sokoloff, Carlin, & Pham, 1984; Stauffer, 1991).

Before 1975 immigrants encountered difficulty in preparing traditional dishes, especially in areas with no established Vietnamese community. Even then, the determined housewife could assemble most necessary ingredients through judicious selection at ethnic American, Chinese, Korean, and Indian groceries. Today, nearly all common Vietnamese foods are available at reasonable costs in the United States, except perhaps for certain native fruits and vegetables. In addition, Vietnamese-Americans have changed their diet to a degree, often increasing their fat intake (Stauffer, 1991).

## PREGNANCY AND CHILDBEARING PRACTICES

### Fertility Practices and Views toward Pregnancy

Indochinese women have children over a longer period of life than European-Americans, evidenced by females aged 40 to 44 having a birth rate nearly 14 times as great as their European-American counterparts (Hopkins & Clarke, 1983). Their fertility rate is about three times that of American women, and generally, they know little about contraception (D'Avanzo, 1992a). Abortions are commonly performed in their homeland, because pregnancy outside of marriage is considered a disgrace to the family.

After arriving in the United States, women often desire information on contraception but are afraid to ask. The problem stems in part from their cultural background and emphasis on premarital modesty and virginity (Sutherland et al., 1983). However, when contraception was addressed and information made available at the Mayo Clinic, 80 percent of Vietnamese women chose some method of contraception. Practitioners should avoid forceful family planning indoctrination on the first encounter, but such information is usually well received on subsequent visits (Hoang & Erickson, 1982).

Women over age 40 years have an average of six pregnancies and four births, representing losses due to spontaneous and induced abortions and stillbirths. With a correction for a 6 percent reported rate of induced abortions, fetal death rates appear to be as high as 44 per 1000 live births, whereas in California the death rate is 8 per 1000. The neonatal death rate reported by one group was 184 per 1000 live births, in contrast to the California rate of 14 per 1000 (Minkler, Korenbrot & Brindis, 1988).

## Prescriptive, Restrictive, and Taboo Practices in the Childbearing Family

Prescriptive food practices for a healthy pregnancy include noodles, sweets, sour foods, and fruit but avoidance of fish, salty foods, and rice (Calhoun, 1986). To restore equilibrium and provide adequate warmth to the breast milk, women consume soups with chili peppers, salty fish and meat dishes, and wine steeped with herbs (Fishman, Evans, & Jenks, 1988). In addition to hot and cold, foods are classified as tonic and wind. Tonic foods include animal protein, fat, sugar, and carbohydrates; they are usually also hot and sweet. Sour and sometimes raw and cold foods are classified as antitonic. **Wind** foods, often classified as cold, include leafy vegetables, fruit, beef, mutton, fowl, fish, and glutinous rice. It is considered critical to increase or decrease foods in various categories to restore bodily balances upset by unusual or stressful conditions such as pregnancy. While the balance of foods may be followed, the terminology is not consistently used (Wadd, 1983).

During the first trimester, the expectant mother is considered to be in a weak, cold, and antitonic state. She therefore should correct the imbalance by eating hot foods, such as ripe mangoes, grapes, ginger, peppers, alcohol, and coffee. To provide energy and food for the fetus, she is prescribed tonic foods, including a basic diet of steamed rice and pork. Cold foods, including mung beans, green coconut, spinach, and melon, and antitonic foods, such as vinegar, pineapple, and lemon, are avoided during the first trimester.

In the second trimester, the pregnant woman is considered to be in a neutral state. Cold foods are introduced and the tonic diet is continued.

During the third trimester, when the woman may feel hot and suffer from indigestion and constipation, cold foods are prescribed and hot foods are avoided or strictly limited. Tonic foods, which are believed to increase birth weight, are restricted to reduce the chances of a large baby, which would make birthing difficult. Wind foods are generally avoided throughout pregnancy, as they are associated with convulsions, allergic reactions, asthma, and other problems. This regimen may appear more complex and restrictive than it actually is in practice. Most women use it only as a general guide, commonly restricting rather than totally abstaining from the proscribed foods. A great variety of food, including rice, many kinds of vegetables and fruits, various seasonings, and certain meats and fish are generally permissible throughout pregnancy.

Intensive prenatal care is not the norm in Southeast Asia. Many women do not seek medical attention until the third trimester due to cost, fear, or lack of perceived need (D'Avanzo, 1992a). Vietnamese women who are generally better educated seek early prenatal care more than other Southeast Asians (Hopkins & Clarke, 1983). Of the Vietnamese-American women interviewed by Calhoun (1985), 75 percent thought that monthly examinations were important; however, for obstetric and gynecologic matters, they tended to feel more comfortable with a female physician or midwife.

Traditionally, Vietnamese women maintain physical activity to keep the fetus moving and to prevent edema, miscarriage, or premature delivery. Prolonged labor may result from idleness, and an undesirable large baby may result from afternoon napping (Manderson & Mathews, 1981). Additional restrictive beliefs include avoiding heavy lifting and strenuous work, raising the arms above the head, which pulls on the placenta causing it to break, and sexual relations late in pregnancy, which may cause respiratory stress in the infant (D'Avanzo, 1992a). In Vietnam, many consider it taboo for pregnant women to attend weddings or funerals. However, they often look at pictures of happy families and healthy children, believing that it helps give birth to healthy babies (Calhoun, 1986).

In Vietnam, most children are delivered in a screened off portion of the home, or in a special birth house by certified midwives, although some are born in hospitals with Western-trained physicians in attendance. Invasive procedures, such as episiotomies, cesarean sections, circumcisions, nasal oxygen, and intravenous fluids are generally disliked by Southeast Asians. However, unlike some women of other ethnic groups, Vietnamese women may ask for anesthesia during labor and delivery. Otherwise, once in labor the Vietnamese woman tries to maintain self-control and may even smile continuously (D'Avanzo, 1992a). Her period of labor is usually short, and there may be no warning of impending delivery. Although a special bed may be available, the mother may prefer walking around during labor and squatting during the birth process. This position is less traumatic than others, both for mother and baby and results in fewer and less serious lacerations.

Because the head is considered sacred, neither that of the mother nor of the infant should be touched or stroked. Removal of vernix from the infant's head can cause distress. The American practice of inserting intravenous devices into infants' scalps can be particularly stressful to Vietnamese families. The health-care provider needs to stress the importance and necessity of this invasive procedure and select other venous routes if possible.

Customary practices include clearing the neonate's throat using the finger, cutting the umbilical cord with a nonmetal instrument, quickly burying the placenta to protect the infant's health, and ritual cleansing for the mother that does not involve actual bathing with water. In the United States, Vietnamese husbands may be present during the birthing process, although they may not assist (Calhoun, 1986; D'Avanzo, 1992a; Mathews & Manderson, 1981; Muecke, 1983b; Nelson & Hewitt, 1983; Wadd, 1983).

Because body heat is lost during delivery, Vietnamese women avoid cold foods and beverages and increase consumption of hot foods to replace and strengthen their blood. Ice water and other cold drinks are usually not welcome, and most raw vegetables, fruits, and sour items are taken in lesser amounts. Prescriptive foods include steamed rice, fish sauce, pork, chicken, eggs, soups with chili or black peppers, other highly seasoned and salty items, wine, and sweets (Calhoun, 1985; Fishman, Evans, & Jenks, 1988; Mathews & Manderson, 1981; Wadd, 1983).

Because water is cold, women traditionally do not fully bathe, shower, or wash their hair for a month after delivery. Some Vietnamese women have complained that they were adversely affected by showering shortly after delivery in American hospitals. Others, however, have welcomed the opportunity to shower and seem willing to give up other traditional practices (Calhoun, 1986; D'Avanzo, 1992a; Mathews & Manderson, 1981; Wadd, 1983). Postpartum women also avoid drafts and strenuous activity, wear warm clothing, stay in bed, indoors, or both for about a month, and avoid sexual intercourse for months. In the past, postpartum women remained in a special bed above a slow burning fire. This practice still continues with the use of hot water bottles or electric blankets.

Other women in the family assume responsibility for the baby's care. The mother's inactivity and dependence on others may be incorrectly interpreted by health-care workers as apathy or depression. A newborn is often dressed in old clothes, it is considered taboo to praise the child lest jealous spirits steal the infant. The mother may be reluctant to cut the child's hair or nails for fear that this might cause illness. The infant is generally maintained on a diet of milk for the first year, with the introduction of rice gruel at around 6 months. There is little formal toilet training; the child usually learns by imitating an older child (Calhoun, 1986).

Breast-feeding is customary in Vietnam, but since resettlement some variations on this practice have been instituted. Some Southeast Asian women discard colostrum and feed the baby rice paste or boiled sugar water for several days. This does not indicate a decision against breast-feeding. After the milk comes in, both mother and young benefit from the hot foods consumed by the mother for the first month. Then, however, a conflict arises: the mother believes that hot foods benefit her health but that cold foods ensure healthy breast milk. This dilemma can be easily solved by having the mother change from breast-feeding to formula. However, if the mother cannot afford formula, she may use fresh milk or rice boiled with water, which may result in anemia and growth retardation. Some health-care professionals, concerned about these developments and their impact on the infant's health, have recommended programs that might restore conditions conducive to traditional breast-feeding (D'Avanzo, 1992a; Fishman, Evans, & Jenks, 1988; Muecke, 1983a; Serdula et al., 1991; Wadd, 1983).

# DEATH RITUALS

## Death Rituals and Expectations

Vietnamese accept death as a normal aspect of the life process. The traditional stoicism of the Vietnamese, the influence of Buddhism with its emphasis on cyclic continuity and reincarnation, and the pervading association of current activities with ancestral spirits and burial places contribute to attitudes toward death.

Most Vietnamese have an aversion to hospitals and prefer to die at home. Some believe that a person who dies outside the home becomes a wandering soul with no place to rest. Family members think that they can provide more comfort to the dying person at home. Sixty percent of women in one survey said that if someone in their family were dying, they would not want that person told; 95 percent said that they would want a priest or minister with them when they died, and 95 percent indicated a belief in life after death (Calhoun, 1985, 1986). Ancestors are commonly honored and worshipped and are believed to bestow protection on the living. Southeast Asians tend not to want to artificially prolong life and suffering, but it may still be difficult for relatives to consent to terminating active intervention, which might be viewed as contributing to the death of an ancestor who would shape the fates of the living (Muecke, 1983a).

Few consent to autopsy unless they know and agree with the reasons for it (Nguyen, 1985). Older Vietnamese, on realizing the inevitability of death, sometimes purchase coffins in advance, display them beneath the household altar, and choose burial sites with a favorable position. Although much Vietnamese custom is associated with proper burial practices and maintenance of ancestral tombs, cremation is an acceptable practice to some families.

## Responses to Death and Grief

Vietnamese families may wish to gather around the body of a recently deceased relative and express great emotion. Traditional mourning practices include the wearing of white clothes for 14 days, the subsequent wearing of black arm bands by men and white head bands by women, and the yearly celebration of the anniversary of a person's death (Calhoun, 1985). Such observances, together with ritual cleaning and worship at ancestral graves, help reinforce family ties and are deeply woven into Vietnamese culture (Stauffer, 1991). Departure from Vietnam has greatly curtailed the observance of these practices, leaving a painful void for many refugees.

Priests and monks should only be called at the request of the client or family. Clergy visitation is usually associated with last rites by the Vietnamese, especially those influenced by Catholicism, and can actually be upsetting to hospitalized clients. Sending flowers may be startling, as flowers usually are reserved for the rites of the dead (Stauffer, 1991).

# SPIRITUALITY

## Religious Practices and Use of Prayer

The major religions practiced by Vietnamese are Buddhism, Confucianism, and Taoism, and 5 percent of Vietnamese are Christians, most of whom are Catholic. There are a number of other religions, and these are basically offshoots and combinations of the major faiths. Animism is found mainly among the highland tribes. Many Vietnamese believe that deities and spirits control the universe and that the spirits of dead relatives continue to dwell in the home (Calhoun, 1986).

Most Vietnamese are Buddhists but some almost never visit temples or perform rituals. Others, both Buddhist and Christian, may maintain a religious altar in the home and conduct regular religious observances. In cases of severe illness, prayers and offerings may be made at a temple (Calhoun, 1985, 1986).

## Meaning of Life and Individual Sources of Strength

While the wish to bring honor and prosperity to the family remains a dominant force for most Vietnamese, many find meaning in life from the practice of Buddhism or other religions. Some are driven by the desire to learn, to relieve suffering, to produce beauty, to assist the progress of civilization, and to gain strength from participating in ethnic community activities.

"The family is the main reference point for the individual throughout his life, superseding obligations to country, religion, and self. The family is responsible for all decisions and individual actions" (Calhoun, 1986, p. 15). The family is the fundamental social unit and the primary source of cohesion and continuity (Nguyen, 1985).

## Spiritual Beliefs and Health Practices

Vietnamese religious practices are influenced by the Eastern philosophies of Buddhism, Confucianism, and Taoism. Central to Buddhism is the concept that suffering is caused by desire, can be eliminated by following the correct path of life, and that the world is a cycle of ordeals: to be born, grow old, fall ill, and die. In addition, people's present lives predetermine their own and their dependents' future lives.

Confucianism stresses harmony through maintenance of the proper order of social hierarchies, ethics, worship of ancestors, and the virtues of chastity and faithfulness. Taoism teaches harmony, allowing events to follow a natural course that one should not attempt to change. These beliefs have contributed to an attitude, which may be perceived as passive by westerners, characterized by maintenance of self-control, acceptance of one's destiny, and fatalism towards illness and death.

## HEALTH-CARE PRACTICES

### Health-seeking Beliefs and Behaviors

One dominant theory influencing health-care practices among Vietnamese is a metaphysical explanation that views health as but one facet of a comprehensive scheme of life. Good health is achieved by having harmony and balance with the two basic opposing forces, *am* (cold, dark, female) and *duong* (hot, light, male). An excess of either force may lead to discomfort or illness.

Naturalistic explanations for poor health include eating spoiled food and exposure to inclement weather. The natural element known as *cao gio* is associated with bad weather and cold drafts and causes problems such as the common cold, mild fever, and headache. Countermeasures involve dietary, herbal, hygienic, and simple medical practices. Collectively, these measures are categorized as *thuoc nam*, the traditional southern medicine of Vietnam, and *thuoc bac*, the more formal northern or Chinese medicine. One final explanation for illness places blame on supernaturalistic causes, such as gods, spirits, or demons. Illness may be seen as a punishment for offending such an entity or violating some religious or moral code.

The belief that life is predetermined is a deterrent to seeking health care. For many Vietnamese, diagnostic tests are baffling, inconvenient, and often unnecessary.

Procedures such as circumcision or tonsillectomy, which biomedicine considers simple, are generally unknown to Vietnamese. Invasive procedures are frightening. The prospect of surgery can be terrorizing. A great fear of mutilation stems from widespread beliefs among non-Christians that souls are attached to different parts of the body and can leave the body, causing illness or death. Loss of blood from any route is feared, and the Vietnamese may refuse to have blood drawn for laboratory tests (Calhoun, 1985). The client may complain, though not to the health-care worker, of feeling weak for months. A Vietnamese-American client may feel that any body tissue or fluid removed cannot be replaced, and the body suffers the loss in this life and into the next life (Stauffer, 1991).

The concept of long-term medication for chronic illnesses and acceptance of unpleasant side effects and increased autonomic symptoms, which are standard components of modern Western medicine, are not congruent with traditional notions of safe and effective treatment of illnesses.

## Responsibility for Health Care

In Vietnam, the family is the primary provider of health care, even in hospitals. This practice survives because of tradition and a shortage of professional personnel (Graaf, 1979). Hospitalized clients are attended by their own families day and night. Lin and Shen (1991) stressed the importance of including family members in all major treatment decisions regarding physical and mental health. Elder family members or clan leaders must always be consulted before a client agrees to a medical treatment (Felice, 1986).

Health care in Vietnam is crisis oriented, with symptom relief as the goal. Vietnamese typically deal with illness by means of self-care, self-medication, and the use of herbal medicines. Facsimiles of Western prescription drugs are sold over the counter throughout Southeast Asia (D'Avanzo, 1992a), which may explain the increasing resistance of bacteria to several readily available antibiotics (Nguyen, 1985). In addition, cases of agranulocytosis develop with overuse of antibiotics (Stauffer, 1991).

Many Vietnamese believe that Western medicine is very powerful and cures quickly, but few understand the risks of overdosages or underdosages. Some believe that Asians have a different physical constitution than European-Americans, so that Western drugs and drug dosages that are appropriate for European-Americans may not be appropriate for Asians. Consequently, they may politely accept the prescription, but not fill it. If they have filled it, they may not take the medicine, or they may adjust the dosage without telling the health-care provider to avoid hurting or embarrassing anyone (Uba, 1992). Clients being treated for depression who fail to take their antidepressants evidence improvement after receiving instructions for taking their medication (Lin & Shen, 1991). Vietnamese clients may not follow prescribed schedules of medication for the treatment and prevention of tuberculosis. Extensive education, repetition of instructions, and home visitation are necessary.

## Folklore Practices

The forces of *am* (cold) and *duong* (hot) are pervasive forces in the practice of traditional Vietnamese medicine. **Am** represents factors that are considered negative, feminine, dark, and empty, whereas **duong** represents those that are positive, masculine, light, and full. These terms are applied to various parts, organs, and processes of the body. For example, the inside of the body is *am,* and the surface is *duong.* The front part of the body is *am,* and the back is *duong.* The liver, heart, spleen, lungs, and kidneys are *am*, and the gallbladder, stomach, intestines, bladder, and lymph system are *duong*. *Am* stores strength, and care must be taken not to use it up too quickly. *Duong* protects the body from outside forces, and if not cared for, the organs are thrown into disorder. Proper balance of these two life forces ensures the correct circulation of blood and good health. If the balance is not proper, life is short (Calhoun, 1986; Mathews & Manderson, 1981; Spector, 1991).

Diseases and other debilitating conditions result from either cold or hot influences. For example, diarrhea and some febrile diseases are due to an excess of cold, whereas pimples and other skin problems result from an excess of hot. Countermeasures involve using foods, medications, and treatments that have properties opposite those of the problem, and avoiding those foods that would intensify the problem. Asian herbs are cold and Western medicines are hot (Nguyen, 1985; Spector, 1991; Stauffer, 1991).

A widely held belief among Vietnamese refugees is that Asian medicine relieves symptoms of a disease more quickly than Western medicine, but that Western medications can actually cure the illness. Almost all prefer Asian methods for children (Goldfield & Lee, 1982). Reliance on traditional folk medicine is declining in the United States, partly because of the unavailability of suitable shamans and traditional herbs (Uba, 1992).

Some of the common treatments practiced in Vietnam and continued to some degree in the United States are described below.

*Cao gio*, literally meaning "rubbing out the wind" is used for treating colds, sore throats, flu, sinusitis, and similar ailments. An ointment or hot balm oil is spread across the back, chest, or shoulders and rubbed with the edge of a coin (preferably silver) in short, firm strokes. This technique brings blood under the skin, resulting in dark ecchymotic stripes, so the offending wind can escape. Healthcare professionals must be careful not to interpret these ecchymotic areas as evidence of child abuse. However, dermabrasion may provide a portal for infection.

*Be bao* or *bar gio*, skin pinching, is a treatment for headache or sore throat. The skin of the affected area is repeatedly squeezed between the thumb and forefinger of both hands, as the hands converge towards the center of the face. The objective is to produce ecchymoses or petechiae.

*Giac*, cup suctioning, another dermabrasive procedure, is used to relieve stress, headaches, and joint and muscle pain. A small cup is heated and placed on the skin with the open side down. As the cup cools, it contracts the skin and draws unwanted hot energy into the cup. This treatment leaves marks that may appear as large bruises.

*Xong*, an herbal preparation relieves motion sickness or cold related problems. Herbs or an agent such as Vicks Vaporub, is put into boiling water and the vapor is inhaled. Small containers of aromatic oils or liniments are sometimes carried and inhaled directly.

Acupuncture, acupressure, and acumassage relieves symptomatic stress and pain. (See Glossary for a description).

**Moxibustion** is used to counter conditions associated with excess cold, including labor and delivery. Pulverized wormwood or incense is heated and placed directly on the skin at certain meridians.

Balms and oils, such as Red Tiger balm available in Asian shops, are applied to affected areas for relief of bone and muscle ailments.

Herbal teas, soups, and other concoctions are taken for various problems, generally in the sense of using cold measures to overcome hot illnesses.

Eating organ meats such as liver, kidneys, testes, brains, and bones of an animal is said to increase the strength of the corresponding human part (Buchwald, Panwala, & Hooton, 1992; Calhoun, 1986; Chow, 1976; Feldman, 1984; Muecke, 1983a; Nguyen, 1985; Spector, 1991; Stauffer, 1991).

Two additional practices in Vietnam are consuming gelatinized tiger bones to gain strength (Nguyen, 1985) and taking powdered rhinoceros horn to reduce fever

(Calhoun, 1985). At least 430 folk medicines used by Vietnamese contain ingredients from endangered, threatened, or protected species (Gaski & Johnson, 1994).

## Barriers to Health Care

Barriers to adequate health care for Vietnamese include:

1. Subjective beliefs and the cost of health care

2. Lack of a primary provider

3. Differences between Western and Asian health care

4. Caregivers judging Vietnamese as deviant and unmotivated because of noncompliance with medication schedules, diagnostic tests, and follow-up care and failure to keep appointments

5. Inability to communicate effectively in the English language with recent immigrants who lack confidence in their ability to communicate their needs (D'Avanzo, 1992b); failure of providers to communicate

6. Avoiding Western practitioners out of a fear that traditional methods will be criticized

7. Fear of conflicts and ridicule resulting in loss of face

8. Lack of knowledge of the availability of resources (Uba, 1992)

Additional barriers exist for Vietnamese when seeking mental health care. These include the fear of stigmatization, difficulty locating agencies that can provide assistance without distorted professional and cultural communication (Gold, 1992), and unwillingness to express inner feelings (Buchwald et al., 1993).

## Cultural Responses to Health and Illness

Fatalistic attitudes and the belief that problems are punishment may reduce the degree of complaining and expression of pain among the Vietnamese, who view endurance as an indicator of strong character. One accepts pain as part of life and attempts to maintain self-control as a means of relief. Deep cultural restraints against showing weakness limits the use of pain medication (Nguyen, 1985). However, the sick person is allowed to depend on family and receives a great deal of attention and care (Calhoun, 1985).

Many Vietnamese believe that mental illness results from offending a deity and that it brings disgrace to the family and therefore must be concealed. A shaman may be enlisted to help, and additional therapy is sought only with the greatest discretion and often after a dangerous delay (Calhoun, 1985, 1986). Emotional disturbance is usually attributed to possession by malicious spirits, the bad luck of familial inheritance, or for Buddhists, to bad karma accumulated by misdeeds in past lives (Muecke, 1983b). The term *psychiatrist* has no direct translation in Vietnamese and may be interpreted to mean nerve physician or specialist who treats crazy people. The nervous system sometimes is seen as the source of mental problems, neurosis being thought of as "weakness of the nerves" and psychosis as "turmoil of the nerves" (Stauffer, 1991).

To overcome these problems, Kinzie et al. (1982) and Buchwald et al. (1993) developed a Vietnamese depression scale, which uses terms that allows an English-speaking practitioner to make a cross-cultural assessment of the clinical characteristics of depressed Vietnamese clients. The health-care provider working with Vietnamese clients may find this scale useful when providing mental health services.

Physically disabled persons are common and readily seen in Vietnam. To the extent that resources allow, they are treated well and cared for by their families and the government. In contrast, a mentally disabled person may be stigmatized by the family and society and can jeopardize the ability of relatives to find marriage partners. The mentally disabled are usually harbored within their families unless they become destructive; then they may be admitted to a hospital (Calhoun, 1985; Fabrega & Nguyen, 1992; Muecke, 1983b; Timberlake & Cook, 1984).

## Blood Transfusion and Organ Donation

Because many Vietnamese believe that the body must be kept intact even after death, they are averse to blood transfusions and organ donation. Many Vietnamese, even those whose families have long been Christian, may object to removal of body parts or organ donation (Stauffer, 1991). However, some staff in a rural hospital in Vietnam donated blood after learning that the body replenished its blood supply. The smaller size of Vietnamese adults makes many of them ineligible to donate a full unit of blood. Other Vietnamese preferring cremation will donate body parts under certain circumstances.

## HEALTH-CARE PRACTITIONERS

## Traditional Versus Biomedical Practitioners

Four kinds of traditional and folk practitioners exist in Vietnam (Burney et al., 1985). The first group are Asian physicians who are learned individuals and employ herbal medication and acupuncture. The second group are more informal folk healers who use special herbs and diets as cures based on natural or pragmatic approaches. The secrets of folk medicine are passed down through the generations. The third group comprises various forms of spiritual healers, some with a specific religious outlook and others with powers to drive away malevolent spirits. The fourth are magicians or sorcerers who have magical curative powers but no communication with the spirits. Many Vietnamese consult one or more of these healers in an attempt to find a cure.

While many Vietnamese have great respect for professional, well-educated persons, they may be distrustful of outside authority figures. Most Vietnamese have come to American to escape oppressive authority. Refugees generally expect health-care professionals to be experts (Muecke, 1983a). A common suspicion is that divulging personal information for a medical history could jeopardize their legal rights. Respect and mistrust are not mutually exclusive concepts for Vietnamese seeking care from Western practitioners.

Acknowledgment and support of traditional belief systems are important in building a trusting relationship. Traditional healers often provide Vietnamese with necessary social support (Lay & Faust, 1987).

Traditional Asian male practitioners do not usually touch the bodies of female clients and sometimes use a doll to point out the nature of a problem. While most Vietnamese might no longer insist on the use of the practice, adults, particularly young and unmarried women, are more comfortable with health-care providers of the same gender. Pelvic examinations on unmarried women should not be made on the first visit or without careful advanced explanation and preparation. When such an examination is necessary, the woman may want her husband present. If possible, the practitioner and any interpreter should both be female. Women may not want to even discuss sexual problems, reproductive matters, and birth control techniques until after an initial visit and confidence has been established in the practitioner (Felice, 1986; Hoang & Erickson, 1982; Muecke, 1983a).

## Status of Health-care Providers

Because of the shortage of physicians in Vietnam, Western medicine is practiced by medical assistants, nurses, village health-care workers, self-trained individuals, and injectionists. Paralleling these approaches are the traditional systems of Asian and folk medicine. All are respected and have high status and may be used concurrently or separately, according to the illness and varying beliefs of each individual (Hoang & Erickson, 1982).

---

**CASE STUDY**

Colonel Tran Van Minh, aged 54 years, arrived in Arlington, Virginia, about a year ago directly from Vietnam under the Orderly Departure Program. Colonel Minh had been the commander of a tank battalion in the old South Vietnamese army in 1975. After a desperate battle against the advancing North Vietnamese forces, during which he saw many of his men and friends die horribly, Colonel Minh was taken prisoner. Incarcerated for over a decade under extremely harsh conditions, he again witnessed the brutalization and death of many associates. After his release, he was still kept under close observation, not allowed to work professionally, and lived mostly on the charity of remaining family members. After a lengthy process, involving bribery and pressure from the U.S. government, he was finally allowed to leave the country.

When South Vietnam fell in 1975, Colonel Minh's brother, Toan, was able to get out of the country with his wife, mother, and several other family members and immigrate to the United States. In 1987, after much effort, they arranged for more of the family to come, including Colonel Minh's wife Cao Thi Xuan, aged 45 years, her son Danh, aged 23 years, and her daughter Tuyet, aged 21 years. The last three family members were supported by the rest of the family for a while, but Xuan found a succession of jobs to support her children and lately has been earning a reasonably good salary as a check-out clerk in a supermarket. Danh, or "Danny," as he is known to American friends, has adapted well to the United States, speaks English fluently, has completed college, and has an excellent job as a computer programmer, contributing extensively to the support of the family. In contrast, Tuyet, sometimes called "Sally," drifts back and forth, has dropped out of school, has no steady employment, and often accompanies members of a local Vietnamese gang. When she returns home, she is subjected to criticism from other family members, especially her 75-year-old paternal grandmother, Lan.

Initially delighted at being reunited with his loved ones and full of hope for the future, Colonel Minh has become confused and morose. He has found no permanent employment and has been reluctant to undergo job retraining but, at the same time, is upset about his wife having to work. While pleased with the success of his son, there have been disputes between the two regarding disposition of family funds and the amount of time Danny spends away from the family. Minh has been somewhat protective of Sally, but he has been pressured by Lan and Toan to totally disown her. Minh, weakened by his long imprisonment, is under intensive medication for tuberculosis. He seems somewhat distrustful of Western health care, is careless about following directions, and is reluctant to return for follow-up examinations. Despite repeated advice, he has continued to smoke heavily.

Lately, Colonel Minh seems to have lost interest in day-to-day matters, constantly speaks with remorse of the old times in Vietnam and all of those who died

*continued on page 474*

there, and has experienced nightmares and much trouble sleeping. Partly at the instigation of Lan, he has begun to visit an elderly local Vietnamese woman reputed to be a traditional "healer" and has been given various herbal concoctions. Just in the last few days, Minh has complained of overall weakness, "heart pains," and headaches. At the urging of Xuan and Danny, he finally has agreed to return to a Western clinic, where he has again described the symptoms.

## STUDY QUESTIONS

1. What is the preferred form of address for Minh and Xuan, and how should their names be recorded?

2. Identify the most critical cultural factors affecting Vietnamese people after immigration.

3. What information can be provided to Minh and his family to help improve medication compliance and other aspects of physical health?

4. If Minh's immediate physical complaints are found to lack substance, what process might be suspected and what measures should be taken?

5. What questions should be asked regarding Minh's traditional treatments?

6. Explain some of the major religious factors influencing the Vietnamese outlook toward health care.

7. Distinguish "ethnic Vietnamese" from other Southeast Asian groups.

8. What is generally considered the most serious health problem for Vietnamese refugees?

9. What is the role of the family in Vietnamese health care?

10. Explain the connotations of "hot" and "cold" in traditional Vietnamese health care.

11. Discuss some of the customary practices in a Western hospital that might be upsetting to a pregnant or postpartum Vietnamese woman.

12. Name three traditional Vietnamese treatments and their connotations to Western professionals.

## References

August, L. R. (1987). Symptoms of war trauma induced psychiatric disorders: Southeast Asian refugees and Vietnam veterans. *International Migration Review, 21*(3), 820–831.

Baron, R.C., Thacker, S. B., Gorelkin, L., Vernon, A. A., Taylor, W. R., & Choi, K. (1983). Sudden death among Southeast Asian refugees. *Journal of the American Medical Association, 250*(21), 2947–2951.

Barry, M., Craft, J., Coleman, D., Coulter, H., & Horowitz, R. (1993). Clinical findings in Southeast Asian refugees. *Journal of the American Medical Association, 249*(23), 3200–3203.

Beiser, M. (1988). Influences of time, ethnicity, and attachment on depression in Southeast Asian refugees. *American Journal of Psychiatry, 145,* 46–51.

Beiser, M., Turner, R., & Ganesan, S. (1989).

Catastrophic stress and factors affecting its consequences among Southeast Asian refugees. *Social Science Medicine, 28*(3), 183–195.

Buchwald, D., Panwala, S. & Hooton, T. M. (1992). Use of traditional health practices by Southeast Asian refugees in a primary care clinic. *Western Journal of Medicine, 156*(5), 507–511.

Buchwald, D., Manson, S. M., Dinges, N. G., Keane, E. M., & Kinzie, J. D. (1993). Prevalence of depressive symptoms among established Vietnamese refugees in the United States. *Journal of General Internal Medicine 8*(2), 76–81.

Burney, L. R., Dumara, K. W., Chea, C. S., Nguyen, H. D., & Bustillo, M. (1985). The Southeast Asian refugee: The impact of cultural variation on the genetic counseling process. In B. B. Biesecker, P. A. Magyari, & N. W. Paul (Eds.), *Strategies in genetic counseling: Religious, cultural and ethnic influences on the counseling process* (pp. 239–244). White Plains, NY: March of Dimes Birth Defects Foundation.

Calhoun, M. A. (1985). The Vietnamese woman: Health/illness attitudes and behaviors. *Health Care for Women International, 6*(1–3), 61–72.

Calhoun, M. A. (1986). Providing health care to Vietnamese in America: What practitioners need to know. *Home Healthcare Nurse, 4*(5), 14–22.

Canadian abstracts: Ethnic origins (1993). Ottowa, Canada: Ministry of Industry, Science and Technology.

Catanzaro, A., & Moser, R. J. (1982). Health status of refugees from Vietnam, Laos, and Cambodia. *Journal of the American Medical Association, 247*(9), 1303–1308.

Centers for Disease Control (1990). Update: Sudden unexplained death syndrome among Southeast Asian refugees—United States. *Journal of the American Medical Association, 260*(14), 2033.

Chen, M. S., Kuun, P., Guthrie, R., Li, W. & Zaharlick, A. (1991). Providing heart health for Southeast Asians: A database for planning interventions. *Public Health Reports, 106*(3), 304–309.

Chow, E. (1976). Cultural health traditions: Asian perspectives. In M. F. Branch & P. P. Paxton (Eds.), *Providing safe nursing care for ethnic people of color.* New York: Appleton-Century-Crofts.

Chung, R. C., & Kagawa-Singer, M. (1993). Predictors of psychological distress among Southeast Asian refugees. *Social Science Medicine, 36*(5), 631–639.

Cochran, S. D., Mays, V. M. & Leung, L. (1991). Sexual practices of heterosexual Asian-American young adults: Implications for risk of HIV infection. *Archives of Sexual Behavior, 20*(4), 381–391.

Dao, A. H., Gregory, D. W., & McKee, C. (1984). Specific health problems of Southeast Asian refugees in middle Tennessee. *Southern Medical Journal, 77*(8), 995–997.

D'Avanzo, C. E. (1992a). Bridging the cultural gap with Southeast Asians. *American Journal of Maternity and Child Nursing, 17*(4), 204–208.

D'Avanzo, C. E. (1992b). Barriers to health care for Vietnamese refugees. *Journal of Professional Nursing, 8*(4), 245–253.

Eyton, J., & Neuwirth, G. (1984). Cross-cultural validity: Ethnocentrism in health studies with special reference to the Vietnamese. *Social Science Medicine, 18*(5), 447–453.

Fabrega, H., & Nguyen, H. (1992). Culture, social structure, and quandaries of psychiatric diagnosis: A Vietnamese case study. *Psychiatry, 55*(3), 230-249.

Feldman, K. W. (1984). Pseudoabrasive burns in Asian refugees. *American Journal of Diseases of Children, 138*(8), 768–769.

Felice, M. E. (1986). Reflections on caring for Indochinese children and youths. *Developmental and Behavioral Pediatrics, 7*(2), 124–130.

Fishman, C., Evans, R., & Jenks, E. (1988). Warm bodies, cool milk: Conflicts in post partum food choice for Indochinese women in California. *Social Science Medicine, 26*(11), 1125–1132.

Fitzpatrick, S., Johnson, J., Shragg, P., & Felice, M. E. (1987). Health care needs of Indochinese refugee teenagers. *Pediatrics, 79*(1), 118–124.

Fox, P. G. (1991). Stress related to family change among Vietnamese refugees. *Journal of Community Health Nursing, 8*(1), 45–56.

Franks, A. L., Berg, C. J., Kane, M. A., Browne, B. B., Sikes, R. K., Elsea, W. R., & Burton, A. H. (1988). Hepatitis B virus infection among children born in the United States to Southeast Asian refugees. *New England Journal of Medicine, 321*(19), 1301–1305.

Gaski, A. L., & Johnson, K. A. (1994). *Prescription for extinction: Endangered species and patented Oriental medicines in trade.* Washington, DC: Traffic USA.

Gold, S. J. (1992). Mental health and illness in Vietnamese refugees. *Western Journal of Medicine, 157*(3), 290–294.

Goldenring, J. M., Davis, J., & McChesney, M. (1982). Pediatric screening of Southeast Asian immigrants. *Clinical Pediatrics, 21*(10), 613-616.

Goldfield, N., & Lee, W. (1982). Caring for Indochinese refugees. *American Family Physician, 26*(3), 157–160.

Graaf, J. K. (1979). Vietnam revisited: A transcultural reassessment. In M. Leininger (Ed.), *Transcultural nursing.* New York: Masson International Nursing Publications.

Guerrero, I. C., Chin, W., & Collins, W. E. (1982). A survey of malaria in Indochinese refugees arriving in the United States, 1980. *American Journal of Tropical Medicine and Hygiene, 31*(5), 897–901.

Hinton, W. L., Chen, Y. J., Nang, D., Tran, C. G., Lu, F. G., Miranda, J. & Faust, S. (1993). DSM-III-R disorders in Vietnamese refugees. *Journal of Nervous and Mental Disease, 181*(2), 113–122.

Hoang, G. N., & Erickson, R. V. (1982). Guidelines for providing medical care to

Southeast Asian refugees. *Journal of the American Medical Association, 248*(6), 710–714.

Hopkins, D. D., & Clarke, N. G. (1983). Indochinese refugee fertility rates and pregnancy risk factors: Oregon. *American Journal of Public Health, 73*(11), 1307–1309.

*Information please: Almanac.* (1995). Boston: Houghton Mifflin.

Jenkins, C. N. H., McPhee, S. J., Bird, J. A., & Bonilla, N. H. (1990). Cancer risks and prevention practices among Vietnamese refugees. *Western Journal of Medicine, 153*(1), 34–39.

Jenkins, C. N. H., McPhee, S. J., Fordham, D. C., Hung, S., Nguyen, K. P., Ha, N. T., Saika, G., Chen, A., Lew, R., Thai, V., Ko, K. L., Okahara, L., Hirota, S., Chan. S., Wong, W. F., Snider, J., Littlefield, D., Quan, D., Folkers, L. F., & Marquez, B. (1992). Cigarette smoking among Chinese, Vietnamese, and Hispanics: California, 1989–1991. *Morbidity and Mortality Weekly Report, 41*(20), 362–367.

Kinzie, J. D. (1986). Indochinese psychiatric clinic. *Hospital and Community Psychiatry, 37*(11), 1144–1147.

Kinzie, J. D., Manson, S. M., Vinh, D. T., Tolan, N. T., Anh, B., & Pho, T. N. (1982). Development and validation of a Vietnamese-language depression rating scale. *American Journal of Psychiatry, 139*(10), 1276–1281.

Kleinman, S. B. (1990). Terror at sea: Vietnamese victims of piracy. *American Journal of Psychoanalysis, 50*(4), 351–362.

Lay, P. D. & Faust, S. (1987). Depression in Southeast Asian refugees. *American Family Physician, 36*(4), 179–184.

Leininger, M. (1970). *Nursing and anthropology: Two worlds to blend.* New York: John Wiley & Sons.

Levy, R. A. (1993). Ethnic and racial differences in response to medicines: Preserving individualized therapy in managed pharmaceutical programmes. *Pharmaceutical Medicine, 7,* 139–165.

Lin, K., & Finder, E. (1983). Neuroleptic dosage for Asians. *American Journal of Psychiatry, 140*(4), 490–491.

Lin, K., & Shen, W. W. (1991). Pharmacotherapy for Southeast Asian psychiatric patients. *Journal of Nervous and Mental Disease, 179*(6), 346–350.

Manderson, L., & Mathews, M. (1981). Vietnamese behavioral and dietary precautions during pregnancy. *Ecology of Food and Nutrition, 11*(1), 1–8.

Mathews, M., & Manderson, L. (1981). Vietnamese behavioral and dietary precautions during confinement. *Ecology of Food and Nutrition, 11*(1), 9-16.

McKelvey, R. S., Webb, J. A., & Mao, A. R. (1993). Premigratory risk factors in Vietnamese Amerasians. *American Journal of Psychiatry, 150*(3), 470–473.

Minkler, D. H., Korenbrot, C., & Brindis, C. (1988). Family planning among Southeast Asian refugees. *Health Care Delivery, 148*(3), 349–354.

Muecke, M. A. (1983a). Caring for Southeast Asian refugee patients in the USA. *American Journal of Public Health, 73*(4), 431–438.

Muecke, M. A. (1983b). In search of healers: Southeast Asian refugees in the American health care system. *Western Journal of Medicine, 139*(6), 835–840.

Nelson, C. C., & Hewitt, M. A. (1983). An Indochinese refugee population in a nurse-midwife service. *Journal of Nurse-Midwifery, 28*(5), 9–14.

Nguyen, D. (1985). Culture shock: A review of Vietnamese culture and its concepts of health and disease. *Western Journal of Medicine, 142*(3), 409–412.

Nguyen, N. A., & Williams, H. L. (1989). Transition from east to west: Vietnamese adolescents and their parents. *Journal of the American Academy of Child and Adolescent Psychiatry, 28*(4), 505–515.

Olsen, S. J., & Frank-Stromborg, M. (1993). Cancer prevention and early detection in ethnically diverse populations. *Seminars in Oncology Nursing, 9*(3), 198–209.

Overfield, T. (1977). Biological variation. *Nursing Clinics of North America, 12*(1), 19–27.

Paxton, P., Ramirez, M. C., & Walloch, E. C. (1976). Nursing assessment and intervention. In M. F. Branch & P. P. Paxton (Eds.), *Providing safe nursing care for ethnic people of color.* New York: Appleton-Century-Crofts.

Pickwell, S. M. (1982). Primary health care for Indochinese refugee children. *Pediatric Nursing, 8*(2), 104–107.

Roberts, N. S., Copel, J. A., Bhutani, V., Otis, C. & Gluckman, S. (1985). Intestinal parasites and other infections during pregnancy in Southeast Asian refugees. *Journal of Reproductive Medicine, 30*(10), 720–725.

Robinson, C. (1980). Special report: Physical and emotional health care needs of Indochinese refugees. Washington, DC: Indochina Refugee Action Center.

Rosenblat, R., & Tang, S. W. (1987). Do Oriental psychiatric patients receive different dosages of psychotropic medication when compared with Occidentals? *Canadian Journal of Psychiatry, 32,* 270–273.

Ross, T. F. (1982). Health care problems of Southeast Asian refugees. *Western Journal of Medicine, 136*(1), 35–43.

Serdula, M. K., Cairns, K. A., Williamson, D. F., & Brown, J. E. (1991). Correlates of breast-feeding in a low income population of Whites, Blacks, and Southeast Asians. *Journal of the American Dietetic Association, 91*(1), 41–45.

Sokoloff, B., Carlin, J., & Pham, H. (1984). Five-year follow-up of Vietnamese refugee children in the United States. *Clinical Pediatrics, 23*(10), 565–570.

Spector, R. E. (1991). *Cultural diversity in health and illness* (3rd ed.). Norwalk, CT: Appleton and Lange.

*Statistics Canada: Ethnic Origin.* (1993). Ottawa, Canada: Ministry of Industry, Science and Technology.

Stauffer, R. Y. (1991). Vietnamese Americans. In

J. N. Giger & R. E. Davidhizar (Eds.), *Transcultural nursing, assessment and intervention* (pp. 402–434). St. Louis: Mosby Year Book.

Stavig, G. R., Igra, A., & Leonard, A. R. (1988). Hypertension and related health issues among Asians and Pacific Islanders in California. *Public Health Reports, 103*(1), 28–37.

Stehr-Green, J. K., & Schantz, P. M. (1986). Trichinosis in Southeast Asian refugees in the United States. *American Journal of Public Health, 76*(10), 1238–1239.

Strand, P. J., & Jones, W. (1983). Health service utilization by Indochinese refugees. *Medical Care, 21*(11),1089–1098.

Sutherland, J. E., Avant, R. F., Franz, W. B., III, Monzon, C. M., & Stark, N. M. (1983). Indochinese refugee health assessment and treatment. *Journal of Family Practice, 16*(1), 61–67.

Sutter, R. W., & Haefliger, E. (1990). Tuberculosis morbidity and infection in Vietnamese in Southeast Asian refugee camps. *American Review of Respiratory Disease, 141*(6), 1483–1486.

Takaki, R. (1991). *Strangers from a different shore: A history of Asian Americans.* Boston: Little, Brown & Co.

Timberlake, E. M., & Cook, K. O. (1984). Social work and the Vietnamese refugee. *Social Work, 29*(2), 108–113.

Tobin, J. J., & Friedman, J. (1983). Spirits, shamans, and nightmare death: Survivor stress in a Hmong refugee. *American Journal of Orthopsychiatry, 53*(3), 439–448.

Tran, T. V. (1991). Family living arrangement and social adjustment among three ethnic groups of elderly Indochinese refugees. *International Journal of Aging and Human Development, 32*(2), 91–102.

Uba, L. (1992). Cultural barriers to health care for Southeast Asian refugees. *Public Health Reports, 107*(5), 544–548.

U.S. Bureau of the Census (1992). *Statistical abstract of the United States.* Washington, DC: Author.

Wadd, L. (1983). Vietnamese postpartum practices: Implications for nursing in the hospital setting. *Journal of Obstetrical, Gynecological, and Neonatal Nursing, 12,* 252–258.

Yu, E. S. H. (1991). The health risks of Asian Americans. *American Journal of Public Health, 81*(11), 1391–1393.

# Glossary

The Glossary also includes terms found only on the disk version of this book. Educators who adopt the book for course instruction receive the disk free of charge. The disk is available for purchase along with individual copies of the book.

***Aagwachse*** (Chap. 4): An Amish folk illness, referred to in English as *livergrown,* with symptoms of abdominal distress thought to be caused by too much jostling, especially of infants, during buggy rides.

***Abnemme*** (Chap. 4): An Amish folk illness characterized by "wasting away," usually affecting infants or young children who seem to be too lean and inactive.

***Abwaarde*** (Chap. 4): Amish term meaning care for, attend in the sense of being present to minister to the needs of another person.

**Acadia** (Chap. 11): Part of the Canadian Maritime provinces.

**Acadian** (Chap. 11): Early French settler of Acadia. A French dialect spoken by people in Acadia.

**Acculturate** (Chap. 1): To modify the culture of a group or individual as a result of contact with another group or individual.

***Achtgewwe*** (Chap. 4): Amish term meaning care for, attend in the sense of being aware of and responding to the need for care in another person; in some way helping or doing for another person.

***Adab*** (Chap. 9): Egyptian word for politeness.

**African-American** (Chap. 3): An American who self-identifies with an ancestry from Africa and/or shares the values, beliefs, lifeways, and practices that are rooted in both the African and American cultures.

***Ainu*** (Japanese chapter on disk): Indigenous people of uncertain origin in northern Japan.

**Allah** (Chap. 6): The greatest and most inclusive of the names for God. An Arabic word used to describe the God worshipped by Muslims, Christians, and Jews.

***Am*** (Chap. 18): A pervasive force in Vietnamese traditional medicine associated with cold conditions and things that are dark, negative, feminine, and empty.

***Amal*** (Chap. 9): Egyptian voodoo-like action done to bring bad luck or illness to an unloved person.

***Americanos*** (Puerto Rican chapter on disk): Hispanic name given to people from the European-American culture.

***Amor propio*** (Chap. 10): Filipino term for saving face.

**Anabaptist** (Chap. 4): Adherent of radical wing of the Protestant Reformation who espouses the baptism of adult believers.

***Andarun*** (Chap. 13): Iranian term meaning inner self.

***Antyesti*** (Hindu chapter on disk): Hindu equivalent of last rites.

**Appalachian Regional Commission** (Chap. 5): Federal commission established in the 1960s for the purpose of improving economic conditions in Appalachia. This commission approves appropriations for improving and building roads, establishing loans for small businesses, and attracting industry to the area.

**Arabic** (Chap. 6): The Semitic language of the Arabs.

*Arwah* (Chap. 9): Egyptian word for the spirits.

**Asafetida bag** (Chap. 5): Odorous combination of roots and herbs, usually made into a poultice, enclosed in a bag, and worn around the neck or some other part of the body to ward off contagious illnesses.

**Ashkenazi** (Chap. 15): Descended from Eastern Europe and Russia.

**Assimilate** (Chap. 1): To gradually adopt and incorporate the characteristics of the prevailing culture.

*Ataque de nervios* (Chap. 16 and Puerto Rican chapter on disk): A hyperkinetic spasmodic activity common in Spanish-speaking groups. The purpose is to express anger or deep sadness.

*Atma* (Hindu chapter on disk): Eternal soul in Hindu.

*Atary* (Chap. 13): An Iranian herb shop.

**Attitude** (Chap. 1): A state of mind or feeling with regard to some matter of a culture.

**Augmented family** (Chap. 3): A term for one form of the African-American extended family that refers to children raised in a household in which they are unrelated to the head of household.

*Ay bendito!* (Puerto Rican chapter on disk): A frequently used Puerto Rican expression that expresses astonishment, surprise, lament, or pain.

*Ayurveda* (Hindu chapter on disk): Traditional Asian Indian medicine.

**Baklava** (Turkish chapter on disk): Turkish pastry with nuts and honey.

**Baltics** (Baltic chapter on disk): The countries of Estonia, Latvia, and Lithuania.

*Barrenillos* (Chap. 8): Spanish word for obsessions.

*Baten* (Chap. 13): Iranian term for inner self.

*Bathala* (Chap. 10): Filipino ancestral religion.

*Be bao* (Chap. 18): Also *bat gio*. Vietnamese folk practice where the skin is pinched with the objective of producing ecchymosis and petechiae. This practice is believed to relieve sore throats and headaches.

**Bedouins** (Chap. 9): Egyptian desert inhabitants.

**Behçet's disease** (Turkish chapter on disk): Endemic disease in Turkey characterized by chronic inflammatory disorders of the blood vessels, with recurrent ulceration of the oral and pharyngeal mucous membranes and the genitalia, skin lesions, severe uveitis, retinal vasculitis, and optic atrophy.

**Being** (Chap. 5): Essence of existence in an unqualified state and conceived as an essential state of nature where one does not need to be actively engaged in an activity.

**Belief** (Chap. 1): Something accepted as true, especially as a tenet or a body of tenets accepted by an ethnocultural group.

*Bisprechung* (German chapter on disk): German term for formal conversation and discourse.

**Black Americans** (Chap. 3): A term used to describe African-Americans.

**Black English** (Chap. 3): A dialect used by African-Americans.

**Boat People** (Haitian chapter on disk): Haitian or Cuban immigrants who arrive in small boats. They are usually of undocumented status.

**Boricua** (Puerto Rican chapter on disk): Puerto Rican term used with great pride. Name given to Puerto Rico by the Taino Indians.

**Botanica** (Chap. 8): Traditional Cuban or other Spanish store selling a variety of herbs, ointments, oils, powders, incenses, and religious figurines used in Santería.

**Brauche** (Chap. 4): Folk healing art common among Pennsylvania Germans.

**Braucher** (Chap. 4): Amish practitioner of *brauche*, a folk healer.

*Briefe zum Himmel* (German chapter on disk): German term for chain letter, a letter sent to a specific number of people with a request that it be passed on to the same number of people.

**Bris or Brit Milah** (Chap. 15): Ritual circumcision of male Jewish children.

*Bruderschaft-trinken* (German chapter on disk): An old German custom symbolizing the two friends' shift to a less formal address. The friends lock arms and sip from a raised glass, after which they shake hands and announce their first names.

**Bureau of Indian Affairs** (BIA, Chap. 17): Federal agency responsible for ensuring services to American Indians, Alaskan Indians, and Eskimo tribes.

**Butsudan** (Japanese chapter on disk): The Japanese term for a Buddhist altar in the home.

**Caida de la mollera** (Chap. 16): A condition of fallen fontanel that is thought to occur because the infant was withdrawn too harshly from the nipple. Common among some Spanish-speaking populations.

**Cao gio** (Chap. 18): Vietnamese practice of placing ointments or hot balm oil across the chest, back, or shoulders and rubbing with a coin. It is used to treat colds, sore throats, flu, and sinusitis.

**Capo de famiglia** (Italian chapter on disk): Italian word for head of the family.

**Cariñoso(a)** (Puerto Rican chapter on disk): Hispanic term denoting caring in both verbal and nonverbal communications.

**Catimbozeiros** (Brazilian chapter on disk): Portuguese word for sorcerer. A *catimbozeiros* can be a folk practitioner.

**Celtic** (Chap. 14): Belonging to a group of Indo-European languages: Irish, Welsh, or Breton.

**Chesm-i-bad** (Chap. 13): Iranian term meaning evil eye.

**Chicano(a)** (Chap. 16): A Mexican-American.

**Choteo:** Cuban term for a lighthearted attitude, with teasing, bantering, and exaggerating.

**Chundo Kyo** (Korean chapter on disk): Korean naturalistic religion that combines Confucianism, Buddhism, and Daoism.

**Clan** (Chap. 17): A division of a tribe tracing descent from a common ancestor.

**Colored** (Chap. 3): A term used to describe African-Americans.

**Comadre** (Brazilian chapter on disk): Portuguese word for godmother.

**Community** (Chap. 2): A group or class of people having a common interest or identity living in a specified locality.

**Compadre** (Brazilian chapter on disk): Portuguese term for godfather.

**Compadrazgo** (Chap. 8): Spanish for a system of personal relationships in which friends or relatives are considered part of the family whether or not there is a blood relationship.

**Confianza** (Puerto Rican chapter on disk): Hispanic term for trust developed between individuals, which is essential for effective communication and interpersonal interactions in health-care settings.

**Conservative** (Chap. 15): Branch of Judaism between Reform and Orthodox with regard to religious practice.

**Contadino** (Italian chapter on disk): Italian word for peasant.

**Copts** (Chap. 9): Christian Egyptians.

**Cornicelli** (Italian chapter on disk): Italian red horns, represent a symbol for good luck.

**Cosmology** (Chap. 17): A branch of philosophy that deals with the origin, processes, and structure of the universe.

**Creole** (Chap. 3 and Haitian chapter on disk): Rich and expressive language derived from the African tongue Fon.

**Crystal Gazer** (Chap. 17): A Navajo folk healer that interprets dreams.

**Cultural competence** (Chap. 1): Having the knowledge, understanding, and skills regarding a diverse culture that allows one to provide acceptable, congruent care.

**Cultural diversity** (Chap. 1): Representing a variety of different cultures.

**Culture** (Chap. 1): Totality of socially transmitted behavior patterns, arts, beliefs, values, customs, lifeways, and all other products of human work and thought characteristics of a population that guides its worldview and decision making. These patterns may be explicit or implicit, are primarily learned and transmitted within the family, and are shared by the majority of the culture.

**Curandeiro** (Brazilian chapter on disk): Portuguese folk practitioner whose healing powers are divinely given.

*Curandero* (Chap. 16): A traditional folk practitioner common in Spanish-speaking communities. This folk practitioner treats traditional illness not caused by witchcraft.

*Daadihaus* (Chap. 4): Amish grandparents' cottage adjacent to farmhouse.

*Dainas* (Baltic chapter on disk): Latvian term for songs.

*Dainos* (Baltic chapter on disk): Lithuanian term for songs.

*Dan wei* (Chap. 7): Functional unit of Chinese society. The work or the neighborhood unit that is responsible to and for the Chinese people's way of life.

*Dao* (Chap. 7): Balance between the ying and yang.

*Dayah* (Chap. 6): Arabic word for midwife.

*Decaimientos* (Chap. 8): Cuban condition related to tired blood.

*Decensos* (Chap. 8): Spanish term for fainting spells.

*Deitsch* (Chap. 4): Pennsylvania German, sometimes incorrectly anglicized as Pennsylvania Dutch. An American dialect derived from several upland and Alemannic German dialects, with an admixture of American English vocabulary.

*Diet* (Japanese chapter on disk): Japanese parliament.

*Demut* (Chap. 4): Amish word for humility or meekness.

**Doing** (Chap. 5): Being actively engaged in an activity for the purpose of accomplishing something.

*Doog* (Chap. 13): Iranian term for yogurt soda.

**The Dozens** (Chap. 3): A joking relationship between two African-Americans in which each is permitted to make fun of the other without taking offense.

**Dulse** (Chap. 14): Also known as Irish moss. Iodine-rich edible seaweed used in clarifying beer and wine and as a suspension medium in some medicines.

*Duong* (Chap. 18): Vietnamese force used in traditional health practice that is associated with things positive, masculine, light, and full.

*Ebo* (Chap. 8): The sacrificial offering made to establish communication between the spirits and human beings in the Santería religion.

*Eid* (Chap. 13): Iranian term for celebration of a feast, for example, *Eid Gorgan* (day or feast ending pilgrimage to Mecca), or *Eid Fetr* (last day of the month of Ramadan).

**Eire** (Chap. 14): Gaelic name for Ireland.

*Empacho* (Chap. 16): A condition common among some Spanish-speaking populations that is believed to be caused by a bolus of food stuck in the gastrointestinal tract. Massage of the abdomen is thought to relieve the condition.

*Endropi* (Chap. 12): Greek word for shame.

*Escondido* (Brazilian chapter on disk): Portuguese term that means hidden. It refers to undocumented aliens who remain hidden.

*Espirituista* (Chap. 16 and Brazilian chapter on disk): Also *espiritualista*. A Spanish or Portuguese folk practitioner who receives talent from God. This folk practitioner treats conditions thought to be caused by witchcraft.

**Ethnic** (Chap. 1): A group of people who has had different experiences from those of the dominant culture by status, background, residence, religion, education, or other factors that functionally unify the group and act collectively on its members. The term pertains to a religious, racial, national, or cultural group.

**Ethnic identity** (Chap. 6): A subjective sense of social boundary (social emphasis) or self-definition that answers the question "Who am I" (Meleis, Lipson, & Paul, 1992).

**Ethnocentrism** (Chap. 1): The tendency for human beings to think that their ways of thinking, acting, and believing are the only right, proper, and natural ones and to believe that those who differ greatly are strange, bizarre, or unenlightened.

**Ethnocultural** (Chap. 1): A group of people who have had different experiences from the dominant culture by status, ethnic background, residence, religion, education, or other factors that functionally unify the group and act collectively on each member.

*Evli* (Turkish chapter on disk): Turkish word for marriage.

**Falling out** (Chap. 3): A sudden collapse, paralysis, and inability to see or speak. This behavior is noted among African-Americans during a funeral or other tragic experiences.

**Familism** (Chaps. 6 and 16): A social pattern in which family solidarity and tradition assume a superior position over individual rights and interests.

**Family** (Chap. 2): Two or more people who are emotionally involved with each other. They may, but not necessarily, live in close proximity to each other.

**Fatalism** (Chap. 5): Acceptance that life occurrences are predetermined by fate and cannot be changed by human beings.

**Fatback** (Chap. 3): A term for salted pork in the African-American culture.

*Fayots* (Chap. 11): Canadian pea soup in Acadia.

**Francophone** (Chap. 11): Canadians using French as their first language.

**Frau** (German chapter on disk): German title for Mrs.

**Fraulein** (German chapter on disk): German title for an unmarried woman.

*Freindschaft* (Chap. 4): Amish three-generational extended family network of relationships.

*Freundschaftkarten* (German chapter on disk): German word for Valentine Day's card.

*Galang* (Chap. 10): Filipino term for respect.

*Garm* (Chap. 13): Iranian term meaning hot.

*Garmie* (Chap. 13): Iranian digestive problem caused from eating too much hot food.

*Gelassenheit* (Chap. 4): Amish term for submission, yieldingness, surrender of self and ego to the higher will of the group or a deity.

*Gemerschaft* (German chapter on disk): German term for community.

**Generalization** (Chap. 1): Reducing numerous characteristics of an individual or group of people to a general form that renders them indistinguishable.

**Geophagia** (Chap. 3): Eating of nonfood substances such as clay, cornstarch, or charcoal during pregnancy.

*Gesprach* (German chapter on disk): German term used for casual conversation.

*Ghalbam gerefteh* (Chap. 13): Iranian term for distress of the heart.

*Giac* (Chap. 18): Vietnamese dermabrasive procedure with cup suctioning.

*Giagia* (Chap. 12): Greek word for grandma.

*Giri* (Japanese chapter on disk): Japanese term for the sense of obligation that exists between people who are socially interconnected.

**Global society** (Chap. 2): Seeing the world as one large community of multicultural people.

**Gohan** (Japanese chapter on disk): Japanese term for rice, particularly the sticky rice that is preferred by Japanese.

*Gol-i-gov zabon* (Chap. 13): Iranian term for foxglove flowers.

**Great Eid** (Chap. 9): Egyptian feast of 4 days.

**Great Potato Famine** (Chap. 14): Time in Ireland from 1848 through the 1850s when the main crop, potatoes, failed and resulted in many Irish emigrating.

*Guan xi* (Chap. 7): Chinese form of social exchange whereby help is received or given by members of Chinese society. A form of barter and exchange.

**Gullah** (Chap. 3): A creole language spoken by African-Americans who reside on or near the Sea Islands off Georgia (for example, Hilton Head and Myrtle Beach).

*Hadith* (Chap. 6): Oral tradition of the Prophet Muhammad; collection of words and deeds that form the basis of Muslim law.

**Haitians** (Haitian chapter on disk): People from the Caribbean Island of Haiti.

*Halakhah* (Chap. 15): Jewish laws or commandments.

*Halal* (Chaps. 6 and 13): The lawful; that which is permitted by Allah. Also, the term used to describe ritual slaughter of meat.

**Han** (Chap. 7): Largest ethnic group of Chinese.

**Hand trembler** (Chap. 17): A Navajo traditional healer.

*Hanyak* (Korean chapter on disk): Korean traditional herbal medicine used to create harmony between oneself and the larger cosmos and a healing method for body and soul.

*Haram* (Chaps. 6 and 13): The unlawful; that which is prohibited by Allah. Anyone who engages in what is prohibited is liable to incur punishment in the Hereafter, as well as punishment under the legal system in countries that incorporate Islamic law into legal codes.

**Hasidic**, *also* **Chasidic** (Chap. 15): An ultra-Orthodox movement within Judaism.

**Health** (Chap. 2): A state of wellness as defined by an ethnocultural group and generally including physical, mental, and spiritual states as they interact with the family, community, and global society.

**Hebrew** (Chap. 15): Language of Israel and Jewish prayer.

*Hegab* (Chap. 9): Egyptian amulet kept close to the body to protect against evil eye and bad spirits.

*Hejab* (Chap. 13): Iranian term for any behavior that expresses modesty in public; for example, in women, modest attire (loose dress or head scarf) or shy, self-limiting behavior in relating to the other gender.

**Herr** (German chapter on disk): German title for Mr.

**High blood** (Chaps. 3 and 5): Too much blood in circulation in the body or too high pressure. Term commonly is used by African-Americans and Appalachians.

*Hijab* (Chap. 6): Modest covering of a Muslim woman; concealing the head and the body except for the hands and face with loose-fitting, nontransparent clothing.

*Hilot* (Chap. 10): Filipino folk healer and massage therapist.

*Hindi ibang tao* (Chap. 10): Filipino term for insider.

**Hinduism** (Hindu chapter on disk): Predominant religion of Asian Indians.

**Hispanic** (Chap. 16): An American of Spanish or Latin American origin.

*Hiya* (Chap. 10): Filipino word for shame.

**Hogan** (Chap. 17): An earth-covered Navajo dwelling.

**Home** (Chap. 5): In the Appalachian context, a connectedness to the land more than a physical dwelling.

**Honor** (Chap. 8): Spanish term for goodness or virtue that can be diminished or lost by an immoral or unworthy act.

**Hot and cold theory** (Chap. 16 and Hiatian chapter on disk): Hispanic concept that illness is caused when the body is exposed to an imbalance of hot and cold. Foods are also classified as hot or cold.

*Hwanbyung* (Korean chapter on disk): Korean traditional illness that occurs from repressing anger or other strong emotions.

*Hwangap* (Korean chapter on disk): At the age of 60 years, a person starts the calendar cycle over again. This milestone becomes a significant celebration in Korean society.

*Ibang tao* (Chap. 10): Filipino term for outsider.

**Ideology** (Chap. 1): Principles and rules that guide the thoughts of an individual, family, or group.

*Il mal occhio* (Italian chapter on disk): Italian word for evil eye.

*Imam* (Chap. 6): Muslim leader of prayer; usually the most learned member of the local Islamic community.

**Indian Health Service** (IHS, Chap. 17): Federal agency that has the responsibility for providing health services to American Indians.

**Indochinese** (Chap. 18): Individuals originating from Vietnam, Cambodia, or Laos.

*Inshallah* (Chap. 6): Arabic word meaning "if God wills."

**Insider** (Chap. 5): Someone known to and accepted by the group who usually has special knowledge regarding the values and beliefs of the group.

*Insullah* (Turkish chapter on disk): Turkish phrase meaning "God willing."

**Islam** (Chap. 6): A monotheistic religion in which the supreme deity is Allah. According to Muslim belief, God imparted His final revelations, the *Holy Qur'an,* through His last prophet, Muhammad, thereby completing Judaism and Christianity.

**Issei** (Japanese chapter on disk): A first-generation Japanese immigrant.

**Itami** (Japanese chapter on disk): The Japanese term for pain.

**Itkhad** (Chap. 9): Egyptian word for respect.

**Jenn** (Chap. 9): Egyptian word for the devil.

**Jerbero** (Chap. 16): See *yerbero.*

**Jing** (Chap. 7): Chinese term for body passages that are interrelated and interconnected. It includes the 14 Meridians called the *jing luo.*

**Jing ye** (Chap. 7): Chinese term for body fluids, including the *jing,* or the clear, thin fluids that moisturize the skin and warm the muscles, and the *ye,* or the thicker and heavier fluids that moisten the joints.

**Jinn** (Chap. 6): Spirits created by God from smokeless fire that inhabit a world parallel to that of humans. According to *Qur'anic* teachings, God sent His message to both worlds that He created. Some *jinn* are righteous, whereas others are evil.

**Joual** (Chap. 11): French dialect incorporating English words into a syntax and grammar that is essentially French.

**Kaddish** (Chap. 15): Jewish prayer said for the dead.

**Kaffeeklatsch** (German chapter on disk): German custom of gathering over coffee to talk.

**Kampo** (Japanese chapter on disk): Japanese term for East Asian or Chinese medical practices and botanical therapies.

**Kango-san** (Japanese chapter on disk): Also *kango-fu.* The Japanese term for registered nurse.

**Karma** (Hindu chapter on disk): Hindu term for actions performed in the present life and the accumulated effects from past lives.

**Kashk** (Chap. 13): Iranian term for milk by-product, sour in flavor.

**Kashrut** (Chap. 15): Also **kashrus.** Jewish dietary laws, derived from the Books of Leviticus and Deuteronomy in the Bible. They designate which foods and food combinations are permissible (*see* **Kosher**) and describe the method for slaughtering animals to be cooked and eaten. Jewish scholars believe that these laws are primary commandments for serving God and only secondarily promote healthy eating.

**Khakshir** (Chap. 13): Iranian term for flat black rocket seed that is used for stomach ailments.

**Ki** (Japanese chapter on disk): The Japanese term for the energy that flows through living creatures.

**Kibun** (Korean chapter on disk): Korean term related to mood, current feelings, and state of mind.

**Kippah** (Chap. 15): Also, *yarmulka.* Jewish head covering.

**Koran:** See *Qur'an.*

**Kosher** (Chap. 15): Literally, "properly preserved" or "fit for eating." It does not signify a brand name or form of cooking but designates those foods that may be eaten by Jews. Prepared foods have symbols on their packaging that indicate the food is kosher. Use of these symbols is regulated by religious authorities (*see* **Kashrut**).

**Koumbari** (Chap. 12): Greek word for coparents.

**Lace-Curtain Irish** (Chap. 14): Name given to Irish in America who left inner-city enclaves and moved to the suburbs.

**La gente de la raza** (Chap. 16): A phrase that denotes a genetic determination to which all Spanish-speaking people belong, regardless of class differences or place of birth.

**Ladino(a)** (Chap. 16): A person of Jewish and Spanish background.

**Latino(a)** (Chap. 16): A person from Latin America.

**Lavash** (Chap. 13): Iranian flat, thin bread made with wheat.

**Laying on of hands** (Chap. 3): A spiritual practice of placing one's hands on an individual for the purpose of healing.

**Lien** (Chap. 18): Vietnamese concept that represents control over and responsibility for moral character.

**Limerick** (Chap. 14): An Irish humorous poem receiving its name from the county of Limerick in Ireland.

**Low blood** (Chaps. 3 and 5): Too little blood, too low blood count, or too thin blood. Term is commonly used by African-Americans and Appalachians.

**Maalesh** (Chap. 6): Arabic word meaning never mind, it doesn't matter.

**Machismo** (Chaps. 8, 16, and Puerto Rican chapter on disk): A sense of masculinity that stresses virility, courage, and domination of women. The need to display physical strength, bravery, and virility.

**Madichon** (Haitian chapter on disk): Haitian term used to indicate that a child's future will be marred by misfortune because the child has disrespected elders.

**Magissa** (Chap. 12): Greek folk healer.

**Mai** (Chap. 7): One of the elements of traditional Chinese medicine that encompasses the Chinese pulses and vessels.

**Mal ojo** (Chap. 16): Also *mal de ojo*. Spanish for the evil eye, a hex condition with unspecified signs and symptoms thought to be caused by an older person admiring a younger person. The condition can be reversed if the person doing the admiring touches the person being admired.

**Manong** (Chap. 10): Filipino term for older brother or old-timer.

**Marianismo** (Puerto Rican chapter on disk): Hispanic term that represents women as being self-sacrificing, submissive, respectful, and obedient to men.

**Marielitos** (Chap. 8): Cuban immigrants who arrived in 1980 on a massive boat lift from Muriel Harbor to Key West, Florida.

**Masallah** (Turkish chapter on disk): Turkish word meaning may "God bless and protect."

**Matiasma** (Chap. 12): Greek word for the evil eye.

**Matka Boska** (Polish chapter on disk): Poland's patroness to help in time of need. Literally means "mother of God."

**Mestizo(a)** (Chap. 16): A person of mixed Spanish and Native-American heritage.

**Métis** (Chap. 11): Ancestry that includes French Canadian and Native-American or other ancestry.

**Mezaj** (Chap. 13): Iranian term for a person's humoral temperament.

**Mezuzah** (Chap. 15): A container with Biblical writings placed on the doorpost of Jewish homes or hung around the neck on a necklace.

**Mezzogiorno** (Italian chapter on disk): Region in Southern Italy.

**Mien** (Chap. 18): Vietnamese concept based on wealth and power.

**Mikveh** (Chap. 15): Ritual bath; a natural body of water or bathhouse that fulfills the requirements of Jewish law as to volume and source of water, where Jews immerse themselves for ritual purification on certain occasions such as before the Sabbath or holidays or after menstruation.

**Minyan** (Chap. 15): Ten male adults needed for prayer in the Jewish faith. They must be at least 13 years old and have had their bar mitzvah.

**Mohel** (Chap. 15): Ritual circumciser in the Jewish faith.

**Moreno** (Brazilian chapter on disk): Portuguese person who has black or brown hair and dark eyes.

**Morita therapy** (Japanese chapter on disk): An indigenous Japanese school of psychotherapy.

**Moslem:** See *Muslim.*

**Mosque** (Chap. 6): Muslim place of worship.

**Moxibustion** (Chap. 18): Vietnamese health-care practice in which pulverized wormwood is heated and placed directly on specific meridians of the skin to counter conditions associated with excess cold.

**Muhammad** (Chap. 6): Prophet chosen by God to deliver the religion of Islam.

*Mukruh* (Chap. 6): The detested; that which is disapproved of by Allah, though not very strongly. The punishment for *mukrah* acts is less than that for *haram* acts, except when done excessively or in a manner that leads an individual toward *haram*.

**Mulatto** (Haitian chapter on disk): Individual with mixed European and African blood. The mulatto usually has light skin, refined facial features, and fine hair.

*Mundang* (Korean chapter on disk): Korean folk healer who has special abilities for communicating with the spirits and in treating illnesses after all other means of treatment have been exhausted.

*Muska* (Turkish chapter on disk): Turkish tradition of writing a prayer on a piece of paper and wrapping it in fabric; it is then hidden in the home or worn by a person seeking help for emotional problems.

**Muslim** (Chap. 6): Also *Moslem.* Believers of Islam, the second largest world religion.

*Nabat* (Chap. 13): Iranian concentrated sugar used for treating stomach upsets.

*Naharati* (Chap. 13): Iranian term meaning generalized distress.

**Navajo neuropathy** (Chap. 17): A neurologic condition confined to Navajo Indians characterized by a complete absence of myelinated fibers. The condition results in short stature, sexual infantilism, systemic infection, hypotonia, areflexia, loss of sensation in the extremities, corneal ulceration, acral mutilation, and painless fractures.

*Nazar* (Turkish chapter on disk): Also *nazur.* Turkish word for envy.

*Nazar boncuk* (Turkish chapter on disk): Turkish small, blue bead used to protect a child from the evil eye.

*Nerva* (Chap. 12): Greek folk illness.

*Nervioso(a)* (Chap. 16 and Puerto Rican chapter on disk): Hispanic term used to describe signs and symptoms of nervousness, anxiety, sadness, and grief.

*Neshasteh* (Chap. 13): Iranian term for wheat starch, which is combined with boiling water and drunk for sore throats or coughs; it is also used to stop diarrhea.

*Nguzo Saba* (Chap. 3): Afrocentric principles of *Umojo* (unity), *Kujichagula* (self-determination), *Ujima* (collective work and responsibility), *Imani* (faith), *Nia* (purpose), *Ujamaa* (cooperative economics), and *Kuumba* (creativity).

*Nihonjin* (Japanese chapter on disk): The Japanese term for a native of Japan.

**Nippon** (Japanese chapter on disk): Also *Nihon.* Name for Japan in Japanese.

*Nisei* (Japanese chapter on disk): The Japanese term for the second-generation of immigrant family.

*Niuyorican* (Puerto Rican chapter on disk): Term used to identify the cultural pride of Puerto Rican generations born and reared in New York.

*Norooz* (Chap. 13): Non-Islamic Iranian New Year; first day of spring.

**Nubians** (Chap. 9): Black Egyptians living around and south of Aswan.

*O-bento* (Japanese chapter on disk): The Japanese term for box lunch.

**Obi** (Japanese chapter on disk): Sash for a Japanese kimono or an abdominal binder.

*O-cha* (Japanese chapter on disk): Japanese term for green tea.

**Office lady** (Japanese chapter on disk): A young woman who works in a Japanese office providing hospitality to visitors and performing limited clerical functions.

*O-furo* (Japanese chapter on disk): Japanese bath.

**Old Order Amish** (Chap. 4): Most conservative and traditionalist group among the followers of Jacob Ammann. Today, this group is simply called *Amish,* but technically known as *Old Order Amish Mennonites,* to distinguish this group from other related Amish and Mennonite groups.

*Onore della famiglia* (Italian chapter on disk): Italian term for family honor.

*Opiatek* (Polish chapter on disk): Polish wafer that everyone shares at Christmas time.

*Oppression* (Haitian chapter on disk): Haitian ailment related to asthma characterized by anxiety and hyperventilation.

**Ordnung** (Chap. 4 and German chapter on disk): Codified rules and regulations that govern the behavior of a local Amish church district, or congregation; local consensus of faith and practice. Also, the German term for order.

**Orishas** (Chap. 8): The gods or spirits in Santería.

**Orthodox** (Chap. 15): Traditional Judaism.

**O-shogatsu** (Japanese chapter on disk): Japanese New Year celebrated for several days around January 1.

**Outsider** (Chap. 5): Someone not known to members of the group and assumed not to have the special knowledge regarding the values and beliefs of the group. Opposite of insider.

**Pabasa** (Chap. 10): Filipino term for novena.

**Padrone** (Italian chapter on disk): Italian word for master, head of the family.

**Pappou** (Chap. 12): Greek word for grandfather.

**Patrao** (Brazilian chapter on disk): Portuguese term for employer.

**Pazienza** (Italian chapter on disk): Italian word for patience or long suffering.

**Person** (Chap. 2): A human being; one who is constantly adapting to his or her environment biologically, psychologically, and socially.

**Personalismo** (Chaps. 8, 16, and Puerto Rican chapter on disk): Spanish word for emphasis on intimate, personal relationships as more important than impersonal, bureaucratic relationships.

**Philotimo** (Chap. 12): Greek work for respect.

**Phylactos** (Chap. 12): Greek amulets worn to ward off envy.

**Pidgin** (Chap. 3): A simplified language used for communicating between speakers of different languages.

**Pilipino** (Chap. 10): Filipino word for Filipino.

**Pogrom** (Chap. 15): Organized persecution or massacre of a minority group.

**Polish Question** (Polish chapter on disk): Discussion between Stalin, Churchill, and Roosevelt at the Potsdam and Malta conferences about what to do with Poland after World War II.

**Polonia** (Polish chapter on disk): Communities heavily occupied by Polish immigrants and descendants of Polish Nationals.

**Practika** (Chap. 12): Greek herbal remedies.

**Pseudofamilies** (Chap. 18): Vietnamese households made up of close and distant relatives and friends that share accommodations, finances, and fellowship.

**Pu tong hua** (Chap. 7): Recognized language of China.

**Qi** (Chap. 7): One of five substances or elements of traditional Chinese medicine encompassing the foundation of the energy of the body, environment, and universe. It includes all sources and expenditures of energy.

**Québec** (Chap. 11): Second largest province in Canada and capital of that province.

**Quebecer** (Chap. 11): Also *québécois*. Descendant of early settler from France and living in Quebec, Canada.

**Qur'an** (Chaps. 6 and 9): Also *Koran*. Muslim Holy Book; believed by Muslims to contain God's final revelations to mankind.

**Rabbi** (Chap. 15): Jewish religious leader.

**Ramadan** (Chaps. 6 and 9): Ninth month of the Islamic year during which Muslims are required to fast during daylight hours for 30 days.

**Razianeh** (Chap. 13): Iranian term; shaped like rye, chewed for halitosis.

**Reconstructionism** (Chap. 15): The branch of Judaism founded in the 20th century that views Judaism as an evolving religion and seeks to adapt belief and practice to changes in the contemporary world.

**Refakatci** (Turkish chapter on disk): Turkish word for someone who stays overnight in the hospital with a sick person.

**Reform** (Chap. 15): Liberal or progressive Judaism.

**Refugee** (Chap. 1): A person fleeing from another country because of religious, political, or other ideologic reasons. Refugee status is predetermined by the host country before emigration.

***Remedios caseiros*** (Brazilian chapter on disk): Portuguese (Brazilian) home medicine or remedy.

***Remedios populares*** (Brazilian chapter on disk): Portuguese (Brazilian) folk medicine practitioners.

***Respeto*** (Chap. 16 and Puerto Rican chapter on disk): Hispanic term denoting respect. Term refers to the qualities developed for others, such as parents, the elderly, and educated people, who are expected to be honored, admired, and respected.

***Rūta*** (Baltic chapter on disk): Plant having a special place in Lithuanian gardens.

***Saiidis*** (Chap. 9): Egyptian group living south of Cairo.

**Sake** (Japanese chapter on disk): Japanese rice wine, used ritually as well as socially.

**Salary man** (Japanese chapter on disk): Japanese term for a male white-collar worker or company man.

**Sand painting** (Chap. 17): Navajo art work originally designed on the hogan floor and then destroyed and returned to the earth. Today, sand paintings are created and sold commercially.

***Sansei*** (Japanese chapter on disk): Japanese term for the third generation of an immigrant family.

**Santería** (Chap. 8): A 300-year-old Afro-Cuban religion that combines Roman Catholic elements with ancient Yoruba tribal beliefs and practices.

***Santero*** (Chap. 8): A practitioner of Santería.

***Sard*** (Chap. 13): Iranian term meaning cold.

***Sardie*** (Chap. 13): Iranian digestive problem from eating too much cold food.

**Secondary members** (Chap. 3): African-American family form where other family members besides the nuclear family live together.

***Sensei*** (Japanese chapter on disk): Japanese term for master, used to address teachers, physicians, or those in seniority in a corporate setting.

**Sephardic** (Chap. 15): Term for descendents of Jews from Spain, Portugal, the Mediterranean, Africa, or Central and South America.

**Settlement** (Chap. 4): Aggregation of Amish church districts, usually the result of intentional geographic grouping.

**Severe combined immunodeficiency syndrome (SCIDS)** (Chap. 17): An immunodeficiency syndrome unrelated to AIDS and characterized by a failure of antibody response and cell-mediated immunity.

**Shanty Irish** (Chap. 14): Term describing Irish who live in urban Irish ethnic enclaves.

**Sheikh** (Chap. 6): An Arab term for anyone deserving respect: a teacher, elder, religious leader, or member of a royal family.

***Shen*** (Chap. 7): One of five substances or elements of traditional Chinese medicine encompassing the spirit.

**Shiatsu** (Japanese chapter on disk): Japanese term for acupressure therapy.

**Shinto** (Japanese chapter on disk): Indigenous religion of Japan.

**Shul:** *See* **synagogue.**

***Sikkeenah*** (Chap. 9): Egyptian word for knife.

***Simpátia*** (Chap. 8 and Puerto Rican chapter on disk): Spanish term for smooth interpersonal relationships, characterized by courtesy, respect, and the absence of harsh criticism or confrontation.

**Sit a spell** (Chap. 5): Process of engaging in nonhierarchial relaxed conversation to become familiar with the beliefs and feelings of others.

**Small Eid** (Chap. 9): Egyptian holy feast of 3 days.

***Sobador*** (Chap. 16): A Spanish folk practitioner similar to a chiropractor who treats illnesses and conditions affecting the joints and musculoskeletal system.

**Sojourner** (Chap. 1): Someone who relocates with the intention of remaining only a short time and then returning home.

***Solidao*** (Brazilian chapter on disk): Portuguese word for loneliness.

**Solidarity** (Polish chapter on disk): A union of interests, purposes, and sympathies promoting fellowship with Polish Nationals.

**Soul food** (Chap. 3): Traditional diet of African-Americans.

**Spanglish** (Chap. 8 and Puerto Rican chapter on disk): Sentence structure that includes both English and Spanish words.

**Speaking in tongues** (Chap. 3): Praying in a language that is not understood by anyone except the person reciting the prayer.

**Stereotyping** (Chap. 1): An oversimplified conception, opinion, or belief about some aspect of an individual or group.

*Sto Lat* (Polish chapter on disk): Polish phrase meaning that the celebrant should live a hundred years.

**Subculture** (Chap. 1): A group of people who have had different experiences from those of the dominant culture by status, ethnic background, residence, religion, education, or other factors that functionally unify the group and act collectively on its members.

**Subfamilies** (Chap. 3): African-American family system in which extended relatives life together.

*Susto* (Chap. 16): Known as "magical fright," a condition thought to be caused by witchcraft. Symptoms can vary and include both mental and physical ones.

**Synagogue** (Chap. 15): Also *temple* or *shul.* Jewish house of worship.

*Ta'arof* (Chap. 13): Iranian ritual expressing courtesy.

*Tabi'at* (Chap. 13): Iranian term for a person's makeup, nature, or genetic build.

*Tae Kyo* (Korean chapter on disk): Korean word that literally means "fetus education," with the objective being health and well-being of fetus and mother through art, beautiful objects, and a serene environment.

*Tae Mong* (Korean chapter on disk): Korean term that signifies the beginning of pregnancy. The pregnant woman dreams of conception of the fetus.

**Tagalog** (Chap. 10): Filipino national language.

*Tagdir* (Chap. 13): Iranian term for destiny, future mapped out by powers greater than oneself, beyond individual control.

**Tag-Lish** (Chap. 10): Dialect mixing English and Tagalog.

*Tatami* (Japanese chapter on disk): Traditional Japanese floor coverings made out of straw.

**Temple:** *See* **synagogue.**

*Tet* (Chap. 18): Asian Lunar New Year celebrated in January or February.

**Torah** (Chap. 15): Five books of Moses in the Jewish faith; the Hebrew Bible.

*Treyf* (Chap. 15): Forbidden; unclean; unfit to eat. Opposite of kosher (*see* above).

**Tribe** (Chap. 17): An American Indian social organization comprising several local villages, bands, districts, lineage, or other groups who share a common ancestry, language, and culture.

*Tridosha* (Hindu chapter on disk): Theory that the body is made up of five elements: fire, air, space, water, and earth.

*Turkiye* (Turkish chapter on disk): Turkish word for the country Turkey.

*Tzedakah* (Chap. 15): Literally, "righteousness"; the concept of sharing with others, commonly used to mean charity given to those in need.

**Values** (Chap. 1): Principles and standards that have meaning and worth to an individual, family, group, or community. They are associated with what is important to a cultural or ethnic group or individual.

*Velorio* (Chap. 16): Latin American funeral ceremony usually held in the home or community where participants gather in a time of melancholy, rejoicing, pain, and hopefulness.

*Vendousas* (Chap. 12): Greek practice of cupping.

*Verguenza* (Chap. 8): Spanish term for a consciousness of public opinion and the judgment of the entire community.

*Viandas* (Puerto Rican chapter on disk): Spanish term for root vegetables.

*Via nuova* (Italian chapter on disk): Italian word for new way.

*Via vecchia* (Italian chapter on disk): Italian word for old way.

**Visiting** (Chap. 4): Frequently practiced Amish custom of family-to-family home visits that help to maintain kinship and church ties and the flow of information within the Amish community.

**Voodoo** (Chap. 3 and Haitian chapter on disk): Also *vodou*. Vibrant religion born from slavery and revolt. The word means "sacred" in the African tongue of Fon.

*Waham* (Chap. 9): Egyptian word for cravings during pregnancy.

**Wake** (Chap. 14): A watch over a deceased person before burial that is usually accompanied by a celebration, which may include feasting.

**Warm hands** (Chap. 4): Healing art related to therapeutic touch that is regarded by the Amish as a gift to be applied for the good of others in need of healing. A form of *brauche*.

*Wesel* (Polish chapter on disk): Polish phrase for a wedding sequence.

**Wetback** (Chap. 16): A derogatory term applied to undocumented aliens of Mexican or Latin-American descent.

**Wind** (Chap. 18): A classification for Vietnamese foods that is closely related to cold foods.

**Witchcraft** (Chap. 3): A belief that illness or harm can come to a person by supernatural forces.

**Worldview** (Chap. 1): The way an individual or group of people look at their universe to form values about their life and the world around them.

*Xong* (Chap. 18): Vietnamese herbal preparation that relieves motion sickness or cold-related problems.

*Xue* (Chap. 7): One of five substances or elements of traditional Chinese medicine encompassing the blood.

**Yang** (Chap. 7): Chinese term for one of two opposing principles of the balance of life. It can be either a single phenomenon or a state of being of a phenomenon. It is interdependent on its opposite, the yin.

*Yangban* (Korean chapter on disk): Korean term meaning upper class.

**Yarmulka** (Chap. 15): *See* **kippah.**

*Yerbero* (Chap. 16): Also *Jerbero*. A Spanish folk practitioner who specializes in treating health conditions through the use of herbal therapy.

**Yiddish** (Chap. 15): A language often spoken by elderly Jews.

**Yin** (Chap. 7): Chinese term for one of two opposite principles of the balance of life. It can be either a phenomenon or a state of being of a phenomenon. It is interdependent with its opposite, the *yang*.

*Zaher* (Chap. 13): Iranian term for public persona.

*Zang fu* (Chap. 7): Concept of traditional Chinese medicine, which includes the Chinese organ systems and their interrelationships.

*Zar* (Chap. 9): An Egyptian transmeditative ceremony.

*Zerangi* (Chap. 13): Iranian term for cleverness.

*Zhong guo* (Chap. 7): Principle term used to denote China. Other Chinese words are added to this term to denote Chinese ancestry, the Chinese language, and the Chinese people.

# Index

Numbers followed by an "f" indicate figures; numbers followed by a "t" indicate tabular material.